AIDS: ANTI-HIV AGENTS, THERAPIES, AND VACCINES

ANNALS OF THE NEW YORK ACADEMY OF SCIENCES
Volume 616

AIDS: ANTI-HIV AGENTS, THERAPIES, AND VACCINES

Edited by Vassil St. Georgiev and John J. McGowan

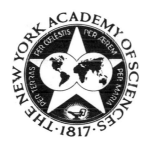

The New York Academy of Sciences
New York, New York
1990

Photo on cover of paperback edition: HIV budding from a T-lymphocyte. See page 5.

Library of Congress Cataloging-in-Publication Data

AIDS : anti-HIV agents, therapies, and vaccines / edited by Vassil St. Georgiev and John J. McGowan.
    p.   cm. — (Annals of the New York Academy of Sciences, ISSN 0077-8923 ; v. 616)
    Contributions presented at the Second International Conference on Drug Research in Immunologic and Infectious Diseases, held in Arlington, Va. on Nov. 6-9, 1989, and sponsored by the New York Academy of Sciences.
    Includes bibliographical references and index.
    ISBN 0-89766-631-3 (cloth : alk. paper). — ISBN 0-89766-632-1 (paper : alk. paper)
    1. AIDS (Disease)—Chemotherapy—Congresses. 2. AIDS (Disease)—Immunotherapy—Congresses. 3. Antiviral agents—Congresses. I. Georgiev, Vassil St. II. McGowan, John J., 1951-　.　III. New York Academy of Sciences. IV. International Conference on Drug Research in Immunologic and Infectious Diseases (2nd : 1989 : Arlington, Va.) V. Series.
    [DNLM: 1. Acquired Immunodeficiency Syndrome—drug therapy—congresses. 2. Antiviral Agents—pharmacology—congresses. 3. Antiviral Agents—therapeutic use—congresses. 4. Immunotheraphy—congresses.　W1 AN626YL v. 616 / WD 308 A28792 1989]
Q11.N5 vol. 616
[RC607.A26]
500 s—dc20
[616.97'92061]
DNLM/DLC
for Library of Congress   91-6884
                                                  CIP

PCP
Printed in the United States of America
ISBN 0-89766-631-3 (cloth)
ISBN 0-89766-632-1 (paper)
ISSN 0077-8923

ANNALS OF THE NEW YORK ACADEMY OF SCIENCES

VOLUME 616
December 26, 1990

AIDS: ANTI-HIV AGENTS, THERAPIES, AND VACCINES [a]

Editors and Conference Chairmen
VASSIL ST. GEORGIEV AND JOHN J. McGOWAN

Session Chairmen
JEROME BIRNBAUM, FRANCIS J. BULLOCK, ROELF DATEMA, THOMAS
KRENITSKY, CARLOS LOPEZ, MARK L. PEARSON, MICHAEL I. SHERMAN,
AND RICHARD TOLMAN

CONTENTS

[a] This volume is the result of a conference entitled **Second International Conference on Drug Research in Immunologic and Infectious Diseases: Acquired Immune Deficiency Syndrome (AIDS)**, held in Arlington, Virginia on November 6-9, 1989, by the New York Academy of Sciences.

Part VII.   Papers from Panel Discussion: Pharmacology and Metabolism
of Anti-HIV Drugs

Part VIII.   Opportunistic Infections in AIDS Patients

Financial assistance was received from:

Major funders
- NATIONAL INSTITUTE OF ALLERGY AND INFECTIOUS DISEASES/NIH
- U. S. ARMY MEDICAL RESEARCH AND DEVELOPMENT COMMAND, DAMD 17-90-Z-0023

Supporters
- BRISTOL-MYERS COMPANY
- E. I. DU PONT DE NEMOURS & COMPANY
- HOFFMANN-LA ROCHE INC.
- SCHERING-PLOUGH CORPORATION
- SMITH KLINE & FRENCH LABORATORIES

Contributors
- ABBOTT LABORATORIES
- BURROUGHS WELLCOME COMPANY
- GENENTECH, INC.
- ELI LILLY AND COMPANY
- MERCK SHARP & DOHME RESEARCH LABORATORIES
- MERRELL DOW RESEARCH INSTITUTE
- PFIZER INC.
- RORER CENTRAL RESEARCH
- G. D. SEARLE AND COMPANY
- STERLING RESEARCH GROUP
- SYNTEX RESEARCH
- THE UPJOHN COMPANY

Preface

VASSIL ST. GEORGIEV [a] AND JOHN J. McGOWAN [b]

[a]Pennwalt Corporation
Philadelphia, Pennsylvania 19102

[b]Basic Research and Development Program
Division of AIDS
National Institute of Allergy and Infectious Diseases
National Institutes of Health
Bethesda, Maryland 20892

This volume contains the proceedings of the Second International Conference on Drug Research in Immunologic and Infectious Diseases: AIDS. The conference, which was organized under the auspices of the New York Academy of Sciences and the National Institutes of Health, was dedicated to recent advancements in drug research and treatment of the acquired immune deficiency syndrome (AIDS). The topics discussed include the latest developments in design and synthesis of anti-HIV agents, their preclinical and clinical investigation, and new therapies involving both known and experimental drugs and vaccines against AIDS and AIDS-associated opportunistic infections. At the conference, leading experts on AIDS shared their views and expectations of how to meet the challenge to society posed by this disease and how to combat most effectively what now appears to be a truly global epidemic.

Current statistics indicate that whereas tens of thousands of cases in five continents have been reported to the World Health Organization, in reality, hundreds of thousands of additional cases still remain unreported and thus represent a threat to society. In addition, there are an estimated 5 to 10 million more people worldwide who are infected with HIV but who show no symptoms of the disease. It is from this pool of asymptomatic carriers that the virus undoubtedly will be transmitted to many thousands of healthy individuals. If not resolved quickly, the social, economic, and political impacts of AIDS will create an enormous burden on society.

The aim of the conference upon which this *Annal* is based was to bring together scientists from all areas of drug research—from design and synthesis to preclinical and clinical evaluation. It is hoped that such an interdisciplinary approach will provide an impetus for the examination and exchange of knowledge, helping to generate new insights and ideas that will set new directions for future AIDS research. To this end, we gratefully acknowledge the contributions of the two guest speakers, Anthony S. Fauci (National Institute of Allergy and Infectious Disease, NIH) on the immuno-pathogenesis of HIV infection, and Gary R. Noble (Centers for Disease Control) on the epidemiology of the AIDS epidemic. Their excellent presentations were certainly well-appreciated by the large audiences attending their lectures.

We trust that this volume will not only serve as a useful resource for both established investigators and new researchers in the field, but will also facilitate the understanding of those areas that are still not well-understood. Our aim is to encourage scientists to explore new avenues in their search for novel and more effective drugs against AIDS.

In conclusion, we would like to express our gratitude to the Conference Committee and the Conference Department of the New York Academy of Sciences for their help in organizing this conference, and to the Editorial Department of the Academy, which saw the proceedings to print.

Acquired Immune Deficiency Syndrome (AIDS)

Progress in Drug Research and Therapeutic Potential

VASSIL ST. GEORGIEV [a,c] AND
JOHN J. MCGOWAN[b,d]

[a]Pennwalt Corporation
Philadelphia, Pennsylvania

[b]Basic Research and Development Program
Division of AIDS
National Institute of Allergy and Infectious Diseases
National Institutes of Health
Bethesda, Maryland 20892

The human immunodeficiency virus (HIV) is the causative agent of the acquired immunodeficiency syndrome (AIDS). The virus is classified as member of a rare but highly organized group of retroviruses that possess, in addition to *trans*-acting cellular genes, their own set of regulatory elements.[1] After invading the human body, HIV will gradually erode the ability of the immune system to resist various pathogens, thus making the patient increasingly vulnerable to a number of opportunistic infections and cancers. With the lack of any meaningful treatment, death from AIDS will occur within 2 to 4 years of its clinical diagnosis.

Currently, three major ways of transmitting AIDS are known: by sexual intercourse, by transfusion of contaminated blood or sharing of tainted needles, and through one's progeny. Although presently very small, the risk of contracting AIDS through occupational exposure by health care workers is still real and should not be overlooked. In general, high-risk groups for HIV infection include: (a) homosexual and bisexual men as well as heterosexuals who maintain sexual contacts with HIV-infected persons; (b) intravenous drug abusers who share needles; and (c) patients receiving blood transfusions or clotting factors. In the latter case, the thorough screening of blood supplies for HIV antibody would, essentially, eliminate the risk of infection. Because of better education about prevention, the spread of AIDS among homosexual and bisexual men is believed to have leveled off. However, transmission of the virus to newborn infants by HIV-infected mothers (most likely intravenous drug abusers) has been on the rise.

[c]Address for correspondence: Division of Life Sciences, Orion Research and Technologies Corporation, P.O. Box 463, Tampa, FL 33601-0463.
[d]Address for correspondence: National Institute of Allergy and Infectious Diseases, NIH, 6003 Executive Blvd., Room 247P, Bethesda, MD 20892.

1

Although early cases of AIDS in the United States have largely been identified with adult male population, in many underdeveloped nations men and women have been equally affected by the syndrome.

Current information indicates that, worldwide, through March 1989, 146,569 cases of AIDS from 148 countries have been registered with the Global Programme on AIDS at the World Health Organization (WHO/GPA). In reality, however, literally hundreds of thousands of additional cases remain unreported, thus representing an awesome threat to society as one continuing source of spreading AIDS. This is true not only for the United States but also for Europe and especially for developing nations of Asia and Africa where the AIDS epidemic is taking devastating proportions. Because of lack of access to health-care and proper (or limited) disease surveillance, in Latin America alone 50% of all AIDS cases are usually not reported, whereas in many African countries only one in every five or ten cases is believed to be reported. According to estimates by WHO/GPA, presently there are over 450,000 cases of AIDS worldwide, and between 5,000,000 and 10,000,000 more people are infected with the virus but showing no symptoms of the syndrome. It is from this pool of asymptomatic carriers of HIV that the virus would, potentially, be transmitted to many more healthy individuals. Again, WHO/GPA estimates that within the next five years, approximately 1,000,000 new cases of AIDS can be expected. If not resolved in proper time, the social, economic, and political impact of AIDS will create an enormous burden on any society. The lack of an effective vaccine or anti-HIV drug, coupled with the high cost of present treatment available and a fatality rate of over 90% after four years from the time of clinical diagnosis, would be hard to contain and control not only in the advanced nations of the industrialized world but even more so in the economically poor and underdeveloped countries of the Third world. These are grim statistics that not only illustrate the seriousness of the problem of AIDS but that also serve as a reminder that this problem is still with us and will stay with us for some time to come before it is resolved.

A schematic representation of HIV is depicted in FIGURE 1. Two glycoproteins, gp120 and gp41 are embedded in the lipid bilayer. gp120, which is the major extracellular envelope glycoprotein, is located over the coat, whereas the gp41 transmembrane glycoprotein passes through the coat. Within the outer coat there is a protein core containing the two stranded viral RNAs and the reverse transcriptase (RT) enzyme.

Structurally, the HIV genome (FIG. 2) encodes all of the proteins required for retrovirus replication; that is, the four capsid proteins derived from the *gag* gene, the three enzymes (protease, reverse transcriptase, and endonuclease) derived from the *pol* gene, and the major exterior glycoprotein and transmembrane protein, both derived from the *env* gene. In addition, the HIV genome was found to possess at least five other

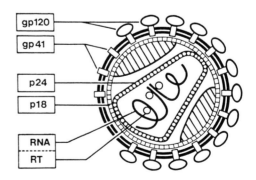

FIGURE 1. Schematic depiction of HIV. gp120 = major extracellular envelope glycoprotein; gp41 = transmembrane envelope glycoprotein; p24 = major core antigen; p18 = myristylated *gag* protein; RT = reverse transcriptase.

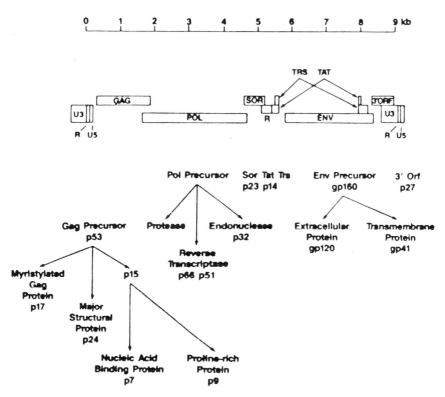

FIGURE 2. Structure of the HIV genome.[1]

accessory genes, namely, *sor, 3'orf, tat, trs* (also known as *art*), and the *R* gene.[1] All of the HIV genes are immunogenic and therefore able to trigger the production of corresponding antibodies. Among the HIV genes, *sor* is a unique protein that is not only critical for the formation of infectious particles,[2] but together with the envelope proteins determines the infectivity of the virus particles. The *tat* gene product, on the other hand, seems to activate the expression from the long terminal repeat (LTR) at both transcriptional and posttranscriptional stages and is considered absolutely essential for the viral reproduction.[1]

As with other retroviruses, the replication cycle of HIV (FIG. 3) is regulated by cellular factions. In addition, the expression of HIV is facilitated by a complex regulatory pathway involving virus-encoded genes.[1]

The immunosuppressive effect associated with HIV is largely based on its ability to destroy a subpopulation of T lymphocytes, the host CD4 helper cells. It is thought, however, that the immunosuppressive action of HIV is controlled by at least two of its accessory genes, *trs* and *3'orf*, which may serve as down-regulators of the viral expression. From an evolutionary standpoint this is understandable inasmuch as such functions would be directly related to the need for the virus to preserve (or at least delay) the destruction of the host T cells in order to promote its own replication cycle and survive. Therefore, the viral survival would necessitate a symbiotic existence with the host cell for at least some period of time.[1] Alternatively, there is experimental evidence

suggesting the opposite: some environmental agents have been actually shown to enhance HIV expression by stimulating the transcription from viral LTR.[3-5] Also, Siekevitz et al.[5] have reported that some *trans*-activating genes [such as those of the human
T-cell lymphotropic virus type I (HTLV-I) and perhaps of HTLV-II] were capable of
trans-activating HIV transcription. Because HIV, HTLV-I, and HTLV-II may also
attack the same host cells and because coinfections with these viruses are known to
exist among some risk groups, *trans*-activation of HIV expression may become a factor
of great practical relevance.[1]

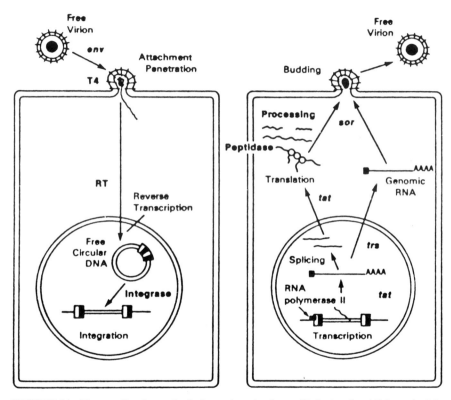

FIGURE 3A. Virus replication cycle. Left panel: early phase of infection (establishment); right
panel: late phase of infection (expression).[1]

It is postulated that initially, the human immunodeficiency virus infects the monocyte, producing chronic or latent infections without destroying the cell.[6] Subsequently,
the infected monocyte by acting as an antigen-presenting cell may come into contact
with an antigen-specific CD4 lymphocyte. During the antigen-induced activation, the
CD4 cell will bind the monocyte-processed viral antigen, causing monocyte-derived
interleukin-1 (IL-1) to interact with the CD4 cell. The activated T lymphocyte will
become highly susceptible to infection by HIV, which, in turn, is being released in large
numbers by the already infected monocyte (FIG. 4).[6] The gp120 envelope glycoprotein

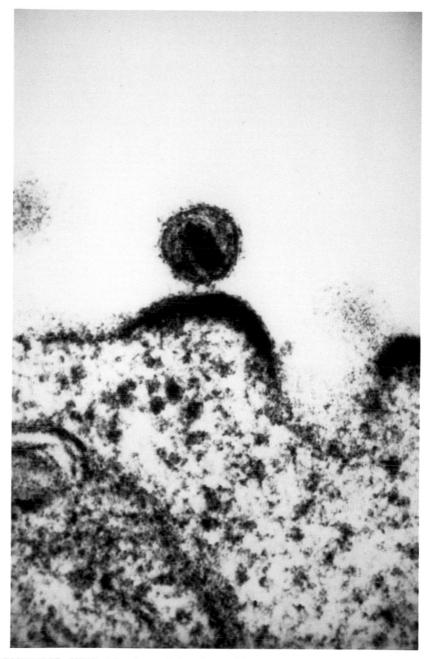

FIGURE 3B. HIV budding from a T lymphocyte (electron micrograph by Tom Folks, NIH).

of HIV that binds to the CD4 receptor of the CD4 helper cell is crucial to the entry of the virus into the host cell.[7,8] It is clear that HIV, which appears to elude the human immune system through a highly variable envelope, cannot afford to vary the gp120 domain that recognizes and binds to the CD4 complex of the T lymphocyte.

Research on HIV directed towards the prevention and treatment of people suffering from AIDS has led to a renewed interest in antiviral drug development in academic, private, and governmental sectors. The work presented at the Second International Conference on Drug Research in Immunologic and Infectious Diseases, Acquired Immune Deficiency Syndrome (AIDS) is a culmination of research efforts aimed at the rapid identification of new potential therapies for the treatment of HIV infection. New anti-HIV drugs have been identified by the design, application, and implementation of

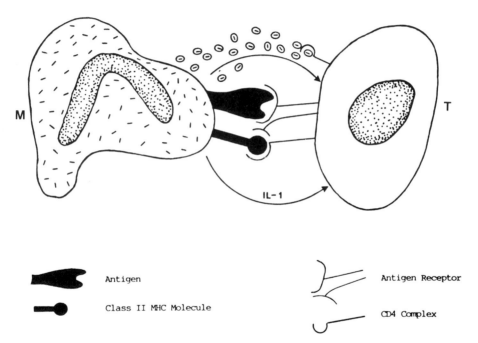

FIGURE 4A. A hypothetical model for the antigen-specific T-cell defect in AIDS;[6] M, virus-infected monocyte/macrophage; T, antigen-specific T4 lymphocyte.

HIV molecular biology either to rational drug screening programs or through targeted drug design and development programs.

The successes and failures of candidate drugs for HIV treatment in both kinds of programs will be discussed in detail by invited speakers. In particular, this volume presents detailed discussions on points in the viral replication cycle that have been targeted for attack (FIG. 5).

The HIV reverse transcriptase and protease have been the most intensively studied viral targets for the development of anti-HIV drugs. These two enzymes are attractive targets since their specificities for HIV replication are unique compared to analogous proteins found in the human cell. In addition, a large base of information on the reverse

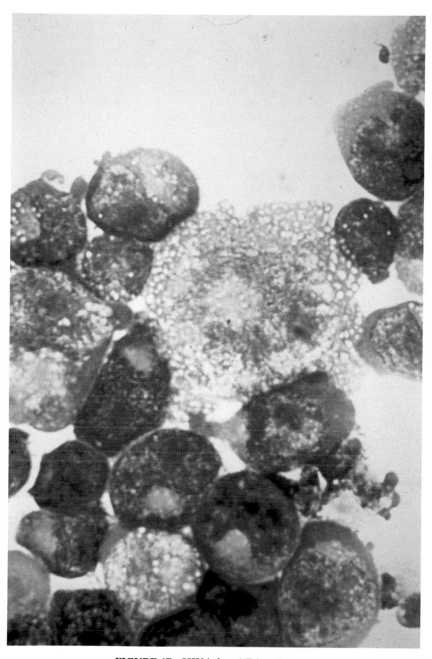

FIGURE 4B. HIV-infected T lymphocytes.

transcriptase and protease of other animal retroviruses or human cells is available. Knowing the differences between the viral and cellular enzymes would lead to the design of drugs that are specific for the virus and less toxic to the host cell.

Considerable progress was made by the early identification of drugs such as 3'-azido-3'-deoxythymidine (AZT, zidovudine). Zidovudine was the first drug discovered and shown to be effective in blocking HIV in cell cultures as well as in animals and humans infected with the virus. The rapid clinical development and licensure of AZT have established criteria by which other nucleosides are compared for efficacy and

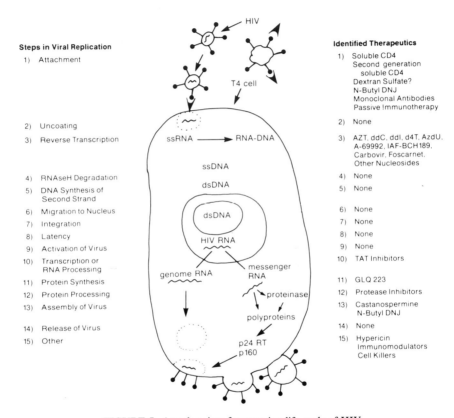

Steps in Viral Replication
1) Attachment
2) Uncoating
3) Reverse Transcription
4) RNAseH Degradation
5) DNA Synthesis of Second Strand
6) Migration to Nucleus
7) Integration
8) Latency
9) Activation of Virus
10) Transcription or RNA Processing
11) Protein Synthesis
12) Protein Processing
13) Assembly of Virus
14) Release of Virus
15) Other

Identified Therapeutics
1) Soluble CD4
   Second generation soluble CD4
   Dextran Sulfate?
   N-Butyl DNJ
   Monoclonal Antibodies
   Passive Immunotherapy
2) None
3) AZT, ddC, ddI, d4T, AzdU, A-69992, IAF-BCH189, Carbovir, Foscarnet, Other Nucleosides
4) None
5) None
6) None
7) None
8) None
9) None
10) TAT Inhibitors
11) GLQ 223
12) Protease Inhibitors
13) Castanospermine N-Butyl DNJ
14) None
15) Hypericin Immunomodulators Cell Killers

FIGURE 5. Attack points for stopping life cycle of HIV.

toxicity in both preclinical and clinical studies. Already novel nucleosides that have potentially more desirable characteristics to treat HIV infections have been identified (*e.g.* AzDU, D4T, ddI, and BCH-189). It is hoped that each of these new drugs will possess a wide cytotherapeutic index, high bioavailability, a broad spectrum of antimicrobial activity, an ability to cross the blood-brain barrier, and a more convenient dosing schedule. It is important that the AZT-resistant viral isolates are not cross-resistant towards the new anti-HIV drugs.

With regard to HIV protease, the three-dimensional structure of the enzyme is already known, and inhibitors have been identified by several research groups. It is expected that HIV protease-specific inhibitors will enter clinical trials within the next year.

Viral attachment as a potential target for anti-HIV therapy has been most aggressively pursued. First generation drugs have been produced and shown to block viral attachment. Of particular interest is the use of a portion of the cellular receptor for the virus (CD4 protein) as a therapy. Recombinant production of soluble CD4 is aimed primarily at preventing viral attachment. Second generation molecules of soluble CD4 linked to toxins or antibodies were reported capable of not only blocking the viral attachment but also of targeting and killing those cells already infected with HIV.

The HIV reverse transcriptase, the protease, and viral attachment are but three of the attack points in the HIV replication cycle. Other targets in the viral life cycle that hold promise in controlling HIV replication in people with AIDS will be the subject of discussion by various contributors to this volume.

Because of their impaired immune responses, patients with AIDS are subject to attack by various opportunistic pathogens. With the reclassification of *Pneumocystis carinii* as a member of the fungi, fungal infections now account for over 80% of all opportunistic infections, a major factor for morbidity and mortality in the acquired immune deficiency syndrome. The obligate intracellular parasite *Toxoplasma gondii* is another leading cause of opportunistic infection among AIDS patients. As compared to immunocompetent hosts, treatment of such infections in immunocompromised patients is often inadequate, difficult to manage, and may require a long-term therapy in order to maintain remission. In recent years, pentamidine has been increasingly used as the drug of choice in the treatment of pneumocystic pneumonia. In the case of toxoplasmosis and other parasitic infections, combination therapy with antifolate drugs and sulfonamides (or trisulfapyrimidines) is considered the most efficient today. With the exception of amphotericin B, the majority of systemic antifungal agents are azole compounds that act by the fungistatic mechanism of action. Current efforts are directed at the discovery of less toxic and fungicidal antimycotic drugs with a broad spectrum of activity. Various pentamidine analogues are also being synthesized in order to broaden their activity. These and other aspects of drug development and therapy in the area of opportunistic infections in AIDS patients will be discussed at length by a number of authors in this volume.

Our hope is that the present *Annal* will serve as a forum for discussion and sharing of knowledge and experience. Novel directions for future research, it is hoped, will emerge as a result of it.

REFERENCES

1. WONG-STAAL, F. 1988. The human immunodeficiency virus genome: structure and function. *In* Immunobiology and pathogenesis of persistent virus infections. C. Lopez, Ed.: 171-179. American Society of Microbiology. Washington, D.C.
2. FISHER, A., B. ENSOLI, L. IVANOFF, S. PETTEWAY, M. CHAMBERLAIN, L. RATNER, R. C. GALLO & F. WONG-STAAL. 1987. The *sor* gene of HIV is essential for efficient virus transmission *in vitro.* Science **237:** 888-893.
3. ZAGURY, D., J. BERNARD, R. LEONARD, R. CHEYNIER, M. FELDMAN, P. S. SARIN & R. C. GALLO. 1986. Long-term culture of HTLV-III infected T-cells: a model of cytopathology of T-cell depletion in AIDS. Science **231:** 850-853.
4. NAHEL, G. & D. BALTIMORE. 1987. An inducible transcription factor activates expression of human immunodeficiency virus in T-cells. Nature **326:** 711-713.

5. SIEKEVITZ, M., S. F. JOSEPHS, M. DUKOVICH, N. PEFFER, F. WONG-STAAL & W. GREENE. 1987. Activation of the HIV LTR by T-cell mitogens and the transactivating protein of HTLV-I. Science **238:** 1575-1578.
6. FAUCI, A. S., S. A. ROSENBERG, S. A. SHERWIN, C. A. DINARELLO, D. L. LONGO & H. C. LANE. 1987. Immunomodulators in clinical medicine. Ann. Intern. Med. **106:** 421-433.
7. SMITH, D., R. A. BYRN, S. A. MASTERS, T. GREGORY, J. E. GROOPMAN & D. J. CAPON. 1987. Blocking of HIV-1 infectivity by a soluble, secreted form of the CD4 antigen. Science **238:** 1704-1707.
8. MCDOUGAL, J., M. S. KENNEDY, J. M. SLIGH, S. P. CORT, A. MAWLE & J. K. A. NICHOLSON. 1986. Binding of HTLV-III/LAV to T4+ T cells by a complex of the 110K viral protein and the T4 molecule. Science **231:** 382-385.

Structure-Function Studies of HIV Reverse Transcriptase[a]

VINAYAKA R. PRASAD AND STEPHEN P. GOFF

Department of Biochemistry and Molecular Biophysics
College of Physicians and Surgeons
Columbia University
New York, New York 10032

Reverse transcriptase (RT) plays a central role in the retroviral life cycle, copying the genetic information in the genomic RNA into a double-stranded DNA form. The process of DNA synthesis is complex, involving several steps unique to the viral life style and not normally occurring in host cellular processes.[1] Soon after infection and entry into a cell, the reverse transcriptase enzyme begins the synthesis of a complementary DNA copy of the viral genome using a cellular tRNA as a primer. During DNA synthesis, the RNA genome of the RNA·DNA duplex is degraded by a special ribonuclease activity, termed RNAse H, associated with the reverse transcriptase molecule. As synthesis of the first strand of DNA occurs, a portion of the RNA that is resistant to RNAse H cleavage—the so-called polypurine tract—serves as primer for the synthesis of the second strand of the DNA. This process requires the DNA-dependent polymerase activity of the RT enzyme. Thus, RT is a multifunctional protein consisting of RNA-dependent DNA polymerase, DNA-dependent DNA polymerase, and ribonuclease H activities.[2]

Due to the pivotal role of RT in retroviral replication, the enzyme is an attractive target for antiretroviral therapy.[3] To develop better drugs targetted to RT, we need to understand the structure and function of this enzyme and the organization of the various catalytic domains on the molecule. We have initiated a series of genetic studies directed towards delineating the various functional domains of HIV RT.

BACTERIAL EXPRESSION OF HIV-1 RT

The RT enzyme of all retroviruses is synthesized as a part of a large gag-pol polyprotein precursor that is initially translated and incorporated into assembling virions. During the maturation of virion particles, the gag-pol polyprotein is processed by the viral protease into its individual components. The mature RT of different viruses shows considerably different structures (FIG. 1). The murine and feline retroviruses encode a simple monomeric enzyme, produced by complete cleavage of the precursor. The avian viruses encode a heterodimeric enzyme consisting of a large beta subunit

[a] This work was supported by Public Health Service Grant 1 U01 AI 24845 and by a Grant from the American Foundation for AIDS Research.

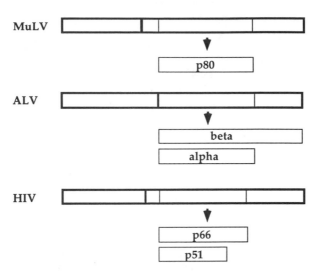

FIGURE 1. Biosynthesis and structure of various reverse transcriptase enzymes. Schematic structures of the gag-pol precursor and the mature RT derived by proteolysis for each of the three major classes of retroviruses are shown. Boxes with heavy outlines denote the gag and pol regions; thin vertical lines mark the boundaries in the pol gene products between the PR, RT, and IN domains. (S. P. Goff.[2] With permission from the *Journal of AIDS.*)

and a smaller alpha subunit. The larger subunit is formed by incomplete cleavage between the RT and IN domains of the precursor. The HIV enzyme is also a hetero-dimer, but of different structure: the RT domain is separated from the PR and IN domains by complete cleavage but then undergoes an additional cleavage in one of its two subunits near the C terminus, forming a 66 kDa subunit and a 51 kDa subunit. Thus, the two polypeptides of the HIV-1 RT, the p66 and p51 kDa proteins, share a common N terminus and differ at their C termini.[4,5]

Although all of these enzymes have been isolated from virion particles, only very limited quantities can be obtained. To facilitate the isolation of large quantities of enzyme, we have expressed the RTs of Moloney murine leukemia virus (M-MuLV),[6] of the HIV-1,[7] and of simian immunodeficiency virus (SIV) 251mac (Prasad and Goff, in preparation) in bacterial expression systems. In each case, we overexpressed the pol region of the relevant virus as a fusion protein with a fragment of the bacterial trpE enzyme in *E. coli.* The large polyprotein encoded by the HIV fusion gene, in crude extracts, displayed the characteristic Mg^{2+}-dependent RNA-directed DNA polymerase activity of HIV RT. This construct was then subsequently optimized by removal of pol sequences flanking RT to produce a highly active and very stable fusion protein that corresponds to the p66 version of the HIV RT found in the virions.[8] All the subsequent mutagenesis studies were performed on this construct.

DOMAIN STRUCTURE OF HIV REVERSE TRANSCRIPTASE

We wished to localize the RNA-dependent DNA polymerase and RNAse H activities of HIV-1 RT. We resorted to linker insertion mutagenesis of HIV RT as a probe of the domain structure of the protein. To introduce defined localized alterations in the HIV RT molecule, we created a battery of in-frame Eco RI linker insertion mutants at various positions along the RT coding region.[9] A total of 21 distinct mutations with net insertions ranging in length from 6 to 24 base pairs were obtained and mapped (FIG. 2). To test the variants for enzymatic activity, cultures of *E. coli* containing each mutant plasmid were starved for tryptophan to induce expression of the fusion protein, and the cells were harvested and lysed. Crude lysates were assayed for the stable accumulation of fusion protein by SDS polyacrylamide gel electrophoresis and then for the level of RNA-dependent DNA polymerase and ribonuclease H activities.

Testing Mutants for DNA Polymerase Activity

The RNA-dependent DNA polymerase activities were measured on homopolymer substrates (poly(rC) primed with oligo(dG)) with magnesium as the divalent cation.

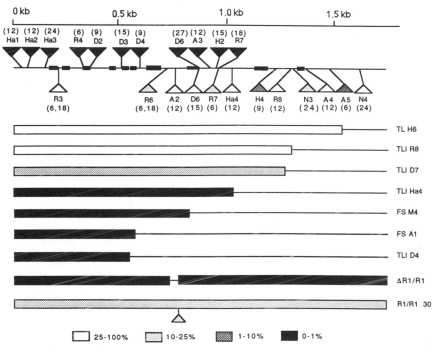

FIGURE 2A. Positions of linker insertion and deletion mutations and the effects of these mutations on DNA polymerase activity of HIV RT. The line at the top represents the sequences of the HIV pol gene encoding the p66 RT (nucleotides 2583-4262 of clone HXB2, numbered from the left edge of the left LTR). The position of each triangle indicates the position of a linker insertion mutation; the size of the insertion in base pairs is indicated in parentheses. Lower lines indicate the structures of proteins encoded by various deletion mutants; boxed areas represent the retained sequences. The level of DNA polymerase activity demonstrated by each mutant is indicated by the shading of the triangle or box, ranging from wild-type (white) to inactive (black), as keyed at the bottom of the FIGURE.

The results showed that most insertions mapping to the N-terminal part of the protein abolished DNA polymerase activity, whereas most mapping to the C terminal part did not (FIG. 2). These results are similar to those obtained for the M-MuLV RT,[10] and they suggest that the DNA polymerase function is similarly localized to the N-terminal region. There were several exceptions, however, to this general behavior. For HIV RT, we noticed several mutations in the N-terminal region that did not have any effect on the polymerase function. Furthermore, the boundary between the two domains was only poorly defined.

To confirm the localization of the polymerase domain to the N-terminal region, we created a series of deletion mutants from the linker insertions. Analysis of these mutants showed that the C-terminal region could be trimmed away substantially without loss of polymerase activity; specifically, constructs that include only the N terminal 50 kDa of the RT protein retained the activity. These results suggest that the p51 subunit of natural RT contains sufficient sequence information necessary for polymerase function and therefore should be active. Deletions that intruded further into the p51 region abolished polymerase activity. Thus, as for the M-MuLV RT, virtually all of the N-terminal region of the protein is essential for DNA polymerase activity.

One mutant with an unusual phenotype was obtained. This mutation, A5, a 6 base insertion located in the presumed RNAse H domain, profoundly affected the polymerase function. Deletions of the entire C-terminal region spanning this mutant, however, displayed wild type levels of activity. Therefore, this mutation showed a sort of dominant disruptive effect on the polymerase domain in the context of the complete p66 molecule.

Testing Mutants for RNAse H Activity

In an attempt to localize the RNAse H domain, we assayed all the mutants for RNAse H activity using an *in situ* gel electrophoresis assay.[11] Radiolabeled RNA in RNA·DNA hybrid form was uniformly distributed in the gel matrix of a polyacrylamide gel before polymerization, extracted proteins were applied and fractionated by electrophoresis, and the enzyme was allowed to renature and digest the substrate in the gel. Active species were identified by their ability to form zones of clearing in the uniform label, visualized by autoradiography. In this assay, the protein is initially denatured and must renature to recover an active site. As was found for the murine enzyme,[10] most insertions in the C-terminal region eliminated the RNAse H activity, whereas many insertions in the N-terminal region had little or no effect on the activity (FIG. 2B). The results are consistent with the notion that much of the C-terminal region is important for the RNAse H activity. Many mutations in the N-terminal region did affect the RNAse H activity, however. Thus, we conclude that alterations in many parts of the RT protein, at both N and C termini, can affect the recovery of this activity. Deletions of the N-terminal region, which we expected to express the RNAse H domain separately, abolished the RNAse H activity (FIG. 2B). This result suggests that, at least in the context of this expression system, the RNAse H domain requires the full protein for its proper folding or for its activity.

In summary, the mutagenesis studies have showed that the N-terminal 50 kDa of the p66 subunit of HIV-1 RT is necessary and sufficient for the RNA-dependent DNA polymerase function. A number of insertions in this region are tolerated, however. In addition, one mutation, localized in the C-terminal region dispensable for polymerase activity, was found to affect the polymerase function. Such "folding" mutants may be useful for genetic reversion studies. The studies have also shown that the RNAse H function was often affected by mutations in the C terminal 15 kDa region. Interestingly, many insertions in the N-terminal region also abolished the RNAse H activity. Furthermore, efforts to localize the RNAse H domain by N-terminal deletions were unsuccessful. These studies indicate that the RNAse H domain is dependent on the N-terminal domain either for folding or for its activity.

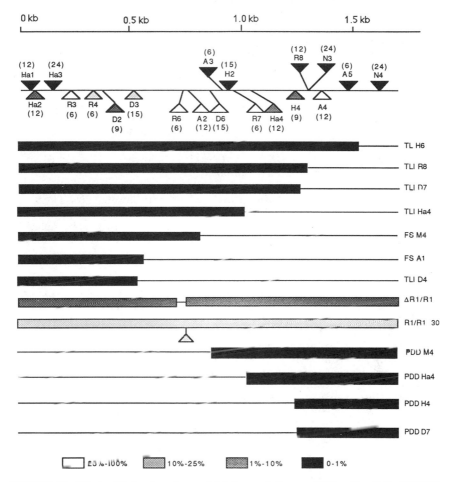

FIGURE 2B. Effects of linker insertion and deletion mutations on RNAse H activity HIV RT. The levels of RNAse H activity of each mutant, as judged from the *in situ* gel assay, are indicated by the shading. (Prasad & Goff.[9] From *Proceedings of the National Academy of Sciences USA*.)

In Situ COLONY SCREENING FOR HIV RT

Linker insertion mutagenesis studies coupled to biochemical analyses have helped us understand the gross localization of the polymerase and RNAse H domains. To obtain further insights, however, into the organization of the polymerase domain—the spatial arrangements of binding sites for various substrates, viz., dNTPs, primer and template RNA, and DNA—it would be helpful to be able to carry out more extensive genetic studies. For instance, the isolation of intragenic second site revertants of the linker insertion mutants would be of great help. The identity and position of the change present in the revertant often reveal important features of a protein and can pinpoint sites of contact between regions located at a distance in the primary sequence of the protein. To isolate such pseudorevertants, it is necessary to examine a large number of clones arising after mutagenesis, selecting or screening for an active variant. Because a biological selection for HIV RT is not available, we developed a screening technique for HIV RT.[12]

The screening method is based on the detection of the enzymatic activity of HIV RT expressed in bacteria, in situ, in a replica of the colonies. We begin with the HIV RT expression plasmid in bacteria grown on ordinary petri plates and prepare a lift of the colonies on a nitrocellulose filter. The expression of the fusion protein is induced in situ in the colonies on the filter, followed by lysis of the bacteria in the colonies and immobilization of the proteins released. The filter is then directly incubated in RT reaction cocktail, yielding an assay for the synthesis, on RNA templates, of radioactively labeled complementary DNA. The labeled reaction product is retained on the filter until fixation and is detected by autoradiography.

Methods were devised for inducing the expression of the enzyme, lysing the bacteria, and fixing the proteins present within each colony onto nitrocellulose filters. The detailed procedure is as follows (FIG. 3): Bacteria carrying the HIV RT expression plasmid were plated on M9 plates with casamino acids (5 mg/mL) and tryptophan (20 μg/mL) to form about 10^3 colonies per 10 cm dish. After incubation at 37°C for 12-14 h, at a time when the colonies were still very small (diameter < 1 mm), the colonies were lifted onto nitrocellulose filter circles, and the filters were placed, colony side up, on M9 plates containing casamino acids but lacking tryptophan. The colonies were incubated for 2 h at 37°C. The filters were then transferred to M9 plates containing casamino acids plus 10 μg/mL 3β-indole acrylic acid, and the colonies were incubated an additional 6 h at 37°C to induce the tryptophan operon. The filters were then placed, colony side up, on 0.4 mL drops of lysozyme solution, and then on detergent solutions to lyse the bacteria. The proteins were linked to the filters under a hand held UV torch set at long wavelength for 10 minutes. Then the filters were soaked in a solution of bovine serum albumin to saturate nonspecific binding sites. The excess debris was removed by washing the filters overnight. The filters were soaked for 30 min in RT reaction mixture containing template and primer but lacking triphosphates, and then the reaction was initiated by transfer of the filters to RT mixture containing triphosphates (10 μM [α-^{32}P]dGTP; 1 Ci/mmol) and was allowed to proceed for 30 min at room temperature. Finally, the filters were fixed in 10% trichloroacetic acid, air-dried, and exposed to X-ray film for 3-4 hours. An autoradiogram of a typical screening is shown in FIGURE 4.

The success of this protocol is partly due to the fact that under the conditions in which the HIV RT activity is assayed, the endogenous DNA polymerase I enzyme is not active. The DNA polymerase I of E. coli displays RNA-dependent DNA polymerase activity in poly(rA)·oligo(dT) template primers with manganese as the divalent cation. In this procedure, however, the HIV RT is assayed with poly(rC)·oligo(dG), with magnesium as the source of divalent cation.

Several applications of this technique can be foreseen: (1) isolation of second-site revertants of linker insertions of HIV RT; (2) isolation of drug-resistant variant reverse transcriptase molecules; (3) isolation of enzymatically active hybrid RT molecules, starting with overlapping, inactive fragments of RT genes from different retroviruses, forcing homologous recombination in bacteria to form active recombinants. We will discuss below our efforts to achieve some of these goals.

ISOLATION OF INTRAGENIC REVERTANTS

We first applied the *in situ* screening method to the isolation of an intragenic suppressor mutation capable of restoring activity to an inactive mutant of HIV-1 RT.[12] The procedure involved *in vitro* mutagenesis of a selected inactive mutant to generate

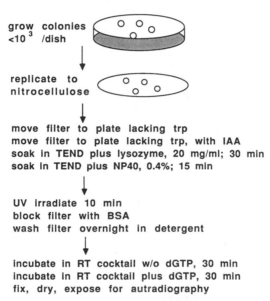

FIGURE 3. Flow chart for the *in situ* screen for HIV RT activity in bacterial colonies. (Prasad & Goff.[12] With permission from the *Journal of Biological Chemistry.*)

a pool of random mutations, followed by screening among the collection of mutagenized clones for the presence of a rare, active variant.

We selected the mutant A5 as parent because this mutant has an interesting phenotype (see above): the mutant shows very low DNA polymerase activity (about 1% of wild-type), though the only change is an insertion in the C-terminal domain. The ability of this mutation to affect the polymerase function despite its localization in the RNAse H domain indicates an interaction of the RNAse H domain with the upstream sequences in some way. The mutant plasmid was subjected to mutagenesis with ethyl methanesulfonate (EMS), and the pool of mutant plasmids was transformed into HB101 and plated for screening. Upon screening 50,000 colonies, one revertant was obtained. This revertant, termed A5rev, displayed 10-20% of the wild-type level of activity, a significant increase above that of the original mutant. Analysis of fusion protein encoded

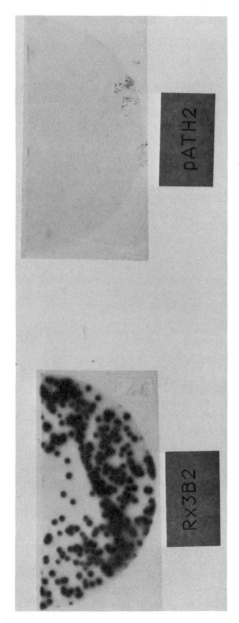

FIGURE 4. Example of *in situ* screen for HIV RT activity. Bacteria carrying the pHRTRX2 plasmid (Rx3B2) expressing the wild-type HIV RT, or pATH2 vector alone, as indicated, were plated and processed for detection of RT activity. (Prasad & Goff.[12] With permission from the *Journal of Biological Chemistry*.)

by the mutant plasmid showed a 100 kDa protein, much smaller than the parental 110 kDa protein. Examination of the A5rev DNA by restriction analysis showed no gross rearrangement or deletions, and the Eco RI site of the A5 was retained in the A5rev. The results suggest that a small change made in the RT sequence resulted in a shorter and more active protein.

To identify the region in which the second genetic change had occurred, we generated hybrid constructs containing various regions of the A5 and A5rev clones. In one pair of constructs, the HIV RT insert region was exchanged between the two clones (ex1 and ex2); in another pair the small fragment downstream of the Eco RI site was swapped (ex3 and ex4). Bacteria carrying each construct were grown and induced for the expression of the hybrid protein, and lysates were assayed for the RT activity. The increased RT activity of the A5rev correlated with the HIV RT sequences and not with the vector; the critical area was the small region 3' to the insertion.

To identify the mutation precisely, we determined the nucleotide sequence of clone A5rev in the vicinity of the original A5 mutation. A single nucleotide change, a C to T transition, was found just 3' of the original insertion (FIG. 5); all the remaining sequences matched that of the parent. The new base change resulted in the conversion of a glutamine codon into a terminator codon. The encoded protein would be 79 amino acids shorter than the parental protein, the missing residues accounting for loss of about 9 kDa, in good agreement with the observed shift in the migration of the A5rev protein.

The result, first, supports our initial finding that the C terminus is not essential for polymerase activity. Second, it suggests that the original A5 mutation blocks polymerase activity only when present in the full RNAse domain. It is noteworthy that the truncation occurred 3' to the parental linker insertion mutation; the A5rev protein actually retains the inserted amino acids present in the A5 parent, residues that in the context of the whole protein were profoundly inhibitory. This suggests that they could act to reduce the activity strongly only when embedded in the complete C-terminal domain. We have previously described a similar mutant, A23, in this region in the M-MuLV RT;[10] when the two genes are aligned, the HIV A5 and M-MuLV A23 mutations map only 8 residues apart. Thus, this region of RNAse H domain may be able to interact with the polymerase domain in several different RT enzymes.

ISOLATION OF DRUG-RESISTANT HIV RT VARIANTS

Recent reports of isolation of AZT-resistant HIV variant viruses from patients receiving therapy against AIDS have important implications in the design of treatments.[13] It has been shown that these AZT-resistant viruses contain specific genetic alterations in the RT gene.[14] Therefore, it appears that during replication, mutations are introduced into the genome that can confer selective growth advantages to the virus. Rare variants containing an appropriate mutation in the reverse transcriptase gene produce an altered enzyme that can function in the presence of a nucleoside analogue inhibitor. The strong selection operating in patients receiving long-term therapy would favor the growth of the resistant variant.

We have employed the *in situ* screening assay for HIV RT in combination with *in vitro* mutagenesis to isolate drug-resistant reverse transcriptases. The technique involves the mutagenesis of the HIV RT expression plasmid to generate a pool of random mutations and then to screen several thousand colonies for enzymatic activity in the presence of inhibitory concentrations of nucleoside analogue drug. In our initial studies

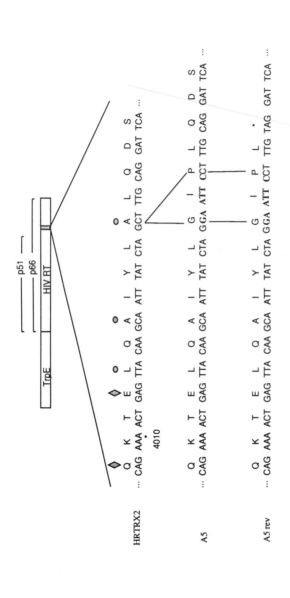

FIGURE 5. Nucleotide sequence around the site of reversion in revertant A5rev. The bar at the top represents the trpE-RT gene fusion; the small shaded area represents the region expanded below. The sequences of the wild-type HRTRX2, the parental A5 mutant, and the A5rev revertant are indicated below. The reversion event was a C-to-T change that created a stop codon soon after the A5 insertion mutation. (Prasad & Goff.[12] With permission from the *Journal of Biological Chemistry*.)

we employed dideoxyguanosine triphosphate as the inhibitor, and by screening approximately 50,000 colonies, we obtained one clone exhibiting significantly higher activity in the presence of the inhibitor than the wild-type enzyme (Prasad and Goff, in preparation). The mutant enzyme was found to exhibit a normal specific activity in the absence of the inhibitor and to be capable of extensive synthesis. Tests of the enzyme in standard assays showed that it was indeed altered in its sensitivity to ddGTP; the concentration required for half-maximal inhibition was approximately 10-fold higher than for the wild-type enzyme. Further analysis of this mutant should allow us to determine the nature and location of the mutation responsible for the resistance and to test the mutant for cross-resistance to other compounds.

The ease with which resistant enzymes such as this one are isolated bodes ill for the development of drug resistance in patients undergoing treatment with similar antiviral compounds.

SUMMARY AND CONCLUSIONS

The retroviral RT is properly under intensive study as the major target of antiviral therapy. The enzyme exhibits a number of features that make it an attractive target: it is crucial for viral replication; its RNA-dependent DNA polymerase activity is probably unique to viral replication, or if not unique, is generally unimportant in host cell function; its activities are readily monitored; and powerful lead compounds in the form of nucleotide analogues are already in hand. Our laboratory has been involved in studies to elucidate the structure and function of the HIV-1 RT and to develop a formal genetics of the enzyme. Working with constructs expressing RT in bacteria, we have been able to use *in vitro* mutagenesis to localize functions on the molecule; by coupling mutagenesis with high-throughput screening of colonies, we have been able to isolate mutants with specific, rare, phenotypes. We believe that extensions of these efforts will help us to understand the functions of the protein and, coupled to a detailed three-dimensional structure, should facilitate the development of new and better inhibitors.

REFERENCES

1. GILBOA, E., S. W. MITRA, S. P. GOFF & D. BALTIMORE. 1980. Cell **18**: 93-100.
2. GOFF, S. P. 1990. J. AIDS **3**: 817-831.
3. CHANDRA, P., A. VOGEL & T. GERBER. 1985. Cancer Res. (suppl.) **45**: 4677s-4684s.
4. LIGHTFOOTE, M. M., J. E. COLIGAN, T. M. FOLKS, A. S. FAUCI & A. M. MARTIN. 1986. J. Virol. **60**: 771-775.
5. DI MARZO VERONESE, F. D., T. D. COPELAND, A. L. DEVICO, R. RAHMAN, S. OROSZLAN, R. C. GALLO & M. G. SARNGADHARAN. 1986. Science **231**: 1289-1291.
6. TANESE, N., M. ROTH & S. P. GOFF. 1985. Proc. Natl. Acad. Sci. USA **82**: 4944-4948.
7. TANESE, N., J. SODROSKI, W. HASELTINE & S. P. GOFF. 1986. J. Virol. **59**: 743-745.
8. TANESE, N., V. R. PRASAD & S. P. GOFF. 1988. DNA **7**: 407-416.
9. PRASAD, V. R. & S. P. GOFF. 1989. Proc. Natl. Acad. Sci. USA **86**: 3104-3108.
10. TANESE, N. & S. P. GOFF. 1988. Proc. Natl. Acad. Sci. USA **85**: 1777-1781.
11. RUCHETON, M., M. N. LELAY & P. JEANTEUR. 1979. Virology **97**: 221-223.
12. PRASAD, V. R. & S. P. GOFF. 1989. J. Biol. Chem. **264**: 16689-16693.
13. LARDER, B. A., G. DARBY & D. RICHMAN. 1989. Science **243**: 1731-1734.
14. LARDER, B. A. & S. D. KEMP. 1989. Science **246**: 1155-1158.

Comparative Studies of 2',3'-Didehydro-2',3'-Dideoxythymidine (D4T) with other Pyrimidine Nucleoside Analogues

JOHN C. MARTIN,[a] MICHAEL J. M. HITCHCOCK,
ARNOLD FRIDLAND,[b] ISMAIL GHAZZOULI,
SANJEEV KAUL, LISA M. DUNKLE,
ROMAN Z. STERZYCKI, AND
MUZAMMIL M. MANSURI

Bristol-Myers Squibb
Wallingford, Connecticut 06492
and
[b]*St. Jude Children's Research Hospital*
Memphis, Tennessee 38101

Subsequent to the discovery of the potent activity of 3'-azido-3'-deoxythymidine (AZT) against human immunodeficiency virus (HIV),[1] dideoxynucleoside analogues as a class were discovered to possess anti-HIV activity.[2] As a result, we and many other institutions embarked on research programs directed towards the identification of nucleoside analogues with optimal therapeutic potential. The disclosure that AZT is not only efficacious in patients with AIDS[3] but is also substantially toxic[4] provided additional momentum to this research. Finally, the recent report of AZT resistance[5] provided a further urgency to the search for new therapeutic agents. A major portion of our research has been focused on the synthesis and evaluation of compounds in the pyrimidine series, analogues of 2'-deoxycytidine and thymidine. Comparative studies led to the selection of 2',3'-didehydro-2',3'-dideoxythymidine (D4T) as a candidate for clinical development.

RESULTS AND DISCUSSION

Cytidine analogues prepared included 2'-fluoro-2',3'-dideoxycytidine (FddC), 3'-hydroxymethyl-2',3'-dideoxycytidine (HMddC), and 2',3'-didehydro-2',3'-dideoxycytidine (D4C), which were evaluated in comparison to 2',3'-dideoxycytosine (ddC),[2] FIGURE 1. The synthesis and evaluation of FddC has been reported by three other

[a] Present address: Gilead Sciences, 346 Lakeside Dr., Foster City, CA 94404.

groups.[6-8] We prepared FddC by deoxygenation and amination of 1-(2-deoxy-2-fluoro-β-D-arabinofuranosyl)uracil (FAU).[9] The novel analogue HMddC, not previously reported in the literature, was synthesized from a ribose homologue precursor.[10] Our evaluation of D4C was carried out in a collaborative effort with Dr. Lin and Professor Prusoff of Yale University.[11,12] Other groups have reported on the anti-HIV activity of D4C,[13,14] the synthesis of which was first described by Horwitz.[15]

The *in vitro* antiviral potencies of the cytidine analogues are compared to that of ddC in TABLE 1, where ID_{50} is the 50% inhibitory dose. Although all were found to

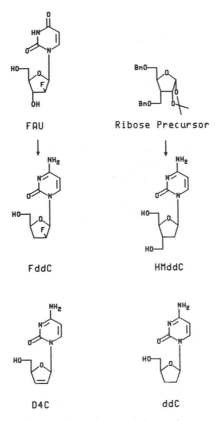

FAU

Ribose Precursor

FddC

HMddC

D4C

ddC

FIGURE 1. 2'-Deoxycytidine analogues.

be active against HIV, none of these analogues showed a potency comparable to that of ddC. HMddC is unique among the compounds discussed in this article in that it exhibited *in vitro* activity against herpes simplex virus types 1 and 2 (HSV 1 and HSV 2) and human cytomegalovirus (HCMV). Because severe herpesvirus infections are a common consequence of the immunosuppression in AIDS patients, such a broad spectrum activity may offer an intriguing therapeutic opportunity.

Because these cytidine analogues were found to be less active than ddC *in vitro* against HIV, they might offer a more narrow therapeutic index. The clinical evaluation

TABLE 1. Antiviral Activity of Cytidine Analogues

Compound	ID_{50}, $\mu g/mL$			
	HSV 1	HSV 2	HCMV	HIV
FddC	—	—	—	0.6
D4C	—	—	—	0.4
HMddC	2.8	1.4	1.7	0.6
ddC	—	—	—	<0.05

of ddC has been difficult because of the dose-limiting toxicity of peripheral neuropathy.[16] The lack of a predictive animal model for this toxicity is of concern when considering the further evaluation of the less active cytidine analogues. Therefore, we turned our attention to the evaluation of thymidine derivatives. Inasmuch as AZT was already proven efficacious,[3] our goal was to identify a substance that would rely on the same enzymes for its metabolism but have an improved therapeutic index.

The thymidine analogues chosen for comparison with AZT were D4T and FddT, FIGURE 2. Like D4C, the substance D4T was identified through the collaboration with Yale,[12,17,18] and others have also noted the activity of D4T.[14,19] Although a synthesis of D4T has been known for some time,[20] we optimized the earlier route[18] and then developed new approaches[21] to allow for the efficient preparation of this substance. Our evaluation of FddT[22] followed the observation of its activity by the Max-Planck Institute.[23] Several other reports of the activity of FddT also have been published.[24,25]

In vitro data have shown that D4T and AZT have comparable potency against HIV, but FddT was at least tenfold more potent.[26] Against human bone marrow stem cells, D4T was substantially less toxic than the other two thymidine analogues.[26] These results led to the prediction that D4T would be less likely than the other two analogues to show dose-limiting bone marrow suppression.

In order to follow up on the *in vitro* observation that D4T might not be as toxic to bone marrow stem cells, the thymidine analogues were evaluated in a one month mouse study.[26] The three substances were given orally to mice once a day for 30 days. The dose levels were 100, 250, 500, and 1000 mg/kg/day. AZT and FddT did show similar spectra of hematopoietic toxicities. With FddT, these toxicities occurred at a much lower dose than with AZT, indicating that FddT may not have a therapeutic advantage over AZT. By contrast, the dose-limiting toxicity of D4T in mice was hepatotoxicity, which was observed at a higher dose level than bone marrow toxicity due to AZT. Because D4T has an *in vitro* antiviral potency comparable to that of AZT, these results indicated that D4T might offer a superior therapeutic index relative to AZT and led to the decision to evaluate this thymidine analogue further in clinical trials.

Because no animal model is available that would be predictive for clinical efficacy, biochemical and pharmacokinetic studies were initiated in order to provide a scientific basis for the clinical development of D4T. These studies were carried out to furnish predictions for efficacious dose levels and dosing frequencies. The biochemical studies were performed to compare the cellular metabolism of D4T with that of AZT. To exert an antiviral effect these substances are first enzymatically phosphorylated in cells to their corresponding triphosphates, which then block virus replication by inhibition of the viral enzyme reverse transcriptase. Inasmuch as triphosphates of D4T and AZT were shown to be comparable inhibitors of reverse transcriptase,[18] predictions of efficacy could be derived by comparing the levels of triphosphate metabolites in cells.

AZT had already been shown to be rather inefficiently metabolized to its corresponding triphosphate because the conversion of the mono- to the diphosphate proceeded poorly.[27] This led to excessive accumulation of AZT monophosphate. Recent results have shown that the cellular pharmacology of D4T differs favorably from that of AZT.[28] The rate-limiting step in D4T metabolism is the initial phosphorylation to the monophosphate, and unlike AZT, excessive quantities of D4T metabolites do not accumulate in cells. In large quantities, such metabolites could interfere with normal cellular metabolism, a phenomenon that has been postulated to be responsible in part for the toxicity seen with AZT.[27]

Another important feature of the cellular metabolism of D4T is that the level of D4T triphosphate increases in proportion to the concentration of the nucleoside analogue incubated with the cells. This contrasts with AZT where the monophosphate increases in a dose-proportional manner, but the level of triphosphate remains relatively constant. Because the active form of a nucleoside drug is the triphosphate, these results predicted that D4T would be more likely to provide a clinical benefit proportional to dose administered.

A final point is that the triphosphates of both D4T and AZT have long intracellular half-lives (3.5 hours).[28] This result lead to a prediction that dosing less frequently than the 5 or 6 times a day currently used for AZT could have utility.[28,29] To gain the benefit of less frequent dosing, more drug would be given per dose; therefore, the possibility of less frequent dosing for D4T depends on the proportion of the triphosphate formed in cells relative to the dose administered.

Differences in the cellular pharmacology between D4T and AZT have been observed by others[30] and recently extended in experiments carried out at St. Jude Children's Research Hospital, TABLE 2. CEM cells were incubated with D4T or AZT over a concentration range of 5 to 50 μM and the levels of metabolites measured. Over this range, the concentration of D4T triphosphate (D4T-TP) produced increased from 5.5 to 22.5 pmol/10^6 cells. By contrast, the amount of AZT triphosphate (AZT-TP) produced was lower and relatively constant, 2.5 to 3.2 pmol/10^6 cells. Additionally, AZT monophosphate (AZT-MP) accumulated to excessive levels whereas D4T monophosphate (D4T-MP) did not.

Before initiating pharmacokinetic studies, the stability of D4T was assayed in acidic solutions inasmuch as instability could lead to poor or variable oral bioavailability. In spite of the allylic acetal functionality in the D4T sugar that might be expected to be acid-sensitive, this compound was found to be quite stable at pH 2, a result recently observed by others.[31]

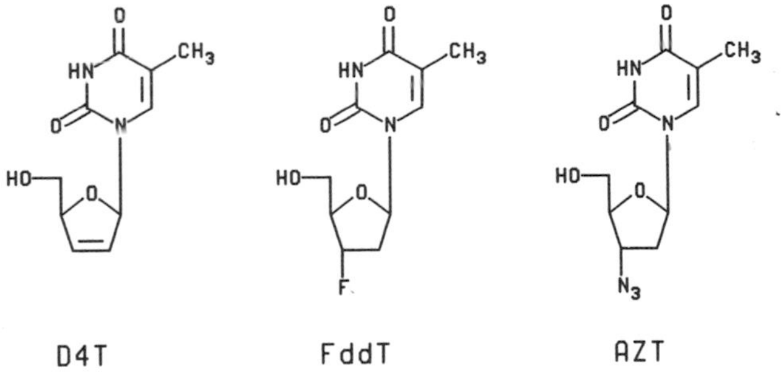

FIGURE 2. Thymidine analogues.

TABLE 2. Metabolism of D4T and AZT in CEM Cells

| Metabolite | pmol/10^6 cells of metabolite at nucleoside concentrations in μM | | | |
	5	10	25	50
D4T-MP	1.7	3.3	6.6	11.5
D4T-TP	5.5	7.3	14.5	22.5
AZT-MP	165	261	465	742
AZT-TP	2.5	2.9	3.1	3.2

Pharmacokinetic studies were carried out in mouse, rat, dog, and monkey by Russell et al.[32,33] The oral bioavailability of D4T in the rat was found to be 98%, and the pharmacokinetic parameters were similar to that of AZT. In the mouse, D4T and AZT were shown to cross the blood-brain barrier to about the same extent. Most important was the discovery that D4T, unlike AZT, was not glucuronidated in the dog or monkey. Because AZT is glucuronidated in humans, this result led to the prediction that D4T would have a greater oral bioavailability and area under the curve (AUC) in humans than does AZT.

The phase I clinical trials of D4T were initiated recently. The compound is being evaluated at dosing intervals of 6 and 8 hours. Some initial pharmacokinetic data are now available and summarized in TABLE 3. These results have confirmed the prediction[32,33] that the oral bioavailability (F, %) of D4T would be greater than that of AZT, 86% and 65%, respectively.[34] The AUC for D4T is also approximately fourfold that seen with comparable doses of AZT. Inasmuch as D4T and AZT have similar in vitro antiviral potencies, these pharmacokinetic data indicate that a therapeutic benefit might be achieved with D4T at lower doses. These favorable results have led to the decision to include lower doses and less frequent dosing (twice a day) in the phase I studies.

The limited clinical experience to date has provided some preliminary indications of efficacy at doses as low as 2 and 4 mg/kg/day. These doses are lower than the therapeutic doses for AZT. The prediction that bone marrow toxicity would not be the dose-limiting toxicity did prove accurate. The major toxicity seen to date, however, has been peripheral neuropathy, which was not predicted. Because this toxicity has now also been observed with ddC[16] and ddI,[35] peripheral neuropathy appears to be an

TABLE 3. Human Pharmacokinetic Data on D4T

| Parameter | Patient 1 | | Patient 2 | |
	i.v.	p.o.	i.v.	p.o.
dose, mg	70.5	280	69	250
C_{max},[a] μg/mL	1.31	3.76	1.38	5.22
T_{max},[b] h	0.75	1.50	1.00	0.50
T_{half},[c] h	1.09	1.11	1.03	1.26
AUC, h.μg/mL	2.22	7.60	2.07	6.55
F, %		86		87

[a] Maximal concentration.
[b] Time that maximal concentration is achieved.
[c] Elimination half-life.

adverse effect common to this class of compounds. Research on the mechanism by which dideoxynucleoside analogues induce this toxicity is important to enable development of predictive assays for the peripheral neuropathy. These assays could then be used to enable selection of new compounds for clinical development.

The selection of D4T as a clinical candidate was based on comparative preclinical studies with other dideoxynucleoside analogues, including AZT. These studies also led to successful predictions for the evaluation of this substance in humans. The results of the ongoing clinical studies with D4T are expected to provide useful information for feedback into our preclinical research process to help improve the correlation between preclinical data and clinical efficacy and safety.

REFERENCES

1. MITSUYA, H., K. J. WEINHOLD, P. A. FURMAN, M. H. ST. CLAIR, S. NUSINOFF LEHRMAN, R. C. GALLO, D. BOLOGNESI, D. W. BARRY & S. BRODER. 1985. Proc. Natl. Acad. Sci. USA **82:** 7096-7100.
2. MITSUYA, H. & S. BRODER. 1986. Proc. Natl. Acad. Sci. USA **83:** 1911-1915.
3. FISCHL, M. A., D. D. RICHMAN, M. H. GRIECO, M. S. GOTTLIEB, P. A. VOLBERDING, O. L. LASKIN, J. M. LEEDOM, J. E. GROOPMAN, D. MILDVAN, R. T. SCHOOLEY, G. G. JACKSON, D. T. DURACK & D. KING. 1987. N. Engl. J. Med. **317:** 185-191.
4. RICHMAN, D. D., M. A. FISCHL, M. H. GRIECO, M. S. GOTTLIEB, P. A. VOLBERDING, O. L. LASKIN, J. M. LEEDOM, J. E. GROOPMEN, D. MILDVAN, M. S. HIRSCH, G. G. JACKSON, D. T. DURACK & S. NUSINOFF-LEHRMAN. 1987. N. Engl. J. Med. **317:** 192-197.
5. LARDER, B. A., G. DARBY & D. D. RICHMAN. 1989. Science **243:** 1731-1734.
6. ZEIDLER, J., L. C. CHEN, J. MATULIC-ADAMIC & K. A. WATANABE. 1988. Abstracts 196th ACS Meeting. Carbohydrate Division Abstract 4. Los Angeles, CA.
7. MACHIN, P. J., J. A. MARTIN & G. J. THOMAS. 1988. European Patent Application 292,023.
8. DE CLERCQ, E., A. VAN AERSCHOT, P. HERDEWIJN, M. BABA, R. PAUWELS & J. BALZARINI. 1989. Nucleosides & Nucleotides **8:** 659-671.
9. WATANABE, K. A., U. REICHMAN, K. HIROTA, C. LOPEZ & J. J. FOX. 1979. J. Med. Chem. **22:** 21-24.
10. ACTON, E. M., R. N. GOERNER, H. S. UH, K. J. RYAN, D. W. HENRY, C. E. CASS & G. A. LEPAGE. 1979. J. Med. Chem. **22:** 518-525.
11. LIN, T. S., R. F. SCHINAZI, M. S. CHEN, E. KINNEY-THOMAS & W. H. PRUSOFF. 1987. Biochem. Pharmacol. **36:** 311-316.
12. LIN, T. S., M. S. CHEN, C. MCLAREN, Y. S. GAO, I. GHAZZOULI & W. H. PRUSOFF. 1987. J. Med. Chem. **30:** 440-444.
13. BALZARINI, J., R. PAUWELS, P. HERDEWIJN, E. DE CLERCQ, D. A. COONEY, G. J. KANG, M. DALAL, D. G. JOHNS & S. BRODER. 1986. Biochem. Biophys. Res. Commun. **140:** 735-742.
14. HAMAMOTO, Y., H. NAKASHIMA, T. MATSUI, A. MATSUDA, T. UEDA & N. YAMAMOTO. 1987. Antimicrob. Agents Chemother. **31:** 907-910.
15. HORWITZ, J. P., J. CHUA, M. NOEL & J. T. DONATTI. 1967. J. Org. Chem. **32:** 817-818.
16. YARCHOAN, R., R. V. THOMAS, J. P. ALLAIN, N. MCATEE, R. DUBINSKY, H. MITSUYA, T. J. LAWLEY, B. SAFAI, C. E. MYERS, C. F. PERNO, R. W. KLECKER, R. J. WILLS, M. A. FISCHL, M. C. MCNEELY, J. M. PLUDA, M. LEUTHER, J. M. COLLINS & S. BRODER. 1988. Lancet i: 76-81.
17. LIN, T. S., R. F. SCHINAZI & W. H. PRUSOFF. 1987. Biochem. Pharmacol. **17:** 2713-2718.
18. MANSURI, M. M., J. E. STARRETT, JR., I. GHAZZOULI, M. J. M. HITCHCOCK, R. Z. STERZYCKI, V. BRANKOVAN, T. S. LIN, E. M. AUGUST, W. H. PRUSOFF, J. P SOMMADOSSI & J. C. MARTIN. 1989. J. Med. Chem. **32:** 461-466.
19. BABA, M., R. PAUWELS, P. HERDEWIJN, E. DE CLERCQ, J. DESMYTER & M. VANDEPUTTE. 1987. Biochem. Biophys. Res. Commun. **142:** 128-134.

20. HORWITZ, J. P., J. CHUA, M. A. DA ROOGE, M. NOEL & I. L. KLUNDT. 1966. J. Org. Chem. **31:** 205-211.
21. MANSURI, M. M., J. E. STARRETT, JR., J. A. WOS, D. R. TORTOLANI, P. R. BRODFUEHRER, H. G. HOWELL & J. C. MARTIN. 1989. J. Org. Chem. **54:** 4780-4785.
22. STERZYCKI, R., M. MANSURI, V. BRANKOVAN, R. BUROKER, I. GHAZZOULI, M. HITCH-COCK, J. P. SOMMADOSSI & J. C. MARTIN. 1989. Nucleosides & Nucleotides **8:** 1115-1117.
23. HARTMANN, H., M. W. VOGT, A. G. DURNO, M. S. HIRSCH, G. HUNSMANN & F. ECKSTEIN. 1988. AIDS Res. Hum. Retroviruses **4:** 457-466.
24. MATTHES, E., C. LEHMANN, D. SCHOLZ, H. A. ROSENTHAL & P. LANGEN. 1988. Biochem. Biophys. Res. Commun. **153:** 825-831.
25. BAZIN, H., J. CHATTOPADHYAYA, R. DATEMA, A. C. ERICSON, G. GILLIAM, N. G. JOHANSSON, J. HANSEN, R. KOSHIDA, K. MOELLING, B. OBERG, G. REMAUD, G. STENING, L. VRANG, B. WAHREN & J. C. WU. 1989. Biochem. Pharmacol. **38:** 109-119.
26. MANSURI, M. M., M. J. M. HITCHCOCK, R. A. BUROKER, C. L. BREGMAN, I. GHAZZOULI, J. V. DESIDERIO, J. E. STARRETT, R. Z. STERZYCKI & J. C. MARTIN. 1990. Antimicrob. Agents Chemother. **34:** 637-641.
27. FURMAN, P. A., J. A. FYFE, M. H. ST. CLAIR, K. WEINHOLD, J. L. RIDEOUT, G. A. FREEMAN, S. NUSINOFF LEHRMAN, D. P. BOLOGNESI, S. BRODER, H. MITSUYA & D. W. BARRY. 1986. Proc. Natl. Acad. Sci. USA **83:** 8333-8337.
28. HO, H. T. & M. J. M. HITCHCOCK. 1989. Antimicrob. Agents Chemother. **33:** 844-849.
29. MARTIN, J. C., M. M. MANSURI, J. E. STARRETT, JR., J. P. SOMMADOSSI, V. BRANKOVAN, I. GHAZZOULI, H. T. HO & M. J. M. HITCHCOCK. 1989. Nucleosides & Nucleotides **8:** 841-844.
30. BALZARINI, J., P. HERDEWIJN & E. DE CLERCQ. 1989. J. Biol. Chem. **264:** 6127-6133.
31. KAWAGUCHI, T., S. FUKUSHIMA, M. OHMURA, M. MISHIMA & M. NAKANO. 1989. Chem. Pharm. Bull. (Tokyo) **37:** 1944-1945.
32. RUSSELL, J. W., V. J. WHITEROCK, D. MARRERO & L. J. KLUNK. 1989. Nucleosides & Nucleotides **8:** 845-848.
33. RUSSELL, J. W., V. J. WHITEROCK, D. MARRERO & L. J. KLUNK. 1990. Drug Metab. Dispos. **18:** 153-157.
34. BLUM, M. R., S. H. T. LIAO, S. S. GOOD & P. DE MIRANDA. 1988. Am. J. Med. **85**(S2A): 189-194.
35. YARCHOAN, R., H. MITSUYA, R. V. THOMAS, J. M. PLUDA, N. R. HARTMAN, C. F. PERNO, K. S. MARCZYK, J. P. ALLAIN, D. G. JOHNS & S. BRODER. 1989. Science **245:** 412-415.

Correlation of Molecular Conformation and Activity of Reverse Transcriptase Inhibitors[a]

PATRICK VAN ROEY,[b] E. WILL TAYLOR,[c]
CHUNG K. CHU,[c] AND RAYMOND F. SCHINAZI [d]

[b]Molecular Biophysics Department
Medical Foundation of Buffalo, Inc.
Buffalo, New York 14203

[c]Department of Medicinal Chemistry
College of Pharmacy
The University of Georgia
Athens, Georgia 30602

[d]Department of Pediatrics
Emory University School of Medicine
and Veterans Administration Medical Center
Atlanta, Georgia 30033

The enzyme reverse transcriptase (RTase) of the human immunodeficiency virus type 1 (HIV-1) is an attractive target for the treatment of AIDS[1,2] because of its role in the introduction of the viral genetic material into the genome of the host cell. The retroviral RTase displays transcriptase, RNase H, and DNA-polymerase activity in producing DNA from the viral RNA template. Nucleoside analogues have long been known as antiviral agents because of their ability to interfere with DNA synthesis by inhibiting DNA polymerases.[3] It is therefore not surprising that the first effective agent against HIV-1 was the nucleoside analogue 3'-azido-3'-deoxythymidine[4-6] (AZT, retrovir, zidovudine) and that much effort in AIDS research has been focussed on the search for more effective analogues.[7-9] No rational approach to the design and development of these analogues has emerged, however. Large numbers of analogues have been synthesized and tested, but very few have been proven to be viable candidates for clinical testing, either for lack of activity or for excessive toxicity. Much effort has been devoted to compounds that lack the 3'-hydroxyl substituent of the natural nucleoside because they can act as chain terminators after incorporation into the DNA chain being formed. Although chain termination by AZT has been demonstrated, however, it has not been fully established that it is an essential requirement for activity or that, alternatively, binding of the inhibitor to RTase, at least temporarily blocking the active site, is sufficient for activity.

The design of RTase inhibitors is complicated by the intricate process of drug activation, the need for selectivity for RTase over other DNA polymerases, the lack of

[a]This research was supported in part by Grants RR-05761 (P. Van Roey), AI-26055, and AI-25899 (C. K. Chu and R. F. Schinazi) of the National Institutes of Health, DHHS, and the Veterans Administration (R. F. Schinazi).

29

knowledge of properties of the active site of RTase or other polymerases, and the conformational flexibility of the nucleoside molecule. The nucleoside analogues need to be converted to their respective 5'-triphosphate nucleotides by nucleoside and nucleotide kinases of the host cell.[3,10] Different enzymes are involved in the phosphorylation of nucleosides with different bases. Hoe *et al.*[11] have shown that the rates of phosphorylation differ for nucleosides with different bases, leading to differences in apparent RTase activity because of differences in the pool size of the 5'-triphosphates rather than in RTase binding efficiency. Therefore, structure-activity studies of the nucleosides need to take the phosphorylation process into account.

Because of the large number of nucleoside analogues synthesized and tested and the extensive literature on the conformational properties of nucleosides, the database required for structure-activity studies is available. FIGURE 1 shows the basic template and numbering scheme of pyrimidine nucleosides. The nucleoside analogues that have been studied most thoroughly as potential anti-HIV-1 drugs include various 2',3'-dideoxyribose,[12] 2'3'-didehydro-2',3'-dideoxyribose,[13] and 3'-substituted 2',3'-dideoxyribose[14] analogues of thymidine, uridine, 5-alkyluridine, 5-halouridine, cytidine, adeno-

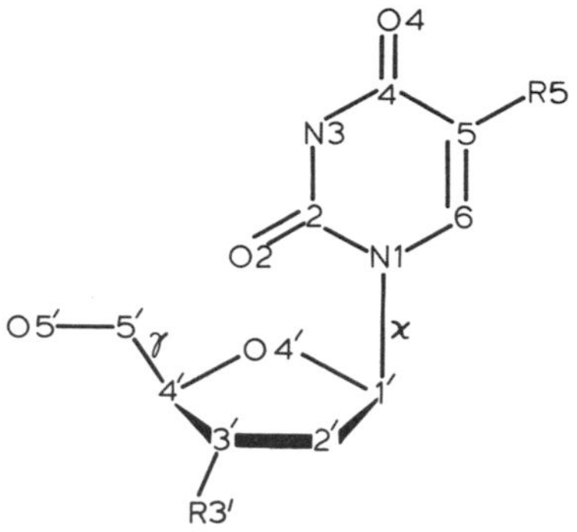

FIGURE 1. Schematic diagram showing the essential components and numbering scheme used for the description of thymidine and uridine analogues.

sine, inosine, and guanosine. Other analogues with modified ribose moieties include compounds in which a methylene group replaces O4'[15] or where oxygen or sulfur is substituted for C3'.[16] More novel compounds are adenallene and cytallene,[17] shown in FIGURE 2, where the ribose ring is replaced by a rigid allene group. Closely related compounds from this list can differ greatly in anti-HIV-1 activity levels.[18] The 2',3'-dideoxy and 2',3'-didehydro-2',3'-dideoxy analogues of thymidine, adenosine, and cytidine are very active but not those of uridine. 2',3'-Dideoxy analogues of 5-ethyluridine, 5-halouridine, 5-aminouridine, inosine, and guanosine are active but much less so. 2',3'-Didehydro-2',3'-dideoxyguanosine and inosine have poor activity. The 3'-azido derivatives of 2',3'-dideoxyuridine, 3'-deoxythymidine, 2',3'-dideoxy-5-ethyluridine, and 2',3'-dideoxycytidine are more active than their unsubstituted analogues. Other 3'-substitutions of thymidine or uridine have very different effects: the fluoro derivative is very active but the activity of the other 3'-halo compounds decreases with size of the substituent. 3'-Amino, cyano, methoxy, and alkyl analogues are inactive. TABLE 1 lists the potency and toxicity determined *in vitro* in infected peripheral blood mononuclear cells (PBM) for the 2',3'-dideoxypyrimidine and 3'-substituted 2',3'-dideoxypyrimidine analogues for which the crystal structures are available.

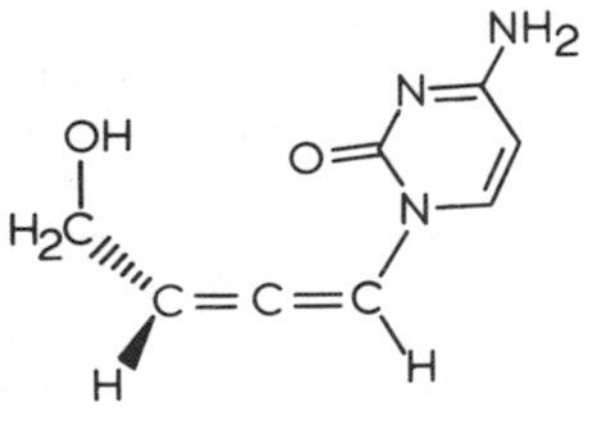

FIGURE 2. Schematic diagram of the rigid analogue cytallene.

Substantial modification of the base reduces the activity, which is not surprising given the base specificity of the nucleoside and nucleotide kinases. Many compounds with identical sugar moieties but different natural bases, however, are often similar in activity. For example, 2',3'-dideoxythymidine, -cytidine, and -adenosine are all very active. For 3'-substituents two effects can be observed: highly electronegative substituents enhance and electropositive substituents reduce the activity. This would suggest that one should be able to correlate the effect of the substitutions with the activity differences. The goal of our study is to determine if these activity properties can be correlated with conformational features of the nucleoside. This would then become a parameter in the rational approach to the design of new compounds. The study of the causes for the toxicity and the specificity for RTase over DNA polymerases of the host cell are, however, beyond the scope of the present study.

No detailed structural information, such as the active site geometry or details of the protein-substrate interactions, is presently available for the nucleoside and nucleotide kinases or for RTase. In the absence of detailed information about the mechanisms of action of the various kinases, one must assume that the active sites are similar, except for the area that accommodates the base, that the mechanisms of phosphorylation are similar, and thus that the intermediate state and binding conformations of the ribose part of the substrates are to be similar. The basic assumption of this analysis is that,

TABLE 1. Potency (EC_{50}, 50% efficiency) and Toxicity (IC_{50}, 50% inhibitory cytotoxicity) in Infected PBM Cells of the Nucleoside Analogues Included in This Study

		R_5	$R_{3'}$	EC_{50} (μM)	IC_{50} (μM)
2',3'-Dideoxynucleosides					
Uridine	ddU	H	H	96.8	ND[a]
Thymidine	ddT	CH_3	H	0.17	> 100
5-Ethyluridine	dd$_e$U	CH_2CH_3	H	4.90	> 100
Cytidine	ddC	H	H	0.011	ND
3'-Substituted 2',3'-dideoxynucleosides					
Azido uridine	N_3ddU	H	N_3	0.18-0.46	1000
Azido thymidine	N_3ddT	CH_3	N_3	0.002-0.009	200
Azido 5-ethyluridine	N_3dd$_e$U	CH_2CH_3	N_3	0.056-1.00	1000
Propylene uridine	peddU	H	CH_2-CH=CH_2	> 100.	ND
Fluoro thymidine	FddT	CH_3	F	0.0089	> 100
Amino thymidine	NH_2ddT	CH_3	NH_2	> 100.	> 100

[a] Not done.

among closely related nucleosides, those that most easily adopt the ligand conformation will be preferentially phosphorylated. This would build a larger pool of 5'-triphosphates of these compounds, leading to apparent higher RTase inhibition activity without necessarily better RTase interaction. This would require this ligand conformation to be a low energy conformation of the nucleoside. The conformations observed in crystal structures are low energy conformations, within the limitation of the crystal constraints—an environment that is determined by favorable intermolecular interactions such as hydrogen bonds and hydrophobic contacts. The high flexibility, especially of the ribose ring, of the nucleoside molecules is well-documented.[19–21] Barriers to rotation between different low energy conformations often do not exceed 5 kcal/mole. This conformational freedom precludes conclusions from a single crystal structure because packing effects may influence the conformation, but analysis of a larger sample of compounds should indicate trends that certain conformations may be favored.

RESULTS

Nucleoside Conformation

The conformations of nucleosides and their analogues have been extensively reviewed by Sundaralingam,[19] by Saenger,[20] and by Pearlman and Kim.[21] Structural data are available from X-ray crystallographic studies of more than two hundred nucleoside analogues, NMR studies, and molecular energy calculations. The three parameters that are essential for the description of the nucleoside conformation are the geometry of the glycosyl link between the base and the ribose ring, the rotation about the exocyclic C4'-C5' bond, and the puckering of the ribose ring. FIGURE 3 illustrates the definitions of the three parameters. The torsion angles χ (C2-N1-C1'-O4') and γ (C3'-C4'-C5'-O5') describe the orientations of the base and the 5'-hydroxyl group relative to the ribose ring. The puckering of the five-membered ribose ring is a continuous displacement of one (envelope) or two atoms (twist) out of the plane of the others. This puckering can be described by two parameters:[22] the pseudorotational phase angle P, which depends on all endocyclic torsion angles and indicates which atoms are displaced out of the plane and the direction of the displacement, and the maximum torsion angle ν_{max}, which corresponds to the magnitude of the displacement.

Detailed analysis of the preferred conformations has led to the following observations: (1) Glycosyl link: preference for an *anti* conformation $-180 < \chi < -115°$ in pyrimidine analogues with high *anti* ($\chi = -60°$) allowed for purine analogues. These conformations are preferred over *syn* conformations in which the base would have possible steric contacts with the ribose ring. (2) Ribose ring puckering: two conformations are preferred: C3'-*endo* ($0 < P < 18°$) and C2'-*endo* ($162 < P < 180°$). *Endo* and *exo* refer to displacement of the atom above or below the plane of the other atoms in the five-membered ring, respectively. 2'-Deoxyribose analogues have a strong preference for C2'-*endo*. These preferences are in general caused by steric effects of the substituents and the *gauche* effect.[23] (3) O5'-hydroxyl group: three possible orientations have been observed: *ap*, +*sc*, and −*sc*, with γ angles of approximately 180°, 60°, and −60°, respectively. Pyrimidine analogues have a strong preference for +*sc*, whereas purine analogues are about equal *ap* or +*sc*. All three conformational parameters are correlated, the strongest link being between the glycosidic link and the ring puckering: C3'-*endo* with $-180 < \chi < -138°$ and C2'-*endo* with $-144 < \chi < -115°$.

Observed Conformations of Anti-HIV-1 Nucleosides

TABLE 2 lists the conformational parameters for ten compounds studied by X-ray crystallographic analysis and that are included in this analysis. The set includes four 2′,3′-dideoxypyrimidines, three active and one inactive, and six 3′-substituted 2′,3′-

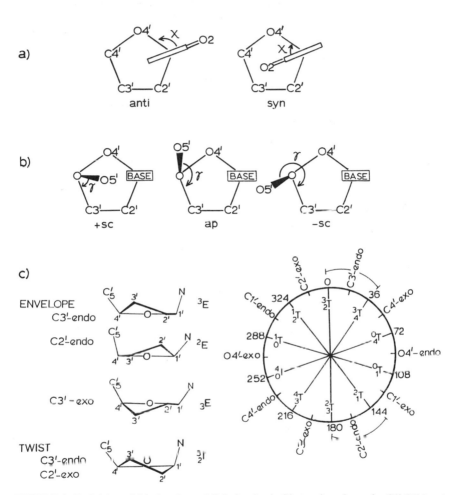

FIGURE 3. Definition of (**a**) the glycosyl link (angle χ), (**b**) rotation about the C4′-C5′ bond (angle χ), and (**c**) the ribose ring puckering (angle P) of nucleosides.

dideoxypyrimidines, four active and two inactive. Details of the crystal structure analysis of these compounds have been published elsewhere.[24–26] Many of these compounds crystallize with two or four independent molecules in the asymmetric unit. Therefore, there are seven independent observations of the 2′,3′-dideoxypyrimidines and 13 observations of 3′-substituted 2′,3′-dideoxypyrimidines. FIGURE 4 shows histograms for all three parameters for the nucleoside analogues included in this study compared with those of all 2'-deoxyuridine and thymidine analogues found in the Cambridge Crystallographic Database.[27] Inasmuch as only one 2',3'-dideoxypurine analogue (adenosine) has been included in our study so far, this analysis will be focused on pyrimidine analogues.

Two *anti* conformations are observed for the glycosyl link: one group of seven observations have a χ angle of approximately $-125°$, and the other 12 have a χ angle

TABLE 2. Conformational Characteristics of Nucleoside Analogues Used in This Study[a]

Compound	Activity	χ	γ	P	
2',3'-Dideoxynucleosides					
ddC	0.011	−156.9	164.5	208.2	$_3E$
ddT A	0.17	−170.2	63.5	12.8	$_2^3T$
B		−128.9	66.0	166.0	^2E
ddU	96.8	−163.5	177.9	7.2	$_2^3T$
dd$_e$U A	4.9	−129.7	−78.2	186.8	$_3^2T$
B		−167.4	57.8	12.5	$_2^3T$
3'-Substituted 2',3'-dideoxynucleosides					
N$_3$ddT A	0.002	−124.4	50.9	174.9	$_3^2T$
B		−173.6	173.4	215.3	$_3^4T$
N$_3$dd$_e$U A	0.56	−129.9	54.0	169.3	$_3^2T$
B		−170.8	175.1	203.3	$_3E$
C		−108.8	48.6	168.5	$_3^2T$
D		−170.6	49.6	209.6	$_3E$
N$_3$ddU	0.18	−159.8	57.3	176.3	$_3^2T$
PeddU	> 100.	−161.6	179.4	15.8	^3E
FddT A	0.0089	−153.2	51.9	175.2	$_3^2T$
B		−149.4	50.6	176.3	$_3^2T$
C		−137.6	48.3	173.5	$_3^2T$
D		−129.5	45.8	171.1	$_3^2T$
NH$_2$ddT	> 100.	−167.4	57.0	3.8	$_2^3T$

[a] Letters A through D following the compound name indicate multiple independent molecules observed in the crystal structure. In the last column, codes E and T refer to envelope or twist conformations. Superscript or subscript number refers to *endo* and *exo*, respectively, for example, $_2^3T$ means C2'-*exo*/C3'-*endo* twist.

of about $-165°$. The former conformation is more common than the latter. No direct correlation between this conformation and biological activity is observed.

The orientation about the C4'-C5' bond is primarily $+sc$ (13 observations), but the *ap* conformation is more populated (5 observations against only one for $-sc$) than expected on the basis of previous observations. The *ap* conformation appears to be observed mostly when the pseudorotation angle P is greater than 180°.

A correlation between the deoxyribose ring puckering and the biological activity becomes apparent when the sample of compounds is reviewed. Although for 2'-deoxy-

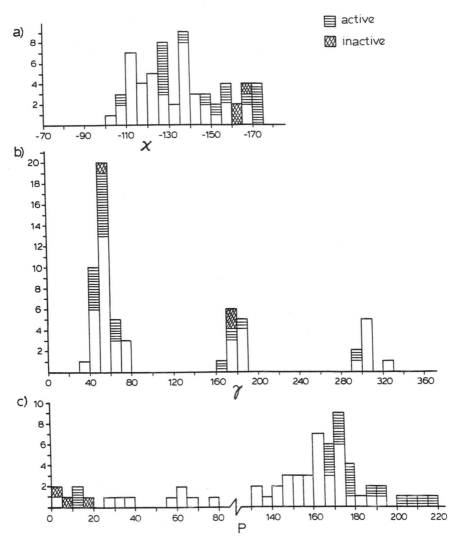

FIGURE 4. Histograms showing comparisons of the characteristics of the molecular conformations of the nucleoside analogues included in this study compared with those of other 2'-deoxyuridines and thymidines in the Cambridge Crystallographic database: (**a**) glycosyl link, (**b**) C4'-C5' rotation, and (**c**) ribose ring puckering. Analogues included in this study are indicated by horizontal shadings (active compounds) or crossed diagonal shading (inactive compounds). Note the large number of χ angles in the range of 150 to 175° and especially the large number of active conformations with $170 < P < 220°$ and inactive compounds with $0 < P < 20°$.

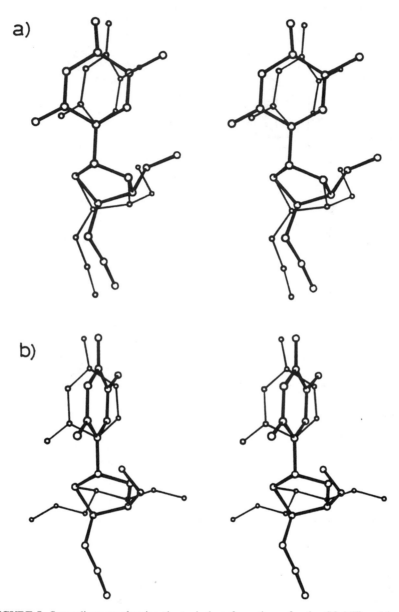

FIGURE 5. Stereodiagrams showing the typical conformations of active (N_3ddT) and inactive (peddU) anti-HIV nucleosides: **(a)** overlap of both conformations of N_3ddT (AZT) (molecule A bold, molecule B fine), **(b)** PeddU (bold) overlapped on N_3ddT molecule A, and **(c)** peddU overlapped on N_3ddT molecule B.

pyrimidines one would expect to find most conformations in the C2'-*endo*/C3'-*exo* twist conformation (P = 162°), there is a strong tendency among active compounds towards C3'-*exo* envelope (P = 198°) or the extreme C3'-*exo*/C4'-*endo* twist conformations (P > 198°). Furthermore, the three inactive compounds 2',3'-dideoxyuridine, 3'-(propyl-2-ene)-2',3'-dideoxyuridine (peddU), and 3'-amino-3'-deoxythymidine have the opposite C3'-*endo* conformations. Only two of the 16 observations of active compounds have this conformation: one of the two observations of 3'-deoxythymidine and one of the two observations of 2',3'-dideoxy-5-ethyluridine. FIGURE 5 shows the comparison of the molecular conformations of the most and least active compounds included in this study: AZT and peddU. These stereodiagrams show the molecules superimposed by the least-squares fitting of the respective N1,C1',C2', and O4' atoms, thereby emphasizing the differences in the ribose ring puckering.

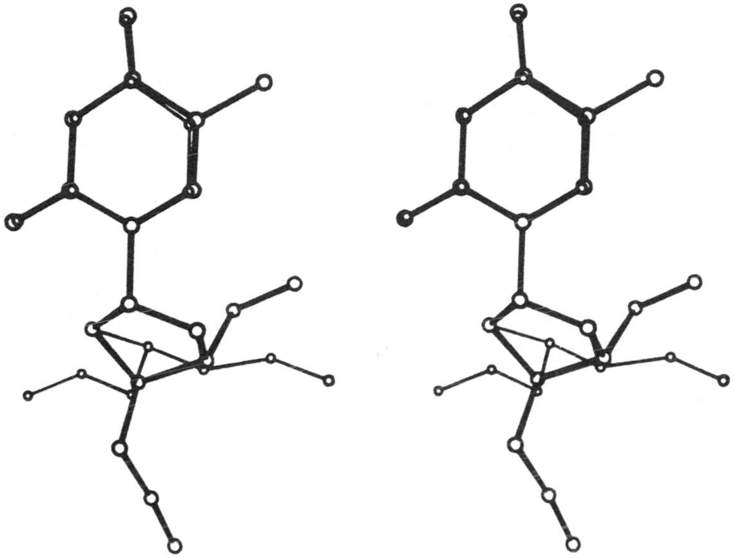

FIGURE 5c. See legend on p. 36.

DISCUSSION

Effect of Conformation on Molecular Properties

The active anti-HIV-1 nucleosides studied show a strong preference for a C3'-*exo* sugar ring conformation with a tendency towards the unusual C3'-*exo*/C4'-*endo* conformation. Associated with this extreme sugar ring conformation is a tendency to a glycosyl link geometry ($\chi \sim -170°$) that nearly eclipses C6 of the base with O4' of the ribose ring and an *ap* C5-O5' orientation. Taylor *et al.*[28] have demonstrated, on the basis of molecular mechanics calculations, that these C3'-*exo* conformations are the minimum energy conformations for the 3'-azido compounds. Their analysis of the factors[29] involved in promoting the C3'-*exo* conformation, especially in 3'-substituted analogues, has indicated that highly electronegative substituents, such as the azido and the fluoro groups, promote the C3'-*exo* conformation because of a *gauche*-effect[23] interaction of the 3'-substituent with O4'.

The conformation of the deoxyribose ring determines the relative location of the substituents. Specifically, C3'-*exo* and C3'-*endo* conformations place the C4'-substituent in axial and equatorial positions, respectively. This severely affects the distance between C5' and N1 of the base, as can be seen in FIGURE 6, and the direction of the C5'-O5' bond. The closer contact between C5' and N1 in the C3'-*exo* conformation may be held responsible for the destabilization of the +*sc* conformation about the C4'-C5' bond.

Significance for Anti-HIV-1 Activity

The phosphorylation of nucleoside analogues is known to be essential for their activity as RTase inhibitors. More efficient phosphorylation of one nucleoside may be crucial to the activity of that compound because it allows the formation of a pool of

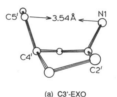

FIGURE 6. Ribose ring conformations of (**a**) N_3ddT, C3'-*exo* and (**b**) ped2U, C3'-*endo*, illustrating the effect of the ribose ring puckering on the relative positions of the base and the C5' substituent.

(a) C3'-EXO   (b) C3'-ENDO

5'-triphosphate substrates for RTase. We have determined that active analogues have a tendency to adopt a specific conformation, namely C3'-*exo* with a trend towards the unusual C4'-*endo*/C3'-*exo* twist conformation. It may well be that this conformation, which is a low energy conformation, is close to the conformation required for binding to the active site of the nucleoside kinases, thereby facilitating phosphorylation of these analogues over those that do not readily adopt this conformation. This preferred conformation differs mainly from the standard 2'-deoxynucleoside conformation by influencing the location of the 5'-hydroxyl group relative to the rest of the molecule: C5'-axial and an *ap* conformation about the C4'-C5' bond. This is consistent with other results. Studies[30] of rigid analogues of adenosine monophosphate have indicated that the *ap* conformation of the C4-C5' rotation is favorable for phosphorylation. The allene analogues of adenosine and cytidine are active anti-HIV compounds[17] and are known to require phosphorylation for activity. The minimum energy conformations of these rigid analogues most closely mimic the C3'-*exo* conformation with an *ap* C4'-C5' conformation.

On the basis of our results, the development of a rational approach to the design of new potentially active anti-HIV-1 nucleosides would need to be based on the search for compounds that have the C3'-*exo* conformation as a low energy conformation and that have the O5'-hydroxyl group in the *ap* conformation.

REFERENCES

1. MITSUYA, H. & S. BRODER. 1986. Proc. Natl. Acad. Sci. USA **83:** 1911-1915.
2. MITSUYA, H. & S. BRODER. 1987. Nature **325:** 773-778.
3. WAQAR, M. A., M. J. EVANS, K. F. MAULY, R. G. HUGHES & J. A. HUBERMAN. 1984. J. Cell. Physiol. **121:** 402-408.
4. MITSUYA, H., K. J. WEINHOLD, P. A. FURMAN, M. H. ST. CLAIR, S. N. LEHRMAN, R. L. GALLO, D. BOLOGNESI, D. W. BARRY & S. BRODER. 1985. Proc. Natl. Acad. Sci. USA **82:** 7096-7100.
5. FISCHL, M. A., D. D. RICHMAN, M. H. GRIECO, M. S. GOTTLIEB, P. A. VOLBERDING, O. L. LASKIN, J. M. LEEDOM, J. E. GROOPMAN, D. MILVAN, R. T. SCHOOLEY, G. G. JACKSON, D. T. DURACK & D. KING. 1987. N. Engl. J. Med. **317:** 185-191.
6. RICHMAN, D. D., M. A. FISCHL, M. H. GRIECO, M. S. GOTTLIEB, P. A. VOLBERDING, O. L. LASKIN, J. M. LEEDOM, J. E. GROOPMAN, D. MILVAN, M. S. HIRSCH, G. G. JACKSON, D. T. DURACK & S. N. LEHRMAN. 1987. N. Engl. J. Med. **317:** 192-197.
7. CHU, C. K., R. F. SCHINAZI, M. K. AHN, G. V. ULLAS & Z. P. GU. 1989. J. Med. Chem. **32:** 612-617.
8. LIN, T. S., J.-Y. GUO, R. F. SCHINAZI, C. K. CHU, J.-N. XIANG & W. H. PRUSOFF. 1988. J. Med. Chem. **31:** 336-340.
9. HERDEWIJN, P., R. PAUWELS, M. BABA, J. BALZARINI & E. DE CLERCQ. 1987. J. Med. Chem. **30:** 2131-2137.
10. ONO, K., H. NAKANE, P. HERDEWIJN, J. BALZARINI & E. DE CLERCQ. 1989. Mol. Pharmacol. **35:** 578-583.
11. HAO, Z., D. A. COONEY, N. R. HARTMAN, C. F. PERNO, A. FRIDLAND, A. L. DEVICO, M. G. SARNGADHARAN, S. BRODER & D. G. JOHNS. 1988. Mol. Pharmacol. **34:** 431-435.
12. HERDEWIJN, P., J. BALZARINI, E. DE CLERCQ, R. PAUWELS, M. BABA, S. BRODER & H. VANDERHAEGHE. 1987. J. Med. Chem. **30:** 1270-1278.
13. MANSURI, M. M., J. E. STARRETT, JR., I. GHAZZOULI, M. J. M. HITCHCOCK, R. Z. STERZYCKI, V. BRANKOVAN, T.-S. LIN, E. M. AUGUST, W. H. PRUSOFF, J.-P. SOMMADOSSI & J. C. MARTIN. 1989. J. Med. Chem. **32:** 461-466.
14. BALZARINI, J., G.-J. KANG, M. DALAL, P. HERDEWIJN, E. DE CLERCQ, S. BRODER & D. G. JOHNS. 1987. Mol. Pharmacol. **32:** 162-167.
15. VINCE, R., M. HUA, J. BROWNELL, S. DALUGE, F. LEE, W. M. SHANNON, G. C. LAVELLE, J. QUALLS, O. S. WEISLOW, R. KISER, P. G. CANONICO, R. H. SCHULTZ, V. L. NARAYANAN, J. G. MAYO, R. H. SHOEMAKER & M. R. BOYD. 1988. Biochem. Biophys. Res. Commun. **156:** 1046-1053.
16. BELLEAU, B., D. DIXIT, N. NGUYEN-BA & J.-L. KRAUS. 1989. 5th Int. AIDS Conf. (Montreal) (Abstract) **5:** 515.
17. HAYASHI, S., S. PHADTARE, J. ZEMLICKA, M. MATSUKURA, H. MITSUYA & S. BRODER. 1988. Proc. Natl. Acad. Sci. USA **85:** 6127-6131.
18. CHU, C. K., R. F. SCHINAZI, B. H. ARNOLD, D. L. CANNON, B. DOBOSZEWSKI, V. B. BHADTI & Z. P. GU. 1988. Biochem. Pharmacol. **37:** 35-43.
19. SUNDARALINGAM, M. 1975. *In* Structure and Conformation of Nucleic Acid and Protein-Nucleic Acid Interactions. M. SUNDARALINGAM & S. T. RAO, Eds.: 487-536. University Park Press, Baltimore, MD.
20. SAENGER, W. 1984. Principles of Nucleic Acid Structure. 9-104. Springer-Verlag. New York.
21. PEARLMAN, D. A. & S.-H. KIM. 1985. J. Biomol. Struct. Dyn. **3:** 99-125.
22. ALTONA, C. & M. SUNDARALINGAM. 1972. J. Am. Chem. Soc. **94:** 8205-8212.
23. OLSON, W. K. 1987. J. Am. Chem. Soc. **104:** 278-286.
24. VAN ROEY, P., J. M. SALERNO, C. K. CHU & R. F. SCHINAZI. 1989. Proc. Natl. Acad. Sci. USA **86:** 3929-3933.
25. BIRNBAUM, G. I., T.-S. LIN & W. H. PRUSOFF. 1988. Biochem. Biophys. Res. Commun. **151:** 608-614.
26. GURSKAYA, G. & E. TSAPKINA. 1988. Dokl. Akad. Nauk. SSSR **303:** 1378-1383.
27. ALLEN, F. H., S. BELLARD, M. D. BRICE, B. A. CARTWRIGHT, A. DOUBLEDAY, H. HIGGS, T. HUMMELINK, B. G. HUMMELINK-PEETERS, O. KENNARD, W. D. S. MOTERHWELL,

J. R. RODGERS & D. G. WATSON. 1979. Acta Crystallogr. Sect. B Struct. Crystallogr. Cryst. Chem. **B35**: 2331–2339.

28. TAYLOR, E. W., B. B. THOMPSON, P. VAN ROEY & C. K. CHU. 1990. J. Am. Chem. Soc. Submitted.
29. TAYLOR, E. W., P. VAN ROEY, R. F. SCHINAZI & C. K. CHU. 1990. Antiviral Chem. Chemother. In press.
30. RALEIGH, J. A. & B. J. BLACKBURN. 1978. Biochem. Biophys. Res. Commun. **83**: 1061–1066.

HIV-1 Protease as a Potential Target for Anti-AIDS Therapy

THOMAS D. MEEK AND GEOFFREY B. DREYER

Department of Medicinal Chemistry
Smith Kline Beecham Pharmaceuticals
King of Prussia, Pennsylvania 19406

Human immunodeficiency virus (HIV), the causative agent of the acquired immune deficiency syndrome (AIDS), is a member of the family of retroviruses, *Retroviridiae*.[1] As the genome of the retroviruses consists of RNA, the hallmark of retroviral infection of a host cell is the conversion of this RNA genome to DNA by virus-mediated reverse transcription, followed by the stable integration of the retroviral DNA genome into the cell's chromosomes.[2] From this point the expression of the integrated retroviral genes, known as the *provirus,* by the replicative machinery of the host cell, produces new retroviral particles that effect either cytopathogenesis or cellular transformation and advance infection to other cells.

Following the installment of the provirus into the host cell genome, the proviral genes of HIV and other retroviruses are expressed, and their products are assembled into new virion particles. The RNA transcripts of the provirus are synthesized by the cellular RNA polymerase II, which then undergo posttranscriptional processing. These primary transcripts serve two functions: as the source of mRNA from which viral proteins are made and as the genomic RNA that is ultimately packaged into new virions. Translation of the proviral mRNA results in the synthesis of viral structural proteins and enzymes, many of which exist as precursors within polyproteins.[3] Post-translational modifications of the proviral gene products are performed by cellular enzymes to prepare the viral proteins for proper packaging within new virions. These processes include myristoylation[4] of the N-termini of the viral polyproteins and glycosylation of the envelope proteins. Virion assembly is initiated within the cell membrane when "immature" particles, composed of a glycoprotein envelope, genomic RNA, and viral polyproteins, begin to form and bud from the cell. Maturation of fully formed immature virion particles that have budded from the cell is effected by the action of a virally encoded enzyme, the retroviral protease.[3,5–9] The protease specifically cleaves the encapsulated viral polyproteins into the functional enzymes and structural proteins of the virion core. The resulting mature virion particles are now able to promote a new infection in an adjacent T lymphocyte.

In retroviruses, the proteins that ultimately make up the virion core and the enzymes essential to viral replication are the respective products of the *gag* and *pol* genes (FIG. 1). Direct translation of *gag* results in a 55 kilodalton (kDa) polyprotein, Pr55^{gag}. This precursor contains the precursor forms of the structural proteins of the virion core in a single polypeptide chain, arranged as H$_2$N-p17-p24-p1-p9(p7)-p6-COOH (FIG. 1).[10–15] The eventual proteolytic processing of Pr55^{gag} generates the gag proteins, each of which has a specific role in the fully formed virion: the matrix protein (p17, MA;[16]) constitutes the membrane-associated outer shell of the virion capsid; the rod-shaped virion capsid itself consists of the capsid protein p24 (CA); and within the capsid, the nucleocapsid protein, NC (p9 or p7) and p6, is associated with the genomic RNA. In the Pr55^{gag} precursor, p9 (NC) is presumably responsible for conveying the genomic RNA from the cytoplasm into the forming virion.[3]

The *pol* reading frame is translated as a fusion polyprotein of both *gag* and *pol* products, which requires evasion of the termination codon of *gag*. In HIV-1, this is accomplished by a ribosomal frameshift to the *pol* reading frame at a specific nucleotide sequence located approximately 230 nucleotides upstream of the termination codon of *gag*.[17] The translated fusion product is a 160 kDa polyprotein, Pr160$^{gag\text{-}pol}$, containing in precursor form the *gag* proteins, the protease (PR), reverse transcriptase-ribonuclease (RT-RN), and endonuclease (integrase, IN) in the sequence, H$_2$N-p17-p24-p15-PR-RT-RN-IN-COOH (FIG. 1).[18–21] This frameshifting occurs with an efficiency of 11%, resulting in a ratio of Pr55^{gag} to Pr160$^{gag\text{-}pol}$ of 8:1.[17]

The assembly of virion particles is apparently initiated by the migration of the myristoylated *gag* and *gag-pol* polyproteins to the cellular membrane.[22,23] Myristoylation of the retroviral polyproteins is essential to their proper assembly into virion particles,[22–24] presumably because this lipid substituent directs the Pr55^{gag} and Pr160$^{gag\text{-}pol}$ polyproteins to the cellular membrane and "anchors" their N-termini into the lipid bilayer[25] (FIG. 2A). Upon concentration, the lipid-embedded polyproteins collect into a crescent shape and begin to bud from the cell beneath the viral envelope.[25] Eventually, a spherical virion particle is formed that contains an annular core composed of the unprocessed polyproteins (FIG. 2B). Retroviral particles of this morphology are considered to be immature[25] and are unable to infect cells.[26–29] Reverse transcriptase in the immature HIV-1 particles is either diminished or almost completely absent,[24,29] indicating that the precursor form of the enzyme within the *gag-pol* polyprotein is in a less active form.

Activation of the retroviral protease within the immature virion apparently occurs following its detachment from the cell membrane. The retroviral protease specifically cleaves Pr55^{gag} and Pr160$^{gag\text{-}pol}$ at discrete sites (FIG. 1) to release and activate the structural proteins and enzymes, thereby rendering the virion replication-competent. This maturation process is manifested in the conversion of the annular virion to one containing a condensed, cone-shaped core,[25] composed of p24, which constitutes the mature virion capsid (FIG. 2C). These virions have the more familiar mature morphology and are infectious and replication-competent. The virion capsid houses the genomic RNA, the nucleocapsid protein p9 and p6, and the retroviral enzymes reverse transcriptase and endonuclease. Recent studies indicate that active protease exists within the capsid of the equine infectious anemia virus and proteolyzes the nucleocapsid proteins after formation of the capsid.[30] The protease may therefore have an important role in early events of the retroviral life cycle, such as destabilization of the virion capsid or activation of the endonuclease, and as such, inhibition of the protease may prevent proviral integration.

In order to study the role of the retroviral protease of HIV-1 on the infection competence of the virus, we prepared several restriction fragments of the BH10 clone of HTLV-III[10] (HIV-1), which encode the protease sequence, and inserted them into a bacterial expression system.[31] Expression of two of these recombinant constructs in *E. coli* resulted in the following observations: (a) apparent autoprocessing at these consensus cleavage sites resulted in the release of an 11 kDa protein fragment from its fusion protein precursors; (b) mutational analysis within the protease coding region confirmed that the recombinant HIV-1 protease was responsible for this autoprocessing; and (c) upon cotranscomplementation of recombinant HIV-1 protease and Pr55^{gag} *in vivo*, the gag precursor was processed into protein fragments of sizes that were consistent with those of the viral gag proteins. The recombinant HIV-1 protease was subsequently purified to apparent homogeneity from bacterial extracts.[32] From elucidation of its primary sequence,[32] it was confirmed that the recombinant HIV-1 protease spans a 99-amino acid sequence between Pro-69 and Phe-167 of the translated *pol* coding region.[11]

Under cell-free conditions, the proteolytic processing of purified, recombinant Pr55^{gag} by the isolated recombinant enzyme[33] was identical to the processing of this precursor in bacteria[31] and in accord with that observed in virions.[34] Acquisition of the recombinant protease in purified form allowed the biochemical characterization of the enzyme.

The complete proteolytic processing of the Pr55^{gag} and Pr160$^{gag-pol}$ substrates by

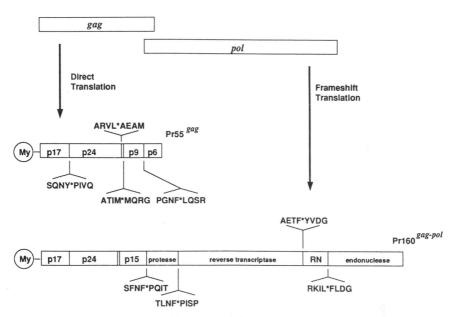

FIGURE 1. The *gag* and *pol* open reading frames of HIV-1, their polyprotein translation products, and the proteolytic cleavage sites. The sequences within the initial translation products that are processed by HIV-1 protease are shown, in which the cleavage is represented by a vertical line in the polyprotein and by * in the amino acid sequence in one-letter code. The gag protein occurring between the L*A and M*M cleavage sites consists of 14 amino acids and is designated p1 in the text. The amino termini of both Pr55^{gag} and Pr160$^{gag-pol}$ are myristoylated (My). The 66 kDa and 51 kDa subunits of reverse transcriptase are both within the region designated, the associated ribonuclease H (RN) activity contained within the carboxyl-terminal region of the 66 kDa subunit.

HIV-1 protease apparently requires only eight discrete cleavages (FIG. 1). This limited digestion of these large polyproteins suggests that HIV-1 protease is a highly specific protease. Three of these cleavage sites (denoted throughout by an asterisk), including the p17-p24 cleavage site of Pr55^{gag} and the termini of the protease, are of the sequence Ser(Thr)-Xaa-Yaa-Phe(Tyr)*Pro. Although unusual for the known endopeptidases, this type of cleavage site is thematic to the retroviral proteases.[35] The other cleavage sites are not conserved (Leu*Ala, Met*Met, Phe*Leu, Phe*Tyr, Leu*Phe) and reflect the general nature of substrates for the retroviral proteases, that is, hydrophobic residues in the P1 and P1′[36] positions. To date, oligopeptides that constitute all eight cleavage sites have been shown to be substrates for HIV-1 protease.[21,37-39] Typically, these peptide substrates consist of six or more amino acids and, depending on the assay conditions, exhibit Michaelis constants in the range of 0.1-10 mM. The most complete set of data, including kinetic studies of the protease, exist for peptide substrates of the "p17-p24" type of cleavage site, -Ser-Gln-Asn-Tyr*Pro-Ile-. Kinetic parameters for some of the oligopeptide substrates of 6-9 amino acids, as determined in our laboratory using chromatographic separation of substrates and products, are as follows: acetyl-Ser-Gln-Asn-Tyr*Pro-NH$_2$, no activity; acetyl-Ser-Gln-Asn-Tyr*Pro-Val-NH$_2$, K_m = 4.9 mM, k_{cat} = 0.44 s^{-1}; acetyl-Ser-Gln-Asn-Tyr*Pro-Val-Val-NH$_2$, K_m = 7.5 mM,

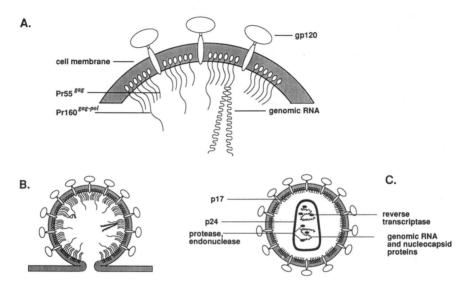

FIGURE 2. Schematic depiction of assembly and maturation of HIV-1 virion in various stages of budding. **(A)** Initiation of virion assembly at the cellular membrane of a T lymphocyte by accumulation of the gag and gag-pol polyproteins and insertion of their N-terminal myristoyl groups (white ellipses) into the membrane. Following cleavage from gp160, the envelope glycoprotein gp120 is situated on the outside of the membrane. The genomic RNA is attached to the nucleocapsid protein domain of Pr55^{gag}. **(B)** An immature virion that has almost completely budded from the cell, containing an annular core of unprocessed polyproteins. **(C)** Morphology of the mature virion core following proteolytic processing. The cone-shaped core, composed of p24, houses the retroviral enzymes, the nucleocapsid proteins, and the RNA genome.

k_{cat} = 54 s^{-1}; acetyl-Ser-Gln-Asn-Phe*Pro-Val-Val-NH$_2$, K_m = 7.5 mM, k_{cat} = 10 s^{-1}; acetyl-Ser-Gln-Asn-Tyr*Pro-Val-Val-Gln-Asn-NH$_2$, K_m = 2.3 mM, k_{cat} = 2.8 s^{-1}; and acetyl-Arg-Ala-Ser-Gln-Asn-Tyr*Pro-Val-Val-NH$_2$, K_m = 5.5 mM, k_{cat} = 59 s^{-1}.[33,38]

As originally observed by Toh et al.,[40] the aspartic proteases of mammalian and microbial origin contain, in duplicate, sequences that are highly homologous to a single conserved domain within the retroviral proteases. The aspartic proteases are "pseudosymmetric" bilobal proteins composed of over 300 amino acids, in which each lobe contains the conserved Asp-Thr-Gly sequence at an active site found at the interface of the lobes.[41,42] In the widely held view of the chemical mechanism of the aspartic proteases,[43–52] the two proximal aspartyl residues assume opposite roles in general acid-general base catalysis: the protonated aspartyl group effects protonation of, or hydrogen-bonding to, the carbonyl oxygen of the scissile amide bond, whereas the unprotonated aspartyl residue deprotonates the lytic water molecule that subsequently attacks the scissile carbonyl as a hydroxide ion. By comparison, the retroviral proteases would constitute only one such "lobe" of the aspartic proteases and would contain only half of the catalytic machinery, namely one aspartyl residue, necessary for cleavage of amide bonds. Based on computer modeling of the primary structures of the proteases of HIV-1 and other retroviruses, Pearl and Taylor have proposed that these proteases would achieve the conserved bilobal structure of the aspartic proteases upon formation of homodimers, in which each monomer contributes an Asp-Thr(Ser)-Gly triad at an active site formed at the subunit interface.[53]

These precepts have been investigated by kinetic studies in numerous laboratories.[28,33,39,53–57] HIV-1 protease is weakly inhibited by pepstatin A ($K_i \leq 2$ μM),[53,56,57] a natural product peptide analogue that typically exerts very potent inhibition of the aspartic proteases and serves to characterize this family of proteases. HIV-1 protease is more strongly inhibited by analogues of pepstatin and by other peptide analogues, which are similar in structure to known potent inhibitors of the aspartic protease renin.[56,57] HIV-1 protease is irreversibly inactivated in a time-dependent manner upon treatment with 1,2-epoxy-(4-nitrophenoxy)propane (EPNP).[33] Tang has demonstrated that this inactivator specifically esterifies one or both of the active-site aspartyl residues in porcine pepsin,[58–60] which has been confirmed by X-ray crystallographic analysis of EPNP-treated penicillopepsin.[43]

The optimal pH for HIV-1 protease activity is 4.5–6.0.[33,53,55,56] Although the aspartic proteases cathepsin D and the pepsins are most active at pH values of less than 4,[44] the operant pH range for HIV-1 protease is reminiscent of that of renin,[61] which is itself only modestly inhibited by pepstatin when compared to that of the other aspartic proteases.[62] The pH dependence of the kinetic constant log k_{cat}/K_m for the oligopeptide substrate of HIV-1 protease, Ac-Arg-Ala-Ser-Gln-Asn-Tyr-Pro-Val-Val-NH$_2$, is a "bell-shaped" curve over a pH range of 3.4–6.5[33,63] and indicates that an unprotonated group of pK = 3.3 and a protonated group of pK = 6.1 are required for catalysis. This pH profile is in accord with the presence of two carboxylic groups of opposite states of protonation in the active site of HIV-1 protease. Moreover, the inactivation of HIV-1 protease by EPNP is dependent on the unprotonated form of an enzymatic residue of pK = 3.8,[33] which again is in concert with the participation of an unprotonated aspartyl residue in the catalytic mechanism.

The native molecular weight of HIV-1 protease was characterized by glycerol density gradient centrifugation, analytical gel filtration, and chemical cross-linking with the amino-specific reagent, dimethylsuberimidate.[33] A molecular weight of 22,000 was derived from an interdependent analysis of the gel filtration and centrifugation data, which was supported by the appearance of a 22 kDa protease-specific band upon NaDodSO$_4$-polyacrylamide gel electrophoresis of the cross-linked enzyme. This molecular weight is twice that observed under denaturing conditions. From these results it was concluded that the active form of HIV-1 protease is a dimer of identical 99-amino acid subunits.

As predicted by Pearl and Taylor,[64] the retroviral proteases are aspartic proteases in which the functional structure of the larger, monomeric aspartic proteases is conserved by simple dimerization of identical polypeptides of considerably smaller size. Recently, the solution of the three-dimensional structure of both recombinant[65,66] and synthetic[67] HIV-1 protease has confirmed the proposed homodimeric structure of this enzyme, and has revealed that their overall molecular architecture is, as expected, very similar to those of the monomeric aspartic proteases.

The indispensable role of HIV-1 protease has been demonstrated in studies in which mutational inactivation of the protease within active proviruses resulted in the formation of replication-incompetent, noninfectious virions.[24-29] These virions were characterized by the presence of unprocessed gag polyproteins and by the diminution or absence of reverse transcriptase activity. The unavailability of protease activity renders these virion particles permanently immature. Recently, similar studies have shown that mutational inactivation of the protease coding region of the HIV-1 provirus,[24,28,29] including a single point mutation of the active site residue, Asp-25,[24,51] results in the formation of noninfectious virions of immature morphology with reduced reverse transcriptase activity.[24,29] In addition, mutational obliteration of either the p17-p24 or p24(p1)-p9 proteolytic cleavage site of Pr55^{gag} within HIV-1 proviruses likewise resulted in noninfectious virions of aberrant morphology.[24] These studies demonstrate that exogenous inhibition of the protease within forming virions of HIV-1 should render these particles incapable of sustaining an active infection within T lymphocytes. Given that HIV-1 protease is a self-generating enzyme, the impact of its inhibition on virion maturation would be all the more dramatic.

Because the HIV-1 protease is an aspartic protease, the rational design of peptide analogue inhibitors of this enzyme could be initiated by the chemical substitution of the scissile dipeptide bond of its oligopeptide substrates with nonhydrolyzable chemical mimics that approximate the structure of an enzymatic transition state or reaction intermediate. One would then expect the resulting peptide analogues to inhibit HIV-1 protease, and given the distinct cleavage sequences of these enzymes, perhaps confer selectivity of inhibition.

Pepstatin A (N-isovaleryl-Val-Val-Sta-Ala-Sta; Sta, statine = 4S-amino-3S-hydroxy-6-methylheptanoic acid), a microbial metabolite that is a generic inhibitor of the aspartic proteases,[68] is, as mentioned above, only a moderately potent inhibitor of HIV-1 protease, yet is illustrative of the development of more potent inhibitors. Inhibition by pepstatin A results from the tetrahedral hydroxyl-bearing carbon in the unusual amino acid statine, which may resemble a transition state or reaction intermediate for proteolysis,[69] or may act as a "bisubstrate" analogue of peptide and H_2O.[70] This concept has inspired a number of other potential transition state analogues for the aspartic proteases, in which the scissile dipeptide has been replaced by a variety of nonhydrolyzable dipeptide isosteres.[71]

For inhibition of HIV-1 protease we sought to compare the inhibitory potency of these known nonhydrolyzable dipeptide isosteres within the context of a single oligopeptide substrate. The proteolytic processing site of choice was Ser(Thr)-Xaa-Yaa-Tyr(Phe)*Pro-Zaa, inasmuch as this type of cleavage site was the most commonly recognized by the retroviral proteases and was thought to maximize inhibitory selectivity for this subset of the aspartic proteases. We synthesized analogues of the substrate acetyl-Ser-Ala-Ala-Tyr-Pro-Val-Val-NH_2 (K_m = 8.6 mM, k_{cat} = 9.5 s^{-1}), in which the hydrolyzable dipeptide linkage was replaced with several such stable mimics, including an analogue of statine,[38] hydroxyethylene isosteres,[72] phosphinic acids,[73] a reduced amide,[38] and an α,α-difluoroketone.[74] These peptide analogues were competitive inhibitors of recombinant HIV-1 protease when assessed in a peptidolytic assay and exhibited a wide range of inhibition constants (apparent K_i = 18-19,000 nM).[57]

Three of the more potent inhibitors were tested as inhibitors of viral proteolytic processing and viral replication in cell culture: compound 1, Cbz-Ala-Pheψ[CH(OH)-CH_2]Gly-Val-Val-OCH_3 (K_i = 120 nM); compound 2, Ala-Ala-Pheψ[CH(OH)CH_2]-Gly-Val-Val-OCH_3 (K_i = 18 nM); compound 3, Cbz-Ala-Ala-Pheψ[CH(OH)CH_2]Gly-Val-Val-OCH_3 (K_i = 48 nM) (Pheψ[CH(OH)CH_2]Gly is the incorporated dipeptide isostere (4S,5S)-4-hydroxy-5-amino-6-phenylhexanoic acid).[75] Using monoclonal antibodies specific for the p17, p24 proteins, and reverse transcriptase of HIV-1, we first employed Western analysis to investigate the effects of these inhibitors on steady-state levels of accumulated viral proteins in chronically infected cells.[75] Seelmeier et al. noted a slight effect of 70 μM pepstatin A on the processing of Pr55^{gag} in infected H9 cells after 48 h, although no change was observed in the steady-state level of p17 or p24.[76] We found compounds 1 and 3 to be significantly more effective than pepstatin A. Treatment of CEM cells chronically infected with HIV-1 (CEM/IIIB cells)[77] with compounds 1 and 3 at 20 μM for 48 h caused a major reduction in the levels of p17, p24, and reverse transcriptase subunits, and a marked buildup of processing intermediates of both Pr55^{gag} (47 kDa and 40 kDa immunoreactive proteins) and Pr160$^{gag\text{-}pol}$ (FIG. 3). Both the 40 kDa and 47 kDa protein intermediates of Pr55^{gag} reacted with either the p17- or p24-specific antibodies, suggesting that these two intermediates could be the result of cleavages at the p24-(p1)*p6 and p6*p9 processing sites, respectively. Reverse transcriptase enzymatic activity was also substantially reduced in the lysates of the inhibitor-treated cells. Compound 2, despite its K_i of 18 nM showed no effect on viral processing or viral morphology after 48 h, suggesting that it is either metabolically unstable or unable to access the protease. The unblocked amino terminus of compound 2 may render it susceptible to metabolic degradation.

These results demonstrated that, as expected, the exogenous inhibition of HIV-1 protease within actively infected cultures of lymphocytes was sufficient to significantly reduce the proteolytic processing of both the Pr55^{gag} and Pr160$^{gag\text{-}pol}$ products. Moreover, perturbations in the levels of these polyproteins and their processing intermediates were accurately reflected in the composition of proteins packaged within virions. Immunoblot analysis verified that purified virus harvested from chronically infected H9/IIIB cells treated with compound 3 contained only incompletely processed gag proteins (Pr55^{gag}, p47, and p40) and no mature p17 or p24.[78] Electron microscopy revealed that the virion particles produced by the inhibitor-treated lymphocytes contained apparently defective core structures; virions processing "crescent-shaped" cores were preponderant, whereas virions containing mature, cone-shaped cores or annular, immature cores represented smaller populations.[79] Given the composition of gag proteins found within the inhibitor-treated virions, this aberrant morphology is suggestive of a stage of polyprotein processing that is intermediate between the annular cores of the immature virions and the cone-shaped cores of the mature virions.

In addition, metabolic labeling of Pr55^{gag} by the "pulse-chase" technique was used to assess the effects of these inhibitors on processing of de novo synthesized viral proteins. Treatment of CEM/IIIB cells with compounds 1-3 resulted in profound inhibition of processing of newly synthesized Pr55^{gag} over a 3 or 6 h period, as seen by immunoprecipitation of viral proteins metabolically labeled with [^{35}S]methionine, followed by electrophoresis and autoradiography.[75] The effects of these inhibitors, added at 0.1-100 μM, were quantified by densitometric analysis of the formation of p24 from Pr55^{gag}. The IC$_{50}$ values for compounds 1 and 3, determined from the densitometry, were approximately 2-5 μM, some 50- to 100-fold higher than their K_i values.[80] Pepstatin A at a concentration as high as 100 μM had little or no discernible effect on Pr55^{gag} processing under these conditions. Although the lack of activity of pepstatin A can be ascribed in part to its micromolar K_i value, its poor ability to enter cells has also been noted.[81]

It remained to be shown whether replication-competent virions could establish an acute infection in T lymphocytes in the presence of a protease inhibitor. Grinde et al.[82] and von der Helm et al.[83] reported that pepstatin A at concentrations of 0.1 mM to 1 mM caused an apparent reduction in the rate of HIV-1 replication in cultures of H9 cells. We treated uninfected Molt 4 cells with HIV-1 strain III$_B$ (200 TCID$_{50}$ per 4 $\times$ 10^4 cells) and then maintained them in culture in the presence of compounds 1-3 at several concentrations. After 7 days the extent of viral replication was determined by p24 radioimmunoassay, by assay for particle-associated reverse transcriptase activity, and by quantification of syncytia. As seen in TABLE 1, although compound 2 showed no effect, compounds 1 and 3 produced dose-dependent reductions in all three measures of viral replication without evidence of cytotoxicity.

The results of reverse transcriptase assays in TABLE 1 are representative and show

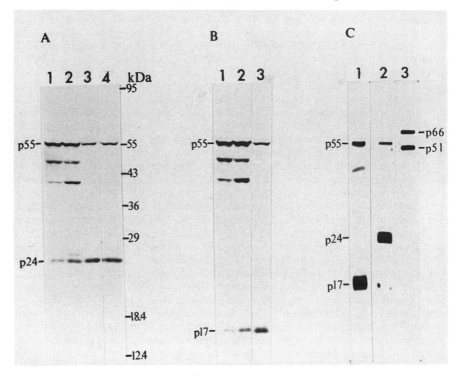

FIGURE 3. Effects of HIV-1 protease inhibitors on processing of *gag* proteins in CEM cells chronically infected with HIV-1, strain III$_B$.[75] Infected cell cultures were treated with either 20 μM of each inhibitor or with 0.2% DMSO (control) approximately every 8 h for a 48 h period. Proteins in cell extracts were separated on NaDodSO$_4$-polyacrylamide (10% polyacrylamide) gels and then electroblotted on to nitrocellulose sheets. Panel A: Western blot protein probed with a monoclonal antibody (mAb) (1:1000) recognizing the Pr55^{gag}/p24 antigen (Beckman AS6). Samples were from cells treated with compound 3 (lane 1), compound 1 (lane 2), pepstatin A (lane 3), and DMSO control (lane 4). Panel B: Western blot probed with mAb (1:1000) specific for Pr55^{gag}/p17 (Beckman AS3). Samples were from cells treated with compound 3 (lane 1), compound 1 (lane 2), and DMSO control (lane 3). Panel C: Western blots of purified HIV-1 virions grown in H9 cells and reacted with mAb against p17 (AS3) (lane 1), p24 (AS6) (lane 2), or RT (AS6) (lane 3). Monoclonal antibodies on all blots were detected with goat anti-mouse IgG covalently linked to alkaline phosphatase (1:1200).

that whereas the solvent dimethyl sulfoxide (DMSO) had a slight inhibitory effect, complete inhibition of infectivity was observed with a single initial dose of 100 μM compound 1 or 25 μM compound 3. This diminution of reverse transcriptase activity was commensurate with a decrease in p24 antigen and in the number of syncytia formed by these cells during the course of the infection. Compound 2, which may be

TABLE 1. Inhibition of Viral Infectivity of HIV-1 by Inhibitors of HIV-1 Protease[a]

Culture Components	Inhibitor (μM) at Day 1/Day 7	RT Activity (avg cpm)		p24 Antigen (avg ng/mL)		Syncytial formation		Percent inhibition of infectivity	
		(A) With Inhibitor	(B) Without Inhibitor	(C) With Inhibitor	(D) Without Inhibitor	With Inhibitor	Without Inhibitor	RT	p24
Molt 4 cells	—	—	1,500	—	0.4	—	—	—	—
Molt 4/virus	—	—	166,600	—	>400	—	+++++	—	—
Molt 4/virus/compound 1	10/1.7	68,000	128,500	>400	>400	+++	+++++	47%	0%
	25/4.2	9,700	78,200	116	>400	++	+++++	88%	>70%
	100/17	2,900	70,400	1.8	>400	—	+++++	96%	>99%
Molt 4/virus/compound 2	10/1.7	93,100	128,500	>400	>400	+++++	+++++	28%	0%
	25/4.2	72,000	78,200	>400	>400	+++++	+++++	8%	0%
	100/17	71,300	70,400	>400	>400	+++++	+++++	0%	0%
Molt 4/virus/compound 3	10/1.7	30,900	128,500	>392	>400	+++++	+++++	76%	>2%
	25/4.2	1,800	78,200	5.4	>400	—	+++++	98%	>99%
	100/17	1,900	70,400	6.8	>400	—	+++++	97%	>98%

[a] Effects of protease inhibitors on HIV-1 infectivity of T lymphocytes.[75] Cultures of uninfected Molt 4 cells were treated with infectious HIV-1, strain III$_B$ (200 infectious units per 40,000 cells). Solutions of compounds 1–3 (10 mM in DMSO) were diluted into medium and added in a single dose to the infected cell cultures to yield concentrations at day 1 of 10 μM, 25 μM, and 100 μM. On day 7, the reverse transcriptase activity and amount of p24 antigen in each culture were determined. Viral infectivity in the absence of the inhibitors was determined from infected cell cultures treated with 0 and 0.1%–1% DMSO, and a control sample contained no virus. Syncytial formation (multinucleated cells of >5 times the diameter of a Molt 4 cell) in each well was scored by microscopic examination (—, no apparent syncytia; +++++, >50 syncytia in a single microscopic field). Percent inhibition of infectivity is expressed as 1−((value in column A)/(value in column B)) × 100 for reverse transcriptase activity and (1−((value in column C)/(value in column D)) × 100 for p24 antigen.

metabolically unstable in cell culture, exerted little or no effect on viral infectivity at any concentration.

In summary, the addition of inhibitors of HIV-1 protease to T-lymphocyte cultures that are either acutely or chronically infected with HIV-1 produces effects on viral protein processing and infectivity that are similar to those observed for protease-deficient mutants of HIV-1 after transfection into cells. Because mutational inactivation of either the protease gene or the p17-p24 cleavage site in Pr55^{gag} resulted in a loss of infectivity of the transfected mutant proviruses, it has been suggested that the maturation of p24 gag is important not only for correct virion assembly from infected cells, but also is necessary for the proper integration of provirus during infection.[24]

Inasmuch as it has been recently demonstrated that T4$^+$ T lymphocytes comprise perhaps the largest reservoir of HIV-1 in the peripheral blood of AIDS patients at various stages of the disease,[84] the demonstration of the effective inhibition of HIV-1 protease within infected T lymphocytes and its attendant effects on viral maturation and infectivity validates this enzyme as a suitable target for the development of novel, rationally designed therapeutic agents for the treatments of AIDS. The apparent ability of these protease inhibitors to block maturation of virions shed from chronically infected T lymphocytes, as well as to attenuate acute infection of uninfected T lymphocytes, suggests that inhibition of this enzyme may have an impact on both early and late stages of the HIV-1 life cycle, such as proviral integration and polyprotein processing, respectively. This may offer a therapeutic advantage over inhibitors of reverse transcriptase such as azidothymidine, which has been recently shown to be more effective against an acute infection than in reducing the population of active virus in chronically infected T lymphocytes.[85] Inhibitors of HIV-1 protease may also prove less toxic than azidothymidine, possibly resulting from their specificity for the retroviral proteases. Indeed, compounds 1–3 were relatively poor inhibitors of the aspartic proteases bovine spleen cathepsin D and human renin. This differential inhibition of the retroviral and mammalian aspartic proteases is clearly a desirable property. We have to date observed no overt cytotoxicity upon treatment of any line of uninfected T lymphocytes studied thus far with these protease inhibitors at concentrations that greatly exceed an efficacious level.

ACKNOWLEDGMENTS

The authors gratefully acknowledge the following individuals for their contributions to the work described in this chapter: T. J. Carr, B. D. Dayton, C. Debouck, J. Gorniak, T. Hart, W. F. Huffman, L. J. Hyland, A. Langlois (Department of Surgery, Duke University), D. M. Lambert, J. J. Leary, V. W. Magaard, T. J. Matthews (Department of Surgery, Duke University), B. W. Metcalf, M. L. Moore, S. R. Petteway Jr., J. E. Strickler, and T. A. Tomaszek Jr. We also wish to thank W. Crowell, R. Assendorf, and C. Del Tito for assistance in production of the figures.

REFERENCES

1. GALLO, R. C. & L. MONTAGNIER. 1988. Sci. Am. **259:** 41–48.
2. VARMUS, H. & R. SWANSTROM. 1982. *In* Molecular Biology of Tumor Viruses. R. Weiss,

N. Teich, H. Varmus & J. Coffin, Eds.: 369-512. Cold Spring Harbor Laboratory. Cold Spring Harbor, NY.

3. DICKSON, C., R. EISENMAN, H. FAN, E. HUNTER & N. TEICH. 1982. *In* Molecular Biology of Tumor Viruses. R. Weiss, N. Teich, H. Varmus & J. Coffin, Eds.: 513-648. Cold Spring Harbor Laboratory. Cold Spring Harbor, NY.

4. SCHULTZ, A. M., L. E. HENDERSON & S. OROSZLAN. 1988. Annu. Rev. Cell Biol. **4:** 611-647.

5. KRAUSSLICH, H.-G. & E. WIMMER. 1988. Annu. Rev. Biochem. **57:** 701-754.

6. KOSTKA, V., Ed. 1989. Proteases of Retroviruses. de Gruyter. Berlin.

7. KRAUSSLICH, H.-G., S. OROSZLAN & E. WIMMER, Eds. 1989. Viral Proteinases as Targets for Chemotherapy. Cold Spring Harbor Laboratory. Cold Spring Harbor, NY.

8. HELLEN, C. U. T., H.-G. KRAUSSLICH & E. WIMMER. 1989. Biochemistry **28:** 9881-9890.

9. KAY, J. & B. M. DUNN. 1990. Biochem. Biophys. Acta. In press.

10. RATNER, L., W. HASELTINE, R. PATARACA, K. J. LIVAK, B. STARCICH, S. F. JOSEPHS, E. R. DORAN, J. A. RAFALSKI, E. A. WHITEHORN, K. BAUMEISTER, L. IVANOFF, S. R. PETTEWAY, JR., M. L. PEARSON, L. A. LAUTENBERGER, T. S. PAPAS, J. GHRAYEB, N. T. CHANG, R. C. GALLO & F. WONG-STAAL. 1985. Nature **313:** 277-284.

11. SANCHEZ-PESCADOR, R., M. D. POWERS, P. J. BARR, K. S. STEIMER, M. M. STEMPIEN, S. L. BROWN SHIMER, W. W. GEE, A. RENARD, A. RANDOLPH, J. A. LEVY, D. DINA & P. A. LUCIW. 1985. Science **227:** 484-492.

12. CASEY, J. M., Y. KIM, P. R. ANDERSEN, K. F. WATSON, J. L. FOX & S. G. DEVARE. 1985. J. Virol. **55:** 417-423.

13. VERONESE, F. D., R. RAHMAN, T. COPELAND, S. OROSZLAN, R. C. GALLO & M. G. SARNGADHARAN. 1987. AIDS Res. Hum. Retroviruses **3:** 253-262.

14. VERONESE, F. D., T. D. COPELAND, S. OROSZLAN, R. C. GALLO & M. G. SARNGADHARAN. 1988. J. Virol. **62:** 795-801.

15. HENDERSON, L. E., T. D. COPELAND, R. C. SOWDER, A. M. SCHULTZ & S. OROSZLAN. *In* Human Retroviruses, Cancer, and AIDS: Approaches to Prevention and Therapy. 135-147. Alan R. Liss, Inc. New York.

16. LEIS, J., D. BALTIMORE, J. M. BISHOP, J. COFFIN, E. FLEISSNER, S. P. GOFF, S. OROSZLAN, H. ROBINSON, A. M. SKALKA, H. M. TEMIN & V. VOGT. 1988. J. Virol. **62:** 1808-1809.

17. JACKS, T., M. D. POWER, F. R. MASIARZ, P. A. LUCIW, P. J. BARR & H. E. VARMUS. 1988. Nature **331:** 280-283.

18. VERONESE, F. D., T. D. COPELAND, A. L. DE VICO, R. RAHMAN, S. OROSZLAN, R. C. GALLO & M. G. SARNGADHARAN. 1986. Science **231:** 1289-1291.

19. LIGHTFOOTE, M. M., J. E. COLIGAN, T. M. FOLKS, A. S. FAUCI, M. S. MARTIN & S. VENKATESAN. 1986. J. Virol. **60:** 771-775.

20. LILLEHOJ, E. P., F. H. R. SALAZAR, R. J. MERVIS, M. G. RAUM, H. W. CHAN, N. AHMAD & S. VENKATESAN. 1988. J. Virol. **62:** 3053-3058.

21. MIZRAHI, V., G. M. LAZARUS, L. M. MILES, C. A. MEYERS & C. DEBOUCK. 1989. Arch. Biochem. Biophys. **273:** 347-348.

22. REIN, A., M. R. MCCLURE, N. R. ROCE, R. B. LUFTIG & A. M. SCHULTZ. 1986. Proc. Natl. Acad. Sci. USA **83:** 7246-7250.

23. RHEE, S. S. & E. HUNTER. 1987. J. Virol. **61:** 1045-1053.

24. GOTTLINGER, H., J. SODROSKI & W. HASELTINE. 1989. Proc. Natl. Acad. Sci. USA **86:** 5781-5785.

25. GONDA, M. A., F. WONG-STAAL, R. C. GALLO, J. E. CLEMENTS, O. NARAYAN & R. V. GILDEN. 1985. Science **227:** 173-177.

26. CRAWFORD, S. & S. P. GOFF. 1985. J. Virol. **53:** 899-907.

27. KATOH, I., Y. YOSHINAKA, A. REIN, M. SHIBUYA, T. ODAKA & S. OROSZLAN. 1985. Virology **145:** 280-292.

28. KOHL, N. E., E. A. EMINI, W. A. SCHLEIF, L. J. DAVIS, J. C. HEIMBACH, R. A. F. DIXON, E. M. SCOLNICK & I. S. SIGAL. 1988. Proc. Natl. Acad. Sci. USA **85:** 4686-4690.

29. PENG, C., B. HO, T. CHANG & N. CHANG. 1989. J. Virol. **63:** 2550-2556.

30. ROBERTS, M. M. & S. OROSZLAN. 1989. Biochem. Biophys. Res. Commun. **160:** 486-494.

31. DEBOUCK, C., J. G. GORNIAK, J. E. STRICKLER, T. D. MEEK, B. W. METCALF & M. ROSENBERG. 1987. Proc. Natl. Acad. Sci. USA **84:** 8903-8906.

32. STRICKLER, J. E., J. GORNIAK, B. DAYTON, T. MEEK, M. MOORE, V. MAGAARD, J. MALINOWSKI & C. DEBOUCK. 1989. Proteins **6:** 139-154.

33. MEEK, T. D., B. D. DAYTON, B. W. METCALF, G. B. DREYER, J. E. STRICKLER, J. G. GORNIAK, M. ROSENBERG, M. L. MOORE, V. W. MAGAARD & C. DEBOUCK. 1989. Proc. Natl. Acad. Sci. USA **86:** 1841-1845.
34. MERVIS, R. J., N. AHMAD, E. P. LILLEHOJ, M. G. RAUM, F. H. R. SALAZAR, H. W. CHAN & S. VENKATESAN. 1988. J. Virol. **62**(11): 3993-4002.
35. PEARL, L. H. & W. R. TAYLOR. 1987. Nature (London) **328:** 482.
36. BERGER, A. & I. SCHECHTER. 1970. Philos. Trans. R. Soc. London Ser. B. Biol. Sci. **257:** 249-264.
37. DARKE, P. L., R. F. NUTT, S. F. BRADY, V. M. GARSKY, T. M. CICCARONE, C.-T. LEU, P. K. LUMMA, R. M. FREIDINGER, D. F. VEBER & I. S. SIGAL. 1988. Biochem. Biophys. Res. Commun. **156:** 297-303.
38. MOORE, M. L., W. M. BRYAN, S. A. FAKHOURY, V. W. MAGAARD, W. F. HUFFMAN, B. D. DAYTON, T. D. MEEK, L. HYLAND, G. B. DREYER, B. W. METCALF, J. E. STRICKLER, J. GORNIAK & C. DEBOUCK. 1989. Biochem. Biophys. Res. Commun. **159:** 420-425.
39. KRAUSSLICH, H.-G., R. H. INGRAHAM, M. T. SKOOG, E. WIMMER, P. V. PALLAI & C. A. CARTER. 1989. Proc. Acad. Natl. Sci. USA **86:** 807-811.
40. TOH, H., M. ONO, K. SAIGO & T. MIYATA. 1985. Nature (London) **315:** 691.
41. TANG, J., M. N. G. JAMES, I.-N. HSU, J. A. JENKINS & T. L. BLUNDELL. 1978. Nature (London) **271:** 618-621.
42. PEARL, L. H. & T. L. BLUNDELL. 1984. FEBS Lett. **174:** 96-101.
43. JAMES, M. N. G., I.-N. HSU & L. T. J. DELBAERE. 1977. Nature (London) **267:** 808-813.
44. FRUTON, J. S. 1976. Adv. Enzymol. Relat. Areas Mol. Biol. **44:** 1-36.
45. ANTONOV, V. K., L. M. GINODMAN, L. D. RUMSH, Y. V. KAPITANNIKOV, T. N. BARSHEV-SKAYA, L. P. YAKASHEV, A. G. GUROVA & L. I. VOLKOVA. 1981. Eur. J. Biochem. **117:** 195-200.
46. BOTT, R., E. SUBRAMANIAN & D. R. DAVIES. 1982. Biochemistry **21:** 6956-6962.
47. RICH, D. H., M. S. BERNATOWICZ & P. G. SCHMIDT. 1982. J. Am. Chem. Soc. **104:** 3535-3536.
48. HOFMANN, T., B. M. DUNN & A. L. FINK. 1984. Biochemistry **23:** 5253-5256.
49. KOSTKA, V., Ed. 1985. Aspartic Proteinases and Their Inhibitors. de Gruyter. Berlin.
50. JAMES, M. N. G. & A. R. SIELECKI. 1985. Biochemistry **24:** 3701-3713.
51. RICH, D. H. 1985. J. Med. Chem. **28:** 263-273.
52. SUGUNU, K., E. A. PADLAN, C. W. SMITH, W. D. CARLSON & D. R. DAVIES. 1987. Proc. Acad. Natl. Sci. USA **84:** 7009-7013.
53. DARKE, P. L., C.-T. LEU, L. J. DAVIS, J. C. HEIMBACH, R. E. DIEHL, W. S. HILL, R. A. F. DIXON & I. S. SIGAL. 1989. J. Biol. Chem. **264:** 2307-2312.
54. SCHNEIDER, J. & S. KENT. 1988. Cell **54:** 363-368.
55. BILLICH, S., M.-T. KNOOP, J. HANSEN, P. STROP, J. SEDLACEK, R. MERTZ & K. MOEL-LING. 1988. J. Biol. Chem. **263:** 17905-17908.
56. RICHARDS, A. D., R. F. ROBERTS, B. M. DUNN, M. C. GRAVES & J. KAY. 1989. FEBS Lett. **247:** 113-117.
57. DREYER, G. B., B. W. METCALF, T. A. TOMASZEK, JR., T. J. CARR, A. C. CHANDLER, III, L. HYLAND, M. L. MOORE, J. E. STRICKLER, C. DEBOUCK & T. D. MEEK. 1989. Proc. Natl. Acad. Sci. USA **86:** 9752-9756.
58. TANG, J. 1971. J. Biol. Chem. **246:** 4510-4517.
59. CHEN, K. C. S. & J. TANG. 1972. J. Biol. Chem. **247:** 2566-2574.
60. HARTSUCK, J. A. & J. TANG. 1972. J. Biol. Chem. **247:** 2575-2580.
61. POORMAN, R. A., D. P. PALERMO, L. E. POST, K. MURAKAMI, J. H. KINNER, C. W. SMITH, I. REARDON & R. L. HEINRIKSON. 1986. Proteins **1:** 139-145.
62. BOGER, J., N. S. LOHR, E. H. ULM, M. POE, E. H. BLAINE, G. M. FANELLI, T.-Y. LIN, L. S. PAYNE, T. W. SCHORN, B. I. LAMONT, T. C. VASSIL, I. I. STABILITO, D. F. VEBER, D. H. RICH & A. S. BOPARI. 1983. Nature (London) **303:** 81-84.
63. HYLAND, L. J., T. A. TOMASZEK, JR., M. L. MOORE & T. D. MEEK. Unpublished results.
64. PEARL, L. H. & W. R. TAYLOR. 1987. Nature **329:** 351-354.
65. NAVIA, M. A., P. M. D. FITZGERALD, B. M. MCKEEVER, C.-T. LEU, J. C. HEIMBACH, W. K. HERBER, I. S. SIGAL, P. L. DARKE & J. P. SPRINGER. 1989. Nature **337:** 615-620.
66. LAPATTO, R., T. BLUNDELL, A. HEMMINGS, J. OVERINGTON, A. WILDERSPIN, S. WOOD,

J. R. MERSON, P. J. WHITTLE, D. E. DANLEY, K. F. GEOGHEGAN, S. J. HAWRYLIK, S. E. LEE, K. G. SCHELD & P. M. HOBART. 1989. Nature (London) **342:** 299-302.

67. WLODAWER, A., M. MILLER, M. JASKOLSKI, B. K. SATHYANARAYANA, E. BALDWIN, I. T. WEBER, L. M. SELK, L. CLAWSON, J. SCHNEIDER & S. B. H. KENT. 1989. Science **245:** 616-621.

68. AOYAGI, T. 1978. *In* Bioactive Peptides Produced by Microorganisms. H. Umezawa, T. Takita & T. Shiba, Eds.: 129-151. Halsted Press.

69. MARCINISZYN, J., JR., J. A. HARTSUCK & J. TANG. 1976. J. Biol. Chem. **251:** 7088.

70. RICH, D. H., E. T. O. SUN & E. ULM. 1980. J. Med. Chem. **23:** 27-33.

71. FISCHER, G. 1988. Nat. Prod. Reports **5:** 465-495.

72. SZELKE, M. 1985. *In* Aspartic Proteinases and Their Inhibitors. V. Kostka, Ed.: 412-441. de Gruyter. Berlin.

73. BARTLETT, P. A. & W. B. KEZER. 1984. J. Am. Chem. Soc. **106:** 4282-4283.

74. GELB, M. H., J. P. SVAREN & R. H. ABELES. 1985. Biochemistry **24:** 1813-1817.

75. MEEK, T. D., D. M. LAMBERT, G. B. DREYER, T. J. CARR, T. A. TOMASZEK, JR., M. L. MOORE, J. E. STRICKLER, C. DEBOUCK, L. J. HYLAND, T. J. MATTHEWS, B. W. METCALF & S. R. PETTEWAY. 1990. Nature (London) **343:** 90-92.

76. SEELMEIER, S., H. SCHMIDT, V. TURK & K. VON DER HELM. 1988. Proc. Natl. Acad. Sci. USA **85:** 6612-6616.

77. MATTHEWS, T. J., K. J. WEINHOLD, H. K. LYERLY, A. J. LANGLOIS, H. WIGZELL & D. BOLOGNESI. 1987. Proc. Natl. Acad. Sci. USA **84:** 5424.

78. MATTHEWS, T. J. *et al.* Unpublished results.

79. HART, T. K. *et al.* Unpublished results.

80. LAMBERT, D. M. *et al.* Unpublished results.

81. CAMPBELL, P., G. I. GLOVER & J. M. GUNN. 1980. Arch. Biochem. Biophys. **203:** 676.

82. GRINDE, B., O. HUNGNES & E. TJOTTA. 1989. AIDS Res. Hum. Retroviruses **5:** 269.

83. VON DER HELM, K., L. GURTLER, J. EBERLE & F. DEINHARDT. 1989. FEBS Lett. **247:** 349.

84. SCHNITTMAN, S. M., M. C. PSALLIDOPOULOS, H. C. LANE, L. THOMPSON, M. BASELER, F. MASSARI, C. H. FOX, N. P. SALZMAN & A. S. FAUCI. 1989. Science **245:** 305-308.

85. POLI, G., J. M. ORENSTEIN, A. KINTER, T. FOLKS & A. S. FAUCI. 1989. Science **244:** 575-577.

Molecular Interactions between Human Immunodeficiency Virus Type 1 and Human Cytomegalovirus[a]

PETER A. BARRY, ELISSA PRATT-LOWE,
DONALD J. ALCENDOR, RONALD E. UNGER, AND
PAUL A. LUCIW

Department of Medical Pathology
University of California, Davis
Davis, California 95616

INTRODUCTION

In humans infected with human immunodeficiency virus type 1 (HIV-1) and in rhesus macaques infected with simian immunodeficiency virus (SIV), the cause of death appears not to be a direct result of infection by either lentivirus; instead, fatality is due to any of a variety of secondary infectious agents brought about by the ablation of the host's immune system.[1] Persistent infections by these heterologous viral, bacterial, or fungal pathogens are a characteristic of individuals suffering from acquired immune deficiency (AIDS).[2] One such viral pathogen, cytomegalovirus (CMV), is a member of the herpesvirus family of viruses and is a frequent pathogen in HIV-infected humans.[3] A large percentage of dually infected individuals suffer life-threatening complications as a direct result of CMV pathogenesis.[4,5] A critical point that requires further investigation is whether infections by heterologous pathogens are merely an opportunistic response to deterioration of the host's immune system, or whether these agents might be important cofactors in the onset of AIDS. The issue of cofactors is vitally important because therapeutic agents directed against these secondary agents will not only alleviate suffering of the individuals, but also might delay onset of frank AIDS. A potential role for heterologous cofactors is not unique to humans infected with HIV. Rhesus macaques experimentally infected with SIV suffer an AIDS-like disease,[6] and rhesus CMV in terminally ill SIV-infected macaques appears to contribute to pathogenesis (A. Lackner & P. Vogel, unpublished results). We have been examining molecular interactions of CMV with HIV-1 and SIV using *in vitro* transient expression assays to

[a]The research in this report was supported in part by Grants from the American Foundation for AIDS Research and the National Institute for Allergy and Infectious Diseases (RO1-AI25109 and PHS-AI27732). P. A. Barry is a recipient of a National Research Service Award, and P. A. Luciw is a recipient of an investigator award from the California Universitywide Task Force on AIDS.

assess the potential consequences of *in vivo* interactions involving CMV with lentiviruses.

MATERIAL AND METHODS

Cell cultures of MRC-5 cells (diploid human fetal lung fibroblast), NIH 3T3 cells (murine fibroblast), L929 cells (murine fibroblast), and Hela cell (human cervical carcinoma), and an isolate of rhesus CMV were obtained from the American Type Culture Collection (ATCC) (Rockville, MD) and grown according to the supplier's recommendations. We used transient transfection assays to measure the ability of CMV to potentiate, or transactivate, expression from the HIV and SIV long terminal repeats (LTR). The protocol for DEAE-dextran transfection has been described.[7] Chloramphenicol acetyltransferase (CAT) enzymatic activity was assayed according to the method of Nordeen *et al.*[8]

The wild-type HIV-1 LTR/CAT plasmid (pHIV LTR/CAT) and the HIV-1 TAT expression plasmid,[9] and the plasmids bearing mutations within the HIV-1 LTR (mutations $(+4/+9)$ and $(+14/+18)$,[10] TATA, $(-16/-12)$, $(-11/-7)$, $(-6/-1)$, pTriple/CAT, $(+4/+8)$, $(+24/+27)$, and $(+30/+33)$,[11,12] Sp1-dpm (III) and Sp1-dpm (I,II,III),[13] NF-κB,[14] $\Delta(-453/-76)$,[15] and $\Delta(+24/+38)$[7]) have been described previously. The numbers refer to the starting and ending nucleotides for clustered site mutations, or to the ends of a deletion. The plasmid expressing the major protein products of the human CMV immediate early (pSVIE) genes contains the transcription units for CMV immediate early regions IE1 and IE2[16] under the transcriptional control of the SV40 early region promoter.[7] Plasmids expressing the immediate early (IE) genes of rhesus CMV (pRhIE 9.4-2)[17] and African green monkey (AGM) CMV (pTJ148)[18] were constructed with the rhesus CMV IE and AGM CMV IE coding regions, respectively, under the transcriptional control of their autologous promoter. A restriction fragment containing the 5′ LTR of SIV was generated by the polymerase chain reaction using a biologically active molecular clone of SIV as template[19] and subcloned into an expression vector for the CAT gene (pSIV LTR/CAT).

RESULTS

Transactivation of the HIV-1 LTR by TAT and CMV IE in L929 Cell Cultures

A plasmid containing the CAT gene under the transcriptional control of the HIV-1/SF2 LTR (pHIV LTR/CAT)[9] was cotransfected into L929 cell cultures with either a plasmid expressing HIV-1 TAT (pSVTAT)[9] or with a plasmid expressing the CMV immediate early (IE) gene products (pSVIE).[7] Expression of both TAT and CMV IE was under the transcriptional control of the SV40 early region promoter. A constant amount of pHIV LTR/CAT (2 micrograms) was cotransfected with increasing amounts of either pSVTAT or pSVIE. In addition, constant amounts of pHIV LTR/CAT (2 micrograms) and pSVTAT (3 micrograms) were cotransfected with an increasing amount of pSVIE. For each transfection, CAT enzymatic activity was assayed with whole cell extracts by the method of Nordeen et al.[8]

In L929 cell cultures, cotransfection of pHIV LTR/CAT with either pSVTAT or pSVIE resulted in large increases in the level of CAT activity (FIG. 1). These results are in agreement with published reports for experiments in other cell types.[7,17,20,21] In general, the response of the LTR to transactivation was linear up to a level of three micrograms of cotransfected transactivator plasmid, whereupon the level of CAT activity reached a plateau. In this particular experiment the increase in CAT activity with 5 micrograms of pSVTAT was an aberration from the majority of experiments. When pHIV LTR/CAT was cotransfected with both pSVIE and pSVTAT, the resultant CAT activities were greater than the sum of CAT activities achieved with each transactivator alone; the level of transactivation approached the product of both transactivators (FIG. 1). CAT activities for cotransfection with both pSVIE and pSVTAT increased linearly to over 1100-fold above basal CAT activities (FIG. 1). Similar results have been presented for experiments in cultures of MRC-5 cells;[7] thus, the mechanisms of transactivation by pSVIE and pSVTAT are different.

Differential Transactivation of the HIV-1 LTR by TAT and CMV IE

In L929 cells cotransfection of pHIV LTR/CAT with pSVTAT resulted in higher levels of CAT activity than cotransfection of pHIV LTR/CAT with pSVIE (FIG. 1). pSVTAT transactivated the HIV-1 LTR to 2-3-fold higher levels than did pSVIE. This ability of TAT to transactivate more efficiently than CMV IE in L929 cultures was in contrast to published results for experiments in MRC-5 in which CMV IE transactivated the HIV-1 LTR more than did TAT.[7] We examined in greater detail the apparent differential abilities of these two transactivators to function in different cell types. We transfected pHIV LTR/CAT in the presence or absence of pSVIE and pSVTAT into cultures of NIH3T3, MRC-5, L929, and Hela cells, and measured CAT activities. As can be seen in TABLE 1, there were dramatic differences between these four cell types in the relative activities of pSVIE and pSVTAT to transactivate the HIV-1 LTR. One way we chose to illustrate this difference was to calculate the ratio of the level of transactivation of the HIV-1 LTR by pSVIE to the level of transactivation by pSVTAT. This ratio, represented as pSVIE/pSVTAT, varied over 7000-fold between the four cell types. Thus, in NIH3T3 cells, pSVIE transactivated the HIV-1 LTR to 70-fold higher levels than did pSVTAT, whereas in Hela cells, pSVIE transactivated the LTR 100-fold less efficiently than did pSVTAT. Experiments in MRC-5 and L929 gave intermediate ratios of 7.0 and 0.3, respectively.

These ratios have been relatively constant between experiments[17] and were not artefacts of the experimental procedure. We have altered transfection conditions and time of harvesting cells after transfection, and the ratio of transactivation by pSVIE and pSVTAT has not changed.

The Mechanism of Transactivation by CMV IE Is the Same in Different Cell Types

Previous reports in MRC-5 cell cultures have demonstrated that the region of the HIV-1 LTR responsive to transactivation by CMV IE was contained within a regulatory domain between nucleotides -6 and $+24$ of the HIV-1 LTR, relative to the start site of transcription at $+1$.[7] The mechanism of transactivation by CMV IE appeared to involve an increase in the frequency of initiation of transcription of the HIV-1 LTR. Because there was a dramatic difference in the abilities of pSVIE and pSVTAT to transactivate the HIV-1 LTR in different cell types (TABLE 1), we examined whether the mechanism of transactivation by CMV IE might be different in different cell types. We determined this by localizing mutations within the HIV-1 LTR that abrogated responsiveness to transactivation by pSVIE in L929 cell cultures. Accordingly, mutated HIV-1 LTR/CAT constructions (see MATERIALS AND METHODS) were transfected into L929 cell cultures, and the responsiveness of each to pSVTAT and pSVIE was determined by measuring CAT activity.

An HIV-1 LTR with mutations either in the three Sp1 sites (Sp1-dpm (I,II,III)),[13] the binding sites for the cellular protein designated LBP-1,[11] or in the TATA sequence[11]

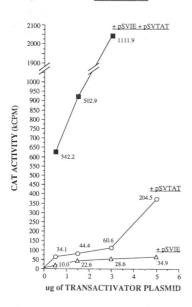

L929 Cells

FIGURE 1. Transactivation of the HIV-1 LTR by plasmids expressing the immediate early genes of CMV or HIV-1 TAT. pHIV LTR/CAT (2 μg) was cotransfected into cultures of L929 cells with increasing amounts of pSVIE, expressing CMV IE (triangle), or with pSVTAT, expressing HIV-1 TAT (circle). CAT activity was assayed with whole cell extracts, as described in MATERIALS AND METHODS, and is expressed in kilocounts per minute (kCPM). In addition, 2 μg of pHIV LTR/CAT plus 3 μg of pSVTAT were cotransfected with increasing amounts of pSVIE (square). The numbers next to each datum point represent the relative increase in CAT activity above basal levels for each concentration of transactivator plasmid. Each value represents the average of duplicate transfections; variability between replicate cultures was less than 10%.

abolished transactivation by both pSVIE and pSVTAT (TABLE 2). Mutations between nucleotides -6 and $+24$ in the HIV-1 LTR resulted in differential responses to transactivation by pSVIE and pSVTAT. The mutation $(-6/-1)$ retained only 14% of wild-type levels of transactivation by pSVIE, whereas it remained fully responsive to transactivation by pSVTAT. Mutations extending out to nucleotides $(+24/+27)$ resulted in lowered level of transactivation by pSVIE, although mutations more distal from the start site (*e.g.,* $\Delta(+24/+38)$ and $(+24/+27)$) had less of an impact on transactivation by pSVIE than mutations immediately closer to the start site of transcription (*e.g.,* $-6/-1$). The phenotype of these mutations on transactivation by pSVTAT was such that mutations downstream of nucleotides $(+4/+9)$ (with the exception of pTriple/CAT) resulted in lowered levels of transactivation by pSVTAT. Mutation $(+24/+27)$ retained less than 8% of wild-type levels of transactivation by

TABLE 1. Transactivation of the HIV-1 LTR by pSVIE and pSVTAT in Different Cell Types[a]

| | Transfected Plasmids | | | | | | |
| | pHIV LTR/ CAT | | pHIV LTR/CAT + pSVIE | | pHIV LTR/CAT + pSVTAT | | |
Cell Type	cpm	Relative Activity	cpm	Relative Activity	cpm	Relative Activity	pSVIE/ pSVTAT
NIH3T3	627	1	537,053	856.5	7660	12.2	70.2
MRC-5	1010	1	56,968	56.4	8155	8.1	7.0
L929	1030	1	32,993	32.0	112,672	109.3	0.3
HeLa	1562	1	5666	3.6	584,749	374.4	0.01

[a] Transfections into L929 cell cultures were performed as described in MATERIAL AND METHODS. CAT enzymatic activities of transfected cell extracts are given in kilocounts per minute (cpm). Relative activity represents the relative levels of stimulation in CAT activity by pSVIE and pSVTAT compared to transfection with pHIV LTR/CAT alone (set at 1). The ratio of the level of transactivation of pHIV LTR/CAT by pSVIE to the level of transactivation by pSVTAT is given as pSVIE/pSV/TAT. Values represent the average of two transfections.

pSVTAT, yet resulted in higher than wild-type levels for transactivation by pSVIE. This region of responsiveness to CMV IE (nucleotides −6 to +24) in L929 cells was the same as that identified in MRC-5 cells.[7] Similar results have been obtained for experiments in Hela cell cultures.

Transactivation of the SIV LTR by Rhesus CMV

Rhesus macaques experimentally inoculated with SIV suffer similar pathologies to humans infected with HIV.[22] In order to use rhesus macaques as a model for investigating the role that CMV may play in augmenting HIV gene expression, we determined whether rhesus CMV could potentiate SIV gene expression. CMV from a rhesus macaque experimentally infected with SIV was isolated. A molecular CMV genomic library was prepared, and a full-length clone containing the rhesus CMV immediate early gene was isolated.[17] Using transient expression assays as before, we examined the ability of CMV to transactivate the SIV LTR.

An SIV LTR/CAT plasmid was transfected into cultures of MRC-5 cells. At 24 hours posttransfection the cells were either mock-infected or infected with rhesus CMV at a multiplicity of infection (MOI) equal to 1 (TABLE 3A). Superinfection of transfected cells with CMV dramatically stimulated CAT expression from the SIV LTR, increasing CAT activity over 100-fold above that observed for SIV LTR/CAT alone. This increase in CAT activity was due, at least in part, to the rhesus IE gene products activating SIV gene expression.

Cultures of L929 cells were transfected with SIV LTR/CAT alone or cotransfected with either pSVIE (containing the human CMV IE under the transcriptional control of the SV40 promoter), AGM CMV IE, or Rh CMV IE (the latter two containing immediate early genes of AGM CMV or rhesus CMV, respectively, under the transcriptional control of their autologous promoters). Both the AGM CMV IE and Rh CMV IE stimulated SIV gene expression (26- and 39-fold, respectively) above the level with SIV LTR/CAT alone (TABLE 3B). The lower level of transactivation with these two constructs compared with pSVIE was, most likely, a result of autoregulation by these transactivators on their autologous promoters.[23] Thus, the rhesus system *in vitro* paralleled the results with the human counterparts.

DISCUSSION

The time course between infection with HIV or SIV and the onset of full-blown AIDS is variable. After infection of a cell by either virus (FIG. 2), the retroviral RNA is reverse-transcribed by the viral-encoded reverse transcriptase. After integration of the double-stranded linear viral DNA into cellular DNA, the provirus can remain latent or be expressed at a very low but persistent level. At some point expression of the virus is stimulated to resume the viral replication cycle. Conditions that stimulate viral replication include activation signals for T cells, brought about by the recognition of antigen in the context of the major histocompatibility complex.[10,24] Additional factors may activate viral expression.

TABLE 2. Transactivation of Plasmids with Mutations in the HIV-1 LTR by pSVIE and pSVTAT Relative to the Wild-Type LTR[a]

| | Relative Activity | |
Plasmid	+pSVIE	+pSVTAT
pHIV LTR/CAT	100	100
Δ-76	229	63
NFKB	460	60
SpI-dpm (III)	27	41
SpI-dpm (I,II,III)	4	1
TATA	3	<1
−16/−12	54	71
−11/−7	189	258
−6/−1	14	154
pTriple/CAT	9	1
+4/+8	37	36
+4/+9	42	37
+14/+18	40	3
Δ+24/+38	68	5
+24/+27	205	8
+30/+33	119	29

[a] Each plasmid containing mutated and wild-type HIV-1 LTR/CAT sequences was cotransfected with either pSVIE or pSVTAT into cultures of L929 cells. The levels of transactivation of the mutated plasmids by pSVIE and pSVTAT are presented relative to the levels of transactivation of the wild-type LTR (arbitrarily set at 100). The mutations and transfection protocols are described in MATERIAL AND METHODS. Each value represents the average of two parallel transfections. Variability was less than 10%.

In humans infected with HIV, and in rhesus macaques experimentally infected with SIV, secondary infectious agents cause serious medical complications; many coinfected individuals suffer from CMV-induced sequelae.[3,4,22] Serologic evidence and *in vitro* experiments[7,14,17,20,21,25-35] provide support for a model in which heterologous infectious agents, including CMV, may play a direct role in altering the pathogenesis of HIV and SIV. An essential element in the model that CMV could affect directly HIV (and SIV) replication is that the two classes of virus would have to coinfect the same cell. Evidence for this has been presented; examination of cells from the central nervous system of AIDS patients, who also presented with CMV pathology, revealed that individual cells harbored both HIV and CMV.[36]

The data presented in this report describe a molecular explanation for events that might occur in coinfected cells. The immediate early gene products of CMV are strong transactivators of HIV (and SIV) gene expression (FIG. 1, TABLES 1,2, and 3). For human CMV IE, at least, the mechanism of transactivation in L929 cell cultures involves a regulatory domain located between nucleotides -6 and $+24$ of the HIV-1 LTR (relative to the start site of transcription at $+1$). This is the same domain that was identified in cultures of MRC-5 cells[7] and in Hela cells (data not shown). Thus, in different cell types the mechanism of transactivation of the HIV-1 LTR by pSVIE involves the same cis-acting element, and, thus, the same trans-acting factors are implicated. Transactivation of the HIV-1 LTR by CMV IE and HIV-1 TAT, however, was cell-type specific, as documented by the different ratios of the level of transactivation by pSVIE to the level of transactivation by pSVTAT (TABLE 2). The evidence for transactivation by CMV IE is consistent with the observation that CMV IE functions to increase the frequency of transcription initiation.[7] We speculate that the reason for the cell-type specificity of transactivation (TABLE 2) involves differences in the state of the transcription complex in the different cell types. Extrapolating this to *in vivo* situations, the consequences of coinfection of the same cell by CMV and HIV would

TABLE 3. Transactivation of the SIV LTR by the Immediate Early Gene Products of Rhesus Cytomegalovirus[a]

A

Plasmid	CAT Activity (cpm)	Relative Activity
SIV LTR/CAT	1,418	1
SIV LTR/CAT + Rh CMV (MOI=1)	151,866	107

B

Plasmid	CAT Activity (cpm)	Relative Activity
SIV LTR/CAT	4,640	1.0
SIV LTR/CAT + pSVIE	859,411	185.0
SIV LTR/CAT + AGM CMV IE	120,975	26.1
SIV LTR/CAT + Rh CMV IE (p9.4-2)	181,548	39.1

[a] Cultures of MRC-5 (part A) were transfected with SIV LTR/CAT and either mock-infected or infected with rhesus CMV at an MOI of 1 at 24 hours posttransfection. Cultures of L929 cells (part B) were transfected with SIV LTR/CAT in the absence or presence of plasmids expressing human CMV IE (pSVIE), AGM CMV IE, or rhesus CMV IE. Cells were analyzed as before.

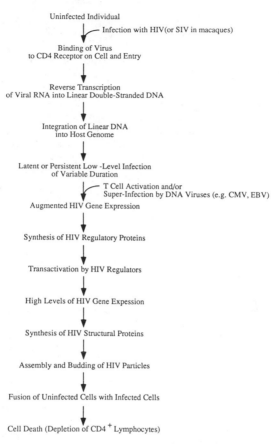

FIGURE 2. Replication cycle of HIV. This figure represents the major events in the life cycle of HIV. The same general features apply to the life cycle of SIV.

depend on the cell type that harbors both viruses. In addition, the state of cell growth at the time of coinfection is likely to be a significant factor in the extent of heterologous viral transactivation. Future plans are aimed at using the rhesus macaque model to investigate the role of CMV in altering pathogenesis of SIV and to examine antiviral (*i.e.*, anti-SIV and anti-CMV) therapeutic agents that might alter the course of pathogenesis.

REFERENCES

1. ROSENBERG, Z. F. & A. S. FAUCI. 1989. The immunopathogenesis of HIV infection. Adv. Immunol. **47:** 377-431.
2. NELSON, J. A., P. GHAZAL & C. A. WILEY. 1990. Role of opportunistic viral infections in AIDS. AIDS **4:** 1-10.

3. DREW, W. L. 1988. Cytomegalovirus infection in patients with AIDS. J. Infect. Dis. **158:** 449-456.
4. REICHERT, C. M., T. J. O'LEARY, D. L. LEVENS, C. R. SIMRELL & A. M. MACHER. 1983. Autopsy pathology in the acquired immunodeficiency syndrome. Am. J. Pathol. **112:** 357-382.
5. PEDERSON, C., J. GERSTOFT, P. TAURIS, J. D. LUNDGREN, P. C. GØTZSCHE, M. BUHL, Y. SALIM & K. SCHMIDT. 1990. Opportunistic infections and malignancies in 231 Danish AIDS patients. AIDS **4:** 233-238.
6. GARDNER, M. B. & P. A. LUCIW. 1989. Animal Models of AIDS. FASEB J. **3:** 2593-2606.
7. BARRY, P. A., E. PRATT-LOWE, B. M. PETERLIN & P. A. LUCIW. 1990. Cytomegalovirus activates transcription directed by the long terminal repeat of human immunodeficiency virus type 1. J. Virol. **64:** 2932-2940.
8. NORDEEN, S. K., P. P. I. GREEN & D. M. FOWLKES. 1987. A rapid, sensitive, and inexpensive assay for chloramphenicol acetyltransferase. DNA **6:** 173-178.
9. PETERLIN, B. M., P. A. LUCIW, P. J. BARR & M. D. WALKER. 1986. Elevated levels of mRNA can account for the trans-activation of human immunodeficiency virus. Proc. Natl. Acad. Sci. USA **83:** 9734-9738.
10. TONG-STARKSEN, S. E., P. A. LUCIW & B. M. PETERLIN. 1987. Human immunodeficiency virus long terminal repeat responds to T-cell activation signals. Proc. Natl. Acad. Sci. USA **84:** 6845-6849.
11. JONES, K. A., P. A. LUCIW & N. DUCHANGE. 1988. Structural arrangements of transcription control domains within the 5' untranslated leader regions of the HIV-1 and HIV-2 promoters. Genes & Dev. **2:** 1101-1114.
12. SELBY, M. J., E. S. BAIN, P. A. LUCIW & B. M. PETERLIN. 1989. Structure, sequence, and position of the stem-loop in TAR determine transcriptional elongation by TAT through the HIV-1 long terminal repeat. Genes & Dev. **3:** 547-558.
13. JONES, K. A., J. T. KADONAGA, P. A. LUCIW & R. TJIAN. 1986. Activation of the AIDS retrovirus promoter by the cellular transcription factor, Sp1. Science **232:** 755-759.
14. NABEL, G. & D. BALTIMORE. 1987. An inducible transcription factor activates expression of human immunodeficiency virus in T cells. Nature (London) **326:** 711-713.
15. MUESING, M. A., D. H. SMITH & D. J. CAPON. 1987. Regulation of mRNA accumulation by a human immunodeficiency virus trans-activator protein. Cell **48:** 691-701.
16. HERMISTON, T., C. L. MALONE, P. R. WITTE & M. F. STINSKI. 1987. Identification and characterization of the human cytomegalovirus immediate-early region 2 gene that stimulates gene expression from an inducible promoter. J. Virol. **61:** 3214-3221.
17. BARRY, P. A., E. PRATT-LOWE, R. E. UNGER, M. MARTHAS, D. J. ALCENDOR & P. A. LUCIW. 1990. Molecular interactions of cytomegalovirus and the human and simian immunodeficiency viruses. J. Med. Primatol. **19:** 327-337.
18. JEANG, K.-T., M.-S. CHO & G. S. HAYWARD. 1984. Abundant constitutive expression of the immediate-early 94K protein from cytomegalovirus (Colburn) in a DNA-transfected mouse cell line. Mol. Cell. Biol. **4:** 2214-2223.
19. MARTHAS, M. L., B. BANAPOUR, S. SUTJIPTO, M. E. SIEGEL, P. A. MARX, M. B. GARDNER, N. C. PEDERSON & P. A. LUCIW. 1989. Rhesus macaques inoculated with molecularly cloned simian immunodeficiency virus. J. Med. Primatol. **18:** 311-319.
20. MOSCA, J. D., D. P. BEDNARIK, N. B. K. RAJ, C. A. ROSEN, J. G. SODROSKI, W. A. HASELTINE, G. S. HAYWARD & P. M. PITHA. 1987. Activation of the human immunodeficiency virus by herpesvirus infection: identification of a region within the long terminal repeat that responds to a trans-acting factor encoded by herpes simplex virus 1. Proc. Natl. Acad. Sci. USA **84:** 7408-7412.
21. DAVIS, M. G., S. C. KENNEY, J. KAMINE, J. S. PAGANO & E.-S. HUANG. 1987. Immediate-early gene region of human cytomegalovirus trans-activates the promoter of human immunodeficiency virus. Proc. Natl. Acad. Sci. USA **84:** 8642-8646.
22. BASKIN, G. B. 1987. Disseminated cytomegalovirus infection in immunodeficient rhesus macaques. Am. J. Path. **129:** 345-352.
23. STENBERG, R. M. & M. F. STINSKI. 1985. Autoregulation of the human cytomegalovirus major immediate early gene. J. Virol. **56:** 676-682.
24. TONG-STARKSEN, S. E., P. A. LUCIW & B. M. PETERLIN. 1989. Signaling through T

lymphocyte surface proteins, TCR/CD3 and CD28, activates the HIV-1 long terminal repeat. J. Immunol. **142:** 702-707.

25. NABEL, G. J., S. A. RICE, D. M. KNIPE & D. BALTIMORE. 1988. Alternative mechanisms for activation of human immunodeficiency virus enhancer in T cells. Science **239:** 1299-1302.

26. GENDELMAN, H. E., W. PHELPS, L. FEIGENBAUM, J. M. OSTROVE, A. ADACHI, P. M. HOWLEY, G. KHOURY, H. S. GINSBERG & M. A. MARTIN. 1986. Transactivation of the human immunodeficiency virus long terminal repeat by DNA viruses. Proc. Natl. Acad. Sci. USA **83:** 9759-9763.

27. OSTROVE, J. M., J. LEONARD, K. E. WECK, A. B. RABSON & H. E. GENDELMAN. 1987. Activation of the human immunodeficiency virus by herpes simplex virus type 1. J. Virol. **61:** 3726-3732.

28. RANDO, R. F., P. E. PELLETT, P. A. LUCIW, C. A. BOHAN & A. SRINIVASAN. 1987. Transactivation of the human immunodeficiency virus by herpesviruses. J. Virol. **1:** 13-18.

29. RICE, A. P. & M. B. MATHEWS. 1988. Trans-activation of the human immunodeficiency virus long terminal repeat sequences, expressed in an adenovirus vector, by the adenovirus E1A 13S protein. Proc. Natl. Acad. Sci. USA **85:** 4200-4204.

30. ENSOLI, B., P. LUSSO, F. SCHACHTER, S. F. JOSEPHS, J. RAPPAPORT, F. NEGRO, R. C. GALLO & F. WONG-STAAL. 1989. Human herpes virus-6 increases HIV-1 expression in co-infected cells via nuclear factors binding to the HIV-1 enhancer. EMBO J. **8:** 3019-3027.

31. TWU, J.-S. & W. S. ROBINSON. 1989. Hepatitis B virus X gene can transactivate heterologous viral sequences. Proc. Natl. Acad. Sci. USA **86:** 2046-2050.

32. SETO, E., T. S. B. YEN, B. M. PETERLIN & J.-H. OU. 1988. Trans-activation of the human immunodeficiency virus long terminal repeat by the hepatitis B virus X protein. Proc. Natl. Acad. Sci. USA **85:** 8286-8290.

33. YUAN, R., C. BOHAN, F. C. H. SHIAO, R. ROBINSON, H. J. KAPLAN & A. SRINIVASAN. 1989. Activation of HIV LTR-directed expression: analysis with Pseudorabies virus immediate early gene. Virology **172:** 92-99.

34. KENNEY, S., J. KAMINE, D. MARKOVITZ, R. FENRICK & J. PAGANO. 1988. An Epstein-Barr virus immediate-early gene product trans-activates gene expression from the human immunodeficiency virus long terminal repeat. Proc. Natl. Acad. Sci. USA **85:** 1652-1656.

35. QUINN, T. C., P. PIOT, J. B. MCCORMICK, F. M. FEINSOD, H. TAELMAN, B. KAPITA, W. STEVENS & A. S. FAUCI. 1987. Serologic and immunologic studies in patients with AIDS in North America and Africa. J. Am. Med. Assoc. **257:** 2617-2621.

36. NELSON, J. A., C. REYNOLDS-KOHLER, M. B. A. OLDSTONE & C. A. WILEY. 1988. HIV and HCMV coinfect brain cells in patients with AIDS. Virology **165:** 286-290.

The Human Immunodeficiency Virus TAT Protein

A Target for Antiviral Agents

IAIN S. SIM

Department of Oncology and Virology
Hoffmann-La Roche Inc.
Nutley, New Jersey 07110

INTRODUCTION

The genome of the human immunodeficiency virus (HIV) encodes three nonstructural, regulatory proteins, TAT, REV, and NEF, in addition to the structural proteins GAG, POL, and ENV that are commonly found in retroviruses, and at least three additional proteins, VIF, VPU, and VPR, the functions of which are not well-understood (FIG. 1a). Of the regulatory proteins, TAT (*trans*-activator of transcription) is of particular interest in the context of antiviral chemotherapy for a number of reasons, not least of which is that it may be regarded as a paradigm for many other viral systems in which *trans*-activators have been found. Virally encoded *trans*-activators play an important role in the replication of several members of the herpesvirus group, the hepadna-, papilloma-, and adenoviruses, as well as in the human retroviruses. The *trans*-activating proteins of each of these viruses can be considered as targets for antagonists, the action of which would be expected to result in the inhibition of viral replication. The potential of such agents remains untested, however, because no inhibitors active by this mechanism have yet been described. The role of TAT in the replication of HIV and its structure, as it relates to function and mechanism of action, are described here. The manner in which antagonists of TAT may be found and evaluated is also discussed.

ROLE OF TAT IN VIRAL REPLICATION

An important feature of the replicative cycle of HIV is the ability of the virus to establish a latent infection of CD4[+] T lymphocytes as a provirus integrated in the chromosome of the host cell,[1] and possibly also as an unintegrated genome.[2] The reactivation of the virus from this latent state and its entry into a destructive, replicative phase are important in the pathogenesis of HIV-induced disease. T-cell activation, by exposure either to specific antigen, cytokine, or heterologous *trans*-activators from a second infecting virus, results in the induction of cellular transcription factors that bind to enhancer elements on the viral long terminal repeat (LTR) (FIG 1b). It would seem that transcription of the viral genome occurs only at a low level at first, the predominant species of mRNAs in the cytoplasm being the doubly spliced forms that encode the regulatory proteins, including TAT. Following the synthesis of TAT, the level of viral gene expression increases substantially and, in time and under the control of the REV protein, longer mRNAs are synthesized that specify the structural proteins of the virus.[3-5]

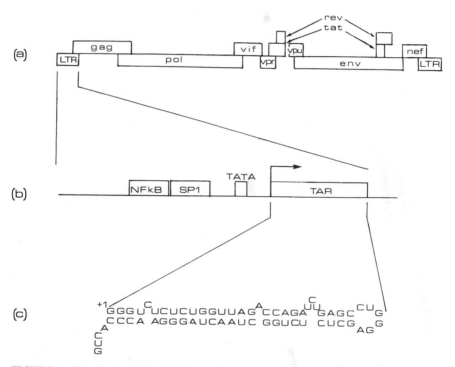

FIGURE 1. Genetic structure of HIV. (a) Alignment of the genes coding for the regulatory proteins (*tat, rev,* and *nef*) and the structural proteins (*gag, pol,* and *env*). The functions of the *vif, vpr,* and *vpu* genes are not well-understood. (b) The long terminal repeat (LTR) contains the regulatory elements NFκB, SP1, and TATA. A reporter gene may be inserted 3' to TAR. (c) The *trans*-activation response region (TAR) located 3' to the start site of transcription (+1) may occur as a RNA stem-loop structure.

Because TAT appears to play a unique and pivotal role in the emergence of HIV from the latent state, antagonists would be very different from antiviral agents directed to other functions of the virus. Inhibitors of viral attachment, such as soluble CD4, and nucleosides that inhibit the viral reverse transcriptase, such as azidothymidine (AZT), dideoxycytidine (ddC), and dideoxyinosine (ddI), may effectively block initiation of infection in a cell freshly exposed to virus. Similarly, antiviral agents that are targeted to events late in the replicative cycle, such as inhibitors of the viral protease and certain glycosidase inhibitors, may also spare fresh cells from infection as a result of blocking the formation of mature, infectious virions. None of these agents, however, would be expected to protect cells, that are already infected with the virus, from the cytopathicity associated with the late phase of HIV replication. By contrast, an antagonist of HIV TAT may effectively suppress transcription of the viral genome in a latently infected host cell, protect the cell from viral cytopathicity, and block the formation of new, infectious virions. It is possible that an antagonist that is highly specific for HIV TAT may suppress viral replication but not inhibit the infected host cell from performing its normal function in the host.

TAT STRUCTURE/FUNCTION

Mechanism of Action: Transcription versus Translation

Full-length TAT is an 86 amino acid protein that is synthesized from a doubly spliced message, although the 72 amino acid form that is derived from the first coding exon appears to be fully functional.[6-8] TAT is a powerful *trans*-activator of the expression of genes under the control of the HIV LTR. In this regard, TAT exerts a positive feedback on its own expression; this presents a particularly difficult challenge in the search for effective antagonists because only partial suppression of TAT activity may not adequately block *de novo* synthesis of TAT protein and thus permit continued *trans*-activation of gene expression.

The action of TAT requires the presence of a sequence, called the *trans*-activation response (TAR) element, that has been mapped to a region encompassing the start site for transcription in the LTR.[9,10] The mechanism(s) by which gene expression is activated by TAT remains unclear, however. Early observations suggested that *trans*-activation could be explained by posttranscriptional events,[4,11] whereas others suggested that the mechanism was bimodal, involving both transcriptional and translational control,[8] or principally at the level of transcription.[10,12,13] A number of studies have suggested that TAT increases the rate of transcription from the viral LTR, rather than stabilizing HIV-specific mRNAs,[14,15] possibly by relieving a block to transcriptional elongation within the TAR region.[16] The use of purified TAT protein, introduced into cells by scrape-loading, has revealed that *de novo* mRNA synthesis is required for *trans*-activation.[17] This observation further supports the hypothesis that TAT does not act directly on mRNA stability, transport, or translation. Although the direct binding of TAT to DNA from the TAR region remains controversial, *trans*-activation can occur in the absence of *de novo* protein synthesis.[18] Thus, the production of new cellular proteins is not required for the action of TAT, although the participation of preexisting host proteins is not eliminated. To the contrary, studies on the DNase-I hypersensitivity of the HIV LTR in the presence or absence of TAT suggest that TAR may be recognized by a host cell-specific DNA-binding protein rather than by TAT.[19]

Functional Domains of TAT

Full-length TAT protein has a number of interesting structural features that ultimately may be of particular significance for the design of specific antagonists (FIG. 2).

Mutational studies and the use of chemically synthesized protein have helped to define domains on the protein that are essential for function. TAT appears to be localized in the nucleus of the cell.[14] Consistent with this observation is the presence of a string of basic amino acids that may serve as a nuclear localization signal in the carboxyterminal half of the molecule. Single amino acid substitutions in this region appear not to markedly affect the *trans*-activating activity of TAT, whereas more extensive deletion of these basic residues has a more profound effect and reduces nuclear accumulation.[20–22]

HIV TAT also contains four Cys-X-X-Cys sequences (where X is a variable amino acid) that participate in the binding of metal ions to form a dimer *in vitro*.[23] Mutation of the cysteine residues markedly reduces TAT function and abolishes virus replication but does not appear to affect metal binding.[20–22] (An exception is the replacement of Cys^{32}, which has a less dramatic effect on function.) Mutation analysis has failed to reveal any single amino acid in the amino terminal region of TAT whose presence is critical for *trans*-activating activity, although the protein has a number of potentially interesting features, such as the clustering of four proline residues. Truncation of the

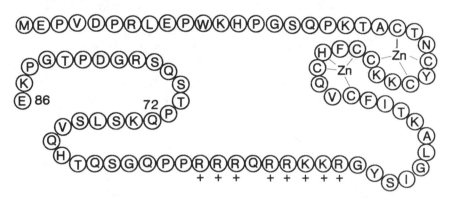

FIGURE 2. HIV TAT. The amino acid sequence is represented by one-letter symbols. The string of basic amino acids (+) may serve as a nuclear localization signal, whereas the cysteine-rich region may complex zinc.

amino terminus by the introduction of new initiating methionine residues downstream, however, does ablate *trans*-activating activity.[22]

ANTIVIRAL AGENTS TARGETED TO HIV TAT

Detection of Antagonists to TAT

In selecting a viral protein as a target for the development of a selective inhibitor that will have antiviral activity, it is important to determine that the molecular target is essential for viral replication. If this condition is not fulfilled, it is likely that drug-resistant viruses will readily arise as a result of gene mutation or deletion. Early studies demonstrated that TAT is required for HIV replication: viral genomes in which the *tat* gene has been mutated or partially deleted are unable to produce new viruses.[24-26] Also important is that the primary structure of the target protein be conserved among many isolates of the virus. A comparison of gene sequences among several isolates suggest that there is a high level of conservation in the *tat* gene; where there are differences in gene sequence, they often give rise to amino acid substitutions that are conservative in nature. It should be noted, however, that full-length TAT appears not to be required for activity: mutation studies have revealed that only the first 58 amino acids are required for function.[27]

The observation that the expression of heterologous genes under the control of the HIV LTR will be *trans*-activated by TAT leads to the design of a relatively simple assay that can be used for the detection of potential inhibitors. A reporter gene under the control of the HIV LTR can be cloned into a plasmid and transfected into a suitable eukaryotic cell, together with a second plasmid that expresses HIV TAT. After an appropriate incubation period, the level of protein synthesized from the reporter gene, in the presence and absence of test substance, can be determined. Chloramphenicol acetyltransferase (CAT) has been widely used as the reporter, although many enzymes, cytokines, or other proteins whose activity can be readily determined, may be used.

In the absence of detailed knowledge of the mechanism of action of TAT, or of known inhibitors of the protein, the design of effective antagonists from a theoretical base is likely to be unproductive. A more practical approach in the search for antagonists is the use of a screen that can rapidly, and in high flux, assess the potential of many thousands of test substances for a possible lead. In this instance, compounds of defined structure, but selected from chemical repositories at random, microbial broths, and plant and marine extracts all represent valuable sources of novel substances for testing. The possible need to assess many substances before an active compound is revealed makes the design of the screen particularly important. The product of the reporter gene should be easy to measure but sufficiently robust that measurement of its biological activity is not greatly impaired by the variety of test substances that are added to the screen. It is likely that a number of the test substances will nonspecifically inhibit the production of the reporter gene product, for example, as a result of a general inhibition of transcription or translation. In the absence of an appropriate control, such substances may erroneously be scored as inhibitors of TAT. For this reason, parallel cultures of cells should be transfected with a second plasmid that expresses the reporter gene independently of HIV TAT (in this context any one of a number of viral promoters may be used). Test substances that are equally inhibitory to the expression of the reporter gene on both plasmids can be eliminated as nonspecific inhibitors that do not act on TAT.

The transcription of genes under the control of the HIV LTR are subject to regulation by cellular factors that bind to the NFκB and SP1 sites of the HIV LTR (FIG. 1b), in addition to TAT that acts through TAR.[28-30] Although one or more of these enhancer-binding sites may be deleted without impairing HIV replication,[31] inhibitors of the corresponding enhancer proteins might be expected to exhibit a generalized inhibition of host cell transcription. For this reason, putative inhibitors of TAT *trans*-activation should also be assessed for activity on basal level expression of the reporter gene in the absence of TAT where no inhibition should be observed with a truly TAT-specific inhibitor.

Further refinement of the cell-based screen for TAT inhibitors is possible, for example, by selecting for cells that express the reporter gene constitutively under the control of HIV TAT. Alternatively, TAT may be supplied exogenously to cells bearing a reporter gene. The uptake of such protein, produced by recombinant DNA methods, and the transactivation of a reporter gene have been described.[17,32] A more direct approach, but one that has proven difficult to implement, would be the use of an *in vitro* assay for TAT activity. Mutagenesis studies have provided considerable insight as to the nature of TAR, the region that is required for TAT action, and binding of TAT protein to TAR RNA *in vitro* has been reported.[33] A particularly striking feature of the TAR RNA is the potential to form a stem-loop structure (FIG. 1c). Mutations that disrupt the stem lead to a loss of responsiveness to TAT, but this may be restored, at least in part, by further mutation to permit reformation of the stem.[34] Mutation of the pentanucleotide, CUGGG, of the loop also results in a loss of responsiveness to TAT.[35] This observation may be particularly relevant because HIV-1 TAT can *trans*-activate HIV-2 gene expression, and the same pentanucleotide can be found in the putative loop(s) of HIV-2 TAR.

Nuclear extracts of HIV-infected cells, but not of uninfected cells, have been reported to stimulate transcription from the HIV LTR *in vitro*.[36] More recently, direct binding of HIV TAT, produced in *Escherichia coli,* to TAR RNA *in vitro* has been demonstrated; TAT did not bind to an RNA in which additional nucleotides were inserted into the loop, nor to an antisense TAR RNA transcript.[33] Although further studies are required, if these observations are confirmed, then a direct binding-inhibition assay for antagonists may become feasible. Moreover, an *in vitro* assay would open the way to a more detailed study of the interaction between TAT and its target site. TAT protein obtained by chemical synthetic means, as well as by recombinant DNA methods, has been reported to be functional in whole cell assays.[37,38]

Antiviral Activity of TAT Antagonists

The antiviral activities of anti-HIV agents have been assessed in a number of cell culture assays, most of which should be as suitable for testing antagonists of TAT as for reverse transcriptase inhibitors, for example. The unique potential of a TAT antagonist will be revealed, however, in its ability to block the reactivation of virus from latently infected cells following stimulation of the cell with mitogen or another appropriate trigger. Although HIV has been found to infect a number of cell types other than just CD4+ T lymphocytes, there is no *a priori* reason why a TAT antagonist should not function equally well in monocytes and microglial cells, for example, as in lymphoctyes.

Retroviruses of animal origin, for example, the murine retroviruses and feline immunodeficiency virus, have been used as models to assess the antiviral activity of anti-HIV compounds such as AZT. Because of the unique nature of HIV TAT, however, these model systems that lack any *trans*-activator are inappropriate for *in vivo* testing of TAT antagonists. Three possible model systems (discounting the use of chimpanzees) can be considered. Simian immunodeficiency virus (SIV) causes severe disease in certain lower primates. Alignment of the amino acid sequences of the SIV and HIV-1 and HIV-2 TAT reveals clusters of high homology among these proteins, especially within the cysteine- and basic amino acid-rich domains.[39] The possibility exists, therefore, that antagonists of HIV TAT may also inhibit SIV TAT.

The transplantation of human immune cells into immunodeficient mice and their infection with HIV is a promising development that may yield a model system for the study of HIV-specific antiviral agents *in vivo*.[40] Third, and unique to the possible assessment of TAT antagonists, is the description of mice that are transgenic for the HIV *tat* gene.[41] TAT mRNA is expressed in the skin cells of these transgenic animals, although the pathological consequences of such expression is observed for the most part only in males. Histological changes in the skin are apparent at approximately four months of age; the lesions progress with time until they take on the appearance of Kaposi's sarcoma-like dermal changes. Tumors are apparent although TAT mRNA is not detected in the tumor cells. Treatment of these TAT-associated lesions with any therapeutic agent has not yet been described. It is possible, however, that an effective TAT antagonist may influence the course of the disease, in which case, mice transgenic for the *tat* gene may represent a very interesting *in vivo* model for drug evaluation.

CONCLUSION

HIV TAT is a unique target for the development of antagonists. The present knowledge base is sufficient to support immediate efforts to discover inhibitors of the protein's function. Meanwhile, the future promises to bring further advances in our understanding of the structure and function of the molecule; this new knowledge will be of major benefit for the design and evaluation of potential antagonists. There is good reason to be optimistic that TAT inhibitors will become available for evaluation in the treatment of HIV-induced disease and that such antagonists will have a useful role in the clinical armory in the fight against AIDS.

REFERENCES

1. PSALLIDOPOULOS, M. C., S. M. SCHNITTMAN, L. M. THOMPSON III, M. BASELER, A. S. FAUCI, H. C. LANE & N. P. SALZMAN. 1989. Integrated proviral human immunodeficiency virus type 1 is present in CD4+ peripheral blood lymphocytes in healthy seropositive individuals. J. Virol. 63: 4626-4631.
2. ZACK, J. A., A. J. CANN, J. P. LUGO & I. S. Y. CHEN. 1988. HIV-1 production from infected peripheral blood T cells after HTLV-I induced mitogenic stimulation. Science 240: 1026-1029.
3. SODROSKI, J., W. C. GOH, C. ROSEN, A. DAYTON, E. TERWILLIGER & W. HASELTINE. 1986. A second post-transcriptional *trans*-activator gene required for HTLV-III replication. Nature 321: 412-417.
4. FEINBERG, M. B., R. F. JARRETT, A. ALDOVINI, R. C. GALLO & F. WONG-STAAL. 1986. HTLV-III expression and production involve complex regulation at the levels of splicing and translation of viral RNA. Cell 46: 807-817.
5. MALIM, M. H., J. HAUBER, R. FENRICK & B. R. CULLEN. 1988. Immunodeficiency virus *rev* *trans*-activator modulates the expression of the viral regulatory genes. Nature 335: 181-183.
6. ARYA, S. K., C. GUO, S. F. JOSEPHS & F. WONG-STAAL. 1985. *Trans*-activator gene of human T-lymphotropic virus type III (HTLV-III). Science 229: 69-73.
7. SODROSKI, J., R. PATARCA, C. ROSEN, F. WONG-STAAL & W. HASELTINE. 1985. Location of the *trans*-acting region on the genome of human T-cell lymphotropic virus type III. Science 229: 74-77.
8. CULLEN, B. R. 1986. *Trans*-activation of human immunodeficiency virus occurs via a bimodal mechanism. Cell 46: 973-982.
9. ROSEN, C. A., J. G. SODROSKI & W. A. HASELTINE. 1985. The location of *cis*-acting regulatory sequences in the human T cell lymphotropic virus type III (HTLV-III/LAV) long terminal repeat. Cell 41: 813-823.

10. MUESING, M. A., D. H. SMITH & D. J. CAPON. 1987. Regulation of mRNA accumulation by a human immunodeficiency virus *trans*-activator protein. Cell **48:** 691-701.

11. ROSEN, C. A., J. G. SODROSKI, W. C. GOH, A. I. DAYTON, J. LIPPKE & W. A. HASELTINE. 1986. Post-transcriptional regulation accounts for the *trans*-activation of the human T-lymphotropic virus type III. Nature **319:** 555-559.

12. PETERLIN, B. M., P. A. LUCIW, P. J. BARR & M. D. WALKER. 1986. Elevated levels of mRNA can account for the trans-activation of human immunodeficiency virus. Proc. Natl. Acad. Sci. USA **83:** 9734-9738.

13. RICE, A. P. & M. B. MATHEWS. 1988. Transcriptional but not translational regulation of HIV-1 by the *tat* gene product. Nature **332:** 551-553.

14. HAUBER, J., A. PERKINS, E. P. HEIMER & B. R. CULLEN. 1987. Trans-activation of human immunodeficiency virus gene expression is mediated by nuclear events. Proc. Natl. Acad. Sci. USA **84:** 6364-6368.

15. JAKOBOVITS, A., D. H. SMITH, E. B. JAKOBOVITS & D. J. CAPON. 1988. A discrete element 3' of human immunodeficiency virus 1 (HIV-1) and HIV-2 mRNA initiation sites mediates transcriptional activation by an HIV *trans* activator. Mol. Cell. Biol. **8:** 2555-2561.

16. KAO, S-Y., A. F. CALMAN, P. A. LUCIW & B. M. PETERLIN. 1987. Anti-termination of transcription within the long terminal repeat of HIV-1 by *tat* gene product. Nature **330:** 489-493.

17. GENTZ, R., C-H. CHEN & C. A. ROSEN. 1989. Bioassay for trans-activation using purified human immunodeficiency virus *tat*-encoded protein: Trans-activation requires mRNA synthesis. Proc. Natl. Acad. Sci. USA **86:** 821-824.

18. JEANG, K-T., P. R. SHANK & A. KUMAR. 1988. Transcriptional activation of homologous viral long terminal repeats by the human immunodeficiency virus type 1 or the human T-cell leukemia virus type 1 tat proteins occurs in the absence of *de novo* protein synthesis. Proc. Natl. Acad. Sci USA **85:** 8291-8295.

19. HAUBER, J. & B. R. CULLEN. 1988. Mutational analysis of the *trans*-activation-responsive region of the human immunodeficiency virus type 1 long terminal repeat. J. Virol. **62:** 673-679.

20. GARCIA, J. A., D. HARRICH, L. PEARSON, R. MITSUYASU & R. B. GAYNOR. 1988. Functional domains required for tat-induced transcriptional activation of the HIV-1 long terminal repeat. EMBO J. **7:** 3143-3147.

21. SADAIE, M. R., J. RAPPAPORT, T. BENTER, S. F. JOSEPHS, R. WILLIS & F. WONG-STAAL. 1988. Missense mutations in an infectious human immunodeficiency viral genome: functional mapping of *tat* and identification of the *rev* splice acceptor. Proc. Natl. Acad. Sci. USA **85:** 9224-9228.

22. RUBEN, S., A. PERKINS, R. PURCELL, K. JOUNG, R. SIA, R. BURGHOFF, W. A. HASELTINE & C. ROSEN. 1989. Structural and functional characterization of human immunodeficiency virus *tat* protein. J. Virol. **63:** 1-8.

23. FRANKEL, A. D., D. S. BREDT & C. O. PABO. 1988. Tat protein from human immunodeficiency virus forms a metal-linked dimer. Science **240:** 70-73.

24. FISHER, A. G., M. B. FEINBERG, S. F. JOSEPHS, M. E. HARPER, L. M. MARSELLE, G. REYES, M. A. GONDA, A. ALDOVINI, C. DEBOUK, R. C. GALLO & F. WONG-STAAL. 1986. The *trans*-activator gene of HTLV-III is essential for virus replication. Nature **320:** 367-371.

25. DAYTON, A. I., J. G. SODROSKI, C. A. ROSEN, W. C. GOH & W. A. HASELTINE. 1986. The *trans*-activator gene of the human T cell lymphotropic virus type III is required for replication. Cell **44:** 941-947.

26. SADIE, M. R., T. BENTER & F. WONG-STAAL. 1988. Site-directed mutagenesis of two trans-regulatory genes (*tat*-III, *trs*) of HIV-1. Science **239:** 910-913.

27. SEIGEL, L. J., L. RATNER, S. F. JOSEPHS, D. DERSE, M. B. FEINBERG, G. R. REYES, S. J. O'BRIEN & F. WONG-STAAL. 1986. Transactivation induced by human T-lymphotropic virus type III (HTLV III) maps to a viral sequence encoding 58 amino acids and lacks tissue specificity. Virology **148:** 226-231.

28. JONES, K. A., J. T. KADONAGA, P. A. LUCIW & R. TJIAN. 1986. Activation of the AIDS retrovirus promoter by the cellular transcription factor, SP1. Science **232:** 755-759.

29. NABEL, G. & D. BALTIMORE. 1987. An inducible transcription factor activates expression of human immunodeficiency virus in T cells. Nature **326:** 711-713.

30. TONG-STARKSEN, S. E., P. A. LUCIW & B. M. PETERLIN. 1987. Human immunodeficiency virus long terminal repeat responds to T-cell activation signals. Proc. Natl. Acad. Sci USA **84**: 6845-6849.
31. LEONARD, J., C. PARROTT, A. J. BUCKLER-WHITE, W. TURNER, E. K. ROSS, M. A. MARTIN & A. B. RABSON. 1989. The NFκB binding sites in the human immunodeficiency virus type 1 long terminal repeat are not required for virus infectivity. J. Virol. **63**: 4919-4924.
32. FRANKEL, A. D. & C. O. PABO. 1988. Cellular uptake of the Tat protein from human immunodeficiency virus. Cell **55**: 1189-1193.
33. DINGWALL, C., I. ERNBERG, M. J. GAIT, S. M. GREEN, S. HEAPHY, J. KARN, A. D. LOWE, M. SINGH, M. A. SKINNER & R. VALERIO. 1989. Human immunodeficiency virus 1 tat protein binds trans-activation-responsive region (TAR) RNA *in vitro*. Proc. Natl. Acad. Sci. USA **86**: 6925-6929.
34. GARCIA, J. A., D. HARRICH, E. SOULTANAKIS, F. WU, R. MITSUYASU & R. B. GAYNOR. 1989. Human immunodeficiency virus type 1 LTR TATA and TAR region sequences required for transcriptional regulation. EMBO J. **8**: 765-778.
35. FENG, S. & E. C. HOLLAND. 1988. HIV-1 tat *trans*-activation requires the loop sequence within *tar*. Nature **334**: 165-167.
36. OKAMOTO, T. & F. WONG-STAAL. 1986. Demonstration of virus-specific transcriptional activator(s) in cells infected with HTLV-III by an *in vitro* cell-free system. Cell **47**: 29-35.
37. GREEN, M. & P. M. LOEWENSTEIN. 1988. Autonomous functional domains of chemically synthesized human immunodeficiency virus tat *trans*-activator protein. Cell **55**: 1179-1188.
38. FRANKEL, A. D., S. BIANCALANA & D. HUDSON. 1989. Activity of synthetic peptides from the Tat protein of human immunodeficiency virus type 1. Proc. Natl. Acad. Sci. USA **86**: 7397-7401.
39. COLOMBINI, S., S. K. ARYA, M. S. REITZ, L. JAGODZINSKI, B. BEAVER & F. WONG-STAAL. 1989. Structure of simian immunodeficiency virus regulatory genes. Proc. Natl. Acad. Sci. USA **86**: 4813-4817.
40. NAMIKAWA, R., H. KANESHIMA, M. LIEBERMAN, I. L. WEISSMAN & J. M. MCCUNE. 1988. Infection of the SCID-hu mouse by HIV-1. Science **242**: 1684-1686.
41. VOGEL, J., S. H. HINRICHS, R. K. REYNOLDS, P. A. LUCIW & G. JAY. 1988. The HIV *tat* gene induces dermal lesions resembling Kaposi's sarcoma in transgenic mice. Nature **335**: 606-611.

A Role for the Aspartyl Protease from the Human Immunodeficiency Virus Type 1 (HIV-1) in the Orchestration of Virus Assembly

MANUEL A. NAVIA [a] AND BRIAN M. MCKEEVER

Merck Sharp and Dohme Research Laboratories
Rahway, New Jersey 07065

Functional HIV-1 protease (PR) is required for the maturation of viral proteins, for the appearance of characteristic structural features in the virion (as determined by electron microscopy), and for the final assembly of mature virus. Most importantly, HIV-1 PR activity is required for the development of infectivity.[1] Still largely undefined, however, is the timing and control of protease action in this assembly process. Based on the three-dimensional structure of HIV-1 PR[2,3] and experimental data reported in the literature, we propose a comprehensive virus assembly model that highlights the role of HIV-1 PR, suggests further experiments to verify the validity of the model, and poses specific questions relevant to the ultimate exploitation of HIV-1 protease as a therapeutic target.

INTRODUCTION

Self-assembly of structural proteins is a genetically economical strategy to follow, although it does raise the possibility of inappropriate or premature aggregation at the time and site of protein synthesis. To prevent this from happening, many viruses, including the picornaviruses and other retroviruses like HIV-1, synthesize their structural proteins and viral-encoded enzymes linked together in polyprotein form. In such systems, internal steric interference between coupled viral components can be designed into the polyprotein in order to prevent aggregation and to assure uneventful synthesis and transport to the site of final assembly. Polyprotein synthesis also implies correct stoichiometry without the need for external direction or control. Once at the site of assembly, however, the inverse problem of decoupling the polyprotein into its independent components must be addressed, as well as the timing of that action within the overall process of viral replication. In HIV-1, this maturation process clearly involves HIV-1 PR in the cleavage of two of the three polyprotein products, *gag* and *gag-pol*, synthesized by the virus.[4] (The third *env* polyprotein is processed by an as yet

---

[a] Present address: Vertex Pharmaceuticals Inc., 40 Allston Street, Cambridge, MA 02139-4211.

uncharacterized enzyme, probably of cellular origin.) The importance of HIV-1 PR activity in virus replication has been demonstrated most elegantly by site-directed mutagenesis of the critical active site residue, Asp25, of the enzyme. Inactivation of this enzyme leads to the production of immature uninfectious virions whose polyproteins remain unprocessed.[1]

That HIV-1 PR was an aspartyl protease had been established early on by systematic comparison of its amino acid sequence (99 residues) with that of the well-studied pepsin-like aspartyl proteases (> 300 residues).[5] Further sequence analysis then showed that the smaller viral enzyme corresponded roughly to one of the two pseudosymmetric domains known to make up the larger aspartyl proteases. These observations led to the suggestion that HIV-1 PR functioned enzymatically when associated as a true dimer.[6] This hypothesis was confirmed by direct visualization of the HIV-1 PR dimer in its X-ray crystal structure.[2]

STRUCTURE OF HIV-1 PROTEASE

Crystals suitable for X-ray diffraction analysis were grown[7] using the hanging drop vapor diffusion method in 250 mM sodium chloride, 100 mM imidazole buffer, 10 mM dithiothreitol, and 3 mM sodium azide at pH 7. The crystals were tetragonal bipyramids in space group $P4_12_12$, with unit cell dimensions a = b = 50.29 Å, c = 106.80 Å. One 99 residue monomer per asymmetric unit was found, implying a strict twofold symmetric structure for the observed (functional) HIV-1 protease dimer.[2] Subsequent native HIV-1 protease structural studies[3] have all been based on these published[7] crystallization conditions. Unfortunately, this crystal form of HIV-1 PR diffracts to little better than 3 Å effective resolution. This resolution limit compares unfavorably, for example, with other crystals of therapeutically interesting proteins, which we have investigated at Merck (e.g. human neutrophil elastase (HNE),[8] 1.7Å; human carbonic anhydrase C (HCAC),[9] 1.6Å, and porcine pancreatic elastase (PPE), 1.3Å)[10,11] and limits fundamentally the degree of detail that can be extracted from the structure. In addition, the high symmetry of the $P4_12_12$ space group combined with the small volume of the unit cell in this crystal form means that the total number of unique reflection data available will be quite small (approx. 2500 reflections vs. 19,000 for HNE, 29,000 for HCAC, and 37,000 for PPE). Operationally, the limit of diffraction reported for a given macromolecular crystal is more important for the implicit number of unique reflections available to the experiment than for the theoretical "resolution" defined by the laws of physical optics. This is so, because the refined structure coordinates we report are, in effect, molecular models constrained to agree (in reciprocal space) with the observed diffraction data collected on our instruments. "Optical resolution" does become a problem, however, when the initial interpretation of the protein model is extracted from the experimentally derived electron density. In our study,[2] modest errors were made in that interpretation, which became evident in the course of refinement, and which have now been corrected.

Within the limitations of HIV-1 PR crystals studied, the structure we first reported[2] has still proven to be quite useful. It confirmed by direct visualization the hypothesis[6] that viral encoded protease monomers would associate to form dimeric structures. It allowed us to quantitate the similarity between the strict viral protease dimer and the pseudo-dimer of a representative pepsin-like aspartyl protease from *Rhizopus chinensis,* whose structure had been solved and refined at high resolution.[12] This similarity was particularly strong in the active site region and implied a corresponding similarity in the mechanism of action. Incidentally, it suggested that the HIV-1 PR dimer observed in the crystal structure was a functional, enzymatically competent dimer and not just an accidental artifact of crystallization. The structure also suggested that the HIV-1 PR monomer would be inactive, inasmuch as it would lack half of the chemical machinery needed to function as an aspartyl protease. In a way, the monomer could be considered a novel kind of zymogen, in that functional enzyme would not, in fact, exist as an entity except at concentrations high enough to assure the formation of dimers with some reasonable probability. Further, the structure implied that dimerization would be necessary for enzyme activity in all instances, both in the free state, and while HIV-1 PR was yet incorporated within the *gag-pol* polyprotein prior to maturation (see FIG. 1). As discussed below, this has a direct bearing on the timing of protease action and on its viability as a therapeutic target. The structure suggested that the symmetric "flap" regions of HIV-1 PR, whose homologues are known crystallographically to close over inhibitors in the active site in the pepsin-like aspartyl proteases,[12–14] would also be flexible, as they are in the larger enzymes.[15] Finally, the structure provided for a direct visualization of the relationship among the various amino acid residues of HIV-1 PR and has served as a guide for understanding and correlating mutagenesis and chemical modification studies of protease function.[16]

ORCHESTRATION OF VIRUS ASSEMBLY BY HIV-1 PROTEASE

FIGURE 2 shows the organization of (and defines the icons used for) the *gag* and *gag-pol* polyprotein products in the subsequent discussion. As mentioned above, linked synthesis in polyprotein form would allow the *gag*-encoded structural proteins, which can self-assemble spontaneously, to be uneventfully synthesized and transported to the site of virus assembly. The *pol*-encoded viral enzymes are similarly transported on the *gag-pol* polyprotein fusion product. Both products are posttranslationally modified by a covalent attachment of a lipophilic myristoyl group (see FIG. 3) onto their shared N-terminal glycine[17] (in the MA (or p17) protein). Subsequently, the myristoylated *gag* and *gag-pol* polyproteins are directed to, and are anchored on, the cytoplasmic side of the host cell membrane. The polyprotein posttranslational modifications are carried out by a preexisting myristoyl transferase enzyme provided by the host cell. The only requirement of the virus is the maintenance of an appropriate recognition sequence for this enzyme (including the critical Gly-1) on the N-terminus of the virus-encoded polyproteins.[17]

By this association of the viral polyproteins with the host cell membrane, a dramatic increase in the effective local concentration of protease monomer can be achieved as a simple consequence of a loss of dimensionality. In other words, the collection of a given number of polyprotein molecules per unit area on the plane of the cell membrane represents a concentration of these versus that same number of polyproteins in the volume of the host cell, and, as a direct consequence of these higher local concentrations, the probability of HIV-1 PR dimer formation (by random collisions) is greatly increased on the host cell membrane,[18] which serves as the site of virus assembly.

Equally critical in this model is the need for HIV-1 PR dimer-mediated proteolysis to take place on the N-terminal side of the PR region of the *gag-pol* polyprotein first. N-terminal cleavage would effectively solubilize the membrane attachment of activated HIV-1 PR dimers formed "early," allowing their passive diffusion (and that of the other C-terminal downstream enzymes) back into the volume of the host cell (see FIG. 4). Shedding-activated HIV-1 PR by this simple device would protect *gag* and *gag-pol* polyproteins collected on the host cell membrane (in anticipation of virus assembly) from premature proteolysis.

As all this is happening, electron microscopy studies[19] show a sequence of protein aggregation and membrane bulging events, leading ultimately to the budding of "immature" viral particles. Neither the trigger, nor the mechanism by which this budding

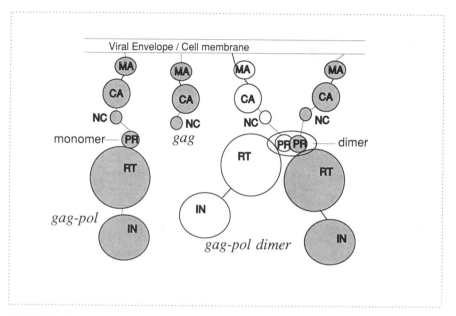

FIGURE 1. Schematic of *gag* and *gag-pol* polyproteins shown anchored to the host cell membrane prior to virus assembly. The component proteins are represented as spheres that correspond roughly in size to their molecular weight. In addition, a *gag-pol* dimer is shown, where the principal interaction between the polyproteins is in the protease (PR) region. As indicated in the text, PR dimers, even within polyprotein as shown, should be enzymatically active. PR monomers should, in all cases, be devoid of enzymatic activity. Proteins incorporated within the *gag* and *gag-pol* polyproteins are identified by the newly standardized nomenclature for retroviruses.[30] MA is the matrix protein (p17), CA the capsid protein (p24), NC the nucleocapsid protein (p7), PR the protease (p11), RT the reverse transcriptase (p66/p51), and IN the integrase (p32).

process is carried out is completely understood. Only after these immature viral particles have budded completely away from the host cell does the final maturation of the virus take place, as evidenced by the appearance of a viral capsid within the viral envelope[19] (see FIG. 5). On this latter point there is considerable confusion, particularly in the popular literature, which often shows the viral capsid being assembled inside the host cell and subsequently forcing the viral envelope to bud. An extensive examination of published micrographs (see, *e.g.* FIG. 3 of ref. 19) shows that this is not the case; virus maturation always seems to take place after budding in HIV-1.

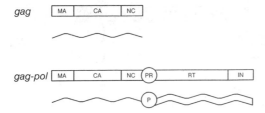

gag

FIGURE 2. Linear organization of the protein components within the *gag* and *gag-pol* polyproteins. Icons used to represent these structures in the subsequent figures are shown below the polyproteins.

Once the nascent virus particle had actually budded away from the rest of the host cell, HIV-1 PR dimers shed from the (now virus) membrane would remain trapped within the greatly reduced volume of the virion, where the continuing "occasional" interaction of *gag-pol* polyprotein would accumulate active protease (see FIG. 6). A cascade of proteolytic events would follow, leading to the liberation of fully functional *gag* and *pol* structural proteins and enzymes (including additional copies of the protease dimer itself). The ensemble of mature viral proteins would then rapidly self-assemble to form the viral capsid, also enclosing within the virus envelope the appropriate stoichiometry of enzymes and RNA to achieve full infectivity. The "occasional" rate at which functional dimers form and cleave themselves away from the cell membrane on the N-terminal side is unknown but has presumably been adjusted in the course of evolution of the virus. (Paradoxically, acceleration of proteolysis might represent an effective therapeutic strategy by depleting the cell membrane assembly site of attached protease prior to virus budding.) Finally, the model presented here questions the notion that the protease monomer encoded by HIV-1 is somehow a "fossil remnant" of the archaic ancestor of the two-domain pepsin-like aspartyl proteases,[20] given the functionally important differences between the HIV-1 PR monomer and dimer states at various points in the viral life cycle.

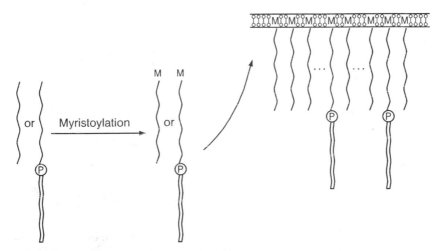

FIGURE 3. N-terminal myristoylation of *gag* and *gag-pol* polyproteins facilitates attachment to membranes. Polyprotein synthesized in the body of the host cell is posttranslationally myristoylated on the N-terminal glycine by a host cell myristoyl transferase enzyme.[17] This lipophilic moiety subsequently mediates anchoring of polyprotein on the inner side of the host membrane in anticipation of the final virus assembly process (see text).

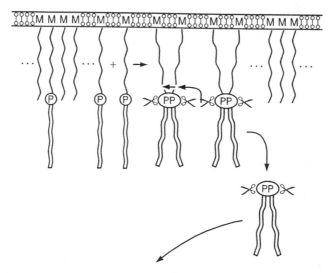

FIGURE 4. Occasional dimerization of PR within the *gag-pol* polyprotein leads to cleavage on the N-terminal side of protease, effectively solubilizing protease (and the downstream RT and IN enzymes) away from the host cell membrane. If activation takes place "early," enzyme activity will diffuse back passively into the body of the host cell, away from the site of viral assembly.

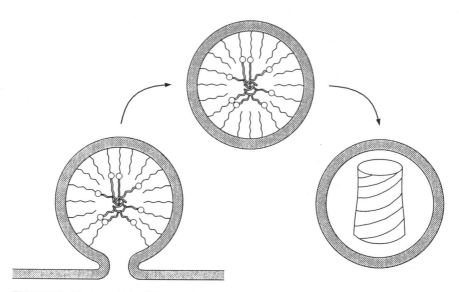

FIGURE 5. Final assembly of HIV-1 takes place only after the immature virion has budded away from the host cell. This observation is confirmed by analysis of published electron micrographs of the budding process (see, *e.g.* Gonda *et al.*[19]). In these studies, mature, infectious HIV-1 is characterized by the appearance of the truncated cone nucleoprotein capsid and the concurrent proteolysis of polyprotein. Note, however, that in the popular science literature, nucleoprotein capsid is often depicted as forming within the infected host cell, often mediating the budding process itself. This view is inconsistent with experimental evidence.

PROTEASE DIMERIZATION AND N-TERMINAL CLEAVAGE

Our initial report[2] of the structure of HIV-1 PR incorporated a misinterpretation of early electron density maps of the enzyme, which led us to believe that the first five residues on the N-terminus of HIV-1 PR were flexible and disordered. This flexibility

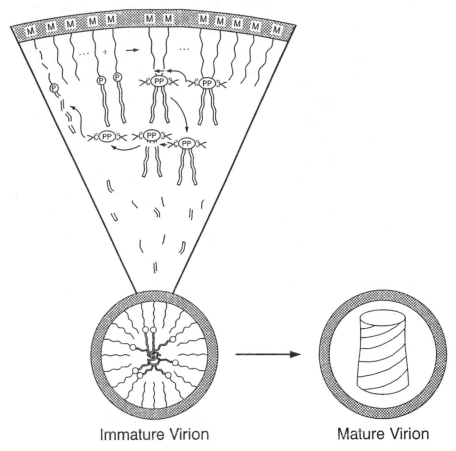

Immature Virion   Mature Virion

FIGURE 6. After budding of the immature virion, any further protease activated and shed from the (now) viral envelope membrane will remain trapped inside the reduced volume of the virion. Accumulated protease will ultimately lead to a proteolytic cascade, which would free structural components and enzymes for the ultimate condensation of mature virus.

would have allowed for the placement of the N-terminal Pro-1 of each of the protease monomer chains into the dimer active site and would have suggested immediately how the enzyme might preferentially excise itself autoproteolytically from the N-terminal side of the *gag-pol* polyprotein. Such an intramolecular (*i.e. cis*) cleavage would be highly favored entropically and would fit the requirements of the model presented above for the cleavage and solubilization of active protease from the polyprotein membrane anchor on the N-terminal side. In the corrected model of the enzyme,[3] however, both the N- and C-terminal of HIV-1 PR are fully ordered. Further, both constitute part of the essential contacts on the backside of the molecule that hold the functional protease dimer together. In this context, any proteolysis of polyprotein would have to take place intermolecularly (*i.e. trans*) and would involve an interaction between at least two HIV-1 PR dimer regions of adjacent *gag-pol* polyproteins. This fact forces us to rationalize in some other way the preference for cleavage on the N-terminal side of the protease region that is required by the proposed virus assembly model and that (fortunately) has now been demonstrated using recombinant *gag-pol* constructs.[21,22] Some of the desired rationalization might be provided by the following observations, all of which are readily subject to further experimental confirmation.

First, the fusion of *gag-pol*, resulting from an infrequent (approx. 1 in 20) ribosomal frameshift from the *gag* to the *pol* reading frame[23] generates a stretch of about sixty amino acids between the frameshift site and the start of the protease (Pro-1 on the N-terminal side), for which no structural or catalytic function is known. We have conducted an analysis of this sequence, using standard methods,[24] which indicates that it is unusually hydrophilic (see, *e.g.* FIG. 7) and lacking in significant secondary structure. This region of the *gag-pol* polyprotein might well serve as a flexible linker, whose evolution has made it particularly susceptible to cleavage, thus facilitating the preferred N-terminal excision of protease required by the model.

In addition to this potential proteolytic hot spot on the N-terminal side of HIV-1 PR, might the reverse transcriptase (RT) regions of adjacent *gag-pol* polyproteins play a role in the assembly process? HIV-1 RT is often isolated in a one-to-one ratio of two forms (of 66 and 51 kDa molecular mass) and is thought to function as a dimer.[25] Given also that pure RT in the 66 kDa form can be isolated and remains stable and functional,[26] one can consider the 51 kDa form an accidental but fortuitous digestion marker indicative of a dimer state. At 66 (or 51) kDa, HIV-1 RT would have the largest cross-section of any of the *gag* or *gag-pol* polyprotein components (see FIG. 8). Even a weak tendency towards dimerization by RT might, in the high concentration environment found on the membrane during virus assembly, serve to prime the formation of the much tighter PR dimer, leading to protease activation. Widespread cross-linking through PR and RT interactions involving different membrane-anchored polyproteins would also be possible and might be involved in driving or triggering the budding process.

Finally, polyprotein, anchored at the N-terminus and interacting at the protease and reverse transcriptase levels, might be so tightly constrained in the high concentration environment on the membrane that little access to the other levels along the polyprotein chain might be available. Protease dimers formed by adjacent polyproteins might be able to reach (and cleave) only the protease regions of its neighbors, much in the way that passengers in a crowded subway car would find it difficult to reach down to tie their shoes.

ALTERNATIVE MODELS FOR PROTEASE INVOLVEMENT IN VIRUS ASSEMBLY

Few models have been proposed to explain the observed protease-orchestrated events in virus assembly. Some of these invoke unspecified conformational changes in the structure of HIV-1 PR. Others suggest that changes in pH or ionic strength (perhaps on budding of the immature virion) might be responsible for triggering protease function.[20] None of these have been spelled out in significant detail, nor have they suggested specific experiments to prove (or disprove) the proposed notion—a hallmark of useful model building. In the former models, it is difficult to imagine how such a minimal macromolecule as HIV-1 PR, even in its dimer form, could muster the necessary machinery to carry out the suggested conformational changes. Nor is the nature of these proposed changes specified. (For a full discussion of models of this type in the context of antibody function, see Klein *et al.*[27]). The latter class of models are better

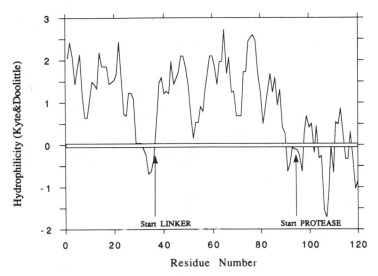

FIGURE 7. Expression of the *pol* gene products (including PR, RT, and IN) proceeds by way of a ribosomal frameshift from the *gag* reading frame to the *pol* reading frame that occurs statistically about 5% of the time.[23] The frameshift eliminates the C-terminal portion of the NC protein in the *gag* polyprotein and creates a linker region of approximately 57 amino acids with unknown structure or function between the frameshift site and the start of the protease monomer on the *gag-pol* polyprotein. An analysis of the 57 amino acid sequence of the linker region created by the frameshift from *gag* to *pol* demonstrates little secondary structure. A hydrophilicity plot, using the algorithm of Kyte and Doolittle[31,24] is shown, which contrasts the extreme hydrophilicity of the linker region with the start of the protease region. These observations suggest that the *gag-pol* linker might, by its flexibility, facilitate the cleavage of polyprotein on the N-terminal side, as required by the proposed virus assembly model.

defined, so that one can ask, for example, for mechanisms that would bring about the required shifts in the properties of the medium trapped with the protease inside the immature virion. Both models fall short, however, in explaining the now widespread[1,16,21,22,28,29] observation that recombinant constructs of HIV-1 polyprotein fragments incorporating the PR monomer can generate active protease dimers that can process polyprotein in turn, and that can, in particular, autoprocess protease. These recombinant products are often observed in high concentration inside inclusion bodies within the producing bacteria. Activation in such a high concentration environment would be a natural consequence of an aggregation model like the one proposed here.

QUESTIONS RAISED BY THE AGGREGATION MODEL

The proposed aggregation model is comprehensive and consistent with the large body of known experimental facts relating to the assembly of retroviruses in general, and HIV-1 in particular. It suggests that these viruses have achieved economy (and elegance) in specifying their assembly by the exploitation of basic underlying physical chemical principles, such as hyperconcentration by loss of dimensionality and self-

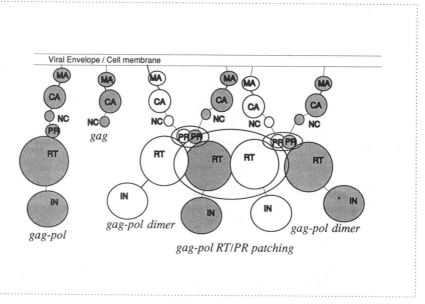

FIGURE 8. Schematic of *gag* and *gag-pol* polyproteins, as in FIGURE 1. Cleavage patterns for HIV-1 reverse transcriptase (RT) suggest that at high concentrations, such as might be found for *gag-pol* polyprotein in the local environment of the host cell/viral envelope membrane, HIV-1 RT might exist in dimer form. Given that RT has by far the largest cross-section of any of the proteins incorporated in *gag* or *gag-pol*, even a modest tendency to dimerize would serve to promote the initial association of *gag-pol* polyprotein prior to the formation of a tighter association between protease monomers. In addition, having two separate binding components on the same *gag-pol* polyprotein molecule opens up the possibility of noncovalent cross-association (one hesitates to use the term cross-linking) to form patches or rafts of polyprotein on the cell membrane. Such rafts are observed on the surface of infected cells and may be related in some way to the actual budding of immature viral particles.

assembly of components driven by liberation of free energy. The model fully explains the active site mutagenesis results of Kohl *et al.,*[1] especially their observation of unprocessed polyprotein in the uninfectious virions produced. It underscores the importance of *gag* and *gag-pol* polyprotein aggregation in the maturation and assembly of virus subsequent to budding and suggests further study of the aggregation process as a possible therapeutic target. It has also proved useful in highlighting and incorporating the existing electron microscopic observations[19] of final viral assembly after budding of immature virions into a consistent scheme. Finally, the model makes predictions that are subject to experimental verification, such as the possible involvement of RT in the assembly process, and raises new questions and issues that are relevant to the exploitation of this enzyme as a therapeutic target.

In this regard, the model points out that the current therapeutic target, that is, the dimeric HIV-1 protease enzyme, does not exist as such over most of its lifetime in the host cell. Most HIV-1 PR exists, in fact, in the form of inactive and uninhibitable monomer within the *gag-pol* polyprotein. Only a small (and unknown) fraction of the total potential pool of enzyme actually dimerizes in the host, for which fraction a simple mechanism is in place (as discussed above) to passively remove activated "early" protease from the site of assembly.

For effective inhibition, the concentration of inhibitor delivered through the host cell, or through the envelope of the immature virus, would have to be high enough to assure the presence of a sufficient number of inhibitor molecules in the budded immature virion to inhibit enzyme dimers as they form at some subsequent time. A novel approach to the problem might involve the inhibition of dimerization, a somewhat problematical task for the tightly associated HIV-1 PR, but perhaps approachable versus dimerization of HIV-1 RT.

ACKNOWLEDGMENTS

This paper is dedicated to the memory of our late colleague, Dr. Irving Sigal, who died tragically in the Pan Am flight 103 disaster in Lockerbie, Scotland. Thanks also go to Drs. J. P. Springer, P. M. D. Fitzgerald, P. L. Darke, and Ms. J. Vanmiddlesworth for their suggestions and assistance.

REFERENCES

1. KOHL, N. E., E. A. EMINI, W. A. SCHLEIF, L. J. DAVIS, J. C. HEIMBACH, R. A. F. DIXON, E. M. SCOLNICK & I. S. SIGAL. 1988. Active human immunodeficiency virus protease is required for viral infectivity. Proc. Natl. Acad. Sci. USA **85:** 4686-4690.

2. NAVIA, M. A., P. M. D. FITZGERALD, B. M. McKEEVER, C.-T. LEU, J. C. HEIMBACH, W. K. HERBER, I. S. SIGAL, P. L. DARKE & J. P. SPRINGER. 1989. Three-dimensional structure of aspartyl protease from human immunodeficiency virus HIV-1. Nature **337:** 615-620.

3. WLODAWER, A., M. MILLER, M. JASKOLSKI, B. K. SATHYANARAYANA, E. BALDWIN, I. T. WEBER, L. M. SELK, L. CLAWSON, J. SCHNEIDER & S. B. H. KENT. 1989. Conserved folding in retroviral proteases: crystal structure of a synthetic HIV-1 protease. Science **245:** 616-621.

4. FARMERIE, W. G., D. D. LOEB, N. C. CASAVANT & C. A. HUTCHISON III. 1987. Expression and processing of the AIDS virus reverse transcriptase in *Escherichia coli.* Science **236:** 305-308.

5. TOH, H., M. ONO, K. SAIGO & T. MIYATA. 1985. Retroviral protease-like sequence in the yeast transposon *Ty1.* Nature **315:** 691.

6. PEARL, L. H. & W. R. TAYLOR. 1987. A structural model for the retroviral proteases. Nature **239:** 351-354.

7. McKEEVER, B. M., M. A. NAVIA, P. M. D. FITZGERALD, J. P. SPRINGER, C.-T. LEU, J. C. HEIMBACH, W. K. HERBER, I. S. SIGAL & P. L. DARKE. 1989. Crystallization of the

aspartyl protease from the human immunodeficiency virus, HIV-1. J. Biol. Chem. **264:** 1919-1921.

8. NAVIA, M. A., B. M. MCKEEVER, J.P. SPRINGER, T.-Y. LIN, H. R. WILLIAMS, E. M. FLUDER, C. P. DORN JR. & K. HOOGSTEEN. 1989. Structure of human neutrophil elastase in complex with a peptide chloromethyl ketone inhibitor at 1.84Å resolution. Proc. Natl. Acad. Sci. USA **86:** 7-11.

9. BALDWIN, J. J., G. S. PONTICELLO, P. S. ANDERSON, M. E. CHRISTY, M. A. MURCKO, W. C. RANDALL, H. SCHWAM, M. F. SUGRUE, J. P. SPRINGER, P. GAUTHERON, J. GROVE, P. MALLORGA, M.-P. VIADER, B. M. MCKEEVER & M. A. NAVIA. 1989. Thienothiopyran-2-sulfonamides: Novel topically active carbonic anhydrase inhibitors for the treatment of glaucoma. J. Med. Chem. **32:** 2510-2513.

10. NAVIA, M. A., J. P. SPRINGER, T.-Y. LIN, H. R. WILLIAMS, R. A. FIRESTONE, J. M. PISANO, J. B. DOHERTY, P. E. FINKE & K. HOOGSTEEN. 1987. Crystallographic study of a beta-lactam inhibitor complex with elastase at 1.84Å resolution. Nature **327:** 79-82.

11. DELUCAS, L. J., C. D. SMITH, H. W. SMITH, S. VIJA Y-KUMAR, S. E. SENADHI, S. E. EALICK, D. C. CARTER, R. S. SNYDER, P. C. WEBER, F. R. SALEMME, D. H. OHLENDORF, H. M. EINSPHAR, L. L. CLANCY, M. A. NAVIA, B. M. MCKEEVER, T. L. NAGABUHUSHAN, G. NELSON, A. MCPHERSON, S. KOSZELAK, G. TAYLOR, D. STAMMERS, K. POWELL, G. DARBY & C. E. BUGG. 1989. Protein crystal growth in microgravity. Science **246:** 651-654.

12. SUGUNA, K., E. A. PADLAN, C. W. SMITH, W. D. CARLSON & D. R. DAVIES. 1987. Binding of a reduced peptide inhibitor to the aspartic proteinase from *Rhizopus chinensis:* Implications for a mechanism of actio. Proc. Natl. Acad. Sci. USA **84:** 7009-7013.

13. JAMES, M. N. G. & A. R. SIELECKI. 1983. Structure and refinement of penicillopepsin at 1.8Å resolution. J. Mol. Biol. **163:** 299-361.

14. FOUNDLING, S. I., J. COOPER, F. E. WATSON, A. CLEASBY, L. H. PEARL, B. L. SIBANDA, A. HEMMINGS, S. P. WOOD, T. L. BLUNDELL, M. J. VALLER, C. G. NOREY, J. KAY, J. BOGER, B. M. DUNN, B. J. LECKIE, D. M. JONES, B. ATRASH, A. HALLETT & M. SZELKE. 1987. High resolution X-ray analyses of renin-inhibitor-aspartic proteinase complexes. Nature **327:** 349-352.

15. JAMES, M. N. G., A. SIELECKI, F. SALITURO, D. H. RICH & T. HOFMANN. 1982. Conformational flexibility in the active sites of aspartyl proteinases revealed by a pepstatin fragment binding to penicillopepsin. Proc. Natl. Acad. Sci. USA **79:** 6137-6141.

16. LOEB, D. D., R. SWANSTROM, L. EVERITT, M. MANCHESTER, S. E. STAMPER & C. A. HUTCHISON III. 1989. Complete mutagenesis of the HIV-1 protease. Nature **340:** 397-400.

17. GRAND, R. J. A. 1989. Acylation of viral and eukaryotic proteins. Biochem. J. **258:** 625-638.

18. GRASBERG, B., A. P. MINTON, C. DELISI & H. METZGER. 1986. Interaction between proteins localized in membranes. Proc. Natl. Acad. Sci. USA **83:** 6258-6262.

19. GONDA, M. A., F. WONG-STAAL, R. C. GALLO, J. E. CLEMENTS, O. NARAYAN & R. V. GILDEN. 1985. Sequence homology and morphologic similarity of HTLV-III and Visna virus, a pathogenic lentivirus. Science **227:** 173-177.

20. BLUNDELL, T. & L. PEARL. 1989. Retroviral proteases, a second front against AIDS. Nature **337:** 596-597.

21. PICHUANTES, S., L. M. BABE, P. J. BARR & C. S. CRAIK. 1989. Recombinant HIV-1 protease secreted by *Saccharomyces cerevisiae* correctly processes myristylated *gag* polyprotein. Proteins: Struct. Funct. Genet. **6:** 324-327.

22. STRICKLER, J. E., J. GORNIAK, B. DAYTON, T. MEEK, M. MOORE, V. MAGAARD, J. MALINOWSKI & C. DEBOUCK. 1989. Characterization and autoprocessing of precursor and mature forms of human immunodeficiency virus type 1 (HIV 1) protease purified from *Escherichia coli.* Proteins: Struct. Funct. Genet. **6:** 139-154.

23. JACKS, T., M. D. POWER, F. R. MASIARZ, P. A. LUCIW, P. J. BARR & H. E. VARMUS. 1988. Characterization of ribosomal frameshifting in HIV-1 *gag-pol* expression. Nature **331:** 280-283.

24. Sequence Analysis Software Package of the Genetics Computer Group of the University of Wisconsin Biotechnology Center; Devereux, Haeberli & Smithies. 1984. Nucleic Acids Res. **12:** 387-395.

25. LOWE, D. M., A. AITKEN, C. BRADLEY, G. K. DARBY, B. A. LARDER, K. L. POWELL, D. J. M. PURIFOY, M. TISDALE & D. K. STAMMERS. 1988. HIV-1 reverse transcriptase:

Crystallization and analysis of domain structure by limited proteolysis. Biochemistry **27:** 8884-8889.

26. HIZI, A., C. McGILL & S. H. HUGHES. 1988. Expression of soluble, enzymatically active, human immunodeficiency virus reverse transcriptase in *Escherichia coli* and analysis of mutants. Proc. Natl. Acad. Sci. USA **85:** 1218-1222.

27. KLEIN, M., N. HAEFFNER-CAVAILLON, D. E. ISENMAN, C. RIVAT, M. A. NAVIA, D. R. DAVIES & K. J. DORRINGTON. 1981. Expression of biological effector functions by immunoglobulin G molecules lacking the hinge region. Proc. Natl. Acad. Sci. USA **78:** 524-528.

28. DEBOUCK, C., J. G. GORNIAK, J. E. STRICKLER, T. D. MEEK, B. W. METCALF & M. ROSENBERG. 1987. Human immunodeficiency virus protease expressed in *Escherichia coli* exhibits autoprocessing and specific maturation of the *gag* precursor. Proc. Natl. Acad. Sci. USA **84:** 8903-8906.

29. GRAVES, M. C., J. J. LIM, E. P. HEIMER & R. A. KRAMER. 1988. An 11-kDa form of human immunodeficiency virus protease expressed in *Escherichia coli* is sufficient for enzymatic activity. Proc. Natl. Acad. Sci. USA **85:** 2449-2453.

30. LEIS, J., D. BALTIMORE, J. M. BISHOP, J. COFFIN, E. FLEISSNER, S. P. GOFF, S. OROSZLAN, H. ROBINSON, A. M. SKALKA, H. M. TEMIN & V. VOGT. 1988. Standardized and simplified nomenclature for proteins common to all retroviruses. J. Virol. **62:** 1808-1809.

31. KYTE, J. & R. F. DOOLITTLE. 1982. A simple method for displaying the hydropathic character of a protein. J. Mol. Biol. **157:** 105-132.

Summary of Part I

Rational Targets for Design and Synthesis of
Anti-HIV Agents

MARK L. PEARSON

Central Research and Development Department
E.I. du Pont de Nemours & Co., Inc.
Experimental Station
Wilmington, Delaware 19880-0328

Can AIDS be cured? Tentative first steps along the path ultimately leading to effective, safe, and specific anti-HIV-1 therapeutics are outlined above in the papers from this initial session of the meeting. Fortunately, the enormous concentration of effort made since 1983 to understand the molecular, cellular, and clinical features of HIV-1 infection in humans has resulted in the identification of a number of potential targets for therapeutic intervention that might—and the operative word is still *might*—allow this disease to be controlled and, indeed, even cured. We are still a long way from achieving either of these objectives, however, as the informed reader will soon appreciate. In late 1989, it remains uncertain if the development of vaccines or more radical immunological approaches have any hope of restoring T-helper cell function in infected individuals. The complexities of the infection process itself, indeed the identification of all the relevant susceptible cell types other than T cells (and macrophages, monocytes, and B cells), remain poorly defined. The involvement of the brain in AIDS-related neuropathy also appears a daunting obstacle, even if we could control the T-helper cell process. A more promising approach—one outlined in the attached manuscripts—is the development of conventional small molecule inhibitors, able to block the activity of one of the several virus-coded proteins on which the HIV-1 replication cycle depends. More radical approaches involving nucleic acids as antisense, triple-strand structures or ribozymes are described elsewhere in this volume.

MOLECULAR TARGETS

What are the molecular structures that might serve as targets for inhibitor design and selection? Haseltine[a] (Harvard) has summarized the life-cycle of the AIDS virus in terms of the synthesis and processing of viral proteins and nucleic acids.[1] The essential nature of the HIV-encoded reverse transcriptase and protease make them attractive substrates for such design efforts. The activity of azidothymidine, AZT, as

---

[a] Not included in this volume.

an inhibitor of reverse transcriptase is well-known; at present this compound is the only widely available anti-HIV therapeutic with an established clinical effectiveness. Other HIV-encoded targets exist as well, notably the *tat* transactivator, which apparently affects both HIV-long terminal repeats (LTR)-initiated transcription and HIV mRNA translation, and the *rev* and *nef* functions, whose molecular mechanisms of action as positive- and negative-acting regulatory factors are somewhat more nebulous. Yet the nagging doubt remains that, even if the acute phase of infection can be blocked by the judicious (or serendipitous) design of an appropriate inhibitor active against any of these targets, somehow the integrated viral DNA itself must also be restricted from even inadvertent "spontaneous" activation at some subsequent time in the patient's lifetime. Thus the viral DNA itself is a target—and one that few have even a glimmer of hope of tackling at the present time, given the absence of good ideas, let alone precedents, in this area. Consequently the papers in this section deal with the more immediate and prosaic task of finding inhibitors of the known *gag-pol* and *tat* gene products, searching for clues to lead compounds that might subsequently be developed into effective anti-AIDS drugs.

INHIBITOR SEARCHES: THE GENETIC AND THE CHEMICAL APPROACH

Reverse Transcriptase

The most obvious place to search for effective anti-AIDS drugs today is in the set of inhibitors that inactivate reverse transcriptase, inasmuch as AZT has been shown to have direct clinical utility. Goff (Columbia) has employed a genetic analysis of the *pol* gene product to dissect the action of protease processing of reverse transcriptase into the p66.p51 heterodimer and RNase H. Site-directed mutagenesis and the selection of mutants resistant to dideoxynucleoside analogue from cloned, bacterially expressed reverse transcriptase has yielded information on the reverse transcriptase's active site. Further genetic analysis of second-site intragenic suppressors of such mutations, and their subsequent biochemical analysis, will shed more light both on the identity of active site residues and the mechanism of action of reverse transcriptase. The results of a screening program by Martin (Bristol-Myers) using a variety of nucleoside analogues to discriminate between antivirals active against HIV-1 versus cytomegalovirus suggests that some of the hematological toxicity and peripheral neuropathy associated with AZT might well be circumvented through the use of other analogues. Especially promising in this regard is 2',3'-didehydro-2',3'-dideoxythymidine (D4T). Related crystallographic and molecular mechanics analysis by Van Roey (Buffalo) on several nucleoside analogues active *in vitro* as reverse transcriptase inhibitors has led to the suggestion that the conformation of the ribose ring may be correlated with their antiviral activity.

Protease

The most exciting place to search for effective anti-AIDS drugs today lies in the inhibitors of the HIV-encoded protease, one of the products of the *gag-pol* region. Ever since the essential requirement of the protease for virus growth was demonstrated by site-directed mutagenesis, it has attracted the attention of many groups as a critical target for drug selection and design. Meek (Smith Kline Beecham, SKB) here summarizes the expression of recombinant HIV-1 protease in *E. coli* as an 11 kDa monomer that dimerizes to form an active aspartyl enzyme. Using synthetic recombinant *gag* substrates and variants thereof, the SKB team has designed inhibitory peptide substrates able to competitively inhibit protease activity. Other proprietary compounds have also been found that block *gag* and *gag-pol* processing in infected cells, allowing the release of noninfectious (presumably structurally defective) virions. This is an exciting development, because it offers a new strategic approach to anti-AIDS therapeutics, one that is independent of the AZT-based reverse transcriptase inhibition approach and its deleterious side effects. As a consequence, protease inhibitors, in addition to their own intrinsic value in monotherapy, also offer the possibility of more effective polytherapies in combination with AZT, or other nucleoside analogues targeted at reverse transcriptase, with the additional benefit of less patient discomfort.

The 3-D crystallographic structure of the HIV-1 protease, a useful guide for the rational design of such inhibitors, is described here by Navia (Merck). This model shows the juxtaposition of the aspartates forming the active site protected by an unusual "flap" structure that limits access to the active site of the processing sequence of the *gag-pol* substrate itself. A provocative model involving membrane-associated subviral structures is presented to account for the formation of the first active protease molecules in the infected cell—clearly a problem because the protease amino acid sequence itself is embedded in the larger *gag-pol* product. This notion also neatly incorporates the likely place of action of the protease: in a partially assembled subviral particle, not the cytoplasm. The challenge now is to exploit this information in the design of better inhibitors: one clearly in the hands of the molecular modelers and the chemists. One can only hope that such information will be rapidly turned into an entire new family of anti-AIDS drugs.

Transactivation of LTR-Initiated Transcription

The last family of targets for rational design considered in this session are the *trans*-acting transcription activators acting on the HIV LTR regulatory region. One of these is tat, the protein that simulates HIV-1 LTR-initiated transcription elongation and also binds HIV mRNA. The others are the immediate-early proteins of cytomegalovirus (CMV), a herpesvirus. Barry (Davis) summarizes the remarkable ability of the cytomegalovirus immediate-early transcription activators to stimulate HIV-1 LTR-initiated transcription in a variety of human cell lines. This appears to be a direct effect of the action of the CMV proteins, based on the use of appropriate plasmid constructs in transfection experiments, one probably involving cooperative interactions with the cellular transcription factors, NK-kB and NFAT-1, which also bind the LTR. The wide variation in responsiveness among different cell types suggests that some of the tropism seen with CMV and HIV for different cell types might be attributable to such effects. The pathological consequence of the transactivation noted here for herpes and HIV is that cooperative infection by other adventitious viruses, such as CMV, likely stimulates further the HIV infectious cycle, thereby exacerbating the AIDS infection. A more direct search for anti-tat compounds is reported by Sim (Hoffmann-La Roche) based on the development of a high-throughput screening assay that relies on a tat-stimulated LTR transcription from a recombinant plasmid carrying alkaline phosphatase as a reporter gene. No active compounds were reported at the meeting, but it is hoped that this approach will be successful in future tests.

The papers in this session illustrate the remarkable power of the molecular technologies currently being directed to the search for rational therapeutics for the treatment of AIDS. Molecular biology has provided a detailed if incomplete view of the molecular interactions governing the life cycle of this virus. Now it is up to the structural biologists, chemists, pharmacologists, and clinical researchers to apply their expertise to the design, synthesis, and clinical testing of inhibitors able to block the action of the several targets currently offering some reasonable hope for new pharmaceutical approaches for the treatment of AIDS.

REFERENCE

1. HASELTINE, W. 1989. Regulation of replication of HIV. *In* V International Conference on AIDS: The Scientific and Social Challenge. R. A. Morisset, Ed. International Development Research Centre. Ottawa, Ontario, Canada.

Inhibition of Glycoprotein Processing and HIV Replication by Castanospermine Analogues

PRASAD S. SUNKARA, MOHINDER S. KANG,

TERRY L. BOWLIN, PAUL S. LIU,

A. STANLEY TYMS,[a] AND ALBERT SJOERDSMA

Merrell Dow Research Institute
Cincinnati, Ohio 45215

[a]*Medical Research Council Collaborative Center*
Mill Hill
London NW71AD, United Kingdom

INTRODUCTION

Recently, antiviral activities of glycoprotein processing enzyme (glucosidase I) inhibitors, castanospermine and deoxynojirimycin, have been demonstrated against Moloney murine leukemia virus (MOLV) and human immunodeficiency virus (HIV).[1-4]

In spite of the potent inhibitory activities of these compounds against the isolated enzyme (IC_{50}: 1×10^{-7} M), the drug concentration required for significant reduction in HIV infectivity is relatively high (1-2 mM). When cells chronically infected with HIV were grown in the presence of either castanospermine or deoxynojirimycin, expression of the mature envelope glycoprotein (gp120) on the cell surface was decreased with a concomitant accumulation of uncleaved precursor gp160.[5,6] These observations may explain the observed decrease in the viral infectivity and inhibition of syncytium formation. Castanospermine, however, showed only moderate *in vivo* activity against Rauscher leukemia virus infections in mice.[7]

Glucosidase I catalyzes the hydrolysis of the outermost α (1 → 2) glucosidic linkages of glycoproteins. O-substitution at the corresponding hydroxyl group (C_6-OH) in castanospermine may lead to inhibitors of higher specificity. We have synthesized a series of acyl derivatives of castanospermine and evaluated these compounds against MOLV and HIV in cell cultures.[8] The data indicated several compounds that showed enhanced potency against the viruses compared to castanospermine, with 6-O-butanoyl castanospermine (B-CAST, MDL 28,574) being the most potent of the analogues so far evaluated.

MATERIAL AND METHODS

Compounds

Castanospermine (1S, 6S, 7R, 8R, 8aR-1, 6, 7, 8 tetra hydroxyindolizidine) was isolated from seeds of the Moreton Bay chestnut, *Castanospermum australe,* as described earlier.[9] 6-*O*-Butanoyl castanospermine (B-CAST, MDL 28,574) and other analogues were synthesized as previously reported.[10] 2′,3′-Dideoxycytidine (ddc) was purchased from Sigma Chemical Co. 3′-Azido-3′-deoxythymidine (AZT) was kindly supplied by Burroughs Wellcome Co., Research Triangle Park, North Carolina.

Moloney Murine Leukemia Virus (MOLV) Plaque Assay

MOLV was obtained from C3H10TY1/2 (clone 8) cells chronically infected with and constitutively producing MOLV.[11] These cells were generously provided by Dr. Max Proffitt (Cleveland Clinic Foundation, Cleveland, Ohio). The XC plaque assay was performed according to the method of Rowe *et al.*[12] Briefly, mouse SC-1 cells (10^5) were seeded into each well of 6-well cluster plates (Costar #3506) in 4 mL MEM with 10% FCS. Following an 18 h incubation period at 37°C, MOLV was then applied at a predetermined titer to give optimal (*i.e.* countable) numbers of virus plaques, that is, 58 ± 15/well. Compounds were added 2 h prior to addition of the virus. Three days later, the culture medium was removed, the SC-1 cell monolayers were exposed to UV irradiation (1800 ergs), and rat XC cells (10^6) were seeded into each well in 4 mL MEM. Following an additional 3-day incubation (37°C), these cells were fixed with ethyl alcohol (95%) and stained with 0.3% crystal violet. Plaques were then counted under low magnification.

Enzyme (Glucosidase I) Inhibition

Mammalian (mouse SC-1) cells were metabolically labeled with [³H]galactose to obtain glucose-labeled glycopeptides during the exponential growth phase. Labeled glycopeptides from control and treated cells were separated on Biogel columns as described earlier.[13] Accumulation of $G_3M_{7-9}N_2$ (glucose (G), mannose (M), and N-acetylglucosamine (N))-containing glycopeptides was measured. Dose response curves were plotted against log 10 drug concentration and the 50% inhibitory dose (IC_{50}) computed after linear regression analysis.

HIV Syncytial Assay in JM Cells

JM (T-cell line) cells were infected with the GB8 strain of HIV-1 to give a multiplicity of infection of 0.02 syncytial-forming units per cell.[14] After a one hour adsorption at room temperature, the cells were washed twice in RPMI and resuspended in fresh medium containing a different concentration of test compounds. The plates were incubated at 37°C in a 5% CO_2 incubator. After two days, syncytia were counted, and the percentage inhibition was calculated.

HeLa T_4 Syncytial Focal Assay for HIV

A HeLa transformant cell line expressing the human T_4 surface protein was kindly provided by Dr. Richard Axel, Columbia University, New York, New York. Cells were exposed to HIV-1 and concentrations of drugs, and to drug alone in triplicates. The cells were incubated at 37°C in a 5% CO_2 incubator for four days. At the end of incubation, the number of syncytia were counted, percent reduction relative to the virus control group was calculated, and the ID_{50} values were determined. Cell viability was determined by quantitation of cell numbers by a Coulter counter, and the concentration of drug ($\mu g/mL$) that reduces cell number by 50% (minimum cytotoxic drug concentration, MTC) was determined. The therapeutic index was obtained by dividing the MTC by the ID_{50}.

Friend Leukemia Viral (FLV) Infections in Mice

Friend leukemia virus was obtained from American Type Culture Collection. The virus was maintained in Swiss mice by injecting 0.2 mL of spleen extract (approx. 50 PFU/mL).[15] Mice were infected on day 0 by i.v. injection of 0.2 mL of infected spleen suspension (1:50,000, w/v). Compounds were mixed in animal feed and were offered to animals *ad libitum* from day 1–day 14. Animals were sacrificed on day 14; spleens were weighed, and the percent inhibition of splenomegaly was determined as follows:

$$\% \text{ inhibition of splenomegaly: } 100 \times \frac{\text{wt. of treated spleen } - \text{ wt. of uninfected spleen}}{\text{wt. of infected spleen } - \text{ wt. of uninfected spleen}}$$

RESULTS

The data presented in TABLE 1 indicate an apparent correlation between MOLV antiviral activity and glucosidase I inhibition by the compounds. The most potent activity against both MOLV (IC_{50}: 0.05 $\mu g/mL$) and HIV-1 (IC_{50}: 0.15 $\mu g/mL$) was observed with B-CAST. A similar trend was observed for activity against HIV, except for MDL 29,435 and MDL 44,370, which showed weak activity against glucosidase I (IC_{50}: 10 $\mu g/mL$), but were at least as active as castanospermine against HIV-1. B-CAST was further evaluated against HIV in HeLa T_4+ assay (TABLE 2) in comparison to reverse transcriptase inhibitors, AZT and ddc. B-CAST is at least 30 times more potent than CAST in this assay, confirming the anti-HIV activity of this compound in JM cells. B-CAST had a cellular "therapeutic index" similar to AZT and ddc (> 1000).

Because of its interesting anti-HIV activity in culture, B-CAST was evaluated *in vivo* against FLV-induced splenomegaly in mice. Treatment with B-CAST produced 66 and 69% inhibition of splenomegaly at dosages of 95 and 159 mg/kg/day, respectively

TABLE 1. Inhibitory Activities of Cast Analogues on Glucosidase I, MOLV, and HIV *in Vitro*[8]

MDL	R	R_1	Glucosidase Inhibition (IC$_{50}$; µg/mL)	MOLV (IC$_{50}$; µg/mL)	HIV-1 (IC$_{50}$; µg/mL)
Castanospermine	H	H	10.0	1.2	6.5
28,574	$CH_3CH_2CH_2-CO-$	H	0.7	0.05	0.15
43,305	[phenyl]–CO–	H	10.0	0.1	1.0
28,653	[furyl]–CO–	H	1.0	0.5	1.0
29,435	[m-H_3C-phenyl]–CO–	H	> 30	> 10.0	7.0
29,204	H_3C–[phenyl]–CO–	H	2.0	0.5	5.8
44,370	Br–[phenyl]–CO–	H	> 30	10.0	0.75
29,270	H	H_3C–[phenyl]–CO–	3.0	1.0	3.4

(TABLE 3). At similar doses, CAST caused a 34 and 53% inhibition of splenomegaly. AZT treatment at 105 mg/kg/day resulted in 66% inhibition of splenomegaly. These data indicate that B-CAST is equipotent with AZT and more active than CAST at similar doses against FLV infections in mice.

DISCUSSION

The data presented indicate a general correlation between anti-MOLV activity and glucosidase I inhibition of a number of castanospermine analogues. A similar trend was also observed for HIV, except for MDL 29,435 and MDL 44,370, which showed weak activity against glucosidase I and MOLV, but were at least as active as castanospermine against HIV-1. Differential uptake of the compounds and/or intracellular conversion to an active metabolite could account for the variable antiviral activity of the compounds. B-CAST was the most potent of the compounds tested. B-CAST was at least 10 times as active against glucosidase I and about 20-fold as potent as an antiretroviral agent against MOLV compared to CAST (TABLE 1). Further, B-CAST was at least 20-30 times more potent than CAST in inhibiting HIV-induced syncytial formation in both HeLa T_4+ and JM cells (TABLES 1 and 2).

Recently, Ruprecht et al.[7] reported the effect of CAST on Rauscher murine leukemia virus in vivo. The treatment of infected mice for 20 days showed a dose-dependent inhibition of splenomegaly. Treatment with CAST, however, showed much less activity compared to AZT. The data presented here in Friend leukemic viral infections in mice show that B-CAST, but not CAST, was as effective as AZT in inhibiting the viral-induced splenomegaly.

The envelope glycoprotein, gp120, plays an important role in the process of HIV infection of CD4+ lymphocytes. The gp120 is synthesized as a result of a cleavage by a host protease of precursor glycoprotein gp160.[5] Preliminary studies on the molecular mechanism of the anti-HIV activity of B-CAST indicate that the compound causes an increase in the apparent molecular weights of gp160 and gp120 viral envelope glycoproteins, presumably due to increased carbohydrate content. More interestingly, a dramatic decrease in the ratio of gp120:gp160 in the B-CAST-treated, HIV-infected H9 cells was observed,[16] indicating blockade of conversion of gp160 to gp120. Similar results were also reported earlier in deoxynojirimycin- and castanospermine-treated HIV-infected cells.[5,6] The unique mechanism of action of B-CAST, desirable therapeutic index in cell cultures, and apparently low animal toxicity (acute oral LD_{50} = >2 g/kg in mice) makes B-CAST an interesting candidate for eventual clinical evaluation in AIDS patients.

TABLE 2. Activity of Selected Agents against HIV in HELA T_4 Cells

Compound	ID_{50}[a] (μg/mL)	MTC[b] (μg/mL)	TI[c]
Castanospermine (CAST)	10.97	> 320	> 29
MDL 28,574 (B-CAST)	< 0.32	> 320	> 1000
ddc	< 0.10	> 100	> 1000
AZT	< 0.001	> 1	> 1000

[a] ID_{50} = The drug concentration (μg/mL) that inhibits the viral cytopathic effect by 50%, calculated by using a regression analysis program for semilog curve fitting.

[b] MTC = The drug concentration (μg/mL) that reduces cell number to 50% in uninfected cultures.

[c] TI = Therapeutic index calculated by dividing the MTC by the ID_{50}.

TABLE 3. Activity of AZT, CAST, and B-CAST against Friend Leukemia Viral Infections in Mice[a]

Treatment	Dose (mg/kg)	Average Spleen Weight (g) (Mean + SE; n = 5)	Percent Inhibition of Splenomegaly[b]
Infected control		0.48 ± 0.08	0
AZT	105	0.23 ± 0.08	66[c]
CAST	91	0.39 ± 0.06	34
CAST	174	0.28 ± 0.09	53[c]
B-CAST	95	0.23 ± 0.04	66[c]
B-CAST	159	0.22 ± 0.06	69[c]

[a] Mice were infected on day 0 by i.v. injection of 0.2 mL of infected spleen suspension (1:50,000, w/v). Compounds were mixed in the feed and were offered to mice on day 1-14, ad libitum. The amount of feed consumed by the animals was used to determine the dose. Animals were sacrificed on day 14, and spleen weights were determined. The unifected control spleens weighed 0.10 ± 0.001 g.

[b] See METHODS for determination of percent inhibition of splenomegaly.

[c] $p < 0.001$ compared to control.

SUMMARY

Inhibitors of glycoprotein processing enzymes have been shown to have activity against HIV. Several analogues of the known glucosidase I inhibitor, castanospermine (CAST), were synthesized and evaluated for their inhibitory effect on glucosidases and for antiviral activity against Moloney murine leukemia virus (MOLV) and HIV-1. The most effective analogue was 6-O-butanoyl CAST (B-CAST, MDL 28,574) with an IC_{50} of 0.05 $\mu g/mL$ against MOLV. A correlation between inhibition of glucosidase I and MOLV replication was observed. This analogue was further evaluated against HIV-induced syncytial formation in HeLa T_4+ cells and against productive infection in JM cells infected with HIV 1 (GB8 strain). B-CAST showed an IC_{50} of 0.3 $\mu g/mL$ in the HeLa T_4+ assay, compared to CAST at 11 $\mu g/mL$. The compound also was more potent (IC_{50}:0.15 $\mu g/mL$) than CAST (4-6 $\mu g/mL$) in JM cells. The antiretroviral activity of B-CAST was further confirmed in Friend leukemia virus (FLV) infection in mice. B-CAST showed equivalent activity to AZT and was more potent than CAST in inhibiting FLV-induced splenomegaly in mice. The data presented herein suggest the potential of these novel glucosidase inhibitors as anti-HIV agents.

ACKNOWLEDGMENTS

The authors would like to thank Dr. W. Shannon and Dr. G. Lavelle of Southern Research Institute, Birmingham, AL, for their help in evaluating compounds in HeLa T_4+ assays.

REFERENCES

1. SUNKARA, P. S., T. L. BOWLIN, P. S. LIU & A. SJOERDSMA. 1987. Biochem. Biophys. Res. Commun. **148:** 1, 206-210.
2. TYMS, A. S., E. M. BERRIE, T. A. RYDER, R. J. NASH, M. P. HEGARTY, D. L. TAYLOR, M. A. MOBBERLEY, J. M. DAVIS, E. A. BELL, D. J. JEFFRIES, D. TAYLOR-ROBINSON & L. E. FELLOW. 1987. Lancet **ii:** 1025-1026.
3. WALKER, B. D., M. KOWALSKI, W. C. GOH, K. KOZARSKY, M. KRIEGER, C. ROSEN, L. ROHRSCHNEIDER, W. A. HASELTINE & J. SODROSKI. 1987. Proc. Natl. Acad. Sci. USA **84:** 8120-8124.
4. GRUTERS, R. A., J. J. NEEFJES, M. TERSMETTE, R. E. Y. DE GOEDE, A. TULP, H. G. HUISMAN, F. MIEDMA & H. L. PLOEGH. 1987. Nature (London) **330:** 74-77.
5. MONTEFIORI, D. C., W. E. ROBINSON & W. M. MITCHELL. 1988. Proc. Natl. Acad. Sci. USA **85:** 9248-9252.
6. PAL, R., T. TAMURA, C. B. BOSCHEK, H. WEGE, R. T. SCHWARZ & H. NIEMAN. 1985. J. Biol. Chem. **260:** 15873-15879.
7. RUPRECHT, R. M., S. MULLANEY, J. ANDERSON & R. BRONSON. 1989. J. AIDS **2:** 2, 149-157.
8. SUNKARA, P. S., D. L. TAYLOR, M. S. KANG, T. L. BOWLIN, P. S. LIU, A. S. TYMS & A. SJOERDSMA. 1989. Lancet **1:** 1206.
9. LIU, P. & B. L. RHINEHART. 1986. Eur. Patent Appl. **EP** 202,661.
10. LIU, P. S., J. K. DANIEL & B. L. RHINEHART. 1989. Eur. Patent Appl. **EP** 297,534.
11. PROFFITT, M. R., M. S. HIRSCH, D. A. ELLIS, B. GHERIDIAN & P. H. BLACK. 1976. J. Immunol. **117:** 11-15.
12. ROWE, W. P., W. E. PUGH & J. W. HARTLEY. 1970. Virology **42:** 1136-1139.
13. SZUMILO, T. & A. D. ELBEIN. 1985. Anal. Biochem. **151:** 32-40.
14. DOWSETT, A. B., M. A. ROFF, P. J. GREENAWAY, E. R. ELPHICK, G. H. FARRAR *et al.* 1987. AIDS **1:** 147-150.
15. FRIEND, C. 1957. J. Exp. Med. **105:** 307-316.
16. SUNKARA, P. S., D. TAYLOR, M. S. KANG, T. L. BOWLIN, P. S. LIU, A. S. TYMS & A. SJOERDSMA. In preparation.

Antimyristoylation of GAG Proteins in Human T-Cell Lymphotropic and Human Immunodeficiency Viruses by *N*-Myristoyl Glycinal Diethylacetal

SHOZO SHOJI,[a] AKIRA TASHIRO,
AND YUKIHO KUBOTA

Department of Biochemistry
Faculty of Pharmaceutical Sciences
Kumamoto University
Kumamoto 862, Japan

Myristate covalently bound through an amide bond to the NH_2-terminal glycine residue of a protein was first discovered in the catalytic subunit of adenosine 3′:5′-phosphate-dependent protein kinase, type II.[1,2] Myristate was found at an NH_2-terminal glycine residue in the following: calcineurin B,[3] precursor polyprotein Pr65[gag] of the murine retrovirus protein,[4] *gag*-onc fusion proteins in mammalian transforming protein,[5a,5b] NADH-cytochrome b_5 reductase,[6] lymphoma tyrosine protein kinase,[7] protein kinase p60[src],[8–10] cellular proteins in the BC_3H muscle cell line,[11] a 36-kilodalton substrate of pp60[v-src],[12] gag protein of the human T-cell lymphotropic virus (HTLV-I),[13] specific proteins[14] of macrophages, insulin receptors,[15] vinculin,[16] structural protein of polymavirus and SV40,[17] preS1 protein of hepatitis B virus,[18] capsid protein VP4 of picornavirus[19] and α subunits of guanine nucleotide-binding regulatory proteins,[20] and human immunodeficiency virus (HIV-1).[21,22] This covalent attachment of myristic acid to select subsets of eukaryotic cellular proteins and viral proteins has been associated with important biological processes such as growth control and morphogenesis, membrane anchorage or fusion, protease protection, and virus replication.[23] Amino-terminal sequences of known *N*-myristoylated proteins are summarized in TABLE 1.

The present study addresses two aspects of protein myristoylation and antimyristoylation in the retrovirus-infected cells. First, two of the most thoroughly studied myristoylated proteins are the transforming protein of the Rous sarcoma virus, pp60[v-src], and the protoncogene product, pp60[v-src].[24–26] These polypeptides are translated on free polysomes and myristoylated before being transported to the plasma membrane.[25,26] Deletion or modification of the first 14 NH_2-terminal amino acids of pp60[v-src] does not affect intrinsic tyrosine src-kinase activity, but prevents myristoylation and membrane association, and abolishes the transforming activity of the protein.[25–28] Together, these observations suggest an important role for myristoylation in targeting proteins to the

[a] Send correspondence to Shozo Shoji, Department of Biochemistry, Faculty of Pharmaceutical Sciences, Kumamoto University, 5-1, Oe-Honmachi, Kumamoto 862, Japan.

TABLE 1. Amino-Terminal Sequences of Myristoylated Proteins

	N-Myristoylated Proteins	References
cAMP-dependent protein kinase	N-Myr-Gly-Asn-Ala-Ala-Ala-Ala-Lys-Lys-	1, 2
Calcineurin B	N-Myr-Gly-Asn-Glu-Ala-Ser-Tyr-Pro-Leu-	3
Cytochrome b_5 reductase	N-Myr-Gly-Ala-Gln-Leu-Ser-Thr-Leu-Gly-	6
LSTRA T-cell-lymphoma kinase pp56^{lsk}	N-Myr-Gly-Cys-Val-Cys-Ser-Ser-Asn-Pro-	7, 48
gag proteins		
Murine leukemia virus p15	N-Myr-Gly-Gln-Thr-Val-Thr-Thr-Pro-Leu-	4
Feline sarcoma virus p15	N-Myr-Gly-Gln-Thr-Ile-Thr-Thr-Pro-Leu-	5a
Baboon endogenous virus p12	N-Myr-Gly-Gln-Thr-Leu-Thr-Thr-Pro-Leu-	5a
Avian reticuloendotheliosis virus p12	N-Myr-Gly-Gln-Ala-Gly-Ser-Lys-	5a
HTLV-I p19	N-Myr-Gly-Gln-Ile-Phe-Ser-Arg-Ser-Ala-	13, 22
HTLV-II p15	N-Myr-Gly-Gln-Ile-His-Gly-Leu-Ser-Pro-	13
HIV-1 p17	N-Myr-Gly-Ala-Arg-Ala-Ser-Val-Leu-Ser-	21, 22
HIV-1 p27 (nef^a)	N-Myr-Gly-Gly-Lys-Trp-Ser-Lys-Arg-Ser-	49
Bovine leukemia virus p15	N-Myr-Gly-Asn-Ser-Pro-Ser-Tyr-Asn-Pro-	5b
Mouse mammary tumor virus p10	N-Myr-Gly-Val-Ser-Ser-Gly-Ser-Lys-Gly-	5a
Mason-Pfizer monkey virus p10	N-Myr-Gly-Gln-Glu-Leu-Ser-Gln-His-Glu-	5a
RSV p60^{b-src}	N-Myr-Gly-Ser-Ser-Lys-Ser-Lys-Pro-Lys-	8
Poliovirus VP 4	N-Myr-Gly-Ala-Gln-Val-Ser-Ser-Gln-Lys-	50
Simian virus (SV) 40 VP2	N-Myr-Gly-Ala-Ala-Leu-Thr-Leu-Leu-Gly-	17
Encephalomyocarditis virus VP 4	N-Myr-Gly-Asn-Ser-Thr-Ser-Ser-Asp-Lys-	19
Foot and mouth disease virus VP 4	N-Myr-Gly-Ala-Gly-Gln-Ser-Ser-Pro-Ala-	19
Pre-S1 protein of hepatitis B virus (HBV)		
Ground squirrel HBV	N-Myr-Gly-Asn-Asn-Ile-Lys-Val-Thr-Phe-	18
Woodchuck HBV	N-Myr-Gly-Asn-Asn-Ile-Lys-Val-Thr-Phe-	18
Duck HBV	N-Myr-Gly-Gln-His-Pro-Ala-Leu-Ser-Met-	18
Human HBV (ayw)	N-Myr-Gly-Gln-Asn-Leu-Ser-Thr-Ser-Asn-	18
Human HBV (adw 2)	N-Myr-Gly-Thr-Ser-Leu-Pro-Ala-	18

^{a} Negative factor.

plasma membrane and in cellular transformation. We show that N-myristoyl-glycinal diethyl acetal (N-Myr-GOA) remarkedly prevents the morphological transformation of chick embryo fibroblasts (CEF) infected with a temperature-sensitive mutant (tsNY68) of Rous sarcoma virus, and that this blockage of transformation appears to be attributed to the inhibition of NH_2-terminal myristoylation of the transforming protein pp60^{v-src} expressed in the infected cells.[29]

Second, the study aimed to establish NH_2-terminal myristoylation of the structure proteins in human T-cell lymphotropic type 1 (HTLV-I)-producing MT-2 cells[30] and human immunodeficiency virus type 1 (HIV-1)-producing CEM/LAV cells,[31] and to determine the NH_2-terminal antimyristoylation with N-myristoyl compounds. N-Myr-GOA and its derivatives were synthesized by the method of Schotten Braumann[32] on the basis of the structure of myristate linked to an NH_2-terminal glycine residue of proteins. The melting points of the diethylacetal form, which is a form of the aldehyde group protected by ethanol, are as follows: N-Myr-GOA, 65-67°C; N-Myr-Gly-GOA, 110-116°C; N-Myr-Gly-Gly-GOA, 103-105°C; and N-Myr-Gly-Gly-Gly-GOA, 87°C. The diethylacetal forms of the N-Myr compounds are slowly converted to the aldehyde forms under an acidic condition.[33] HTLV-I-producing MT-2 and HIV-1-producing CEM/LAV cells were separately cultured with [^{3}H]myristic acid in the presence or absence of N-Myr compounds. The radiolabeled proteins, after immunoprecipitation with an antiserum to adult T-cell leukemia (ATL) or the anti-p17^{gag} monoclonal antibody of HIV-1, were identified as p19^{gag} of HTLV-I and p17^{gag} of HIV-1 by fluorography after SDS-PAGE. Of the N-Myr compounds tested, N-Myr-GOA and N-Myr-Gly-GOA remarkably prevented the myristoylation of p19^{gag} and p17^{gag}, but N-Myr-Gly-Gly-GOA and N-Myr-Gly-Gly-Gly-GOA did not.[22] N-Myr-GOA did not immediately prevent both reverse transcriptase *in vitro* and incorporation of [^{3}H]thymidine by DNA synthesis, but it significantly affected HIV-1 production. Myristoylation of the gag component may be an important participant in virus capsid assembly.

MATERIAL AND METHODS

Reagents used, and their sources, were as follows: anti-p17^{gag} monoclonal antibody of HIV-1, anti-src gene product antibody (antisera from Rous sarcoma virus tumor-bearing rabbits), goat anti-rabbit IgG conjugated with peroxidase, Wako Chemical Co. (Osaka, Japan); minimum essential medium (MEM), Nissui Seiyaku (Tokyo, Japan); [9,10-^{3}H(N)]myristic acid (100 mCi/mg), [1-^{14}C]-leucine (50 mCi/mmol), [γ-^{32}P]ATP (50 Ci/mmol), [^{3}H]thymidine 5'-phosphate, 2-deoxy-D-[^{3}H]glucose, New England Nuclear; protein A-Sepharose, template primer poly(rA)p(dT)$_{12-18}$, Pharmacia Biotechnology International AB (Uppsala, Sweden). N-Myr-GOA and N-Myr-glycyl peptide derivatives were synthesized by the Schotten-Baumann method as described previously.[32] A tsNY68 sample of Rous sarcoma virus was kindly donated by Dr. S. Kawai (University of Tokyo, Japan).

CEF Culture and Analysis of Myristoylated pp60^{v-src}

CEF were prepared from 10-day-old embryonic eggs kindly supplied by the Chemo-Sera Therapeutic Research Institute (Kumamoto, Japan). Cells infected with

Rous sarcoma virus (tsNY68) were grown at 37°C for 48 h in MEM supplemented with 10% tryptose phosphate broth and 5% fetal calf serum in humidified 5% CO_2 atmosphere, as described previously.[34] The cells were labeled with [^{3}H]myristic acid (100 μCi) at 37°C for 24 h, quickly washed five times with PBS($-$), scraped off, and centrifuged at 2700 $\times$ g for 20 min.[35] The pelleted cells were lysed in 1 mL of immunoprecipitation buffer (50 mM Tris-HCl, pH 7.5, 150 mM NaCl, 1% Triton X-100, 1% deoxycholate, 0.1% SDS, 2 mM phenylmethane sulfonylfluoride, 0.001% trasylol, 83 μM antipain, 117 μM leupeptin, 73 μM pepstatin[36]). The radiolabeled lysates were subsequently employed for radioimmunoprecipitation analysis (RIPA)[36] to detect src gene products with the anti-src Gene product antibody, and then the immunoprecipitates were adsorbed by protein A Sepharose, and solubilized with SDS, followed by SDS-PAGE[37] and subsequent fluorography.[38] src Gene product was also confirmed by immunoblotting[39] as described previously.[29]

Usage of N-Myr-GOA and N-Myr Compounds

N-Myr-GOA (1 mg) and the other N-Myr compounds were separately dissolved in 1 mL of chloroform, dried, and suspended in 1 mL of PBS($-$) by sonication under sterile conditions. The N-myristoyl-compound suspension was used by direct addition to the medium at desirable concentrations. The N-myristoyl compound is difficult to solubilize immediately in the medium; therefore, it was encapsulated at appropriate concentrations in a liposome formed with dipalmitoyl phosphatidylcholine(DPPC)-phosphatidic acid(10:1), as described previously.[40] The liposome containing N-Myr-GOA at a desirable concentration was employed for antimyristoylation of the gag protein by addition to the cultured medium.

HTLV-I- or HIV-1-Producing Cell Culture

HTLV-I-producing cell lines MT-2[30] and MT-4,[41] and HIV-1-producing cell line CEM/LAV[31] were cultured in RPMI-1640 medium supplemented with 5% fetal calf serum, penicillin (100 IU/mL), and streptomycin (100 μg/mL). Human T cell line CEM was also cultured under the same conditions. The experimental details of each cell culture condition are described in each result.

Identification of Myristoylated gag Protein in HTLV-I and HIV-1

Identification of N-myristoylated gag proteins in human retroviruses was carried out by RIPA, followed by SDS-PAGE and fluorography in the same basic manner used in tsNY68-infected CEF, as described above. HTLV-I- and HIV-1-producing cells were separately cultured in the medium with ^{14}C- or ^{3}H-labeled myristic acid, and labeled viruses or labeled cells were separated, collected, and lysed with RIPA buffer. Radioactive myristoylated proteins were identified as gag proteins by RIPA, followed by SDS-PAGE and subsequent fluorography, as described previously.[22]

HIV-1 Preparation and Titration

CEM/LAV cells (2×10^5 cells/mL) were cultured for 3 days under the same condition as described above, to prepare HIV-1, and then the supernatant was centrifuged from the cultured medium, filtered (0.45 nm membrane), and used as the HIV-1 virus. The titration (4×10^5 $TCID_{50}$/mL) of the virus was measured by the tissue-culture infectious dose ($TCID_{50}$) method,[42] which is determined with the cytopathic effect (syncytium formation) of MT-4 infected with HIV-1.[41]

Inhibitory Assay of HIV-1 Production by N-Myr-GOA

Infection of MT-4 cells with HIV-1 was performed at a multiplicity of infection (m. o. i.) of 0.1 with incubation for 1 h at 37°C. The virus-infected cells were washed once and resuspended with fresh medium to produce a concentration of 2×10^5 cells/mL. The infected cells were separately cocultured with liposome-encapsulated N-Myr-GOA at final concentrations of 0, 10, 20, and 40 µM. The cultured medium was harvested at days 0, 1, 2, 3, and 4, and virus production of the resulting supernatants was determined with reverse transcriptase activity in virus particles precipitated by polyethylene glycol[43] and syncytium formation of the 4 day cultured cell after inoculation.

Reverse Transcriptase Activity

Reverse transcriptase of virus particles in the supernatant form was determined with template primer, poly(rA)-oligo(dT)$_{12-18}$, and [³H]thymidine triphosphate.[43]

RESULTS AND DISCUSSION

Detection of pp60^{v-src} Nonmyristoylated with N-Myr-GOA

CEF infected with Rous sarcoma virus (tsNY68) were cultured in the presence or absence of N-Myr-GOA (50 µM), as described previously.[29] The infected CEF, treated or untreated with N-Myr-GOA, could be recognized as elongated, parallel-orientated, flattened cells that are the typical morphologic phenotype of normal cells.[29] The infected-transformed cells (5×10^5 cells/5 mL) formed colonies (1413 colonies per 28 cm²) after three weeks of cultivation. On the other hand, the infected cells treated with N-Myr-GOA lost the ability of colony formation.

The infected CEF, treated or untreated with N-Myr-GOA, were separately labeled with either [³H]myristate- or [1-¹⁴C]leucine, collected by centrifugation, as described above, and lysed in RIPA buffer.[36] Each lysate was used separately for analysis of

[³H]myristate- or [1-¹⁴C]leucine-containing proteins by fluorography after SDS-PAGE. Of various [³H]myristate-containing proteins in the cell lysate (FIG. 1, lane A), the major labeled 60 K protein was regarded as pp60[v-src] from immunoblotting analysis (lane A') and RIPA (lane C), because it was immunoprecipitated with anti-src gene product antibody that reacts with pp60[v-src]. The antibody[44] also reacted with other viral proteins and their precursors, intermediates, and mature cleavage products. No [³H]myristate-containing proteins (lane B) were found in the radioactive lysate from

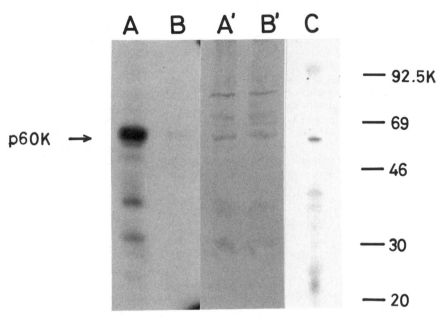

FIGURE 1. Effect of *N*-Myr-GOA on protein myristoylation in CEF infected with tsNY68. The infected CEF were labeled with [³H]myristate in MEM at 37°C for 24 h in the absence (lanes A and A') or presence (lanes B and B') of *N*-Myr-GOA (50 μM), lysed in RIPA buffer, and submitted to SDS-PAGE and processed for fluorography.[38] One-half portion of each lysate, which contained equivalent quantities of protein, were used for analysis of [³H]myristate-containing proteins and src-gene products by fluorography (lanes A and B) and immunoblotting (lanes A' and B') after SDS-PAGE. Lane C represents RIPA of the lysate with anti-src gene product antibody. The arrow indicates p60 K. Molecular weight markers are shown on the right. The experimental details are given in MATERIALS AND METHODS.

the infected CEF treated with *N*-Myr-GOA, but a 60 K protein and a few other proteins, which were invisible in lane B of the fluorogram, were detectable by the immunoblotting analysis with anti-src gene product antibody (lane B'). The results show that a 60 K protein could be identified as nonmyristoylated pp60[v-src]. The p60 K protein corresponding to pp60[v-src] was not detectable in the cell lysates treated with *N*-Myr-GOA by either immunoprecipitation or immunoblotting analyses with nonimmune rabbit serum.

There were no significant differences in [1-^{14}C]leucine incorporation into the p60 K protein or radioactivities of IgG [^{32}P] phosphorylated with src-kinase between *N*-Myr-GOA-treated CEF and untreated cells (data not shown). These results taken together indicate that *N*-Myr-GOA-prevented NH$_2$-terminal protein myristoylation of pp60^{v-src} did not affect protein synthesis or src kinase activity.[29]

The influence of *N*-Myr-GOA on specific localization of pp60^{v-src} in the infected cells was determined by indirect immunofluorescence. Upon immunofluorescence microscopic observation using anti-src gene product antibody, fluorescent grains were localized along the entire circumference of the untreated transformed cells, as well as in its cytoplasmic elements, whereas only the cytoplasm of infected cells treated with *N*-Myr-GOA was stained.[29]

The results suggest that pp60^{v-src} nonmyristoylated with *N*-Myr-GOA did not localize on the plasma membrane compartment of the cell. Judging from these results, *N*-Myr-GOA is an excellent reagent for *in vitro* blocking of NH$_2$-terminal myristoylation. Therefore, *N*-Myr-GOA is used to attempt blockage of NH$_2$-terminal myristoylation of gag proteins in human retroviruses.

Confirmation of NH$_2$-Terminal Myristoylated p19^{gag} of HTLV-I

HTLV-I-producing MT-2 cells (approximately $7 \times 10^6/10$ mL/75cm^2) were grown in RPMI 1640 medium supplemented with 5% fetal calf serum at 37°C under a humidified 5% CO$_2$ atmosphere. The cells were labeled separately with [1-^{14}C]myristate (25 μCi) at 37°C for 0 h, 3 h, 6 h, and 9 h. Cells and virus particles were harvested from the MT-2 cell-cultured medium. The cells were collected by centrifugation (1000 $\times$ g, 10 min), washed twice with cold phosphate-buffered saline, and then lysed in 500 μL of RIPA buffer (50 mM tris-HCl, pH 7.5; 150 mM NaCl; 1% Triton X-100; 1% deoxycholate; 0.1% SDS; and 2 mM phenylmethane sulfonyl fluoride).[36] Prior to collection of the virus particle from the medium-free cells, the medium was submitted to centrifugation (15000 $\times$ g, 30 min) to remove insoluble materials. The virus particles were collected by centrifugation (100,000 $\times$ g, 90 min) and then lysed in 50 μL of a lysis buffer (10 mM phosphate buffer, pH 7.4, 2% SDS). The lysates were treated with 1 M NH$_2$OH[45] in 50 mM Tris buffer, pH 7.4, at room temperature. Equivalent quantities of proteins from each lysate were used for analysis of [1-^{14}C] myristate-bound proteins by SDS-PAGE.

Of the various radiolabeled proteins in the HTLV-I lysates (FIG. 2, lanes A to E), the radioactive proteins (p28 K and p19 K; indicated by arrows in the fluorogram) increased with increasing incubation time (0 h, lane A; 3 h, lane B; 6 h, lane C; and 9 h, lane D), and the same proteins were observed in the MT-2 cell lysates (FIG. 2, lanes F to H). The radioactive proteins were positively identified as NH$_2$-terminal myristoyl proteins, p28^{gag} and p19^{gag}, because both proteins were resistant to NH$_2$OH-treatment (lanes E and G), and radiolabeled proteins that were immunoprecipitated with the antiserum to ATL were detected (lane H). The band observed at a position corresponding to 69 K in the case of the HTLV-I lysate in FIGURE 2, lane D (before NH$_2$OH-treatment), does not seem to be myristate covalently bound through an amide bond because the radioactivity was remarkably decreased after NH$_2$OH treatment (lane E). MT-2[13] and MT-2-related T-cell lines[46,47] produced both p19 K, which is a gag protein of HTLV-I, and p28 K, which was shown to be a fusion product of the gag-Px gene of HTLV-I.

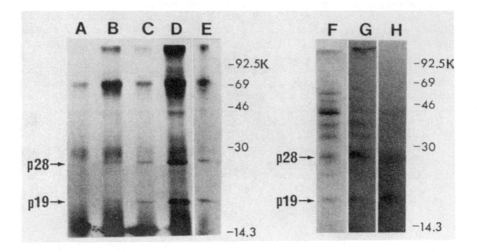

FIGURE 2. Detection of NH$_2$-terminal myristoyl proteins in HTLV-I and MT-2 cell lysates. Virus lysates (lanes A to E; E: NH$_2$OH-treated), cell lysates (lanes F to H; G: NH$_2$OH-treated), and the immunoprecipitate[36] of a cell lysate (lane H) with antiserum to ATL from a patient were analyzed by 14% SDS-PAGE,[37] followed by fluorography.[38] The experimental details are given in the text. The arrows indicate p28 K and p19 K. Molecular weight markers are shown on the right.

Myristoylation of p17^{gag} of HIV-1

CEM/LAV cells were grown under identical conditions as in the case of HTLV-I-producing MT-2 cells. The cells were incubated with either radiolabeled myristate or radiolabeled leucine. The experimental details are given in the legend to FIGURE 3. A protein (p17 K) labeled with [1-^{14}C]myristate (FIG. 3, lane B) and both p17 K and p24 K labeled with [1-^{14}C] leucine (lane C) in HIV can be easily detected in the fluorogram. Alternatively, neither protein myristoylation (lane D) nor synthesis (lane E) of proteins p17K and p24 K, the latter being a processing protein of a precursor gag protein,[36] occurred in CEM cells (non-HIV-1-infected and non-HIV-1-producing cells). Myristoylation of p17 K in the CEM/LAV cell lysate (lane G) was found to be ambiguous in the fluorogram because unknown proteins generated from the CEM cell lysate (lane H) migrated very close to p17^{gag}. A radiolabeled myristoyl protein that was immunoprecipitated with an anti-p17^{gag} monoclonal antibody, however, was clearly detected at a position corresponding to p17 K in the cases of the cells (lane I) and virus lysate (lane J). This protein was also resistant to NH$_2$OH-treatment (lane K). Thus the results revealed that p17^{gag} in HIV-1 is an NH$_2$-terminal myristoyl protein.[22]

Antimyristoylation of p19^{gag} and p17^{gag} with N-Myr-GOA

MT-2 cells and CEM/LAV cells (approximately 1.5 $\times$ 10^6 cells/10 mL/75cm^2) were grown separately in RPMI 1640 medium supplemented with 5% fetal calf serum at 37°C under a humidified 5% CO_2 atmosphere. The cells were precultivated for 15 h with either *N*-Myr-GOA or other *N*-Myr compounds at concentrations of 0, 5, 20, 50, and 100 μM. Further additions of either *N*-Myr-GOA or other *N*-Myr compounds were made to each of the precultured media, which were then allowed to stand for 1 h under the same conditions. The final concentrations of *N*-Myr-GOA or other *N*-Myr compounds were 0, 10, 40, 50, 100, and 200 μM. Each mixture was then incubated separately with [1-^{14}C] myristate (25 μCi) and DL-[1-^{14}C]leucine (5 μCi) for 24 h at 37°C. The cells and virus were harvested separately from the cultured medium.

Protein myristoylation of structure protein p19^{gag} from the HTLV-I and MT-2 cell lysates decreased with increasing concentration (50, 100, and 200 μM) of *N*-Myr-GOA (FIG. 4A, lanes 1 to 8), whereas incorporation of [1-^{14}C]leucine into p19^{gag} and p28^{gag} did not significantly decrease with increasing concentration (FIG. 4A, lanes 9 to 12); p19^{gag} labeled with [^{35}S]methionine was not seen (data not shown) because of the lack of methionine in p19^{gag}. Myristoylation of structure protein p17^{gag} from HIV-1 (FIG. 4B, lanes 13 to 16) and CEM/LAV (FIG. 3B, lanes 17 to 20) was also prevented by increasing the concentration of *N*-Myr-GOA (10, 40, and 200 μM). The NH$_2$-terminal myristoylation of p17^{gag} was strongly inhibited by *N*-Myr-GOA at a concentration of 40 μM (lane 15), whereas the incorporation of [1-^{14}C] leucine into p17^{gag} at various

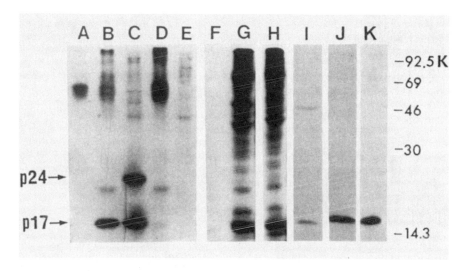

FIGURE 3. Detection of NH$_2$-terminal myristoyl proteins in HIV-1 and CEM/LAV cell lysates. Virus lysates (lanes A to C) from CEM/LAV-cell medium, lysates (lanes D and E) of the fraction corresponding to virus from the CEM-cell medium cultured under identical conditions, the cell lysates of CEM/LAV (lanes F and G) and CEM (lane H), the immunoprecipitates[36] of the CEM/LAV cell lysate (lane I) and the virus lysate (lane J), and the NH$_2$OH-treated virus lysate (lane K) were applied. The arrows indicate p17 K and p24 K. Molecular weight markers are shown on the right. CEM/LAV cells (approximately 1.1×10^7 cells/10 mL/75 cm^2) were grown in RPMI 1640 medium supplemented with 5% fetal calf serum at 37°C for 0 h (lanes A and F) and 24 h (other lanes) under a humidified 5% CO_2 atmosphere. The cells were incubated with either [1-^{14}C]myristate (25 μCi; lanes B and D), [^{3}H]myristate (100 μCi; lanes I to K), or DL-[1-^{14}C]leucine (5 μCi; lanes C and E). The other experimental conditions were the same as in FIG. 2.

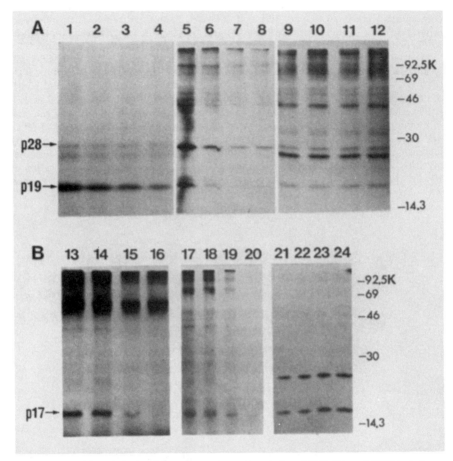

FIGURE 4. Effect of *N*-Myr-GOA on protein myristoylation of HTLV-I and HIV-1. **A** shows the effect of *N*-Myr-GOA on protein myristoylation of HTLV-I (lanes 1 to 4) and MT-2 (lanes 5 to 8), and the incorporation of [1-^{14}C] leucine into HTLV-I (lanes 9 to 12) at various concentrations: 0 μM: lanes 1, 5, and 9; 50 μM: lanes 2, 6, and 10; 100 μM: lanes 3, 7, and 11; 200 μM: lanes 4, 8, and 12. **B** illustrates the effect of *N*-Myr-GOA on the protein myristoylation of HIV (lanes 13 to 16) and CEM/LAV (lanes 17 to 20) and the incorporation of [1-^{14}C]leucine into HIV (lanes 21 to 24) at various concentrations: 0 μM: lanes 13, 17, and 21; 10 μM: lanes 14, 18, and 22; 40 μM: lanes 15, 19, and 23; 200 μM: lanes 16, 20, and 24. The experimental details are given in the text. The other experimental conditions are the same as in Fig. 2.

concentrations (lanes 21 to 24) was not inhibited. *N*-Myr-GOA did not affect the incorporation of [³H]thymidine into the cells under the same conditions. The results revealed that *N*-Myr-GOA prevented the NH₂-terminal myristoylation of structure proteins p19^{gag} in HTLV-I, and p17^{gag} in HIV-1, whereas it did not inhibit protein synthesis in the cultured cells.[22]

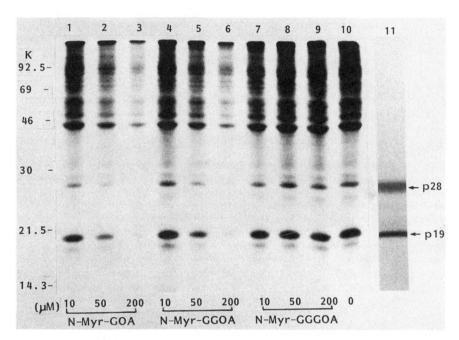

FIGURE 5. Effects of *N*-Myr-glycyl peptide derivatives on *N*-myristoylation of HTLV-I gag proteins. MT-4 cells (approximately 1.5×10^6 cells/10 mL/75 cm²) were grown separately in RPMI 1640 medium supplemented with 5% CO₂ atmosphere. The cells were precultured for 16 h with either *N*-Myr-GOA or *N*-Myr compounds at concentrations of 0, 10, 50, and 200 μM. Lanes 1-3: *N*-Myr-GOA, 10, 50, and 200 μM; lanes 4-6: *N*-Myr-Gly(G)-GOA, 10, 50, and 200 μM; lanes 7-9: *N*-Myr-Gly(G)-Gly(G)-GOA, 10, 50, and 200 μM; lane 10: 0 μM. The other experimental conditions are the same as in FIG. 2.

Effect of N-Myr-glycyl *Derivatives on* NH₂-*Terminal Myristoylation of HTLV-I gag Proteins*

MT-2 cells were cultured under the same condition as above, and after cells were treated or untreated with *N*-Myr-compounds, NH₂-terminal myristoylation was determined as described above. *N*-Myr-GOA and *N*-Myr-Gly-GOA remarkably prevented NH₂-terminal myristoylation of p19^{gag} protein of HTLV-I (FIG. 5) but *N*-Myr-Gly-Gly-GOA and *N*-Myr-Gly-Gly-Gly-GOA did not. A fluorogram of the cell lysate treated with *N*-Myr-Gly-Gly-Gly-GOA is omitted because the result was close to that of *N*-Myr-Gly-Gly-GOA. The cytotoxicity of *N*-Myr-glycyl derivatives against MT-2 was measured with Trypan blue dye exclusion for viability after 24 h under similar conditions but without viral infection (TABLE 2). The viabilities of MT-2 and the incorporation of [^{14}C]myristic acid into the cells were not significantly decreased in the concentration range of 10 to 50 μM N-Myr-GOA derivatives. At a concentration of 20 μM or above, N-Myr-GOA and its derivatives are toxic to the cells, and [^{14}C] myristate uptake decreased apparently in proportion to cytotoxicity.

Effect of N-Myr-glycyl Derivatives on NH₂-Terminal Myristoylation of HIV-1 gag Protein

Prevention by N-Myr-glycyl peptide derivatives against NH$_2$-terminal myristoylation of HIV-1 gag proteins was determined under the same conditions as described above. The cytotoxicity of these compounds against CEM/LAV cells and incorporation of [^{14}C]-myristic acid into CEM/LAV were also investigated. These results are shown in TABLE 3. N-Myr-GOA (50 μM) inhibited NH$_2$-terminal myristoylation of p17^{gag} protein in HIV-1 virus as shown in FIGURE 4B. N-Myr-Gly-GOA also prevented NH$_2$-terminal myristoylation of the proteins (data not shown), but N-Myr-Gly-Gly-GOA and N-Myr-Gly-Gly-Gly-GOA did not. N-Myr-GOA (50 μM) is not cytotoxic and does not affect [^{14}C]myristate uptake.

Prevention of NH₂-Terminal Myristoylation of HTLV-I and HIV-1 gag Proteins with the Liposome-Encapsulated N-Myr-GOA

N-Myr-GOA is a good antimyristoyl reagent, but it is not sufficiently soluble in the culture medium. Therefore, liposome containing appropriate concentrations of N-

TABLE 2. Cytotoxicity of N-Myr-Glycyl Peptide Derivatives to MT-2 Cells

N-Myr-peptides	(μM)	Viable cells[a] ($\times 10^{-5}$/mL)	(Percent)	[^{14}C]Myr uptake[b] into cells (percent)
	0	6.6	100	100
N-Myr-GOA	10	5.3	80	96
	50	6.8	104	96
	200	3.7	57	62
N-Myr-GGOA	10	6.5	99	99
	50	5.7	87	73
	200	3.9	60	60
N-Myr-GGGOA	10	5.6	86	84
	50	6.7	102	93
	200	4.4	66	96
N-Myr-GGGGOA	10	4.8	73	88
	50	4.7	71	88
	200	5.2	79	108

[a] By Trypan blue dye exclusion.
[b] Relative activities (percent) of [^{14}C]myristate uptake into MT-2 cells.

TABLE 3. Prevention of *N*-Terminal Myristoylation with *N*-Myr-Glycyl Peptide Derivatives and Their Cytotoxity

N-Myr-peptides	(μM)	Viable cells[a] ($\times 10^{-5}$/mL)	(percent)	[^{14}C]Myr uptake[b] into cells (percent)	[^{14}C]Myr[c] p17^{gag}
	0	8.0	100	100	100
N-Myr-GOA	10	8.4	103	91	58
	50	7.9	98	80	37
	200	6.0	74	67	25
N-Myr-GGGOA	10	9.2	114	83	101
	50	8.8	109	71	96
	200	7.6	94	74	77
N-Myr-GGGGOA	10	7.8	97	86	94
	50	10.2	127	86	87
	200	6.6	84	95	77

[a] By Trypan blue dye exclusion.
[b] Relative activities (percent) of [^{14}C]myristate into CEM/LAV cells.
[c] Relative activities (percent) of [^{14}C]Myr-p17^{gag} protein were obtained from the densitometric analyses of the X-ray film.

Myr-GOA was prepared, and the liposome-encapsulated *N*-Myr-GOA was used for antimyristoylation of gag proteins in the same manner as described above. NH$_2$-terminal myristoylation of p19^{gag} and p17^{gag} in HTLV-I and HIV-1 was increasingly inhibited by increasing concentration of the liposome-encapsulated *N*-Myr-GOA (FIG. 6). The liposome-encapsulated *N*-Myr-GOA strongly inhibited NH$_2$-terminal myristoylation of gag proteins in HTLV-I and HIV-1 at concentrations in the range of 10 to 25 μM. The radioactivities of p19^{gag} and p17^{gag} remarkably decreased to 11 and 5% of control, respectively (TABLE 4). Therefore, antiviral activity of the compound in the form of a liposome was determined with the cytopathic effects and reverse transcriptase activity of CEM/ LAV treated or untreated with *N*-Myr-GOA, as described below.

Antiviral Activity of N-Myr-GOA

MT-4 cells infected with HIV-1 as described in MATERIAL AND METHODS were cultured at 37°C for 4 days in mediums with liposome-encapsulated *N*-Myr-GOA at concentrations of 0, 10, 20, and 40 μM. The resulting supernatants were harvested at 1, 2, 3, and 4 days, and their antiviral activities were determined with both virus progeny (FIG. 7A) and reverse transcriptase (FIG. 7B).

Virus progeny and reverse transcriptase activity were increasingly depressed by both increasing concentration and prolonged incubation times of the liposome-encapsulated *N*-Myr-GOA compound. Virus progeny treated with the compound at a final concentration of 40 μM was depressed to approximately 2% of untreated virus production (FIG. 7Ac), whereas reverse transcriptase activity (FIG. 7Bc) was depressed as well. In this experiment, remarkable blockage of the NH$_2$-terminal myristoylation of p17^{gag}

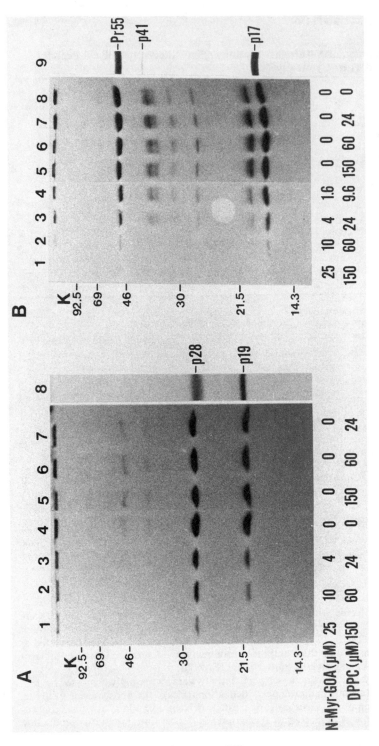

FIGURE 6. Effects of liposome-encapsulated *N*-Myr-GOA on NH$_2$-terminal myristoylation of HTLV-I and HIV-1 gag proteins. MT-4 cells and CEM/LAV were separately preincubated for 6 h at 37°C with liposome-encapsulated *N*-Myr-GOA at concentrations of 0, 1.6, 4, 10, and 25 μM, labeled for 16 h with [^{3}H]myristate, and then harvested. The other experimental conditions are the same as in FIGURES 2 and 3. MT-2 cell lysate (**A**), *N*-Myr-GOA: 0 μM, lane 4 (0), lane 7 (24), lane 6 (60), and lane 5 (150); 4 μM, lane 3 (24); 10 μM, ATL serum. CEM/LAV cell lysate (**B**), *N*-Myr-GOA: 0 μM, lane 8 (0), lane 7 (24), lane 6 (60), and lane 5 (150); 1.6 μM, lane 4 (9.6); 4 μM, lane 3 (24); 10 μM, lane 2 (60); 25 μM, lane 1 (150); lane 9, immunoprecipitated with anti-p17^{gag} monodonal antibody. Concentrations (μM) of liposome (DPPC) are presented in parentheses.

TABLE 4. Blockage of *N*-Myristoylation of gag Proteins in HTLV-I and HIV-1 by Liposome-Encapsulated *N*-Myr-GOA

	cpm[a] of [³H]Myristoylated proteins					
	HTLV-I			HIV-1		
N-Myr-GOA[a]	p19	p28	Pr53	p17	p41	Pr55
0	3,444 (100)	4,198 (100)	1,229 (100)	2,985 (100)	2,700 (100)	2,931 (100)
1.6	ND[b]	ND	ND	2,173 (73)	1,521 (56)	1,778 (61)
4	1,216 (36)	1,719 (41)	594 (48)	1,582 (53)	1,301 (48)	1,560 (52)
10	878 (26)	1,287 (31)	496 (40)	631 (21)	553 (21)	617 (21)
25	375 (11)	642 (15)	156 (13)	157 (5)	161 (6)	205 (7)

[a] Radioactivities of the gag proteins extracted from SDS-PAGE. Relative activity (percent) is represented in parenthesis. The experimental details are given in the text.
[b] ND, not determined.

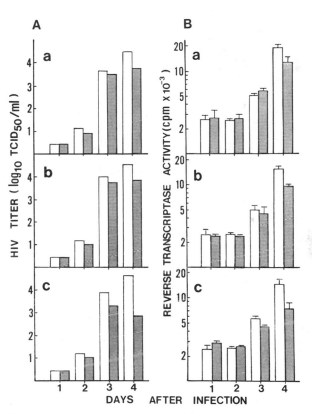

FIGURE 7. Effects of *N*-Myr-GOA on the virus production of HIV-1-infected MT-4 cells. MT-4 cells infected with HIV-1 (m.o.i = 0.1) were treated with the liposome without *N*-Myr-GOA (open column) or with *N*-Myr-GOA (closed column). Virus progeny (**A**) and reverse transcriptase (**B**) in the cell-free supernatant from the cultured medium were determined. The experimental details are given in the text. a: *N*-Myr-GOA, 10 μM (60); b: 20 μM (120); c: 40 μM (240). Concentrations (μM) of the liposome (DPPC) are presented in parenthesis.

was confirmed by fluorography under the identical conditions (FIG. 8). Inhibitory mechanism of virus progeny by N-Myr-GOA was unknown, but the reagent may be an inhibitor for either N-myristoyl transferase or myristoyl CoA synthetase. Mammalian retroviral gag polyproteins and their related gag-fusion proteins possess NH$_2$-terminal N-myristoylated glycine residues.[5b] NH$_2$-terminal myristoylations of the murine leukemia virus Pr65^{gag} precursor and the Mason-Pfizer monkey virus gag-polyprotein precur-

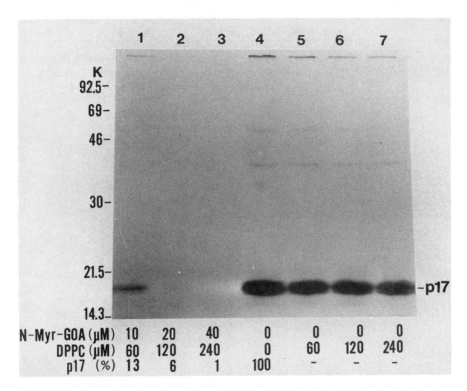

FIGURE 8. Prevention of myristoylation of p17^{gag} in HIV-1-infected MT-4 cells with the liposome-encapsulated N-Myr-GOA. MT-4 cells infected with HIV-1 (m. o. i. $= 0.1$) were cocultured with the liposome without N-Myr-GOA (lane 4 to 7) or with N-Myr-GOA (lane 1 to 3) for 48 h, further incubated with [^{3}H]myristate for 16 h, and harvested. The radiolabeled cell lysates were analyzed by SDS-PAGE and followed by fluorography as described above. The other experimental conditions are the same as in FIG. 2. Concentrations (μM) of both the liposome (DPPC) and its encapsulated N-Myr-GOA, and the relative radioactivities (percent) of p17^{gag}, are presented at the bottom of the FIGURE.

sor are required for retrovirus-matured particle formation.[51,52] Recent studies with an HIV-1 gag-precursor mutant that possesses Met-Ala-Ala- instead of Met-Gly-Ala- at the NH$_2$-terminus of p17^{gag} revealed that this mutant is responsible for the *in vitro* loss of myristoylation and inability to produce infectious virus particles.[53] NH$_2$-terminal myristoylation of gag proteins and their respective gag-fusion proteins may participate in virus assembly; capsid formation, virus maturation, and budding subsequently occur.

Therefore, more attractive and less cytotoxic antimyristoyl reagents should be therapeutic drugs for human immunodeficiency syndrome.

ACKNOWLEDGMENTS

The authors would like to thank S. Araki, Ryukyu University, for the use of the antiserum to ATL, and K. Takatsuki, Kumamoto University, for the human retrovirus-producing cell lines. We thank the Chemo-Sero-Therapeutic Research Institute for use of their radioisotope facilities (P3).

REFERENCES

1. CARR, S. A., K. BIEMANN, S. SHOJI, D. C. PARMELEE & K. TITANI. 1982. n-Tetradecanoyl is the NH$_2$-terminal blocking group of the catalytic subunit of cyclic AMP-dependent protein kinase from bovine cardiac muscle. Proc. Natl. Acad. Sci. USA **79**: 6128-6131.
2. SHOJI, S., L. H. ERICSSON, K. A. WALSH, E. H. FISCHER & K. TITANI. 1983. Amino acid sequence of the catalytic subunit of bovine type II adenosine cyclic 3′,5′-phosphate dependent protein kinase. Biochemistry **22**: 3702-3709.
3. AITKEN, A., P. COHEN, S. SANTIKARN, D. H. WILLIAMS, A. G. CALDER, A. SMITH & C. B. KLEE. 1982. Identification of the NH$_2$-terminal blocking group of calcineurin B as myristic acid. FEBS Lett. **150**: 314-318.
4. HENDERSON, L. E., H. C. KRUTZSCH & S. OROSZLAN. 1983. Myristyl amino-terminal acylation of murine retrovirus proteins: An unusual post-translational protein modification. Proc. Natl. Acad. Sci. USA **80**: 339-343.
5a. SCHULTZ, A. & S. OROSZLAN. 1983. *In vivo* modification of retroviral $_{gag}$ gene-encoded polyproteins by myristic acid. J. Virol. **46**: 355-361.
5b. SCHULTZ, A. & S. OROSZLAN. 1984. Myristylation of *gag-onc* fusion proteins in mammalian transforming retroviruses. Virology **133**: 431-437.
6. OZOLS, J., S. A. CARR & P. STRITTMATTER. 1984. Identification of the NH$_2$-terminal blocking group of NADH-cytochrome b$_5$ reductase as myristic acid and the complete amino acid sequence of the membrane-binding domain. J. Biol. Chem. **259**: 13349-13354.
7. MARCHILDON, G. A., J. E. CASNELLIE, K. A. WALSH & E. G. KREBS. 1984. Covalently bound myristate in a lymphoma tyrosine protein kinase. Proc. Natl. Acad. Sci. USA **81**: 7679-7682.
8. SCHULTZ, A. M., L. E. HENDERSON, S. OROSZLAN, E. A. GARBER & H. HANAFUSA. 1985. Amino terminal myristylation of the protein kinase p60[src], a retroviral transforming protein. Science **227**: 427-429.
9. PELLMAN, D., E. A. GARBER, F. R. CROSS & H. HANAFUSA. 1985. Fine structural mapping of a critical NH$_2$-terminal region of p60[src]. Proc. Natl. Acad. Sci. USA **82**: 1623-1627.
10. PELLMAN, D., E. A. GARBER, F. R. CROSS & H. HANAFUSA. 1985. An N-terminal peptide from p60[src] can direct myristylation and plasma membrane localization when fused to heterologous proteins. Nature **314**: 374-377.
11. OLSON, E. N., D. A. TOWLER & L. GLASER. 1985. Specificity of fatty acid acylation of cellular proteins. J. Biol. Chem. **260**: 3784-3790.
12. SORIC, J. & J. A. GORDON. 1985. The 36-kilodalton substrate of pp60[v-src] is myristylated in a transformation-sensitive manner. Science **230**: 563-566.
13. OOTSUYAMA, Y., K. SHIMOTOHNO, M. MIWA, S. OROSZLAN & T. SUGIMURA. 1985. Myristylation of gag protein in human T-cell leukemia virus type-I and type-II. Jpn. J. Cancer Res. (Gann) **76**: 1132-1135.

14. ADEREM, A. A., M. M. KEUM, E. PURE & Z. A. COHN. 1986. Bacterial lipopolysaccharides, phorbol myristate acetate, and zymosan induce the myristoylation of specific macrophage proteins. Proc. Natl. Acad. Sci. USA **83:** 5817-5821.

15. HEDO, J. A., E. COLLIER & A. WATKINSON. 1987. Myristyl and palmityl acylation of the insulin receptor. J. Biol. Chem. **262:** 954-957.

16. KELLIE, S. & N. M. WIGGLESWORTH. 1987. The cytoskeletal protein vinculin is acylated by myristic acid. FEBS Lett. **213:** 428-432.

17. STREULI, C. H. & B. E. GRIFFIN. 1987. Myristic acid is coupled to a structural protein of polyoma virus and SV40. Nature **326:** 619-622.

18. PERSING, D. H., H. E. VARMUS & D. GANEM. 1987. The preS1 protein of hepatitis B virus is acylated at its amino terminus with myristic acid. J. Virol. **61:** 1672-1677.

19. CHOW, M., J. F. E. NEWMAN, D. FILMAN, J. M. HOGLE, D. J. ROWLANDS & F. BROWN. 1987. Myristylation of picornavirus capsid protein VP4 and its structural significance. Nature **327:** 482-486.

20. BUSS, J. E., S. M. MUMBY, P. J. CASEY, A. G. GILMAN & B. M. SEFTON. 1987. Myristoylated α subunits of guanine nucleotide-binding regulatory proteins. Proc. Natl. Acad. Sci. USA **84:** 7493-7497.

21. VERONESE, F. D. M., T. D. COPELAND, S. OROSZLAN, R. C. GALLO & M. G. SARNGAD-HARAN. 1988. Biochemical and immunological analysis of human immunodeficiency virus gag gene products p17 and p24. J. Virol. **62:** 795-801.

22. SHOJI, S., A. TASHIRO & Y. KUBOTA. 1988. Antimyristoylation of gag proteins in human T-cell leukemia and human immunodeficiency viruses with N-myristoyl glycinal diethyl acetal. J. Biochem. **103:** 747-749.

23. TOWLER, D. A., J. I. GORDON, S. P. ADAMS & L. GLASER. 1988. The biology and enzymology of eukaryotic protein acylation. Annu. Rev. Biochem. **57:** 69-99.

24. BUSS, J. E., M. P. KAMPS & B. M. SEFTON. 1984. Myristic acid is attached to the transforming protein of Rous sarcoma virus during or immediately after synthesis and is present in both soluble and membrane-bound forms of the protein. Mol. Cell. Biol. **4:** 2697-2704.

25. CROSS, F. R., E. A. GARBER, D. PELLMAN & H. HANAFUSA. 1984. A short sequence in the p60^{src} N terminus is required for p60^{src} myristylation and membrane association and for cell transformation. Mol. Cell. Biol. **4:** 1834-1842.

26. KAMPS, M. P., J. E. BUSS & B. M. SEFTON. 1985. Mutation of NH$_2$-terminal glycine of p60^{src} prevents both myristoylation and morphological transformation. Proc. Natl. Acad. Sci. USA **82:** 4625-4628.

27. GARBER, E. A., J. G. KRUEGER, H. HANAFUSA & A. R. GOLDBERG. 1983. Only membrane-associated RSV src proteins have amino-terminally bound lipid. Nature **302:** 161-163.

28. BUSS, J. E., M. P. KAMPS, K. GOULD & B. M. SEFTON. 1986. The absence of myristic acid decreases membrane binding of p60^{src} but does not affect tyrosine protein kinase activity. J. Virol. **58:** 468-474.

29. SHOJI, S., M. MATSUNAGA, R. TSUJITA & Y. KUBOTA. 1989. Blockage of morphological transformation of chick embryo fibroblasts infected with Rous sarcoma virus by N-myristoyl glycinal diethyl acetal in vitro. Biochemistry Int. **18:** 509-518.

30. MIYOSHI, I., I. KUBONISHI, S. YOSHIMOTO, T. AKAGI, Y. OHTSUKI, Y. SHIRAISHI, K. NAGATA & Y. HINUMA. 1981. Type C virus particles in a cord T-cell line derived by cocultivating normal human cord leukocytes and human leukaemic T cells. Nature **294:** 770-771.

31. BARRÉ-SINOUSSI, F., J. C. CHERMANN, F. REY, M. T. NUGEYRE, S. CHAMARET, J. GRUEST, C. DAUGUET, C. AXLER-BLIN, F. VÉZINET-BRUN, C. ROUZIOUX, W. ROZEN-BAUM & L. MONTAGNIER. 1983. Isolation of a T-lymphotropic retrovirus from a patient at risk for acquired immune deficiency syndrome (AIDS). Science **220:** 868-871.

32. SONNTAG, N. O. V. 1953. The reactions of aliphatic acid chlorides. Chem. Rev. **52:** 237-399.

33. KILPATRICK M. 1963. Kinetics of hydrolysis of acetals in protium and deuterium oxides. J. Am. Chem. Soc. **85:** 1036-1038.

34. KAWAI, S. & H. HANAFUSA. 1971. The effects of reciprocal changes in temperature on the transformed state of cells infected with a Rous sarcoma virus mutant. Virology **46:** 470-479.

35. KAWAI, S. & H. HANAFUSA. 1973. Isolation of defective mutant of avian sarcoma virus. Proc. Natl. Acad. Sci. USA **70:** 3493-3497.
36. HATTORI, S., T. KIYOKAWA, K. IMAGAWA, F. SHIMIZU, E. HASHIMURA, M. SEIKI & M. YOSHIDA. 1984. Identification of gag and env gene products of human T-cell leukemia virus (HTLV). Virology **136:** 338-347.
37. LAEMMLI, U. K. 1970. Cleavage of structural proteins during the assembly of the head of bacteriophage T4. Nature **227:** 680-685.
38. CHAMBERLAIN, J. P. 1979. Fluorographic detection of radioactivity in polyacrylamide gels with the water-soluble fluor, sodium salicylate. Anal. Biochem. **98:** 132-135.
39. TOWBIN, H., T. STAEHELIN & J. GORDON. 1979. Electrophoretic transfer of proteins from polyacrylamide gels to nitrocellulose sheets: Procedure and some applications. Proc. Natl. Acad. Sci. USA **76:** 4350-4354.
40. HAUSER, H. O. 1971. The effect of ultrasonic irradiation on the chemical structure of egg lecithin. Biochem. Biophys. Res. Commun. **45:** 1049-1055.
41. HARADA, S., Y. KOYANAGI & N. YAMAMOTO. 1985. Infection of human T-lymphotropic virus type-1 (HTLV-1)-bearing MT-4 cells with HTLV-III (AIDS virus): Chronological studies of early events. Virology **146:** 272-281.
42. WALKER, B. D., M. KOWALSKI, W. C. GOH, K. KOZARSKY, M. KRIEGER, C. ROSEN, L. ROHRSCHNEIDER, W. A. HASELTINE & J. SODROSKI. 1987. Inhibition of human immunodeficiency virus syncytium formation and virus replication by castanospermine. Proc. Natl. Acad. Sci. USA **84:** 8120-8124.
43. POIESZ, B. J., F. W. RUSCETTI, A. F. GAZDAR, P. A. BUNN, J. D. MINNA & R. C. GALLO. 1980. Detection and isolation of type C retrovirus particles from fresh and cultured lymphocytes of a patient with cutaneous T-cell lymphoma. Proc. Natl. Acad. Sci. USA **77:** 7415-7419.
44. BRUGGE, J. S. & R. L. ERIKSON. 1977. Identification of a transformation-specific antigen induced by an avian sarcoma virus. Nature **269:** 346-348.
45. TOWLER, D. & L. GLASER. 1986. Protein fatty acid acylation: Enzymatic synthesis of an *N*-myristoylglycyl peptide. Proc. Natl. Acad. Sci. USA **83:** 2812-2816.
46. TANAKA, Y., Y. KOYANAGI, T. CHOSA, N. YAMAMOTO & Y. HINUMA. 1983. Monoclonal antibody reactive with both p28 and p19 of adult T-cell leukemia virus-specific polypeptides. Jpn. J. Cancer Res. (Gann) **74:** 327-330.
47. KOBAYASHI, N., H. KONISHI, H. SABE, K. SHIGESADA, T. NOMA, T. HONJO & M. HATANAKA. 1984. Genomic structure of HTLV (human T-cell leukemia virus): detection of defective genome and its amplification in MT-2 cells. EMBO J. **3:** 1339-1343.
48. VORONOVA, A. F., J. E. BUSS, T. PATSCHINSKY, T. HUNTER & B. M. SEFTON. 1984. Characterization of the protein apparently responsible for the elevated tyrosine protein kinase activity in LSTRA cells. Mol. Cell. Biol. **4:** 2705-2713.
49. GUY, B., M. P. KIENY, Y. RIVIERE, C. L. PEUCH, K. DOTT, M. GIRARD, L. MONTAGNIER & J.-P. LECOCQ. 1987. HIV F/3' orf encodes a phosphorylated GTP-binding protein resembling an oncogene product. Nature **330:** 266-269.
50. PAUL, A. V., A. SCHULTZ, S. E. PINCUS, S. OROSZLAN & E. WIMMER. 1987. Capsid protein VP4 of poliovirus is N-myristolated. Proc. Natl. Acad. Sci. USA **84:** 7827-7831.
51. REIN, A., M. R. McCLURE, N. R. RICE, R. B. LUFTIG & A. M. SCHULTZ. 1986. Myristylation site in Pr65^{gag} is essential for virus particle formation by Moloney murine leukemia virus. Proc. Natl. Acad. Sci. USA **83:** 7246-7250.
52. RHEE, S. S. & E. HUNTER. 1987. Myristylation is required for intracellular transport but not for assembly of D-type retrovirus capsids. J. Virol. **61:** 1045-1053.
53. GÖTTLINGER, H. G., J. G. SODROSKI & W. A. HASELTINE. 1989. Role of capsid precursor processing and myristoylation in morphogenesis and infectivity of human immunodeficiency virus type 1. Proc. Natl. Acad. Sci. USA **86:** 5781-5785.

The Genetic Analysis of the HIV Envelope Binding Domain on CD4

JAMES ARTHOS,[a,b] KEITH C. DEEN,[a]
ALLAN SHATZMAN,[a] ALEMSEGED TRUNEH,[a]
MARTIN ROSENBERG,[a] AND
RAYMOND W. SWEET[a]

[a]SmithKline Beecham Pharmaceuticals
King of Prussia, Pennsylvania 19479

[b]Department of Biology
University of Pennsylvania
Philadelphia, Pennsylvania 19104

INTRODUCTION

CD4 is a 55 kDa nonpolymorphic glycoprotein expressed predominantly on the surface of a subset of T lymphocytes. On this cell type, CD4 serves to mediate an efficient cellular immune response through association with the major histocompatibility complex (MHC) class II molecules on the surface of antigen-presenting cells (reviewed in ref. 1). In humans, CD4 also serves as a receptor for the human immunodeficiency virus (HIV) (reviewed in refs. 1 and 2). The cellular tropism of HIV for cells bearing the CD4 receptor results from a high-affinity interaction between the HIV external envelope glycoprotein (gp120) and CD4.[3,4] This association appears to induce the release of gp120 from the viral surface, with the consequent exposure of a region of the membrane-anchored gp41 protein implicated in virus/cell fusion (see Hart *et al.*, this volume). The surface domain of CD4 is composed of 372 amino-terminal amino acids organized into four tandem domains, based on sequence homology to immunoglobulin regions.[5,6] The most amino-terminal of these domains, V1, shows particular homology to κ-immunoglobulin light chain variable regions (V_κ). In this report we first summarize the genetic analysis of CD4 by our laboratory and other laboratories.[7–12] These studies localized the gp120 binding site to the V1 domain within residues about 41 to 55. Curiously, a complementing analysis with synthetic CD4 peptides implicates a separate region, residues 81 to 92, in recognition of gp120[13,14] (also see Eiden *et al.*, this volume). The genetic studies also defined, at least partially, the epitopes of more than 60 different anti-CD4 monoclonal antibodies (mAbs).[8,15] The localization of the epitopes of these antibodies is consistent with a structural motif for the V1 domain that is similar to that of V_κ.

Through deletion mutagenesis in the V1 domain, we have further defined the minimal region of the CD4 V1 region, which is required for high-affinity binding to gp120. Soluble V1 domain proteins with small deletions at either the carboxy or amino terminus were constructed and expressed in *E. coli*. These proteins were examined for their ability to recognize HIV gp120 as well as a series of conformation-sensitive mAbs.

We found that sequences near both termini are critical for maintaining the structure of the V1 domain and the proper presentation of the gp120 recognition site.

RESULTS AND DISCUSSION

The gp120 Binding Site Is in the V1 Domain

Through the expression and assay of truncated, soluble CD4 proteins, the high-affinity binding site for gp120 was localized to the most amino-terminal domain of CD4, the V1 region.[11] One of these proteins, sT4, consisted of the entire extracellular domain of CD4; a second protein, V1V2, consisted of the first two extracellular domains; a third protein, V1, contained only the most amino-terminal domain. These soluble proteins, were expressed in mammalian cells and/or in *E. coli,* and their binding to the gp120 was quantitated in a competition radioimmunoassay (RIA). The V1V2 and V1 proteins competed as efficiently as the full-length soluble protein, sT4. In addition, all three proteins inhibited HIV infection and virus-induced syncytium formation at similar molar concentrations.[11] From these results we concluded that the high-affinity binding site for gp120 resided solely within the V1 domain. A similar conclusion was reported by Chao *et al.*[16]

The gp120 Binding Site Overlaps a Region That Aligns with CDR2 of V_κ

The gp120 binding site within the V1 domain was defined by extensive genetic analysis in several laboratories.[7-12] In our studies, we introduced 33 substitutions into V1 using the murine CD4 protein, which does not bind virus, as a template for this mutagenesis.[11] By this approach, we sought to minimize gross structural distortions that could result from mutation. These mutants were expressed in the context of an sT4 protein in mammalian cells or a V1V2 protein in *E. coli.* Binding of the soluble mutant proteins to purified gp120 was quantitated in flow cytometry and RIA assays. Only two closely spaced clusters of mutants, involving residues 41-43 and 51-55, affected the recognition of gp120. Specific mutations within these regions reduced the affinity for gp120 by at least 20-fold. These results, together with the results from other laboratories, are summarized in FIGURE 1. Several features of the gp120 binding region emerge from these combined data. First, substitution mutagenesis places the site between residues 41 and 55. Some multiple substitution mutants that affect binding extend proximal to this region, but they include alterations in the region 41-43 which alone disrupts recognition of gp120. A larger binding region, encompassing residues 32 to 66, is suggested by insertional mutagenesis; however, the potentially disruptive nature of such mutations creates ambiguity in the interpretation of these results. The effect of the short deletions at the extreme amino terminus is discussed below. Second, within the region 41-55, the data do not reveal which side chains contact residues in gp120. For all positions at which there have been multiple substitutions, mutations that disrupt binding are countered by other innocuous side chain alterations. Third, based on the alignment with a V_κ sequence, the binding site encompasses the second

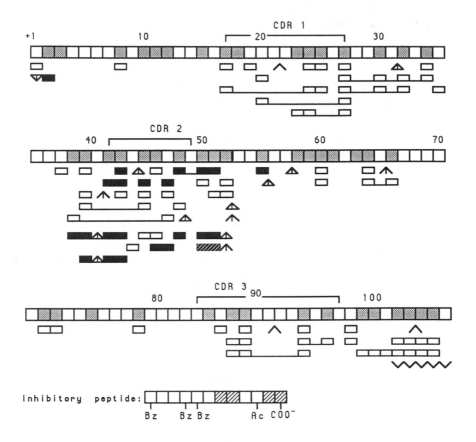

FIGURE 1. Effect of mutations in the V1 domain on binding of gp120. One hundred and six amino acid residues of the V1 domain are shown together with the positions of mutations and their effect on recognition of gp120. These results are compiled from references 8-12. Stippled boxes indicate residues that differ between mouse and human CD4 as previously aligned.[11] Mutants containing multiple substitutions, insertions, or deletions are denoted by connecting lines and symbols. CDR 1, 2, and 3 indicate the regions corresponding to the complementarity-determining regions in V_κ based on a previous sequence alignment.[15] Also shown is a modified synthetic peptide extending from 81 to 92, which inhibits gp120 binding to CD4, virus infection, and virus-mediated cell fusion (see text): shaded boxes indicate acidic residues. Bz, benzyl; Ac, acetyl.

complementarity-determining region (CDR2), one of three such regions in light chain variable domains that contribute to antigen recognition by antibody. Fourth, studies with synthetic peptides have implicated a quite separate region, residues 81-92, in gp120 recognition[13,14] (FIG. 1). Although none of the mutations in this region affected gp120 binding, a single amino acid substitution at position 87 was recently reported to dramatically reduce syncytium formation between CD4+ cells and cells expressing HIV envelope protein.[17] Further analyses are required to unravel the interaction of this region of CD4 with gp120. Finally, mutations that disrupted binding to gp120 had the predicted negative effect on virus infection in cell culture. Soluble CD4 proteins containing mutations that disrupted binding to gp120 failed to inhibit virus attachment, virus infection, and virus-mediated cell fusion.[11] Thus, inhibition of virus by soluble CD4 proteins is strictly dependent upon their association with gp120 at the high-affinity binding site.

V1 Is Structurally Related to V_κ

High-resolution structural analysis of CD4 is in progress in several laboratories. We have indirectly probed, however, the structure of the V1 domain through epitope mapping of 55 anti-CD4 mAbs. The binding sites of the antibodies were first localized to domains of CD4 using the truncated soluble CD4 proteins V1, V1V2, and sT4. The epitopes within the V1 domain were then mapped using the panel of substitution mutants. Four generalizations emerged from these analyses. First, each of the mutations affected only a subset of the antibodies, indicating only local perturbation of structure. Second, many antibodies that recognized V1V2 but not V1 were nonetheless affected by mutations within the V1 region. This result suggests that some segments of the V1 and V2 domains lie close to one another. Third, many of the antibodies were affected by noncontiguous mutations. Fourth, none of the antibodies precisely mimicked the binding of gp120 to CD4. Similar observations were reported by Petersen and Seed.[8]

Among immunoglobulin proteins of known structure, the V1 domain aligns most closely with V_κ of the Bence-Jones protein REI. A schematic α-carbon trace of one variable region from the crystal structure of REI[18] is shown in FIGURE 2. Based on a sequence alignment, we superimposed the positions of amino acid residues in V1 onto this structure.[15] In the context of this structure, the mAb epitopes, as defined by the substitution mutants, were localized to exposed loops, and the noncontiguous residues that comprised many epitopes were close in space. These observations suggest that the V1 domain bears structural similarity to an immunoglobulin V_κ region.

In this model for V1, the gp120 binding site consists of a small loop corresponding to the CDR2 region in V_κ. We have suggested that this small loop may be accommodated by a compact binding pocket in gp120, which by its size excludes recognition by host antibodies,[11] a proposal initially forwarded by Rossman *et al.* for the receptor binding site on rhinoviruses.[19] Protection of the receptor binding site on gp120 in this manner may allow the virus to evade the humoral immune response.

The Minimal Region of V1 Required for High-Affinity Binding to gp120

The soluble V1 protein described in the above studies consisted of residues −2 (2 residues upstream of the mature amino terminus in the leader peptide) to 106 of the mature CD4 receptor. To define the minimal sequence required to maintain the structure of the V1 domain, and the gp120 binding site in particular, a series of amino and carboxy truncated derivatives of the 106 amino acid V1 domain were expressed in *E. coli* (FIG. 3). Using a direct immunoprecipitation assay and a more quantitative competition binding assay, each of the V1 truncated proteins was examined for its ability to recognize gp120. The surface structure of each of these proteins was further examined in similar assays with several CD4 mAbs that recognize conformational epitopes across the V1 domain. Retention of the core β-sheet structure in these proteins was assessed by measuring formation of the single cystine bridge in V1, a conserved

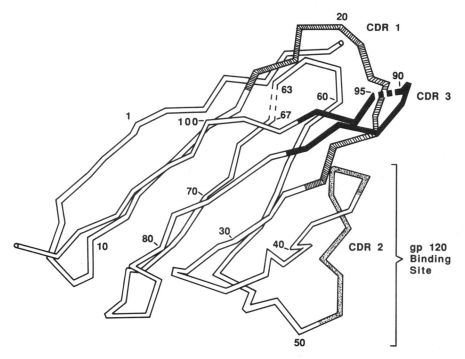

FIGURE 2. Structural model of the V1 domain. Schematic α-carbon trace of one variable region of REI.[18] Numbering is for V1 based on a sequence alignment with REI.[15] Dashes indicate two positions of amino acid insertions in V1 relative to REI. Shaded regions are CDRs 1, 2, and 3. The predicted loop comprising the gp120 binding site (41-55) is indicated.

feature of IgV-like domains. Finally, we have begun to address the relative contributions of side-chain and main-chain interactions at the C terminus through a similar analysis of substitution mutants of the phenylalanine residue at position 98.

At the carboxy terminus, removal of residues 102-106 (V1-101) had little effect on the recognition of gp120 or on overall surface conformation of the V1 domain (TABLE 1). Truncation to position 97, however, markedly disrupted the interaction with gp120 and with the mAbs, an effect that was further exacerbated by deletions to position 93 or 88 (TABLE 1). Yet the intramolecular disulfide bond was formed in even the most

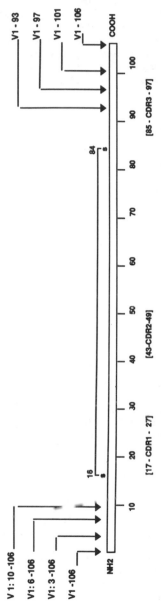

FIGURE 3. Soluble V1 proteins truncated at the amino and carboxy termini. The amino terminal mutants initiate with a methionine residue immediately preceding the indicated amino acid and terminate with residue 106. The carboxy terminal mutants begin at residue 2 (2 residues into the leader peptide of CD4) and terminate following the indicated amino acid. Numbers indicate amino acid positions. CDR 1, 2 and 3 as in FIG. 1.

disordered of these proteins, V1-88, indicating retention of the core β-sheet structure. The region 97-101 contains two residues, phe98 and gly99, which align with invariant residues ($>98\%$ conservation) in immunoglobulin light-chain variable regions. Mutation of gly99, and also the leucine residue in position 100, were previously reported to not affect binding to gp120 and certain anti-CD4 mAbs.[9,12] We thus examined the effect of alteration of the phenylalanine at position 98. As assayed by immunoprecipitation, substitution of either leucine or alanine did not disrupt binding to gp120 or the mAbs (data not shown). In the context of an IgV_κ region structure, the tolerance of these side-chain substitutions in the region 98-101 suggests that the surface distortion induced by the deletion of 101 to 97 results from the loss of main-chain H-bonding between adjacent C-terminal β strands.

TABLE 1. Properties of the Truncated V1 Proteins[a]

V1 Protein	Disulfide bond	gp120	Binding to: Leu3A	OKT4A	IOT4A
C-term					
106	+	+++	+++	+++	+++
101	+	+++	+++	+++	+++
97	+	−	++	++	+
93	+	−	−	−	−
88	+	−	−	−	−
N-term					
3	+	+	+	+	+
6	+	−	−	−	−
10	+	−	−	−	−

[a] Formation of the disulfide bridge was determined by a characteristic shift in mobility in SDS/PAGE under reducing versus nonreducing conditions. Binding to gp120 and the anti-CD4 mAbs was measured qualitatively by immunoprecipitation followed by immunoblotting. Approximate percent precipitation: +++, 100%; ++, 30-50%; +, about 10%; −, undetectable. For the C-terminal truncates, binding was assessed more quantitatively by measuring the ability of these proteins to compete with native, cell-surface CD4 for binding to gp120 and the mAbs. The results of this assay were similar to that above except that the V1-97 protein did not compete appreciably for binding to gp120 or the mAbs.

At the amino terminus, removal of as few as the two amino-terminal residues (lys-lys) affected surface conformation (TABLE 1). Further truncations to residues 6 and 10 ablated binding to gp120 and the mAbs (TABLE 1). Even these severely disruptive deletions, however, did not prevent the formation of the core β-sheet structure, as measured by formation of the cystine bridge.

We conclude that amino acid residues at both the extreme amino and carboxy termini of V1 are important determinants for maintaining the external conformation of this domain and the integrity of the high-affinity binding site for gp120. Considering the predicted structural similarity between V1 and V_κ, similar sequence constraints on conformation may extend to immunoglobulin light-chain variable regions.

SUMMARY

Through mutagenesis, we identified a single high-affinity binding site for gp120 on the human CD4 protein. This site is localized in the V1 domain within residues 41 to 55. The collection of mutants was also used to define the epitopes for 55 anti-CD4 monoclonal antibodies. The locations of these epitopes are consistent with a V_κ-like structure for the V1 domain. In the context of this structure, the gp120 binding site encompasses the small CDR2 loop. Through deletion mutagenesis at the termini of the V1 domain, we further defined the minimal region required to retain high-affinity binding to gp120. Short deletions at both termini disrupt binding to gp120 and recognition by conformation-sensitive anti-CD4 monoclonal antibodies. We conclude that amino acids at both the amino and carboxy termini are critical to the conformation of the V1 domain and, in particular, to the integrity of the gp120 binding site.

ACKNOWLEDGMENTS

The authors gratefully acknowledge our many collaborators, cited in references 11 and 15, in the mapping of the gp120 binding site and the analysis of anti-CD4 mAb epitopes.

REFERENCES

1. PARNES, J. R. 1989. Adv. Immunol. **44**: 265-311.
2. SATTENTAU, Q. J. & R. A. WEISS. 1988. Cell **52**: 631-633.
3. McDOUGAL, J. S., M. S. KENNEDY, J. M. SLIGH, S. P. CORT, A. MAWLE & J. K. A. NICHOLSON. 1986. Science **231**: 382-385.
4. LASKY, L. A., G. NAKAMURA, D. H. SMITH, C. FENNIE, C. SHIMASAKI, E. PATZER, P. BERMAN, T. GREGORY & D. J. CAPON. 1987. Cell **50**: 975-985.
5. MADDON, P. J., D. R. LITTMAN, M. GODFREY, D. E. MADDON, L. CHESS & R. AXEL. 1985. Cell **42**: 93-104.
6. CLARK, S. J., W. A. JEFFERIES, A. N. BARCLAY, J. GAGNON & A. F. WILLIAMS. 1987. Proc. Natl. Acad. Sci. USA **84**: 1649-1653.
7. LANDAU, N. R., M. WARTON & D. R. LITTMAN. 1988. Nature (London) **334**: 159-162.
8. PETERSON, A. & B. SEED. 1988. Cell **54**: 65-72.
9. CLAYTON, L. K., R. E. HUSSEY, R. STEINBRICH, H. RAMACHANDRAN, Y. HUSAIN & E. L. REINHERZ. 1988. Nature (London) **335**: 363-366.
10. MIZUKAMI, T., T. R. FUERST, E. A. BERGER & B. MOSS. 1988. Proc. Natl. Acad. Sci. USA **85**: 9273-9277.
11. ARTHOS, J., K. C. DEEN, M. A. CHAIKIN, J. A. FORNWALD, Q. J. SATTENTAU, P. R. CLAPHAM, R. A. WEISS, J. S. McDOUGAL, C. PIETROPAOLO, R. AXEL, A. TRUNEH, P. J. MADDON & R. W. SWEET. 1989. Cell **57**: 469-481.
12. LAMARRE, D., A. ASKENAZI, S. FLEURY, D. H. SMITH, R. P. SEKALY & D. J. CAPON. 1989. Science **245**: 743-746.
13. LIFSON, J. D., K. M. HWANG, P. J. NARA, B. FRASER, M. PADGETT, N. M. DUNLOP & L. E. EIDEN. 1988. Science **241**: 712-716.
14. NARA, P. J., K. M. HWANG, D. M. RAUSCH, J. D. LIFSON & L. E. EIDEN. 1989. Proc. Natl. Acad. Sci. USA **86**: 7139-7143.

15. SATTENTAU, Q. J., J. ARTHOS, K. C. DEEN, N. HANNA, D. HEALY, C. L. P. BEVERLY, R. W. SWEET & A. TRUNEH. 1989. J. Exp. Med. **170:** 1319-1334.
16. CHAO, B. H., D. S. COSTOPOULOS, T. CURIEL, J. M. BERTONIS, P. CHISHOLM, C. WILLIAMS, R. T. SCHOOLEY, J. J. ROSA, R. A. FISHER & J. M. MARAGANORE. 1989. J. Biol. Chem. **264:** 5182-5186.
17. CAMERINI, D. & B. SEED. 1990. Cell **60:** 747-754.
18. EPP, O., E. E. LATTMAN, M. SCHIFFER, R. HUBER & W. PALM. 1975. Biochemistry **14:** 4943-4952.
19. ROSSMAN, M. G., E. ARNOLD, J. W. ERICKSON, E. A. FRANKENBERGER, J. P. GRIFFITH, H.-J. HECHT, J. E. JOHNSON, G. KRAMER, M. LUO, A. G. MOSSSER, R. R. RUECKERT, B. SHERRY & G. VRIEND. 1985. Nature **317:** 145-152.

Peptides Derived from the CDR3-Homologous Domain of the CD4 Molecule Are Specific Inhibitors of HIV-1 and SIV Infection, Virus-Induced Cell Fusion, and Postinfection Viral Transmission *in Vitro*

Implications for the Design of Small-Peptide Anti-HIV Therapeutic Agents[a]

D. M. RAUSCH,[b,j] K. M. HWANG,[c] M. PADGETT,[b]
A.-H. VOLTZ,[b] A. RIVAS,[d] E. ENGLEMAN,[d]
I. GASTON,[e] M. McGRATH,[e] B. FRASER,[f]
V. S. KALYANARAMAN,[g] P. L. NARA,[h]
N. DUNLOP,[h] L. MARTIN,[i] M. MURPHEY-CORB,[i]
TRACY KIBORT,[c] J. D. LIFSON,[c] AND L. E. EIDEN[b,j]

[a] A portion of this work was supported by Grants CA 24607 and AI 25922 from the National Institutes of Health to the laboratory of E. Engleman and to Genelabs, Inc. L. E. Eiden acknowledges the support of the Intramural AIDS Targeted Antiviral Program, NIH, and additional funding from the Office of the Director, ADAMHA.
[b] Laboratory of Cell Biology, National Institute of Mental Health, Bethesda, Maryland 20892.
[c] Genelabs, Inc., Redwood City, California.
[d] Stanford University Blood Center, Palo Alto, California.
[e] San Francisco General Hospital, University of California at San Francisco, San Francisco, California.
[f] Center for Biologics Evaluation and Research, Food and Drug Administration, Bethesda, Maryland.
[g] Bionetics Research, Inc., Rockville, Maryland.
[h] Laboratory of Tumor Cell Biology, National Cancer Institute, Frederick, Maryland.
[i] Delta Primate Center, Tulane University, Covington, Louisiana.
[j] Address for correspondence: Lee Eiden, Ph.D., and Dianne M. Rausch, Ph.D., Building 36, Room 3A-17, NIMH, Bethesda, MD 20892.

125

INTRODUCTION

The acquired immunodeficiency syndrome (AIDS) is currently epidemic in the United States, Central Africa, Europe, and the Caribbean, and has been reported elsewhere throughout the world.[1,2] AIDS consists in infection by the human immunodeficiency virus (HIV),[3-5] which causes T-helper/inducer cell depletion[6-8] and immune dysfunction leading to increased risk of secondary opportunistic infection, sustained weight loss, and encephalomyelitis manifested in many cases in a change in mental status and motor and cognitive function (AIDS dementia complex; ADC).[6-13] It is now appreciated that the cells infected with the AIDS virus are primarily the T-helper/inducer cell population depleted in the course of the disease,[14,15] and cells of the monocyte/macrophage lineage.[16-18] The latter were identified as a viral reservoir by visualization of viral protein products and viral RNA in situ, and by virus rescue from tissue, including brain and lung, rich in these infected cells.[16-20] Macrophages, like helper-inducer T lymphocytes, possess the surface antigen CD4, which appears to function as the receptor through which HIV gains entry to these two cell populations.[21-25] As proof, the envelope glycoprotein gp120 of HIV binds with relatively high affinity to the CD4 molecule in direct in vitro binding experiments.[26] Also, CD4-directed and gp120-directed antisera that block HIV infection of CD4-positive lymphocytes and monocyte/macrophages block as well the direct binding of gp120 to CD4 on cells or in soluble form.[21-27]

In addition to providing a receptor for viral entry into two critical populations of immune cells, CD4 appears to be important in the cytopathogenic sequelae of HIV infection, namely the formation of multinucleated giant cells through fusion of HIV-infected, gp120-bearing infected cells, and noninfected CD4-positive "bystander" cells.[28,29] Gp120/CD4 interactions may be further involved in HIV-induced immune dysfunction subsequent to infection: in vitro data[30] suggest that gp120 released from HIV may bind to CD4-positive cells and target them for antibody-dependent cell-mediated cytotoxicity. Gp120 may also directly block CD4-dependent immune responses.[31] These include recognition of foreign antigen on the surface of antigen-presenting cells by cytotoxic T cells and by T-helper/inducer cells that stimulate proliferation and antibody production by B lymphocytes.[32,33] Finally, CD4 may be important in the transmission of virus from the monocyte reservoir to activated T lymphocytes at the end of the latency period of HIV infection, and preceding the development of manifest AIDS, because anti-CD4 antibodies are capable of blocking viral transmission from latently infected macrophages to T lymphocytes in culture (M. McGrath et al., unpublished observations).

The CD4 antigen, therefore, has a central role in all stages of HIV infection and disease, and the CD4-gp120 interaction is an important potential therapeutic target. Attacking this interaction from the point of view of CD4 rather than gp120 is a rational strategy because the gp120 protein is highly variable from one infected individual to the next and even across serial viral isolates from the same individual,[34-38] whereas CD4 is constrained from structural mutation by its dominant functional role in the immune system. Therefore an "antireceptor"[39] or "receptor decoy"[40] strategy is appropriate and indeed has been adopted using both CD4-derived synthetic peptides and synthesis of fragments of the CD4 molecule by eukaryotic cells programmed through transfection of appropriate recombinant DNA.[41-50] Although such a strategy could potentially assure a broad spectrum therapy with respect to HIV-1, -2, and variants compared to vaccine-type strategies, the major challenge in antireceptor therapy is achieving specificity in the blockade of viral infection while minimizing interference in CD4 function, which itself could result in iatrogenic immunodeficiency.[51,52] The following report summarizes our progress to date in the characterization of a gp120/CD4 interaction site within a small region of the CDR3-homologous domain of the CD4 molecule, using a synthetic peptide approach. Antiretroviral potency, spectrum, and mechanism(s) of action of several prototype CD4 peptides are described, as well as the relative specificity of these peptides to inhibit virus-CD4 interaction, compared to inhibition of CD4-dependent immune functions such as alloantigen stimulation of T lymphocytes and T-cell mediated cytotoxicity. Finally, we will briefly and preliminarily describe the toxicity, pharmacokinetics, and effects on immune parameters of a prototype CD4 peptide administered during SIV infection of four rhesus macaques.

USE OF SYNTHETIC PEPTIDES TO SCAN THE CD4 MOLECULE FOR gp120 INTERACTION DOMAINS

Our rationale for the synthesis of a set of 10-25-residue peptides comprising the entire extracellular domain of the CD4 molecule was to assay these peptides as inhibitors of HIV-induced cell fusion in order to define the region(s) of CD4 critical for interaction with the HIV gp120 envelope glycoprotein. Identification of peptides derived from CD4 that inhibit HIV infection or fusion would unambiguously identify a gp120 binding site(s) of CD4. By contrast, site-directed mutagenesis of the CD4 molecule, and bioassay of viral receptor patency of the mutagenized receptor molecule, allows identification of regions of the CD4 molecule that are either directly involved in binding of gp120 or are important in maintaining the conformation of the binding site for gp120, which could be physically distant from the site of mutagenesis.[53–59]

We initially tested crude, that is, partially purified synthetic peptides, which contain an array of partially derivatized congeners, more or less randomly constrained in various conformations by the presence of sterically bulky R-protecting groups. When tested as crude (60-90% pure) mixtures, only peptides containing all or most of the CDR3-like region of CD4 [CD4(85-94)] were capable of inhibiting HIV-induced cell fusion and HIV-1 infection (FIG. 1). These peptides, for example, the CD4(74-92) peptide mixture, inhibited fusion only at a relatively high (125 μM) concentration. Inhibition of HIV-induced cell fusion and HIV-1 infection, however, was complete at this concentration, suggesting that competition with cellular CD4 for interaction with the HIV envelope was complete, albeit of relatively low affinity. A peptide of identical amino acid composition but altered sequence, synthesized and partially purified in an identical fashion, was wholly without anti-infective or antifusigenic activity in the two assays employed (FIG. 1). Recently, two separate laboratories, using a similar scanning approach, have identified a unique region of the CD4 molecule from which synthetic peptides that inhibit HIV interaction with CD4 can be derived.[60,61] In each case the active peptide overlapped the CDR3-homologous region of the protein.

CHARACTERIZATION OF A CD4(81-92)-DERIVED PEPTIDE AS AN INHIBITOR OF HIV INFECTION AND HIV-INDUCED CELL FUSION *IN VITRO*

Chromatographic fractionation of the CD4(71-92) peptide mixture revealed that biological activity resided not in the authentic intended peptide, KLIEDSDTYICEV-

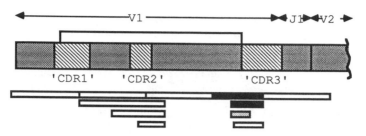

FIGURE 1. Mapping potential sites of CD4/gp120 interaction on the CD4 molecule with CD4-derived synthetic peptides. The N terminus of the CD4 molecule, residues 1-119, comprising the V1J1-homologous region is shown, with the putative cystine bridge between residues 16 and 84 indicated schematically, and the regions analogous to the complementarity-determining hypervariable regions of immunoglobulin light chain indicated with cross-hatching. The V1 region of CD4 shares about 30% sequence identity with human immunoglobulin kappa light chain. Peptides synthesized as semipure, randomly derivatized versions of portions of the CD4 linear sequence are depicted as the narrow bars below the linear sequence of CD4(1-120) and correspond to the region of CD4 directly above them. Bars are clear if the corresponding peptide had no antisyncytial activity (see reference 46) at a concentration of 500 μM, black if the corresponding peptide inhibited HIV-1-induced cell fusion at a nominal concentration of 125 μM or below, and grey if the corresponding peptide had a nominal antiviral potency between 125 and 500 μM.

EDQKEE, but in a side fraction from the synthesis. This fraction was a complex mixture of several peptide components, including peaks upon mass fragmentographic analysis suggestive of contamination with species of molecular weight greater than that of the parent peptide. Such derivatives would be expected from failure to completely remove benzyl or carbobenzoxy protecting groups, among others, from the parent peptide. Two complementary approaches were used to show that partial derivatization of the parent peptide was necessary to impart full biological activity. First, the biologically inactive authentic peptide was deliberately benzylated in solution following synthesis and purification by treatment with alpha-bromoxylene, resulting in restoration of antisyncytial activity comparable to that seen in the initial crude peptide mixture. Second, a deliberately S-benzylated congener of CD4(74-92) was synthesized by employing acid stable benzyl rather than acid-labile para-methylbenzyl protection of cysteine in the tBoc synthesis. Although this peptide was not significantly more potent than the original peptide mixture, it afforded the advantage of a preparation in which oxidation or further reaction of free cysteine in the peptide would not be a complicating factor in stability or postsynthesis generation of additional peptide products. Synthesis of a series of S-benzyl peptides progressively truncated at either the C or N terminus allowed the demonstration of CD4(81-92) as the minimal sequence required for blockade of HIV-induced cell fusion and HIV infection of CD4-positive cells with these crude peptide mixtures. Upon chromatographic fractionation of the S-benzyl-CD4(81-92) peptide mixture, biological activity was again absent from the intended pure peptide TYIC(benzyl)EVEDQKEE, residing instead in a later-eluting peak upon chromatographic development with acetonitrile on a C18 reverse-phase column. Again, the pure, inactive monobenzylated material could be converted to biologically active material by postsynthesis derivatization in solution with alpha-bromoxylene, strongly suggesting that multiple derivatization was required to impart anti-HIV activity to CD4(81-92)-derived peptides.

ANTIVIRAL ACTIVITY OF DERIVATIZED PEPTIDE CONGENERS OF CD4(81-92) IS SEQUENCE AND DERIVATIZED-RESIDUE-SPECIFIC

The requirement for multiple derivatization of the peptide is summarized in FIGURE 2. The most potent compound in this series is derivatized at positions 1,4,5, and 8. The requirements for derivatization are relatively stringent as regards both the nature and position of the derivatized groups. For example, replacement of a benzyl with an acetamidomethyl group at cysteine-4 yields a biologically inactive compound, whereas either acetyl or carbobenzoxy substitution at position 10 enhances activity relative to

	Peptide Sequence	IC100, Fusion
A.	TYICEVEDQKFE	>500 µM
	TYIC$_b$EVEDQKEE	>500 µM
	TYIC$_b$E$_b$VEDQKEE	125 µM
	T$_b$YIC$_b$E$_b$VEDQKEE	63 µM
	T$_b$Y$_b$IC$_b$EVEDQKEE	63 µM
	T$_b$YIC$_b$EVE$_b$DQKEE	>500 µM
	T$_b$YIC$_{acm}$E$_b$VEDQKEE	>500 µM
B.	T$_b$YIC$_b$E$_b$VEDQKEE	63 µM
	T$_b$YIC$_b$E$_b$KVQDEEE	63-132 µM
	T$_b$EYEIKC$_b$QE$_b$DVE	125-250 µM
	T$_b$EVE$_b$IKC$_b$QEDVE	>500 µM
	KEEIC$_b$E$_b$VEDQT$_b$Y	>500 µM
C.	T$_b$YIC$_b$EVE$_b$DQdKEE	32 µM
	T$_b$YdIC$_b$EVE$_b$DQKEE	125 µM
	T$_{bd}$YIC$_b$E$_b$VEDQKEE	250 µM
	acT$_b$YIC$_b$E$_b$VEDQKacEEa	16 µM
	acT$_b$YIC$_b$E$_b$VEDQdKacEEa	16 µM

FIGURE 2. Structure-activity relationships for inhibition of HIV-induced cell fusion in the CD4(81-92) peptide series. Purified (>95%), structurally defined peptides were preincubated with H9 cells chronically infected with HIV-1$_{HXB2}$, and these cells were then cocultured with CD4-positive indicator cells and the extent of cell fusion (syncytium formation) scored as described (see references 28 and 46). Values given are the concentrations of each peptide required to totally abolish syncytium formation in the assay. None of the peptides tested was cytotoxic as assessed by exclusion of vital dye by cells protected from HIV-1 cytopathic effect (syncytium formation) at the end of the assay (24 hours of cocultivation). A. Effects of derivatized residue position, number, and chemical nature on anti-viral potency. B. Sequence specificity of tribenzyl-CD4(81-92) antiviral potency. Shadowed residues are those maintained in the correct sequence relative to CD4(81-92). Note that the degree of peptide sequence "scrambling" progressively increases from the first to the last two members of this series. C. Effects of structural modifications aimed at increasing peptide stability (inhibiting biotransformation) on antiviral potency of tribenzyl-CD4(81-92). Peptide sequences are given in the single-letter amino acid code (T, thr; Y, tyr; I, ile; C, cys; E, glu; V, val; D, asp; Q, gln; K, lys). Other abbreviations: b, benzylation of the preceding amino acid; acm, acetamidomethyl derivatization; D, indicates that the amino acid following is the D isomer; ac, N-acetylation; a, C-terminal amidation. A portion of these data are taken from Kalyanaraman et al.[65a]

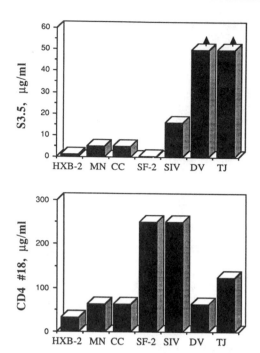

FIGURE 3. Cell fusion induced by various isolates of HIV-1 and by SIV is differentially inhibited by anti-CD4 monoclonal antibody S3.5 and $T_1C_4E_5$-tribenzyl-K_{10}-acetyl-CD4(81-92) [peptide #18]. Human T-lymphoblastoid cell lines chronically infected with HIV-1 isolates HXB-2, MN, CC, SF-2, DV or TJ, or SIV_{SM} were incubated with various concentrations of peptide or monoclonal antibody in a twofold dilution series from less than 0.1 to 50 (antibody) or 1000 (peptide) μg/mL for approximately 30 min at room temperature. Aliquots of 50,000 cells were then added to an equal number of uninfected CD4-positive indicator cells in 96-well culture dishes, and syncytia were scored after 24 hours of coculture exactly as described in reference 28 with the modifications described in 46. Shown is the concentration of antibody or peptide in μg/mL required to give complete blockade of syncytium formation for each isolate tested. Arrows over the bars for DV and TJ in the upper graph indicate that S3.5, which is a Leu3a-directed anti-CD4 monoclonal antibody cross-reacting with anti-Leu3a, completely failed to inhibit syncytium formation at the highest dose tested (50 μg/mL) when syncytium formation was induced by addition of cells chronically infected with the HIV-1 isolates DV and TJ.

the parent tribenzylated compound. It is of interest that with benzylation at positions 1 and 4 fixed, positioning the third benzyl group at either tyrosine-2 or glutamic acid-5 produces equally active compounds, whereas removal of the benzyl group to glutamic acid-7 affords a completely inactive compound. These results suggest that whereas conformation can be optimized by derivatization at multiple residues, some residues, such as the glutamic acid at position 7 (CD4-87), cannot be derivatized at all, perhaps because this residue is directly involved in contact with the gp120 molecule during virus binding and infection of CD4-positive cells.

A second set of syntheses involved altering the primary sequence of CD4(81-92), keeping the amino acid composition, and specific residues derivatized, constant (FIG. 2). These experiments suggest that sequence specificity is most critical in the core sequence TYICEVE. Once again, it is not clear if this is because the N-terminal heptapeptide contains a portion of the gp120 binding site, or if the binding site, within the C-terminal half of the molecule, must be positioned correctly by the derivatized sequence at the N terminus. Currently, the most potent compound examined is $T_1C_4E_5$-tribenzyl, K_{10}-acetyl-CD4(81-92)[peptide #18]. C-terminal amidation, as well as N-terminal acetylation, are maneuvers that should improve peptide stability *in vivo*. Both are tolerated without loss of biological activity relative to the stem compound #18 (D.M. Rausch *et al.*, in preparation). Several d-to-l amino acid substitutions are also tolerated without loss of antiviral potency or efficacy in the stem compound, so that a considerably longer-lived peptide than #18 (serum half-life in rhesus macaque is less than 1 hour) should be obtainable.

CD4(81-92) PEPTIDES EXHIBIT ANTIVIRAL ACTIVITY AGAINST A WIDE VARIETY OF CD4-DEPENDENT RETROVIRUSES

Peptide #18 is a potent inhibitor of fusion for several isolates of HIV-1 as well as SIV_{SM}, a simian CD4-dependent immunodeficiency-inducing retrovirus[62,69] (FIG. 3). Interestingly, peptide #18 blocks cell fusion induced by several isolates of HIV-1 whose cytopathic (syncytial-forming) effects are relatively refractory to blockade by the antibody S3.5, a neutralizing anti-CD4 antibody that recognizes the Leu3a epitope.[63] Peptides in this series are also inhibitors of HIV infection in suspension culture, although in this case peptides clearly block HIV infection more potently than infection with SIV_{SMM} (strain Delta B670) (FIG. 4). Peptides of the CDR3-like domain of human CD4 are also inhibitors of HIV-2 infection *in vitro*.[46] In addition, CD4(81-92) peptide derivatives inhibit fusion between macrophages infected with HIV and lymphocytes, indicating that this aspect of infection and viral transmission, which may be important in the progression of AIDS *in vivo*, is also potentially blockable with these antiviral peptides (TABLE 1). CD4(81-92) peptide derivatives appear to be specific for inhibition of CD4-dependent retroviruses and exhibited little or no inhibition of HTLV-I-induced

TABLE 1. $T_1C_4E_5$-Tribenzyl-CD4(81-92) Inhibits Fusion of Chronically HIV-1 Infected Macrophages with Uninfected T Lymphocytes[a]

	Percent Inhibition of Scored Syncytia	
GLH328, μmol/L	Donor #1	Donor #2
10	0	12
50	12	22
100	97	57
250	100	100
500	100	100

[a] Macrophages isolated from two separate donors were infected with $HIV-1_{DV}$ as described by Crowe *et al.*[19] and maintained in culture for 36 (donor 1) or 42 (donor 2) days. Chronically infected macrophages were then cocultivated with CD4-positive VB lymphoblastoid indicator cells in the presence or absence of peptide. The number of syncytia (multinucleated giant cells) per well were counted, and data were expressed as percent inhibition of scored syncytia, *i.e.*, 100 − [(number of syncytia per experimental well/mean number of syncytia in control wells) × 100)].

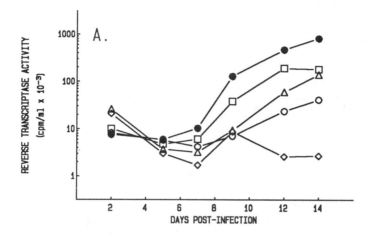

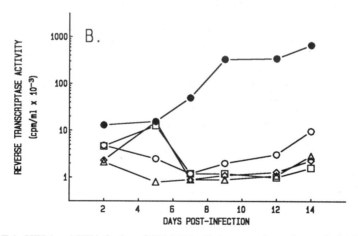

FIGURE 4. HIV-1 and SIV infection of CEM-174 cells in suspension culture: relative inhibition by $T_1C_4E_5$-tribenzyl-CD4(81-92) [GLH328] and $T_1C_4E_5$-tribenzyl-K_{10}-acetyl-CD4(81-92) [#18]. Titered frozen stocks of HIV-1$_{HTLV-IIIB}$ or SIV$_{SM/B670}$ were thawed and used to infect CEM-174 cells previously treated with 25 μg/mL DEAE-dextran and washed with medium. Following a 60 minute viral inoculation period at 37 °C, in the presence or absence of peptide, cells were diluted into fresh culture medium with or without the appropriate concentrations of peptide and aliquoted into 48-well culture dishes. Half of the culture medium was removed every 2-3 days for reverse transcriptase measurement and replaced with fresh medium with or without peptide. Data shown are the mean ± SEM of triplicate determinations. Unconditioned medium spiked with peptide was negative in the reverse transcriptase assay. **A:** SIV$_{B670}$; **B:** HIV-1$_{HTLV-IIIB}$. Closed circles, no peptide; open circles, 250 μM GLH328; diamonds, 250 μM #18; triangles, 125 μM #18; squares, 62.5 μM #18. A portion of these data are taken from Kalyanaraman et al.[65a]

syncytium formation at doses that completely block HIV-1-induced syncytium formation and HIV-1 infection *in vitro* (TABLE 2). These data are consistent with the proposed mechanism of action of CD4(81-92) peptide derivatives, which is blockade of CD4/gp120 interaction by binding to gp120 at the site normally occupied by the CDR3-like domain of CD4 during both infection and HIV-induced cell fusion (see below).

CD4(81-92) PEPTIDES DO NOT INHIBIT CD4-DEPENDENT CELLULAR IMMUNE FUNCTIONS *IN VITRO*

The success of an antireceptor strategy for the design of inhibitors of CD4-dependent retrovirus infection and pathogenesis depends on identifying a peptide region of

TABLE 2. Peptides #18 and #30 Do Not Block HTLV-1-Induced Syncytium Formation at Concentrations That Completely Inhibit HIV-1-Induced Syncytium Formation[a]

Compound	Concentration (μg/mL)	Syncytia/20 fields (200 $\times$)
#18	32	56
	16	90
	8	90
	4	74
#30	32	18
	16	88
	8	80
	4	108
none		64

[a] Chronically HTLV-1-infected lymphoid cells were cocultured with X/C indicator cells for 18-24 hours as described[46] and syncytia per 20 fields counted at 200 $\times$ magnification. Syncytia were defined as multinucleated (4 or more nuclei) structures bounded by a single continuous plasma membrane. Both peptide #18 [$T_1C_4E_5$-tribenzyl-K_{10}-acetyl-CD4(81-92)] and peptide #30 [N-alpha-acetyl-$T_1C_4E_5$-tribenzyl-K_{10}-acetyl-CD4(81-92) amide] inhibit HIV-1$_{HXB-2}$-induced syncytium formation in a dose-dependent manner, with complete inhibition of HIV-1-induced giant cell formation at 32 μg/mL.

the CD4 molecule large enough to mimic the binding domain for gp120, but sufficiently small that other ligands of the CD4 receptor, such as those involved in class II MHC-dependent antigen recognition by T-cell receptor/CD4-positive cells, do not bind the peptide, because this could result in blockade of immune function and potential immunodeficiency even in the absence of HIV infection. Accordingly, the ability of potent peptide inhibitors of HIV infection, such as CD4(81-92) peptides #18 and #30, were assayed for their ability to block a variety of CD4-dependent cellular immune functions. CD4(81-92) peptides do not inhibit the mixed lymphocyte response, which is blocked by the anti-CD4 antibody anti-Leu3a, at doses that effectively block HIV-1 infection and HIV-1-induced cell fusion (TABLE 3). The CD4-dependent cytotoxic T-cell response, also blocked by anti-Leu3a, was likewise unaffected by the presence of peptides

TABLE 3. Peptides #18 and #30 Do Not Block the CD4-Dependent Mixed Lymphocyte Response (MLR)[a]

Peptide/Antibody, μg/mL		Response mean cpm $\times$ 10^{-3}			
		D1 $\times$ S1	D1 $\times$ S2	D2 $\times$ S1	D2 $\times$ S2
none		45.1	57.6	38.5	45.5
#18	3.12	43.9	54.8	37.5	32.5
	6.25	46.6	57.2	32.4	41.6
	12.5	53.8	54.9	35.4	47.4
	25	56.4	60.6	41.5	48.2
	50	45.9	57.0	44.1	47.3
	100	41.7	53.6	28.7	35.8
#30	3.12	48.3	58.9	35.4	45.2
	6.25	47.4	46.2	44.4	46.3
	12.5	41.9	52.3	35.7	40.0
	25	42.6	51.3	38.7	39.8
	50	51.2	59.1	26.5	47.9
	100	43.1	55.3	28.8	36.3
anti-Leu3a	3.12	16.4	39.3	2.5	22.4
	6.25	14.2	37.1	4.7	23.9
	12.5	7.4	40.2	4.9	13.0
	25	7.8	40.4	3.5	15.2
	50	7.1	27.7	3.4	16.1
	100	6.2	29.4	2.4	9.8

[a] Data shown are the proliferative responses ([3H]thymidine incorporation) of nonirradiated PBMCs (donor cells) from each of two individuals, D1 and D2, in the presence of lethally x-irradiated PBMCs (stimulator cells) from each of two additional individuals, S1 and S2, who were MHC-allogeneic to D1 and D2. anti-Leu3a, anti-CD4 monoclonal antibody anti-Leu3a.

#18 and #30 at doses sufficient to block HIV infection and syncytium formation (TABLE 4). These data indicate that administration of CD4(81-92) peptide would not be expected to result in iatrogenic immunodeficiency. In addition, they suggest that passive immunization strategies, or administration of CD4 antibodies to generate an anti-idiotypic antibody response capable of blocking HIV infection by binding gp120 itself, may be better focused on antibodies directed to the CDR3-like domain of CD4, rather than the CDR2-like domain, which is recognized by antibodies like anti-Leu3a that also block CD4-dependent cellular immune responses.

CD4(81-92) PEPTIDES ACT BY INHIBITING gp120/CD4 BINDING AND DEFINE A PROBABLE gp120 BINDING SITE ON THE CD4 MOLECULE

Structure-activity analysis (FIG. 2) has established the sequence- and derivatized residue-specificity of CD4(81-92) peptide action in inhibiting HIV infection and cell fusion. Antiviral potency is also restricted to CD4-dependent retroviruses (TABLE 2). The mechanism by which this specific antiviral effect of CD4(81-92) peptides is exerted is likely to be relevant to understanding the molecular details of CD4/gp120 interaction in HIV infection and pathogenesis. The high-affinity binding of gp120 to CD4-positive cells can be demonstrated using metabolically labeled [^{35}S]gp120 obtained from a cell line that overproduces the envelope glycoprotein or by binding of purified gp120 iodinated by way of the iodogen reaction.[64,65] Using either method, inhibition of gp120 binding to CD4-positive cells by CD4(81-92) peptide derivatives can be demonstrated.[65a] FIGURE 5 shows a typical gp120 blocking experiment employing ^{35}S-labeled gp120 as the CD4 ligand. In these experiments, the gp120 bound to CD4 is rescued after cell solubilization by immunoprecipitation with OKT4, as described originally by McDougal *et al.*,[23] and quantified by autoradiography after electrophoresis on polyacrylamide gels.[65] Peptides that inhibit HIV infection and HIV-induced cell fusion completely (125 and 250 μM T$_1$C$_4$E$_5$-tribenzyl-CD4(81-92) and 250 μM T4DTEbzl) also totally blocked gp120/CD4 interaction. Peptides that inhibit HIV infection and fusion only partially (125 μM T4DTEbzl) also partially blocked gp120/ CD4 binding. Control peptides such as GGa23, a neuropeptide with a net charge similar to that of CD4(81-92) and totally without antiviral activity, also failed to block gp120/CD4 binding (FIG. 5).

In principle, inhibition of CD4/gp120 interaction by CD4(81-92) peptide derivatives could be due either to direct binding to gp120, or to peptide binding to CD4 itself, altering its conformation and indirectly preventing gp120 binding. Preliminary kinetic analysis of inhibition of gp120/CD4 binding by CD4(81-92) peptides suggests competitive kinetics, favoring a model in which peptides bind to gp120 and block its attachment to CD4 (Kalyanaraman *et al.*, submitted). There is no precedent for CD4 intramolecular self-association leading to conformational exclusion of gp120 binding, and if such

TABLE 4. Peptides #18 and #30 Do Not Block CD4-Dependent, MHC Class II-Restricted Cytotoxic T-Lymphocyte Activity

Peptide/Antibody, μg/mL		^{51}Cr release, percent of untreated control
#18	1.56	106
	3.12	109
	6.25	100
	12.5	101
	25	93
	50	104
	100	104
#30	1.56	107
	3.12	108
	6.25	97
	12.5	97
	25	94
	50	93
	100	96
anti-Leu3a	1.56	101
	3.12	101
	6.25	104
	12.5	76
	25	57
	50	29
	100	1.4

a conformational shift occurred, it would be expected to block binding of neutralizing antibodies such as anti-Leu3a and CD4 ligands such as class II MHC to the CD4 molecule. Neither of these things occurs in the presence of even high concentrations of tribenzyl-CD4(81-92). In the absence of direct evidence for CD4(81-92) peptide binding to gp120, and not CD4, the possibility that CD4(81-92) peptides inhibit gp120/CD4 association by binding to CD4 itself remains viable. Nevertheless, it seems most likely that the CDR3-like domain of the CD4 molecule, or the portion of it between residues 85 and 92, constitutes a critical part of the binding surface for gp120 on the CD4 molecule. If so, passive immunization, vaccination, and anti-idiotypic strategies for immune protection from HIV infection and pathogenesis should be focused on this

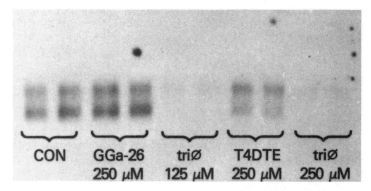

FIGURE 5. Gp120 binding to CD4 is specifically inhibited by $T_1C_4E_5$-tribenzyl-CD4(81-92). HIV-1$_{HTLV-IIIB}$-infected 6D5$_{451}$ cells, which constitutively secrete HIV-1 envelope glycoproteins gp120 and gp160, were metabolically labeled with [^{35}S]methionine, and cell culture medium containing labeled gp120 and gp160 was collected, concentrated, and incubated with CD4-positive CEM$_{50}$ cells as described[64,65] in the presence or absence of the indicated concentrations of peptide. CD4-envelope glycoprotein complexes were solubilized from the cell suspension and collected by immunoprecipitation with OKT4. The precipitate was solubized, denatured, and electrophoresed on a polyacrylamide gel, and the gel was autoradiographed. The intensity of the autoradiographic signal is directly proportional to the amount of gp120 and gp160 specifically bound to CD4, because no signal is detected in the presence of excess unlabeled gp120. CON, no peptide present during the binding experiment; GGa-26, rat pancreastatin, a glutamic acid-rich peptide; triø, $T_1C_4E_5$-tribenzyl-CD4(81-92); T4DTE, partially purified S-benzyl-CD4(81-92). The potencies of these peptides to inhibit HIV-1-induced syncytium formation are > 500 μM (not active), 63 μM, and 200 μM, respectively.

region of the CD4 molecule, in addition to those regions that are defined by *in vitro* mutagenesis studies as being critical for gp120 binding, but not necessarily by constituting a gp120 binding site at the mutagenized locus.

VIROSTATIC ACTIVITY OF CD4(81-92) PEPTIDES

If CD4(81-92) peptide derivatives bind directly to gp120, then these peptides may block other stages of the viral life cycle besides infection and cell fusion. For example, peptide binding to gp120 or gp160 could inhibit viral assembly and decrease the yield of infectious viral progeny from already-infected cells. Peptide effects on postinfection steps in the virus life cycle leading to decreased infectiousness were measured by a modification of the syncytium-forming microassay of Nara *et al.*,[66,67] as depicted in FIGURE 6. Several CD4(81-92) peptide derivatives were tested in this assay and compared to the activity of anti-CD4 antibodies. $T_1C_4E_5$-tribenzyl-CD4(81-92) blocks syncytium formation when added during infection by blocking infection itself, as evidenced by subsequent lack of formation of infectious cell centers (ICCs) from these treated cells, and blocks syncytium formation of already-infected cells when added 48 hours postinfection without decreasing the infectiousness of these cells, as evidenced by high levels of p24 in culture supernatant at the end of the 120 hour culture period and the ability of infected cells to form infectious cell centers on fresh indicator cells once they are washed free of peptide. The anti-CD4 monoclonal antibodies S3.5 and anti-Leu3a, like tribenzyl-CD4(81-92), concomitantly block syncytium formation, p24 production, and infectious cell-center formation when added from 0-48 hours, but block only syncytium formation, without affecting p24 production or infectious cell-center formation, when added from 48-120 (ref. 47 and D. M. Rausch, unpublished observations). By contrast, the CD4(81-92) peptide #18, a charge-modified version of tribenzyl-CD4(81-92), inhibits not only syncytium formation but also formation of infectious cell centers from cells treated with peptide 48 hours postinfection (FIG. 7). This decrease in the infectiousness of already virally infected cells by these CD4(81-92) peptide derivatives is accompanied by a corresponding decrease in release of viral progeny from infected cells (FIG. 7B) and is due neither to toxicity to the CD4+ cells nor to failure to adequately remove the peptide prior to assay for ICCs (see ref. 47 for supporting data). Thus, some analogues in the CD4(81-92) series appear to possess the ability to reduce viral load of already-infected cells. This property correlates in a general way with the hydrophobicity of the compounds, suggesting that the mechanism of this antiviral effect may be peptide binding to gp160 or gp120 within the infected cell, interfering with viral assembly at some as yet unknown stage, and that more hydrophobic versions of CD4(81-92) are more efficient at entering the infected cell than less hydrophobic peptides.

PRELIMINARY TEST OF THE PHARMACOKINETICS, SAFETY, AND EFFICACY OF $T_1C_4E_5$-TRIBENZYL-CD4(81-92) IN SIV-INFECTED RHESUS MACAQUES

CD4(81-92) peptide derivatives inhibit HIV-1, HIV-2, and SIV infection of CD4-positive cells *in vitro* and inhibit HIV-and SIV-induced syncytium formation as well. In addition, CD4(81-92) peptide derivatives appear to have a virostatic component to their antiviral action that is not shared by, for example, antibodies that block both HIV-1 infection and syncytium formation (FIG. 7). Despite their efficacy *in vitro*, however, CD4(81-92) peptide derivatives are active only at relatively high concentrations. In addition, despite the apparent lack of toxicity of prototype compounds such as $T_1C_4E_5$-tribenzyl-CD4(81-92) and $T_1C_4E_5$-tribenzyl-K_{10}-acetyl-CD4(81-92) even at high doses in rodent models (Hwang *et al.*, unpublished observations), toxic effects of peptide administration must be assessed in primates, and if possible, in a primate model approximating the compromised health and potential vulnerability to xenobiotics of the HIV-infected patient. For these reasons, we have preliminarily assessed the tolerance of

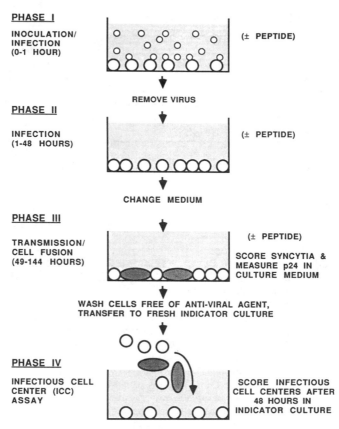

PHASE I

INOCULATION/
INFECTION
(0-1 HOUR)

(± PEPTIDE)

REMOVE VIRUS

PHASE II

INFECTION
(1-48 HOURS)

(± PEPTIDE)

CHANGE MEDIUM

PHASE III

TRANSMISSION/
CELL FUSION
(49-144 HOURS)

(± PEPTIDE)

SCORE SYNCYTIA &
MEASURE p24 IN
CULTURE MEDIUM

WASH CELLS FREE OF ANTI-VIRAL AGENT,
TRANSFER TO FRESH INDICATOR CULTURE

PHASE IV

INFECTIOUS CELL
CENTER (ICC)
ASSAY

SCORE INFECTIOUS
CELL CENTERS AFTER
48 HOURS IN
INDICATOR CULTURE

FIGURE 6. Kinetic phases of CEM-SS quantitative syncytial-forming microassay for HIV infection, transmission, and cell infectiousness. CD4-positive, syncytium-sensitive CEM cells were exposed to a titered inoculum of cell-free virus for one hour, after which virus was removed from the cells and replaced with fresh medium. During the period of inoculation, infection of CEM cells began, and the virus was presumably internalized and reverse-transcribed shortly thereafter. Over the next 48 hours, transcription from the integrated viral genome produced both genomic and messenger RNA, and viral proteins required for virus assembly and packaging were produced. No viral gag protein appeared in cell supernatant at this time, however, and no syncytial centers were visible, indicating that although infection was complete, cell fusion and release of viral progeny from infected cells had not yet occurred.[47,68] At this time, medium was changed, and cells were maintained for an additional 72 hours in culture. During this time, the appearance of the cells was monitored for the appearance of focal syncytia, indicating the presence of single infected cells, beginning the process of syncytium formation with their uninfected neighbors. Simultaneously, p24 core antigen in culture supernatants was measured as an index of the release of infectious viral progeny. Cells were then washed to remove test agents if present, and an aliquot of the cell suspension plated onto fresh indicator cells to assess their ability to form syncytia (infectious cell centers; ICCs). Each syncytium (ICC) thus formed represented a cell originally infected in the 120 hour syncytium-forming assay, which retained its infectiousness, *i.e.,* ability to undergo HIV-induced syncytium formation with neighboring cells. Using this experimental paradigm, peptides (and other antiviral agents) can be added to the cultures during inoculation and infection (0-48 hours) or during viral transmission by way of cell fusion and release of viral progeny (48-120 hours), in order to assess their relative ability to inhibit infection and HIV-induced cell fusion, respectively. By subsequently measuring ICCs in those cultures where inhibition of fusion (following 48-120 hour exposure to antiviral agent) occurred, assessment of virostatic activity (postinfection attentuation of viral transmission by infected cells) can also be made.

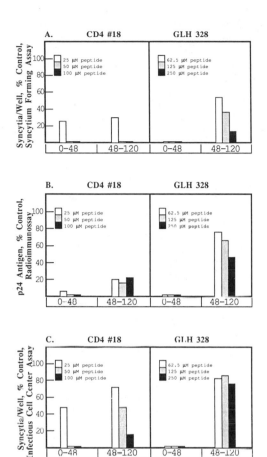

FIGURE 7. Anti-infective, antisyncytial, and virostatic activities of $T_1C_4E_5$-tribenzyl-CD4(81-92) [GLH328] and $T_1C_4E_5$-tribenzyl-K_{10}-acetyl-CD4(81-92) [#18]. CEM-SS cells were treated with CD4 peptide GLH328, or CD4 peptide #18 during the infection (0-48 hours) or transmission (48-120 hours) phases of the syncytium-forming assay. The viral inoculum was a thawed titered stock of HIV-$1_{\text{HTLV IIIB}}$. In **A** the concentration of peptide is plotted against the number of syncytia formed at the end of the assay, which indicates anti-infective potency when the antiviral agent is present during infection (0-48 hours) and indicates antisyncytial potency when the antiviral agent is added postinfection (48-120 hours). In **B** the concentration of peptide is plotted against the amount of p24 released into the cell culture supernatant during the period from 48 hours (when p24 levels are undetectable in control-infected cultures) to 120 hours (when p24 levels are approximately 200 ng/well in control-infected cultures). A decrease in p24 levels caused by peptide present from 0-48 hours indicates a direct anti-infective antiviral activity of the peptide, whereas a decrease in p24 levels caused by peptide present from 48-120 hours indicates a virostatic antiviral activity of the peptide. In **C** the concentration of peptide is plotted against the number of syncytia formed in the infectious cell center assay (ICC) following cell washing and replating on to fresh indicator cells. The ICC confirms the anti-infective potency when the antiviral agent is present during infection (0-48 hours) and indicates the virostatic potency when the antiviral agent is added postinfection (48-120 hours). Values shown are duplicate determinations from two separate experiments. A portion of these data are taken from Nara *et al.*[47]

SIV-infected rhesus macaques to chronic administration of $T_1C_4E_5$-tribenzyl-CD4(81-92) (GLH328). This compound was employed, although it is not the most potent CD4(81-92) peptide derivative screened to date (see FIG. 4), because of availability of rodent toxicity and pharmacokinetic data, and because it was the only CD4(81-92) peptide derivative active against SIV *in vitro* for which a reliable assay for serum peptide concentration was available at the time this study was begun (January 1989). In order to obtain a preliminary assessment of potential efficacy of this compound, GLH328 was administered concomitantly with SIV inoculation in four juvenile rhesus macaques and with three untreated animals serving as age- and inoculum-matched controls. The virus employed was $SIV_{SM/B670}$, an SIV isolate previously characterized as causing AIDS in juvenile rhesus macaques with a fatal outcome within 7 months in the majority of cases when administered at the dose employed in this study.[70,71] Peptide was infused at a basal rate of 200 mg/hour (2.5 kg animals were used) for 10 hours, with bolus injections of 200 mg/8 min immediately before, after, and 1 hour after virus inoculation, which occurred one hour after the beginning of basal peptide infusion. Plasma levels of the compound obtained during the ten-hour period following virus inoculation are shown in FIGURE 8. Peptide was administered as a bolus injection of 200 mg/animal weekly/biweekly for an additional 28 weeks, at which time surviving animals were untreated but monitored for viral antigenemia and signs of viral disease. No untoward effects of peptide infusion attributable to the peptide itself, as assessed by standard blood chemistry profile, were observed during infusion or subsequently (Martin *et al.,* unpublished observations). The course of CD4/4B4$^+$ cell depletion, and viral antigenemia for each of the seven animals in the study, is shown in FIGURE 9, along with the survival curves for the untreated and peptide-treated groups. Animals were euthanized when life expectancy was estimated to be less than one week, due to chronic weight loss or diarrhea due either primarily to virally induced syncytial disease or secondary to severe opportunistic infection (see refs. 71, 72). No evidence for blockade of viral infection was obtained; however, peptide treatment appeared to attenuate the lethal course of B670 infection: the mean individual survival postinoculation for each group is at present 248 days for the peptide-treated and 168 days for the control untreated group. Effectiveness of antiviral therapy with CD4(81-92) peptide derivatives may be a function of several factors, including treatment time following viral inoculation, differential peptide potency in blocking SIV infection of CD4-positive target cells *in vivo* compared to blockade of infection *in vitro,* virostatic as well as anti-infective activity of the peptide employed, and pharmacokinetics of peptide delivery to tissue compartments in which viral infection initially occurs.

FUTURE DIRECTIONS

Administration of tribenzyl-CD4(81-92) concurrently with SIV inoculation increased the mean postinoculation survival time of SIV-infected macaques, but did not block virus infection. The interaction between SIV and the rhesus CD4 receptor may not accurately model the interaction between HIV and the human CD4 receptor in the evaluation of human CD4-based peptide therapy, as indicated by the immunological nonidentity of human and rhesus CD4[72] and the higher concentrations of both CD4(81-92) peptide derivatives and soluble CD4 itself required to block SIV infection, relative to HIV infection, *in vitro* (FIG. 4 and refs. 73 and 74). Nevertheless, the rank order of potency of CD4(81-92) peptides to inhibit both HIV and SIV infection *in vitro* are quite similar (FIG. 4). Thus, evaluation of therapeutic efficacy of antiviral peptides and other agents directed towards disruption of human CD4/HIV gp120 interaction in SIV-infected rhesus macaques appears to be warranted, albeit such potential therapeutics may be predicted to be less efficacious in SIV than in HIV infection. The identification of the CDR3-like domain of CD4 as a likely gp120 binding site for HIV and SIV suggests passive immunization, using antibodies against CD4(81-92), as a potential treatment for HIV and SIV infection. Studies evaluating antibodies directed against the CDR2-like putative gp120-binding domain of CD4 are currently underway in HIV-infected patients.[75] The use of anti-idiotypic antibody immunization, using anti-

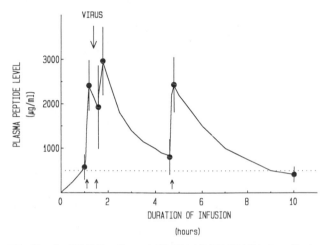

FIGURE 8. Blood levels of $T_1C_4E_5$-tribenzyl-CD4(81-92) [GLH328] in juvenile rhesus macaques during continuous intravenous administration over a ten hour period with intermittent bolus injections of peptide. Two to three kilogram juvenile rhesus macaques were anesthetized and infused intravenously with GLH328 at a rate of 200 mg/hour for ten hours, with additional bolus injections of 200 mg/ 10 min at the times shown (vertical arrows along abscissa), relative to the time of virus inoculation (vertical arrow at top of figure). Blood levels of GLH328 were determined by a quantitative HPLC method after plasma extraction (Hwang *et al.*, in preparation), and are given as the mean ± SEM for three of the four animals simultaneously inoculated with virus and infused with peptide in the experiment depicted in FIG. 9. Peptide plasma levels were not determined for the fourth animal. Note that plasma levels of GLH328 were maintained at or above the dose required to inhibit SIV infection of CEM174 cells *in vitro* (dotted line parallel to abscissa), over a 10 hour period, with this dosage regimen. Animals had been given a 200 mg/kg loading dose over a one hour period the previous day.

CD4(81-92) antibodies in treatment of SIV infection may also bear investigation, especially as CDR2-directed anti-idiotypic antibodies would appear to have only limited potential for successful immunization against HIV, based on the ability to generate anti-HIV neutralizing antibodies through immunization of rodents with the CDR2-directed antibody anti-Leu3a.[76,77] The search for more potent modified analogues of CD4(81-92) is also worthwhile. It is encouraging that a conformationally restricted version of $T_1C_4E_5$-tribenzyl-CD4(81-92) designed by one of us (K. M. Hwang) is potent at submicromolar concentrations to inhibit HIV-1 infection and syncytium formation *in vitro*, using a wide variety of HIV-1 isolates as input virus in the syncytium-forming

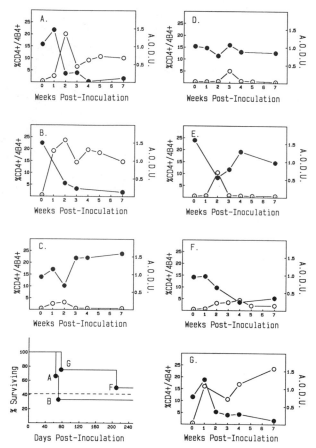

FIGURE 9. Sequelae of SIV inoculation in juvenile rhesus macaques, untreated or concurrently treated with $T_1C_4E_5$-tribenzyl-CD4(81-92). CD4/4B4 double-positive cells as a percentage of $CD4^+$ peripheral blood lymphocytes and serum SIV_{B670} core protein antigenemia (arbitrary optical density units, ELISA) are plotted for the seven individual rhesus macaques (2-3 kg, both sexes) inoculated with SIV_{B670} (10 IC_{50}s, i.v.). The three upper panels on the left show the course of $CD4^+/4B4^+$ cell depletion (closed circles) and viral antigenemia (open circles) in the three untreated, virus-inoculated animals. The four panels on the right show the course of $CD4^+/4B4^+$ cell depletion and viral antigenemia in the four peptide-treated, virus-inoculated animals. The bottom left panel shows the percentage of animals surviving in each group as a function of time (days postinoculation), each symbol representing the time at which each animal was euthanized upon determination of morbidity due to opportunistic infection, gastrointestinal or respiratory syncytial disease, or wasting and loss of appetite, singly or in combination. The letter next to each symbol indicates the corresponding animal whose immunologic parameters are depicted in the other panels.

microassay.[78,79] Finally, the virostatic activity of some CD4(81-92) peptide derivatives may recommend them as adjuncts to antiviral therapy with other therapeutics, especially when penetration to fetus or brain cannot be obtained with other antiviral agents.

SUMMARY

Peptides 12-25 amino acids in length from the V1J1 region of the CD4 molecule (residues 1-120) were synthesized as randomly derivatized, deliberately derivatized, or pure peptide products, and tested for their ability to inhibit HIV-1-induced cell fusion, HIV-1 and SIV infection of CD4-positive human cells, HIV-1 envelope glycoprotein binding to the CD4 molecule, CD4-neutralizing antibody binding to the CD4 holoreceptor, and CD4-dependent cellular immune function in the mixed lymphocyte and cytotoxic T-cell bioassays. Only peptides derived from the complementarity-determining region 3 (CDR3)-homologous domain of CD4, in particular CD4(81-92) and CD4(81-101), were effective antiviral agents. Within the CD4(81-92) series, R-group derivatization of selective amino acid residues was an absolute requirement for biological activity. The prototype compound $T_1C_4E_5$-tribenzyl-K10-acetyl-TYICEV-EDQKEE inhibited HIV-1-induced cell fusion at 32 μM, HIV-1 infection of CEM-SS cells at 10 μM, SIV infection of CEM-174 cells at less than 125 μM, gp120/CD4 binding at 60 μM, and postinfection cell-mediated viral transmission at 10-15 μM. Compounds of identical structure and derivatization, but of altered primary sequence, were substantially less active, or without activity, in these assays. These data indicate that the effect of amino acid derivatization of the CD4(81-92) peptide was most likely restriction of the flexible underivatized peptide backbone to a conformation closely approximating that of the CDR3-homologous gp120 binding site of the native CD4 molecule. Peptide antiviral activity was specific, as judged by lack of cytotoxicity, lack of inhibition of HTLV-1-induced cell fusion, and lack of inhibition of CD4-dependent cellular immune function *in vitro*. Further derivatization of the prototype compound involving the production of cyclic congeners yielded peptides with submicromolar potency to block HIV-1 infection, strengthening the hypothesis that previous peptide derivatizations accomplished partial restriction of the conformation of CD4(81-92) to one favorable for interaction with gp120. Concentrations of the original prototype compound $T_1C_4E_5$-tribenzyl-CD4(81-92) that inhibited infection *in vitro* more than 50% could be achieved for several hours by intravenous infusion in primates and were well-tolerated at these levels. The peptide was not efficacious to inhibit establishment of viral infection at these doses; however, peptide treatment did lower average viral antigenemia and delay the cumulative time to morbidity relative to the control group.

ACKNOWLEDGMENT

The expert technical assistance of Kathy Mishler in carrying out some of the *in vitro* HIV infection assays is gratefully acknowledged.

REFERENCES

1. U.S. Public Health Service. 1986. Public Health Rep. **101**: 341.
2. PIOT, P., F. A. PLUMMER, F. S. MHALU, J.-L. LAMBORAY, J. CHIN & J. M. MANN. 1988. AIDS: An international perspective. Science **239**: 573-579.
3. GALLO, R. C., S. Z. SALAHUDDIN, M. POPOVIC, G. M. SHEARER, M. KAPLAN, B. F. HAYNES, T. J. PALKER, R. REDFIELD, J. OLESKE, B. SAFAI, G. WHITE, P. FOSTER & P. D. MARKHAM. 1984. Frequent detection and isolation of cytopathic retroviruses (HTLV-III) from patients with AIDS and at risk for AIDS. Science **224**: 500-502.
4. BARRE-SINOUSSI, F., J. C. CHERMANN, F. REY, M. T. NUGEYRE, S. CHAMARET, J. GRUEST, C. DAUGUET, C. AXLER-BLIN, F. VEZINET-BRUN, C. ROUZIOUX, W. ROZEN-BAUM & L. MONTAGNIER. 1983. Isolation of a T-lymphotrophic retrovirus from a patient at risk for acquired immune deficiency syndrome (AIDS). Science **220**: 868-871.
5. GALLO, R. C. & L. MONTAGNIER. 1988. AIDS in 1988. Sci. Am. **259**: 41-48.
6. GOTTLIEB, M. S., R. SCHROFF, H. M. SCHANKAR, J. D. WEISMAN, P. T. FAN, R. A. WOLF & A. SAXON. 1981. Pneumocystis carinii pneumonia and mucosal candidiasis in previously healthy homosexual men. N. Engl. J. Med. **305**: 1425-1431.
7. MASUR, H., M. A. MICHELIS, J. B. GREENE, I. ONORATA, R. A. VANDE STOUWE, R. S. HOLZMAN, G. WORMSER, L. BRETTMAN, M. LANGE, H. W. MURRAY & S. CUNNING-HAM-RUNDLES. 1981. An outbreak of community-acquired pneumocystis carinii pneumonia. N. Engl. J. Med. **305**: 1431-1438.
8. SIEGAL, F. P., C. LOPEZ, G. S. HAMMER, A. E. BROWN, S. J. KORNFELD, J. GOLD, J. HASSETT, S. Z. HIRSCHMAN, C. CUNNINGHAM-RUNDLES, B. R. ADELSBERG, D. M. PARHAM, M. SIEGAL, S. CUNNINGHAM-RUNDLES & D. ARMSTRONG. 1981. Severe acquired immunodeficiency in male homosexuals, manifested by chronic perianal ulcerative herpes simplex lesions. N. Engl. J. Med. **305**: 1439-1444.
9. Centers for Disease Control. 1985. Revision of the case definition of acquired immunodeficiency syndrome for national reporting—United States. Morbid. Mortal. Weekly Rep. **35**: 222-223.
10. REDFIELD, R. R., D. C. WRIGHT & E. C. TRAMONT. 1986. The Walter Reed staging classification for HTLV-III/LAV infection. N. Engl. J. Med. **314**: 131-132.
11. REDFIELD, R. R. & D. S. BURKE. 1988. HIV infection: the clinical picture. Sci. Am. **259**: 90-99.
12. EPSTEIN, L. G., L. R. SCHARER, E.-S. CHO & M. MYENHOFER. 1985. HTLV-III/LAV-like retrovirus particles in the brains of patients with AIDS encephalopathy. AIDS Res. **1**: 447-454.
13. NAVIA, B. A., B. D. JORDAN & R. W. PRICE. 1986. The AIDS dementia complex. I. Clinical features. Ann. Neurol. **19**: 517-524.
14. POPOVIC, M., M. G. SARNGADHARAN, E. READ & R. C. GALLO. 1984. A method for detection, isolation, and continuous production of cytopathic human T-lymphotropic retroviruses of the HTLV family (HTLV-III) from patients with AIDS and pre-AIDS. Science **224**: 497-500.
15. SCHNITTMAN, S. M., M. C. PSALLIDOPOULOS, H. C. LANE, L. THOMPSON, M. BASELER, F. MASSARI, C. H. FOX, N. P. SALZMAN & A. S. FAUCI. 1989. The reservoir for HIV-1 in human peripheral blood is a T cell that maintains expression of CD4. Science **245**: 305-308.
16. KOENIG, S., H. E. GENDELMAN, J. M. ORENSTEIN, M. C. DAL CANTO, G. H. PEZESHK-POUR, M. YUNGBLUTH, F. JANOTTA, A. AKSAMIT, M. A. MARTIN & A. S. FAUCI. 1986. Detection of AIDS virus in macrophages in brain tissue from AIDS patients with encephalopathy. Science **233**: 1089-1093.
17. GARTNER, S., P. MARKOVITS, D. M. MARKOVITZ, M. H. KAPLAN, R. C. GALLO & M. POPOVIC. 1986. The role of mononuclear phagocytes in HTLV-III/LAV infection. Science **233**: 215-219.
18. SHAW, G., B. H. HAHN, S. K. ARYA, J. E. GROOPMAN, R. C. GALLO & F. WONG-STAAL. 1984. Molecular characterization of human T-cell leukemia (lymphotropic) virus type III in the acquired immune deficiency syndrome. Science **226**: 1165-1171.
19. CROWE, S., J. MILLS & M. McGRATH. 1987. AIDS Res. Hum. Retroviruses. **3**: 135-145.

20. FAUCI, A. S. 1988. The human immunodeficiency virus: infectivity and mechanisms of pathogenesis. Science **239:** 617-622.

21. KLATZMANN, D., E. CHAMPAGNE, S. CHAMARET, J. GRUEST, D. GUETARD, T. HERCEND, J.-C. GLUCKMANN & L. MONTAGNIER. 1984. T-lymphocyte T4 molecule behaves as the receptor for human retrovirus LAV. Nature **312:** 767-768.

22. DALGLEISH, A. G., P. C. L. BEVERLEY, P. R. CLAPHAM, D. H. CRAWFORD, M. P. GREAVES & R. A. WEISS. 1984. The CD4(T4) antigen is an essential component of the receptor for the AIDS retrovirus. Nature **312:** 763-767.

23. McDOUGAL, J. S., M. S. KENNEDY, J. M. SLIGH, S. P. CORT, A. MAWLE & J. K. A. NICHOLSON. 1986. Binding of HTLV-III/LAV to T4+ T cells by a complex of the 110K viral protein and the T4 molecule. Science **231:** 382-385.

24. MADDON, P., A. G. DALGLEISH, J. S. McDOUGAL, P. R. CLAPHAM, R. A. WEISS & R. AXEL. 1986. The T4 gene encodes the AIDS virus receptor and is expressed in the immune system and the brain. Cell **47:** 333-348.

25. CLAPHAM, P. R., R. A. WEISS, A. G. DALGLEISH, M. EXLEY, D. WHITBY & N. HOGG. 1987. Human immunodeficiency virus infection of monocytic and T-lymphocytic cells: receptor modulation and differentiation induced by phorbol ester. Virology **158:** 44-51.

26. LASKY, L. A., G. NAKAMURA, D. H. SMITH, C. FENNIE, C. SHIMASAKI, E. PATZER, P. BERMAN, T. GREGORY & D. J. CAPON. 1987. Delineation of a region of the human immunodeficiency virus type 1 gp120 glycoprotein critical for interaction with the CD4 receptor. Cell **50:** 975-985.

27. McDOUGAL, J. S., A. MAWLE, S. P. CORT, J. K. A. NICHOLSON, G. D. CROSS, J. A. SCHEPPLER-CAMPBELL, D. HICKS & J. SLIGH. 1985. Cell tropism of the human retrovirus HTLV-III/LAV. J. Immunol. **135:** 3151-3162.

28. LIFSON, J. D., G. R. REYES, M. S. McGRATH, B. S. STEIN & E. G. ENGLEMAN. 1986. AIDS retrovirus induced cytopathology: giant cell formation and involvement of CD4 antigen. Science **232:** 1123-1127.

29. SODROSKI, J., W. C. GOH, C. ROSEN, K. CAMPBELL & W. A. HASELTINE. 1986. Role of the HTLV-III/LAV envelope in syncytium formation and cytopathicity. Nature **322:** 470-474.

30. SILICIANO, R. F., T. LAWTON, C. KNALL, R. W. KARR, P. BERMAN, T. GREGORY & E. L. REINHERZ. 1988. Analysis of host-virus interactions in AIDS with anti-gp120 T cell clones: effect of HIV sequence variation and a mechanism for CD4+ cell depletion. Cell **54:** 561-575.

31. DIAMOND, D. C., B. P. SLECKMAN, T. GREGORY, L. A. LASKY, J. L. GREENSTEIN & S. J. BURAKOFF. 1989. Inhibition of CD4+ T cell function by the HIV envelope glycoprotein, gp120. J. Immunol. **141:** 3715.

32. SATTENTAU, Q. J. & R. A. WEISS. 1988. The CD4 antigen: physiological ligand and HIV receptor. Cell **52:** 631-633.

33. LIFSON, J. D. & E. G. ENGLEMAN. 1989. Role of CD4 in normal immunity and HIV infection. Immunol. Rev. **109:** 93-117.

34. HAHN, B. H., M. A. GONDA, G. M. SHAW, M. POPOVIC, J. HOXIE, R. C. GALLO & F. WONG-STAAL. 1985. Genomic diversity of the AIDS virus HTLV-III: different viruses exhibit greatest divergence in their envelope genes. Proc. Natl. Acad. Sci. USA **82:** 4813-4817.

35. HAHN, B. H., G. M. SHAW, M. E. TAYLOR, R. R. REDFIELD, P. D. MARKHAM, S. Z. SALAHUDDIN, F. WONG-STAAL, R. C. GALLO, E. S. PARKS & W. P. PARKS. 1986. Genetic variation of HTLV-III/LAV over time in patients with AIDS or at risk of AIDS. Science **232:** 1548-1554.

36. STARCICH, B. R., B. H. HAHN, G. M. SHAW, P. D. McNEELY, S. MODROW, H. WOLF, E. S. PARKS, W. P. PARKS, S. F. JOSEPHS, R. C. GALLO & F. WONG-STAAL. 1986. Cell **45:** 637-648.

37. GURGO, C., H.-G. GUO, G. FRANCHINI, A. ALDOVINI, E. COLLALTI, K. FARREL, F. WONG-STAAL, R. C. GALLO & M. S. REITZ, JR. 1988. Envelope sequences of two new United States HIV-1 isolates. Virology **164:** 531-536.

38. Human Retroviruses and AIDS 1989 Database. G. Myers, S. Josephs, J. A. Berzofsky, A. B. Rabson, T. F. Smith & F. Wong-Staal, Eds. Theoretical Biology and Biophysics Group T-10. Los Alamos, New Mexico.

39. EIDEN, L. E. 1991. Pharm. Sci. In press.
40. GERSHONI, J. M. & A. ARONHEIM. 1988. Molecular decoys: ligand-binding recombinant proteins protect mice from curaremimetic neurotoxins. Proc. Natl. Acad. Sci. USA **85:** 4087-4089.
41. SMITH, D. H., R. A. BYRN, S. A. MARSTERS, T. GREGORY, J. E. GROOPMAN & D. J. CAPON. 1987. Blocking of HIV-1 infectivity by a soluble secreted form of the CD4 antigen. Science **238:** 1704-1707.
42. FISHER, R. A., J. M. BERTONIS, W. MEIER, V. A. JOHNSON, D. S. COSTOPOULOS, T. LIU, R. TIZARD, B. D. WALKER, M. S. HIRSCH, R. T. SCHOOLEY & R. A. FLAVELL. 1988. HIV infection is blocked *in vitro* by recombinant soluble CD4. Nature **331:** 76-78.
43. HUSSEY, R. E., N. E. RICHARDSON, M. KOWALSKI, N. R. BROWN, H.-S. CHANG, R. F. SILICIANO, T. DORFMAN, B. WALKER, J. SODROSKI & E. L. REINHERZ. 1988. A soluble CD4 protein selectively inhibits HIV replication and syncytium formation. Nature **331:** 78-81.
44. DEEN, K. C., J. S. MCDOUGAL, R. INACKER, G. FOLENA-WASSERMAN, J. ARTHOS, J. ROSENBERG, P. J. MADDON, R. AXEL & R. W. SWEET. 1988. A soluble form of CD4 (T4) protein inhibits AIDS virus infection. Nature **331:** 82-84.
45. TRAUNECKER, A., W. LUKE & K. KARJALAINEN. 1988. Soluble CD4 molecules neutralize human immunodeficiency virus type 1. Nature **331:** 84-86.
46. LIFSON, J. D., K. M. HWANG, P. L. NARA, B. FRASER, M. PADGETT, N. M. DUNLOP & L. E. EIDEN. 1988. Synthetic CD4 peptide derivatives that inhibit HIV infection and cytopathicity. Science **241:** 712-716.
47. NARA, P. L., K. M. HWANG, D. M. RAUSCH, J. D. LIFSON & L. E. EIDEN. 1989. CD4 antigen-based antireceptor peptides inhibit infectivity of human immunodeficiency virus *in vitro* at multiple stages of the viral life cycle. Proc. Natl. Acad. Sci. USA **86:** 7139-7143.
48. CAPON, D. J., S. M. CHAMOW, J. MORDENTI, S. A. MARSTERS, T. GREGORY, H. MITSUYA, R. A. BYRN, C. LUCAS, F. M. WURM, J. E. GROOPMAN, S. BRODER & D. H. SMITH. 1989. Designing CD4 immunoadhesins for AIDS therapy. Nature **337:** 525-531.
49. TRAUNECKER, A., J. SCHNEIDER, H. KIEFER & K. KARJALAINEN. 1989. Highly efficient neutralization of HIV with recombinant CD4-immunoglobulin molecules. Nature **339:** 68-70.
50. GERETY, R. J., D. G. HANSON & D. W. THOMAS. 1989. Human recombinant soluble CD4 therapy. Lancet **ii:** 1521.
51. WALDOR, M. K., S. SRIRAM, R. HARDY, L. A. HERZENBERG, L. A. HERZENBERG, L. LANIER, M. LIM & L. STEINMAN. 1985. Reversal of experimental allergic encephalomyelitis with monoclonal antibody to a T-cell subset marker. Science **227:** 415-417.
52. SHIZURU, J. A., A. K. GREGORY, C. T.-B. CHAO & C. G. FATHMAN. 1987. Islet allograft survival after a single course of treatment of recipient with antibody to L3T4. Science **237:** 278-280.
53. LAMARRE, D., A. ASHKENAZI, S. FLEURY, D. H. SMITH, R.-P. SEKALY & D. J. CAPON. 1989. The MHC-binding and gp120-binding functions of CD4 are separable. Science **245:** 743-746.
54. CLAYTON, L. K., R. E. HUSSEY, R. STEINBRICH, H. RAMACHANDRAN, Y. HUSAIN & E. L. REINHERZ. 1988. Substitution of murine for human CD4 residues identifies amino acids critical for HIV-gp120 binding. Nature **335:** 363-366.
55. LANDAU, N. R., M. WARTON & D. R. LITTMAN. 1988. The envelope glycoprotein of the human immunodeficiency virus binds to the immunoglobulin-like domain of CD4. Nature **334:** 159-162.
56. PETERSON, A. & B. SEED. 1988. Genetic analysis of monoclonal antibody and HIV binding sites on the human lymphocyte antigen CD4. Cell **54:** 65-72.
57. SATTENTAU, Q. J., J. ARTHOS, K. DEEN, N. HANNA, D. HEALEY, P. C. L. BEVERLY, R. SWEET & A. TRUNEH. 1989. Structural analysis of the human immunodeficiency virus-binding domain of CD4. J. Exp. Med. **170:** 1319-1334.
58. MIZUKAMI, T., T. R. FUERST, E. A. BERGER & B. MOSS. 1988. Binding region for human immunodeficiency virus (HIV) and epitopes for HIV-blocking monoclonal antibodies of the CD4 molecule defined by site-directed mutagenesis. Proc. Natl. Acad. Sci. USA **85:** 9273-9277.

59. ARTHOS, J., K. C. DEEN, M. A. CHALKIN, J. A. FORNWALD, G. SATHE, Q. J. SATTENTAU, P. R. CLAPHAM, R. A. WEISS, J. S. McDOUGAL, C. PIETROPAOLO, R. AXEL, A. TRUNEH, P. J. MADDON & R. W. SWEET. 1989. Identification of the residues in human CD4 critical for the binding of HIV. Cell **57**: 469-481.

60. SHAIRA-NAHOR, O., H. GOLDING, L. K. VUJCIC & F. A. ROBEY. 1989. CD4-derived peptide protects CD4+ T cells from HIV-1 infection. Fifth International Conference on AIDS. Abstracts, 574.

61. HAYASHI, Y., K. IKUTA, N. FUJII, K. EZAWA & S. KATO. 1989. Inhibition of HIV-1 replication and syncytium formation by synthetic CD4 peptides. Arch. Virology **105**: 129-135.

62. LOWENSTEIN, L. J., N. C. PEDERSON, J. HIGGINS, K. C. PALLIS, A. UYEDA, P. MARX, N. W. LERCHE, R. J. MUNN & M. B. GARDNER. 1986. Seroepidemiologic survey of captive Old World primates for antibodies to human and simian retroviruses, and isolation of a lentivirus from sooty mangabeys (*Cercocebus atys*). Int. J. Cancer **38**: 563-574.

63. RIVAS, A., S. TAKADA, J. KOIDE, G. SONDERSTRUP-MCDEVITT & E. G. ENGLEMAN. 1988. CD4 molecules are associated with the antigen receptor complex on activated but not resting T cells. J. Immunol. **140**: 2912-2918.

64. KALYANARAMAN, V. S., R. PAL, R. C. GALLO & M. G. SARNGADHARAN. 1988. A unique human immunodeficiency virus culture secreting soluble gp160. AIDS Res. Hum. Retroviruses **4**: 319-329.

65. KALYANARAMAN, V. S., V. RODRIGUEZ, F. VERONESE, R. RAHMAN, P. LUSSO, A. L. DEVICO, T. COPELAND, S. OROSZLAN, R. C. GALLO & M. G. SARNGADHARAN. 1990. AIDS Res. Hum. Retroviruses. In press.

65a. KALYANARAMAN, V. S., D. M. RAUSCH, J. OSBORNE, M. PADGETT, K. M. HWANG, J. D. LIFSON & L. E. EIDEN. 1990. Evidence by peptide mapping that the region CD4(81-92) is involved in gp120 CD4 interaction leading to HIV infection and HIV-induced syncytium formation. J. Immunol. In press.

66. NARA, P. L., W. C. HATCH, N. M. DUNLOP, W. G. ROBEY, L. O. ARTHUR, M. A. GONDA & P. J. FISCHINGER. 1987. Simple, rapid, quantitative, syncytium-forming microassay for the detection of human immunodeficiency virus neutralizing antibody. AIDS Research and Human Retroviruses **3**: 283-302.

67. NARA, P. & P. J. FISCHINGER. 1988. Quantitative infectivity assay for HIV-1 and -2. Nature **332**: 469-470.

68. NARA, P. 1989. HIV-1 neutralization: evidence for rapid, binding/postbinding neutralization from infected humans, chimpanzees, and gp120-vaccinated animals. *In* Vaccines 89. R. A. Lerner, H. Ginsberg, R. M. Chanock & F. Brown, Eds.: 137-144. Cold Spring Harbor Laboratory.

69. KANNAGI, M., J. M. YETZ & N. L. LETVIN. 1985. *In vitro* growth characteristics of simian T-lymphotropic virus type III. Proc. Natl. Acad. Sci. USA **82**: 7053-7057.

70. MURPHEY-CORB, M., L. N. MARTIN, S. R. S. RANGAN, G. B. BASKIN, B. J. GORMUS, R. H. WOLF, W. A. ANDES, M. WEST & R. C. MONTELARO. 1986. Isolation of an HTLV-III-related retrovirus from macaques with simian AIDS and its possible origin in asymptomatic mangabeys. Nature **321**: 435-437.

71. SCHARER, L. R., G. B. BASKIN, E.-S. CHO, M. MURPHEY-CORB, B. M. BLUMBERG & L. G. EPSTEIN. 1988. Comparison of simian immunodeficiency virus and human immunodeficiency virus encephalitides in the immature host. Ann. Neurol. **23**(Suppl.): S108-S112.

72. McCLURE, M. O., Q. J. SATTENTAU, P. C. L. BEVERLEY, J. P. HEARN, A. K. FITZGERALD, A. J. ZUCKERMAN & R. A. WEISS. 1987. HIV infection of primate lymphocytes and conservation of the CD4 receptor. Nature **330**: 487-489.

73. WATANABE, M., K. A. REIMANN, P. A. DELONG, T. LIU, R. A. FISHER & N. L. LETVIN. 1989. Effect of recombinant soluble CD4 in rhesus monkeys infected with simian immunodeficiency virus of macaques. Nature **337**: 267-270.

74. CLAPHAM, P. R., J. N. WEBER, D. WHITBY, K. McINTOSH, A. G. DALGLEISH, P. J. MADDON, D. C. DEEN, R. W. SWEET & R. A. WEISS. 1989. Soluble CD4 blocks the infectivity of diverse strains of HIV and SIV for T cells and monocytes but not for brain and muscle cells. Nature **337**: 368-370.

75. DHIVER, C., D. OLIVE, S. ROUSSEAU, C. TAMALET, M. LOPEZ, J.-R. GALINDO, M.

MOURENS, M. HIRN, J.-A. GASTAUT & C. MAWAS. 1989. Pilot phase I study using zidovudine in association with a 10-day course of anti-CD4 monoclonal antibody in seven AIDS patients. AIDS 3: 835-842.

76. DALGLEISH, A. G., B. J. THOMSON, T. C. CHANH, M. MALKOVSKY & R. C. KENNEDY. 1987. Neutralisation of HIV isolates by anti-idiotypic antibodies which mimic the T4 (CD4) epitope: a potential AIDS vaccine. Lancet ii: 1047-1050.

77. MCDOUGAL, J. S., J. K. A. NICHOLSON, G. D. CROSS, S. P. CORT, M. S. KENNEDY & A. C. MAWLE. 1986. Binding of the Human Retrovirus HTLV-III/LAV/ARV/HIV to the CD4 (T4) Molecule: Conformation Dependence, Epitope Mapping, Antibody Inhibition, and Potential for Idiotypic Mimicry. J. Immunol. 137: 2937-2944.

78. HWANG, K., D. M. RAUSCH, M. PADGETT, V. S. KALYANARAMAN, P. L. NARA, L. E. EIDEN & J. D. LIFSON. 1990. Use of peptides and peptide derivatives of CD4 to assess the relative contributions of CDR-1, CDR-2 and CDR-3 homology domains of the CD4 molecule to binding of HIV envelope glycoprotein and HIV infectivity in vitro. J. Cell Biochem. (Suppl. 14C): 230.

79. RAUSCH, D. M., K. M. HWANG, M. PADGETT, V. S. KALYANARAMAN, P. L. NARA, D. BUCK, F. CELADA, J. D. LIFSON & L. E. EIDEN. 1990. Peptides spanning the CDR-3-homologous domain of the CD4 antigen [CD4(81-101)] specifically inhibit infection and syncytium formation induced by HIV-1 and SIV. J. Cell Biochem. (Suppl. 14D): 159.

Anti-HIV Effects of CD4-*Pseudomonas* Exotoxin on Human Lymphocyte and Monocyte/ Macrophage Cell Lines

PER ASHORN, BERNARD MOSS, AND
EDWARD A. BERGER[a]

Laboratory of Viral Diseases
National Institute of Allergy and Infectious Diseases
National Institutes of Health
Bethesda, Maryland 20892

INTRODUCTION

The receptor for human immunodeficiency virus (HIV) is CD4, a 55 kDa glycoprotein expressed on the surface of certain human lymphoid and monocytic cell types (reviewed in ref. 1). The finding[2-7] that recombinant soluble forms of CD4 retain the capacity for high-affinity binding to gp120 (the external subunit of the HIV envelope glycoprotein) has suggested potential therapeutic uses of CD4 derivatives. For example, soluble molecules containing CD4 sequences alone are able to neutralize HIV infectivity *in vitro*,[2-6] suggesting they may have specific antiviral activity in HIV-infected individuals. Alternatively, hybrid molecules have been produced containing the gp120-binding region of CD4 linked to other protein sequences possessing specific effector activities.[8-11] In these cases the CD4 moiety serves not only as a neutralizing agent, but also as a targeting agent to direct the novel effector activities of these molecules selectively against HIV-infected cells.

We have previously described a genetically engineered hybrid protein consisting of the gp120-binding region of CD4 linked to active domains of *Pseudomonas aeruginosa* exotoxin A (PE).[8] This protein, designated CD4(178)-PE40, selectively binds to HIV-infected cells due to their surface expression of the HIV envelope glycoprotein (FIG. 1). Based on the known mechanism of action of PE,[12] CD4(178)-PE40 is then presumably translocated to the cytoplasm of the HIV-infected cell where it ADP-ribosylates elongation factor 2, resulting in inactivation of protein synthesis and eventual cell death. As illustrated schematically in FIGURE 2, the domain structure of PE makes this an ideally suited molecule for the construction of hybrid derivatives containing alternative ligands in place of the normal cell binding domain of PE, thereby resulting in novel toxins with new cell type specificities based on binding to cells expressing the appropriate surface molecules.

[a]To whom correspondence should be addressed.

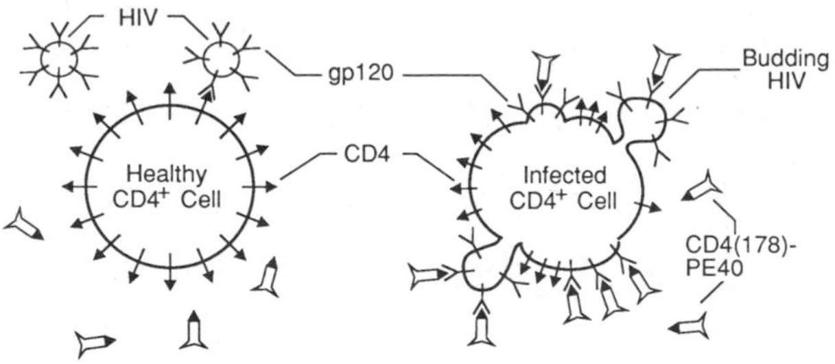

FIGURE 1. Selective binding of CD4(178)-PE40 to HIV-infected cells. When healthy CD4-positive T lymphocytes become infected with HIV, virus replication results in the synthesis and transport of the HIV envelope glycoprotein (gp120/gp41 complex) to the cell surface. This process renders the infected cells sensitive to the CD4(178)-PE40 hybrid protein that, by virtue of its CD4 moiety, can bind selectively to the gp120 molecules on the surface of the infected cell.

Originally, we reported, that CD4(178)-PE40 inhibits protein synthesis in cells expressing the HIV-1 envelope glycoprotein encoded by a recombinant vaccinia virus vector, as well as in a human T-cell line chronically infected with HIV-1.[8] Subsequently, we showed that this protein is a highly potent and selective agent for killing of HIV-1-infected human T-cell lines and that it inhibits HIV-1 spread in cocultures of infected and uninfected T cells.[15] Inasmuch as cells of the monocyte/macrophage lineage may be a major reservoir for HIV in infected individuals,[16,17] we have now analyzed the activity of CD4(178)-PE40 against a human promonocyte cell line chronically infected with HIV-1.

MATERIAL AND METHODS

Cell Lines and Culture Conditions

The cell lines used in this study included U937, a human promonocyte cell line susceptible to HIV infection,[18] and U1, a derivative of U937 chronically infected with the LAV isolate of HIV-1.[19] Cells were cultured at $+37\,°C$ in 5% CO_2 in RPMI-1640 medium containing 10% heat-inactivated fetal calf serum, 10 mM HEPES buffer, 2 mM L-glutamine, 100 U/mL penicillin, and 0.1 mg/mL streptomycin. U937 and U1 cultures were grown in triplicate in 96-well flat-bottom tissue culture plates (Costar, Cambridge, MA).

Reagents

PE was purchased from Swiss Serum and Vaccine Institute. CD4(178)-PE40 was obtained from the Upjohn Co., Kalamazoo, MI, where it was expressed and isolated from *E. coli* as previously described.[8] AZT (3-azido-3′-deoxythymidine or zidovudine),

MTT (3-[4,5-dimethylthiazole-2-yl]-2,5-diphenyltetrazolium bromide; thiazole blue), and PMA (phorbol 12-myristate 13-acetate) were purchased from Sigma Chemical Co., St. Louis, MO.

Viability Assays

The relative numbers of viable cells were determined by the MTT oxidation procedure that has been shown to correlate well with the Trypan blue exclusion assay under the conditions employed in these studies.[20] U937 and U1 cells were grown in 100 μL medium per well in 96-well plates, and the MTT assays were performed directly in the same plates. Reactions were initiated by addition of 10 μL MTT solution (5 mg/mL, w/vol, in PBS). The plates were incubated at $+37\,°C$ for 4 h, and the reactions were terminated with 100 μL per well of 0.01 M HCl containing 10% (w/vol) SDS. Oxidized MTT was allowed to dissolve in medium for 16 h at $+37\,°C$, and the intensity of the blue color was measured at 590 nm with an automated ELISA plate reader (V-max, Molecular Devices, Menlo Park, CA).

RESULTS AND DISCUSSION

Effects of PE Derivatives on Cell Viability of Uninfected and HIV-1-Infected Human T-Cell Lines

Most mammalian cell types express receptor(s) for native PE and are thus sensitive to killing by this toxin.[21] By contrast, CD4(178)-PE40 kills two HIV-infected T-cell lines with IC_{50} values in the range of 100 pM but has no effect on the corresponding uninfected parental cells (TABLE 1 and refs. 15 and 20). Specificity is provided by the CD4 moiety of the hybrid toxin, inasmuch as the control protein PE40 has no effect on infected or uninfected cells. The selective killing of HIV-infected cells is not due to

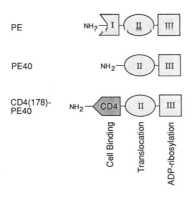

FIGURE 2. Schematic representation of PE derivatives, showing the association of specific structural domains with specific functions.[12–14] Domain I of native PE binds to receptors present on a wide variety of cell types, giving the toxin broad specificity. PE40 lacks domain I and thus serves as a control for nonspecific toxicity. In CD4(178)-PE40, the CD4 region consists of the amino-terminal 178 amino acids, representing the first two immunoglobulin-like domains within which is contained the binding site for gp120.[6,7] This hybrid toxin binds specifically to cells expressing the HIV envelope glycoprotein.[8]

mere interaction of the hybrid toxin with the HIV envelope glycoprotein, as judged by the failure of CD4 derivatives lacking an enzymatically active domain (*i.e.* sCD4 or CD4(178)-PE40$_{asp553}$) to promote killing.

Effect of CD4(178)-PE40 on a Human Monocyte/Macrophage Cell Line Chronically Infected with HIV

Inasmuch as a major reservoir for HIV *in vivo* may be the tissue macrophages,[16,17] it was important to test the ability of CD4(178)-PE40 to selectively kill HIV-infected human cells of monocyte/macrophage lineage. U1 is a chronically latent HIV-1 infected promonocyte cell line, that under normal conditions expresses very low levels of viral proteins. Phorbol esters such as PMA will stimulate these cells to differentiate into macrophage-like cells, with a concomitant induction of HIV expression. To test the susceptibility of these cells to CD4(178)-PE40, we stimulated the cells with PMA, cultured them in the presence of high concentrations of CD4(178)-PE40 or PE, and measured the relative numbers of viable cells after a 4 day culture. Uninduced U1 cells as well as both induced and uninduced U937 cells served as controls. As shown in FIGURE 3, the U1 cells were killed by CD4(178)-PE40 only when induced with PMA. The failure of the hybrid toxin to kill U937 cells even in the presence of PMA indicates that the sensitivity observed for the induced U1 cells is associated with virus expression, presumably gp120, at the cell surface.

Taken together, the *in vitro* results presented in this communication support the potential value of CD4(178)-PE40 in the treatment of HIV-infected individuals. The previously reported selective effects of CD4(178)-PE40 on HIV-infected lymphocytes can now be extended to cells of the monocyte/macrophage lineage. The finding that latently infected lymphoid[20] or myeloid (FIG. 3) cell types are killed by the hybrid

TABLE 1. Sensitivity of HIV-1-Infected and -Uninfected T-Cell Lines to Killing by CD4(178)-PE40 or Control Proteins[a]

Cell Type	HIV-1 Infected	IC$_{50}$ (nM)			
		CD4-PE40	PE40	sCD4	CD4-PE40$_{asp553}$
8E5	yes	0.08	> 10[b]	> 10[b]	> 10[b]
A3.01	no	> 10[b]	> 10[b]	> 10[b]	> 10[b]
H9/HTLVIIB	yes	0.1	> 8[b]	ND[c]	ND
H9	no	> 10[b]	> 8[b]	ND	ND

[a] The cells were plated in 24-well tissue culture plates with serial tenfold dilutions of the indicated proteins. After a 4-5 day culture relative numbers of cells were counted using the MTT method as described in MATERIAL AND METHODS. IC$_{50}$ is the drug concentration required for killing of 50% of cells. PE40[22] and CD4(178)-PE40$_{asp553}$[23] are control recombinant proteins with greatly reduced cytotoxic activity because of the absence of the cell binding domain (PE40) or a mutation abolishing the ADP ribosylation activity [CD4(178)-PE40$_{asp553}$]. In some experiments, lys-PE40, a genetically engineered version of PE40 with an additional lysine residue in the amino-terminal end of the molecule,[24] was used instead of PE40. Some of the results presented in the TABLE have been summarized from data reported in refs. 15 and 20.

[b] No toxicity at this concentration.

[c] ND = Not done.

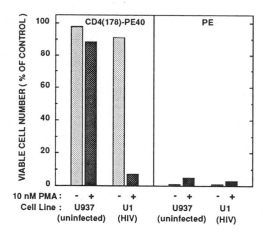

FIGURE 3. Selective killing of HIV-1-infected human monocyte/macrophages by CD4(178)-PE40. Uninfected U937 or HIV-1-infected U1 cells were pretreated for 24 h with or without 10 nM PMA, and washed and plated in triplicate in 96-well flat bottom microtiter plates at a density of 25×10^3 cells/well without PMA. The cells were then cultured for 4 days with 100 nM CD4(178)-PE40 or PE. The relative viable cell numbers are expressed as a percent of the MTT values obtained for corresponding control cultures maintained in the absence of drugs.

toxin only after HIV induction may have important clinical implications, because the presence of latently infected cells is an important characteristic of HIV infection.[25]

SUMMARY

CD4(178)-PE40 is a recombinant protein consisting of the HIV envelope glycoprotein-binding region of human CD4 linked to active domains of *Pseudomonas aeruginosa* exotoxin A. The hybrid toxin selectively kills HIV-infected human T-cell lines and protects against HIV spread in mixtures of uninfected and infected cells. We now report that CD4(178)-PE40 also selectively kills chronically HIV-1-infected cells of monocyte/macrophage lineage. The results provide further support for therapeutic use of this hybrid toxin in the treatment of HIV-infected individuals.

ACKNOWLEDGMENTS

We thank P. Robbins and K. Weih for excellent technical assistance and M. Martin for the use of his equipment.

REFERENCES

1. SATTENTAU, Q. & R. WEISS. 1988. Cell **52:** 631-633.
2. SMITH, D., R. BYRN, S. MARSTERS, T. GREGORY, J. GROOPMAN & D. CAPON. 1987. Science **238:** 1704-1708.
3. FISHER, R., J. BERTONIS, W. MEIER, V. JOHNSON, D. COSTOPOULOS, T. LIU, R. TIZARD, B. WALKER, M. HIRSCH, R. SCHOOLEY & R. FLAVELL. 1988. Nature **331:** 76-78.

4. HUSSEY, R., N. RICHARDSON, M. LOWALSKI, N. BROWN, H-C. CHANG, R. SILICIANO, T. DORFMAN, B. WALKER, J. SODROSKI & E. REINHERZ. 1988. Nature **331:** 78-81.
5. DEEN, K., J. McDOUGAL, R. INACKER, G. FOLENA-WASSERMAN, J. ARTHOS, J. ROSENBERG, P. MADDON, R. AXEL & R. SWEET. 1988. Nature **331:** 82-84.
6. TRAUNECKER, A., W. LUKE & K. KARJALAINEN. 1988. Nature **331:** 84-86.
7. BERGER, E., T. FUERST & B. MOSS. 1988. Proc. Natl. Acad. Sci. USA **85:** 2357-2361.
8. CHAUDHARY, V., T. MIZUKAMI, T. FUERST, D. FITZGERALD, B. MOSS, I. PASTAN & E. BERGER. 1988. Nature **335:** 369-372.
9. TILL, M., V. GHETIE, T. GREGORY, E. PATZER, J. PORTER, J. UHR, D. CAPON & E. VITETTA. 1988. Science **242:** 1166-1168.
10. CAPON, D., S. CHAMOW, J. MORDENTI, S. MARSTERS, T. GREGORY, H. MITSUYA, R. BYRN, C. LUCAS, F. WURM, J. GROOPMAN, S. BRODER & D. SMITH. 1989. Nature **337:** 525-531.
11. TRAUNECKER, A., J. SCHEIDER, H. KIEFER & K. KARJALAINEN. 1989. Nature **339:** 68-70.
12. PASTAN, I. & D. FITZGERALD. 1989. J. Biol. Chem. **264:** 15157-15160.
13. ALLURED, V., R. COLLIER, S. CARROL & D. McKAY. 1986. Proc. Natl. Acad. Sci. USA **83:** 1320-1324.
14. HWANG, J., D. FITZGERALD, S. ADHYA & I. PASTAN. 1987. Cell **48:** 129-136.
15. BERGER, E., K. CLOUSE, V. CHAUDHARY, S. CHAKRABARTI, D. FITZGERALD, I. PASTAN & B. MOSS. 1989. Proc. Natl. Acad. Sci. USA **86:** 9539-9543.
16. GARTNER, S., P. MARKOVITS, D. MARKOVITS, M. KAPLAN, R. GALLO & M. POPOVIC. 1986. Science **232:** 215-219.
17. KOENIG, S., H. GENDELMAN, J. ORENSTEIN, M. DAL CANTE, G. PEZESHPOUR, M. YUNGBLUTH, F. JANETTA, A. AKSAWIT, M. MARTIN & A. FAUCI. 1986. Science **233:** 1089-1093.
18. SUNDSTROM, C. & K. NILSSON. 1976. Int. J. Cancer **17:** 565-577.
19. FOLKS, T., J. JUSTEMENT, A. KINTER, S. SCHNITTMAN, J. ORENSTEIN, G. POLI & A. FAUCI. 1988. J. Immunol. **140:** 1117-1122.
20. BERGER, E., V. CHAUDHARY, K. CLOUSE, D. JARAQUEMADA, J. NICHOLAS, K. RUBINO, D. FITZGERALD, I. PASTAN & B. MOSS. 1989. AIDS Res. Hum. Retroviruses **6:** 795-804.
21. THOMPSON, M. & B. IGLEWSKI. 1982. *Pseudomonas aeruginosa* toxin A and exoenzymes. *In* ADP-Ribosylation Reactions: Biology and Medicine. O. Hagaishi & K. Ueda, Ed.: 641-674. Academic Press. New York.
22. KONDO, T., D. FITZGERALD, V. CHAUDHARY, S. ADHYA & I. PASTAN. 1988. J. Biol. Chem. **263:** 9470-9475.
23. DOUGLAS, C. & R. COLLIER. 1987. J. Bacteriol. **169:** 4967-4971.
24. BATRA, J., Y. JINNO, V. CHAUDHARY, T. KONDO, M. WILLINGHAM, D. FITZGERALD & I. PASTAN. 1989. Proc. Natl. Acad. Sci. USA **86:** 8545-8549.
25. ROSENBERG, F. & A. FAUCI. 1989. AIDS Res. Hum. Retroviruses **5:** 1-4.

Early Events of HIV Infection as Targets for Antiviral Agents

R. DATEMA

Virology Department 106
Bristol-Myers Squibb Company
Wallingford, Connecticut 06492

INTRODUCTION

The early events of HIV infection are defined here as binding of the virus to the cell, followed by fusion of the virus with the cell membrane and entry into the cytoplasm. The viral envelope glycoprotein gp120/41 is the key player in this sequence of events. This glycoprotein is synthesized as a precursor, gp160, cleaved during intracellular transport to gp120 and gp41. These two subunits are held together by noncovalent bonds as a part of a multimeric complex.[1-3] Expression of the glycoprotein is necessary for formation of infectious virus particles and for cytopathic fusion of gp120/41-expressing cells with cells containing the viral receptor, the CD_4 molecule.[1] Thus, gp120/41 is a good target for antiviral therapies.

RECEPTOR BINDING

The first step in the infection of a cell by a virus is the attachment of the virus to the host cell.[4] In this process, in the case of enveloped viruses, the viral envelope glycoprotein binds to a constituent of the host cell membrane. It is possible to design potential antiviral agents by identifying the binding domains of the viral glycoprotein and the cell-surface receptor and studying their interactions. As shown in FIGURE 1, three strategies come to mind immediately: (a) mimics of the [binding site present in the] viral envelope glycoprotein or ligand analogues; (b) mimics of the [binding site present in the] cellular receptor or receptor analogues; and (c) agents binding just offside the receptor or ligand binding site but interfering with ligand-receptor interaction (black structures in FIG. 1). An example of a ligand analogue is an antireceptor monoclonal antibody;[5] soluble forms of the cellular receptor are examples of receptor analogues. Receptor analogues have obtained considerable attention as potential antiviral agents.[6]

RECEPTOR ANALOGUES

The receptor for HIV in most cell types is the CD_4 molecule.[7] Using truncated forms of CD_4 and mutational analyses, it was found that the gp120 binding site is present in the N-terminal part of CD_4, namely the region covered by amino acids 31 to 58.[8] Several truncated forms of CD_4 have been proposed as antiviral agents, and some have entered clinical trials.[9] The soluble derivatives of CD_4 show potent antiviral

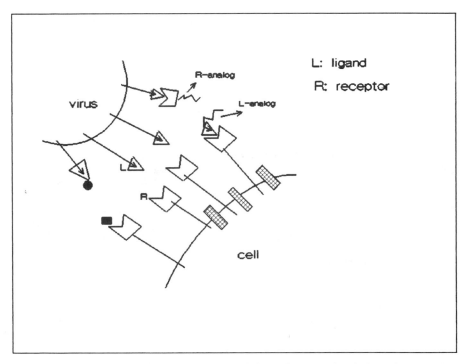

FIGURE 1. The binding of the virus to the cell is mediated by the viral envelope protein (——▷), embedded in the viral membrane, binding to the receptor (——⟨), which is also a transmembrane protein. The picture shows ligand analogues (∿▷), receptor analogues (∿⟨), and other agents (■, ●) interfering with receptor-ligand binding.

effects *in vitro* using laboratory strains of HIV.[10-14] In addition, synergy between sCD_4 and dideoxynucleosides was demonstrated,[15] further emphasizing the usefulness of this class of agents. Nevertheless, potential limitations of the sCD_4 approach are (1) clinical isolates of HIV may have a lower sensitivity to sCD_4 than lab strains;[16] (2) some cells may be infected by HIV through CD_4-independent pathways[17] or by way of virus-immune complexes,[18] that is, through F_c receptors; (3) CD_4 analogues may affect the immune system; and (4) the CD_4 analogues may not have the preferred pharmacokinetic properties. Some of these issues are now being addressed. Thus sCD_4 still blocked infection of monocytes in the presence of enhancing antibodies.[19] Also, the MHC molecule-binding and gp120-binding sites of CD_4 can be separated, allowing synthesis of the CD_4 analogues, possibly not affecting the immune response.[20] Further, hybrid sCD_4-immunoglobulin molecules, fusion proteins of a gp120-binding domain of CD_4 and an IgG heavy-chain constant region, have a long serum half-life.[21,22]

This work clearly shows that it is possible to "engineer" derivatives of CD_4 with additional useful properties.[22] One preferred way is to use CD_4 analogues to target toxins (ricin, *Pseudomonas* exotoxin) to gp120-expressing, that is, infected cells. This can be accomplished by covalent conjugation or by expressing parts of CD_4 and the toxin as a fusion protein[23,24] (this symposium). Another way is to express soluble CD_4 with a C-terminal extension (Lys-Asp-Glu-Leu), thus retaining it in the endoplasmic reticulum.[25,26] In this way, the HIV envelope glycoprotein, when synthesized in infected cells, is retained in the endoplasmic reticulum, preventing cell-surface expression. It remains to be seen whether this leads to effective intracellular immunization.

LIGAND ANALOGUES

The region of gp120 binding to CD_4 is highly conserved among HIV-1 isolates and found in the C-terminal part of gp120.[1,9] The CD_4-binding domain of gp120 resembles, of course, a normal ligand for CD_4. This molecular mimicry, a possible cause of autoimmune disease,[27] is an obvious concern in the design of ligand analogues.

To determine the functional anatomy of the CD_4-binding region of gp120, mutational analyses were performed.[28,29] It is not clear yet whether the CD_4-binding region is present in a "canyon" lined by conserved residues, as shown for some other viral receptor-binding proteins.[30,31] Analysis of tertiary structure determinants of gp120 relevant for CD_4 binding (disulfide bonds,[32,33] glycosylation sites, and glycosylation per se) and analysis of the critical amino acid residues affecting viral tropism[34] are the first steps in the rational design of ligand analogues. X-ray diffraction studies of (truncated forms of) gp120 are to follow. Antiidiotypic antibodies can be obtained, as positive images of the CD_4-binding site, to generate structural information on this target enabling rational drug design.[35]

In retroviral systems glycosylation of the envelope glycoproteins plays an important role in determining viral infectivity,[36] and this also applies to HIV (this symposium). In fact, it is well-established that the protein-bound oligosaccharides play an important role in generation and maintenance of protein conformation.[36,37] Furthermore, several studies suggest involvement of gp120-bound carbohydrates in CD_4 binding[38] but also in binding to cells independent of CD_4.[39]

OTHER INTERACTIONS

Polysulfated polysaccharides, other polysulfated polymers, and certain polyanionic dyes (aurin tricarboxylic acid, for example) effectively block HIV replication in cell cultures by blocking binding of HIV to CD_4^+ cells.[40–42] The mechanism by which these polyanions block infectious cell entry remains to be studied at the molecular level but may be due to "shielding" of gp120.[42]

High-capacity screening systems for compounds blocking gp120/CD$_4$ interaction can be easily designed and will in the near future lead to discovery of new inhibitors. The antiviral potential of such agents and the advantages or disadvantages compared with sCD$_4$ derivatives are of considerable interest.

POSTRECEPTOR-BINDING EVENTS

Following receptor binding a virus is internalized. This is a complex process, involving virus-cell fusion, studied in detail only in a few viral systems,[43] excluding HIV. Clearly, CD$_4$ binding is not sufficient for infectious cell entry. Thus, mouse cells expressing human CD$_4$ are refractory to HIV despite virus binding to CD$_4$ and despite the facts that full-length HIV-cDNA transfected into mouse cells can give rise to infectious progeny or that an HIV pseudotype, wrapped in a VSV-coat, can infect mouse cells (see ref. 7 for a review). Analyses of these systems in fusion assays[44] should lead to a better understanding of post-CD$_4$-binding events in infectious cell entry.

With HIV, internalization is preceded by a fusion of virion with the plasma membrane.[7] Genetic analyses[1,9] suggest involvement of both gp120 and gp41, the transmembrane part of the HIV envelope glycoprotein, in the fusion process. The N terminus of gp41, generated by trypsin-like cleavages of gp160 has the properties of a "fusion peptide" analogous to the fusion peptides of ortho- and paramyxoviruses.[2] Influenza A viruses fuse with the cell membrane in endosomes at pH 5. This low pH triggers a conformation change in the viral hemagglutinin, "exposing" the fusion peptide to participate in fusion.[43] Preventing this conformational rearrangement is an ideal target for antiviral agents. The equivalent reaction in gp120/41 has not yet been identified, however. Thus, whereas the detailed structural information on the influenza virus hemagglutinin would allow rational design of a flu fusion inhibitor, fusion assays have to be used to screen for inhibitors of gp120/41-mediated fusion. These assays, measuring, for example, polykaryon or syncytium formation when cocultivating CD$_4$-expressing cells and gp120/41-expressing cells, identified a trypsin inhibitor,[45] pradimicin A,[46] oxathiin carboxanilide,[47] and α (1,3)- and α (1,6)-D-mannose-specific lectins,[48] as inhibitors of the postreceptor-binding events. The inhibition of tryptic cleavage concerns a cleavage of gp120 (not the cleavage of gp160 to gp120/41) by cell-bound tryptase(s). Both pradimicin A and the lectins have affinity for mannose-containing oligosaccharides. By binding to the highly glycosylated gp120/41, the agents may prevent conformational rearrangements immediately preceding fusion.

PERSPECTIVE

Initial efforts to obtain inhibitors of infectious cell entry concentrated on receptor analogues. As shown above other antiviral strategies are emerging, whereas the receptor analogues become more and more sophisticated in their design. Indeed this area of antiviral research nicely complements the other sophisticated areas: inhibition of HIV reverse transcriptase and inhibition of the HIV protease.

REFERENCES

1. HASELTINE, W. A. 1988. J. AIDS 1: 217-240.
2. MCCUNE, J. M., L. B. RABIN, M. B. FEINBERG, M. LIEBERMAN, J. C. KOSEK, G. R. REYES & I. L. WEISSMAN. 1988. Cell 53: 55-67.
3. SCHAWALLER, M., G. E. SMITH, J. J. SHEKEL & D. C. WILEY. 1989. Virology 172: 367-369.
4. DALES, S. 1973. Bacteriol. Rev. 37: 103-105.
5. MINOR, P. D., P. A. PIPKIN, D. HOCKLEY, G. C. SCHILD & J. W. ALMOND. 1984. Virus Res. 1: 203-213.
6. ROSSMAN, M. G. 1988. Nature 333: 392-393.
7. SATTENTAU, Q. & R. WEISS. 1988. Cell 52: 631-633.
8. ARTHOS, J., K. C. DEEN, M. A. CHAIKIN, J. A. FORNWALD, G. SATHE, Q. J. SATTENTAU, P-R. CLAPHAM, R. A. WEISS, J. C. MCDOUGAL, C. PIETROPAOLO, R. AXEL, A. TRUNEH, P. J. MADDON & R. W. SWEET. 1989. Cell 57: 469-481.
9. HASELTINE, W. A. 1989. J. AIDS 2: 311-334.
10. SMITH, D., R. BYRN, S. MARSTERS, T. GREGORY, J. GROOPMAN & D. CAPON. 1987. Science 238: 76-78.
11. FISHER, R., J. BERTONIS, W. MEIER, V. JOHNSON, D. COSTOPOULOS, T. LIU, R. TIZARD, B. WALKER, M. HIRSCH, R. SCHOOLEY & R. FLAVELL. 1988. Nature 331: 76-78.
12. HUSSEY, R., N. RICHARDSON, M. LOWALSKI, N. BROWN, H-C. CHANG, R. SILICIANO, T. DORFMAN, B. WALKER, J. SODROSKI & E. REINHERZ. 1988. Nature 331: 78-81.
13. DEEN, K., J. MCDOUGAL, R. INACKER, G. FOLENA-WASSERMAN, J. ARTHOS, J. ROSENBERG, P. MADDON, R. AXEL & R. SWEET. 1988. Nature 331: 82-84.
14. TRAUNECKER, A., W. LUKE & K. KARJALAINEN. 1988. Nature 331: 84-86.
15. JOHNSON, V. A., D. P. MERRILL, T. C. CHOU & M. S. HIRSCH. 1990. Abstract F.A. 66, Sixth International Conference on AIDS, San Francisco.
16. DAAR, E. S., X. L. LI, T. MOUDGIL & D. D. HO. 1990. Abstract S.B. 88, Sixth International Conference on AIDS, San Francisco.
17. CLAPHAM, P. R., J. N. WEBER, D. WHITBY, K. MCINTOSH, A. G. DAHLGLEISH, P. J. MADDON, K. C. DEEN, R. W. SWEET & R. A. WEISS. 1989. Nature 337: 368-370.
18. HOMSY, J., M. MEYER, M. TATENO, S. CLARKSON & J. A. LEVY. 1989. Science 244: 1357-1360.
19. PERNO, C-F., M. W. BASELER, S. BRODER & R. YARCHOAN. 1990. J. Exp. Med. 171: 1043-1056.
20. LAMARRE, D., A. ASHKENAZI, S. FLEURY, D. H. SMITH, R-P. SEKALY & D. J. CAPON. 1989. Science 245: 743-746.
21. CAPON, D. J., S. M. CHARNOW, J. MORDENTI, S-A. MARSTERS, T. GREGORY, H. MITSUYA, R. A. BYRN, C. LUCAS, F. M. WURM, J. E. GROOPMAN, S. BRODER & D. H. SMITH. 1989. Nature 337: 525-531.
22. TRAUNECKER, A., J. SCHNEIDER, H. KIEFER & K. KARJALAINEN. 1989. Nature 339: 68-70.
23. TILL, M. A., V. GHETIE, T. GREGORY, E. J. PATZER, J. P. PORTER, J. W. UHR, D. J. CAPON & E. S. VITETTA. 1988. Science 242: 1166-1168.
24. CHAUDHARY, V. K., T. MIZUKAMI, T. R. FUERST, D. J. FITZGERALD, B. MOSS, I. PASTAN & E. A. BERGER. 1988. Nature 335: 369-372.
25. BUONOCORE, L. & J. K. ROSE. 1990. Nature 345: 625-628.
26. PELHAM, H. R. B. 1989. Annu. Rev. Cell Biol. 5: 1-23.
27. OLDSTONE, M. B. A. 1987. Cell 50: 819-820.
28. LASKY, L. A., G. NAKAMURA, D. H. SMITH, C. FENNIE, C. SHIMASAKI, E. PATZER, P. BERMAN, T. GREGORY & D. J. CAPON. 1987. Cell 50: 975-985.
29. KOWALSKI, M., J. POTZ, L. BASIRIPOUR, T. DORFMAN, W. C. GOH, F. TERWILLIGER, A. DAYTON, C. ROSEN, W. HASELTINE & J. SODROSKI. 1987. Science 237: 1351-1355.
30. WEIS, W., J. H. BROWN, S. CUSACK, J. C. PAULSON, J. J. SKEHEL & D. C. WILEY. 1988. Nature 333: 426-431.
31. ROSSMANN, M. G. 1989. J. Biol. Chem. 246: 14587-14590.
32. HEMMING, A., A. BOLMSTEDT, P. FLODBY, L. LUNDBERG, M. GIDLUND, H. WIGZELL & S. OLOFSSON. 1989. Arch. Virology 109: 269-276.

33. TSCHACHLER, E., H. BUCHOW, R. GALLO & M. S. REITZ. 1990. J. Virol. **64:** 2250-2259.
34. CORDONNIER, A., L. MONTAGNIER & M. EMERMAN. 1989. Nature **340:** 571-574.
35. WOLFF, M. E. & A. MCPHERSON. 1990. Nature **345:** 365-366.
36. DATEMA, R., S. OLOFSSON & P. A. ROMERO. 1987. Pharm. Ther. **33:** 221-286.
37. RADEMACHER, T. W., R. B. PAREKH & R. A. DWEK. 1988. Annu. Rev. Biochem. **57:** 785-838.
38. MATTHEWS, T. J., K. J. WEINHOLD, H-K. LYERLY, A. LANGLOIS, H. WIGZELL & D. BOLOGNESI. 1987. Proc. Natl. Acad. Sci. USA **84:** 5424-5428.
39. LARKIN, M., R. A. CHILDS, T. J. MATTHEWS, S. THIEL, T. MIZUOCHI, A. M. LAWSON, J. S. SAVILL, C. HASLETT, R. DIAZ & T. FEIZI. 1989. AIDS **3:** 793-798.
40. ITO, M., M. BABA, A. SATO, R. PAUWELS, E. DE CLERCQ & S. SHIGETA. 1987. Antiviral Res. **7:** 361-367.
41. BABA, M., R. PAUWELS, J. BALZARINI, J. ARNOUT, J. DESMYTER & E. DE CLERCQ. 1988. Proc. Natl. Acad. Sci. USA **85:** 6132-6136.
42. SCHOLS, D., R. PAUWELS, J. DESMYTER & E. DE CLERCQ. 1990. Virology **175:** 556-561.
43. HOEKSTRA, D. & J. W. KOK. 1989. Biosci. Rep. **9:** 273-305.
44. ASHORN, P. A., E. A. BERGER & B. MOSS. 1990. J. Virol. **64:** 2149-2156.
45. HATTORI, T., A. KOITO, K. TAKATSAKI, H. KIDO & N. KATUNUMA. 1989. FEBS Lett. **248:** 48-52.
46. TANABE-TOCHIKURA, A., T. S. TOCHIKURA, O. YOSHIDA, T. OKI & N. YAMAMOTO. 1990. Virology **176:** 467-473.
47. BADER, J. P., J. B. MCMAHON, R. J. SCHULTZ, V. L. NARAYANAN & M. R. BOYD. 1990. Antiviral Res. Suppl. 1, April 1990, Abstr. 6.
48. BALZARINI, J., D. SCHOLS, E. VAN DAMME, W. PEUMANS & E. DE CLERCQ. 1990. Antiviral Res. Suppl. 1, April 1990, Abstr. 65.

Innovations in the Use of Antisense Oligonucleotides

GERALD ZON

Applied Biosystems, Inc.
Foster City, California 94404

INTRODUCTION

The use of antisense oligonucleotides for control of genetic expression has received an increasing amount of attention during the past few years, from both the scientific community and in the area of new business development. Antisense oligomers refers in a general way to synthetic DNA-like molecules that have approximately 10 to 30 nucleobase-like components that can hybridize with complementary bases in RNA in a sequence-specific manner. This binding can in turn either directly inhibit or otherwise interfere with the normal course of production of the specific "target" protein encoded by the intercepted RNA. Pioneering work in this area, which began over 20 years ago, included various lines of investigation: oligodeoxynucleotides with attached alkylating groups,[1,2] nonionic oligomers (with either $CH_2C(O)$[3] or $P(O)CH_3$[4] internucleoside linkages) to interfere with RNA function, and demonstration of antiviral (Rous sarcoma) effects with an unmodified 13-mer oligodeoxynucleotide.[5,6]

Structurally *unmodified* oligodeoxynucleotides, which are now readily obtained by the use of automated DNA synthesizers,[7] have been more or less (depending on the particulars) successfully employed for inhibition of specific protein synthesis *in vitro*, both acellularly and with whole-cell cultures.[8] Due to degradation of oligonucleotides by nucleases, it is generally assumed at this time that effective *in vivo* applications as chemotherapeutic agents require the development of appropriately modified oligonucleotide analogues, which will have suitable stability as well as a desired profile of other drug properties.

Development of antisense oligomer drugs involves considerations that are unique to this entire class of molecules, such as accessibility of either unprocessed RNA or final mRNA, their tertiary structure, sequence-specific hybridization, and optimal kinetics relative to transcriptional and translational events. By contrast, other considerations are unique to subset members of the general class of antisense oligomer molecules. Such analogue-dependent items include stability toward nucleases *in vivo*, pharmacokinetics, cellular uptake, tissue distribution, delivery vehicles, metabolism, toxicity, and other side effects. Finally, superimposed upon the aforementioned factors, there are very practical considerations involving cost of manufacturing, cost of drug needed for treatment, acceptable charges for treatment, available alternative drugs, and risk-versus-benefit analysis associated with any new drugs.

Perhaps the most significant impetus for developing antisense oligomer drugs is the promise of effective therapy for major diseases that have no current treatment but could be combated by inhibiting the expression of specific proteins. Inasmuch as a number of recent review articles[8-13] and a monograph[14] comprehensively cover the state of the art at this time, this report will focus primarily on those antisense oligomer studies that deal with HIV and related topics. Chemical developments are occurring rapidly, and some of the most recent ones are also described, together with relevant analytical methods.

ANTI-HIV STUDIES

In June 1986, Zamecnik and co-workers[15] published the first report on the possibility of using antisense oligomers to inhibit replication of HIV in cultured human cells: transformed T-lymphocyte (H9) cells and peripheral human blood cells. Unmodified oligodeoxynucleotides 12 to 26 residues in length, which were targeted either close to the tRNA Lys primer binding site, or at donor and acceptor splice sites for the tat gene, were incubated with cells plus virus at 5-50 μg/mL, which corresponds to 1-10 μM concentrations of a 15-mer (5000 MW). After 96 h, measurements gave percent inhibition of HIV reverse transcriptase (RT) activity, relative to control cells incubated without oligomer. The percent inhibition of the production of virus-encoded p15 and p24 proteins was also measured. Some level of activity was found for each of the conditions reported, except for a 15-mer that failed to give measurable inhibition, presumably due to its noncomplementarity with HIV sequences. In a subsequent publication,[16] 20 different target sites were selected and studied with unmodified oligo-deoxynucleotides (all 20-mers) and a similar assay: Molt-3 cells + HIV + oligomer (0.6-15 μM) for 96 hours. Activity was scored as percent inhibition of syncytia formation and production of p24, relative to control cells. As before, all of the 20-mers were active to some extent, except for the noncomplementary control. It was stated that different noncomplementary controls had been used in other series of experiments and were uniformly inactive. Shortly thereafter a third report[17] by the Zamecnik group indicated that, in the same assay with Molt-3 cells,[16] unmodified 15-mer homopolymers (dA_{15}, dC_{15}, dG_{15}, and dT_{15}) all showed some activity. This is indicative of a sequence-nonspecific antiviral effect, assuming there is a relatively low degree of complementarity between HIV sequences and these homopolymers (including shorter domains therein). Based on other findings in this report,[17] essentially the same results and conclusion obtain for oligodeoxynucleotides modified throughout with either phosphorothioate [$P(O)S^-$], phosphormorpholidate [$P(O)NR_2$, $R_2 = CH_2\,CH_2\,O\,CH_2\,CH_2$], or phosphorbutylamidates [$P(O)NR'R''$, $R' = CH_2\,CH_2\,CH_2\,CH_3$, $R'' = H$]. Subsequently reported[18] experiments by Zamecnik and coworkers using this same assay[16] have been carried out with oligodeoxynucleotide analogues having methylphosphonate [$P(O)CH_3$] linkages. In each case there was some activity; however, no data was given for controls with noncomplementary sequences, which precludes any conclusion regarding sequence specificity of the observed antiviral effects.

A similar study by Zaia et al.[19] involved H9 cells + HIV + 8-mer test compounds (≤ 100 μM) with measurements of percent inhibition of syncytia formation and RT activity, relative to controls. The three sequences tested were antisense to a splice site of tat, its sense counterpart, and a sequence complementary to herpes simplex virus. Although the antisense construct was the most active, interpretation of the results is complicated by the absence of reported information about the complementarity of these short 8-mer sequences to HIV sequences.

Matsukura *et al.*[20] likewise investigated unmodified and modified antisense oligomers using an infection assay of the sort mentioned above: immortalized T4$^+$ T cells
(ATH8 cells) $\pm$ HIV $\pm$ oligomer (1-25 μM) and measurement of viable cells as a
function of time. Various 14-base target sites were selected, and the sense, noncomplementary, and homooligomers were used as controls for sequence specificity. In contrast
to the aforementioned reports,[16-19] identical sequence anti-*rev*[21] phosphodiester [unmod-
ified, P(O)O$^-$] and methylphosphonate 14-mer oligomers failed to show statistically
significant levels of activity, whereas the corresponding phosphorothioate had 70%
antiviral activity at 10 μM. On the other hand, the control phosphorothioate oligomers
clearly revealed that there were sequence-nonspecific antiviral effects. This sequence
nonspecificity has been confirmed by more recent and extensive experiments.[22] Southern
blot analysis was used by Matsukura *et al.*[20] to establish that, at 1 μM for 7 days, a
28-base phosphorothioate homooligomer of dC prevented detectable levels of *de novo*
viral DNA synthesis. This observation implied that a mechanism (or mechanisms) of
action was (were) operative at an early stage of the infection process.

In summary, the collective data in these several initial reports[15-20] indicated that
unmodified oligonucleotides and various different modified oligomer analogues can all
exhibit sequence-nonspecific antiviral effects as measured in a virus-challenge (*de novo*
infection) assay. By its very nature, such an assay allows a test compound to potentially
interfere with any critical process within the virus life cycle. Consequently, *de novo*
infection assays are efficient for initial screening of compounds for antiviral activity but
are inappropriate for establishing mechanisms of actions, including whether antiviral
activity exhibited by an intended antisense oligomer actually derives from an antisense
process.

This ambiguity and the relatively potent anti-HIV effects found for phosphorothioate oligomers prompted Matsukura and co-workers[23] to use chronically HIV-III$_B$-in-
fected H9 cells as the basis for assays aimed at establishing, in a convincing manner,
whether a phosphorothioate oligomer was capable of exhibiting sequence-specific suppression of viral expression. In these investigations, which used an extended (28-mer)
version of the previously described[20] anti-*rev* sequence, antiviral activity (measured by
[^{3}H]nucleotide uptake and p24 levels at 10 μM oligomer) was found for the phosphorothioate but not the unmodified (phosphodiester) control. More importantly, in a series
of control phosphorothioates, neither the sense, random, dC$_{28}$, nor anti-*rev* with N^3-
dT residues showed statistically significant levels of activity. The latter control compound has no measurable duplex formation with model DNA target. The altered HIV
mRNA profile induced by the anti-*rev* phosphorothioate oligomer was consistent with
a sequence-specific antiviral effect derived from interference with the regulatory gene,
rev, by some form of "translation arrest." It is unclear at this time whether this
mechanism accounts for the anti-HIV effects observed by Shibahara *et al.*[24] for ana
logues closely related to these phosphorothioates, *viz* oligo (2'-*O*-methyl) ribonucleoside
phosphorothioates. The ambiguity arises from a lack of irrelevant control sequences
and, moreover, use of a *de novo* infection assay.[24]

SEQUENCE-NONSPECIFIC EFFECTS OF THE OLIGOMERS

As noted above, anti-HIV testing[15-20,22] of unmodified oligonucleotides and analogous modified oligomers has revealed sequence-nonspecific activity in *de novo* infection
assays. This conclusion has been supported by more recent data also obtained with the
de novo infection assay.[25] Interestingly, 3' attachment of a cholesteryl group had an

enhancing effect, possibly due to more favorable interaction of the polyanionic oligomers (phosphodiesters and phosphorothioates) with cell membranes.[25] Perhaps the most significant "spin-off" discovery to date regarding sequence-nonspecific biological activity of the phosphorothioates is the finding by Mitsuya (personal communication) that the 28-mer dC homopolymer protects against dysfunction of accessory (antigen-presenting) cells following exposure to HIV *in vitro*. Dextran sulfate also had a protective effect, whereas DNA-chain terminators 3'-azido-2', 3'-dideoxythymidine (AZT), 2', 3'-dideoxyadenosine (ddA), and 2', 3'-dideoxycytidine (ddC) did not provide statistically significant protection.

Formal analogy with the long-known[26] inhibitory properties of synthetic thiol-containing DNAs toward polymerases suggests the possibility of a similar mode of action for phosphorothioates and perhaps other types of oligonucleotides. This has now been found in several cases. Wilson and co-workers[27] determined that purified HIV RT is inhibited by 28-mer oligodeoxycytidine as well as its phosphorothioate analogue, with the later (K_i = 2.8 nM) being 200-fold more potent that the former. This phosphorothioate also inhibited murine leukemia virus (MuLV) RT and cellular α- and γ-polymerases, but not DNA polymerases β and Pol I. Cheng and coworkers[28] subsequently reported that this phosphorothioate (and related homooligomers) strongly inhibited herpes simplex virus type 2 (HSV-2) DNA polymerase, but showed less inhibition of human DNA polymerase α, β, and γ, as well as HSV-1. More recently the 2', 5'-phosphorothioate tetramer 5'-monophosphate analogues of 2-5A were found to be effective inhibitors of HIV RT.[29] Phosphodiester-linked α-anomeric oligonucleotides likewise inhibit both HIV RT and MuLV RT.[30]

Stein and coworkers (private communication) have used a gel retardation assay to obtain evidence for binding of soluble recombinant CD4 to both phosphodiester and phosphorothioate 28-mer homooligomers of dC, with the latter being more effective than the former. These investigators also found that both oligomers could be displaced by a fluoresceinated (FITC) derivative of gp120, the envelope protein of HIV that binds to CD4, which suggests that sequence-nonspecific blockage of gp120 binding to cellular CD4 may be one of the mechanisms by which phosphorothioate (and other) oligomers protect cells from this virus. It is unclear at this time whether such *in vitro* binding phenomena are related to those reported for polyanionic sulfonated carbohydrates such as dextran sulfate.[31]

Sequence-nonspecific inhibition of protein translation by phosphorothioate oligomers in acellular systems[32,33] and in microinjected *Xenopus* oocytes[32] has been reported recently. Adventitious binding of oligomers to either ribosomal components, or an antitemplate-like effect,[26–28] are possibilities for consideration. In any event, the more localized negative charge distribution on sulfur in internucleoside $O = P - S^-$ linkages, and the lower electronegativity (polarizability) of sulfur compared to oxygen, could lead to stronger electrostatic interactions between phosphorothioate groups and positively charged amino acid residues in proteins, especially those that "recognize" polynucleotides through phosphate contacts. Investigations of the influence of thiophosphate substitution on various different nucleases,[34,35] RNA-protein (bacteriophage R17 coat protein) interaction,[36] duplex DNA structure,[35] and autolytic processing of RNA[37] are worth noting in this connection.

OLIGONUCLEOTIDE UPTAKE BY CELLS

The cellular uptake of intended antisense oligomers is obviously a subject of great importance for effective use of these compounds as inhibitors of gene expression.

Zamecnik and co-workers[15] investigated the uptake of ^{32}P-labeled unmodified oligonucleotides and suggested that cells exposed to a 20 μM solution of a 20-mer for 15 min
acquired an apparent intracellular concentration of 1.5 μM. More recently Loke et
al.[38] reported that oligonucleotides are taken up in a saturable, size-dependent manner
compatible with receptor-mediated endocytosis. It was further noted that methyl-
phonate-linked oligo(dT)$_7$ did not block uptake of oligo(dT)$_8$, whereas oligo (dT)$_{12}$
and phosphorothioate-linked oligo (dT)$_7$ efficiently inhibited uptake, which led to the
suggestion that the ionic character of the oligomer backbone may be a critical determinant of the mechanism of uptake, given Ts'o and Miller's earlier data[9] on passive
uptake of methylphosphonates. Using oligo (dT)-cellulose for affinity purification, Loke
et al.[38] identified an 80-kDa surface protein that may mediate transport. Yakubov et
al.[39] shortly thereafter described the use of alkylating oligonucleotides to detect 79-
and 90-kDa proteins in mouse fibroblasts that apparently undergo alkylation upon
exposure to these reactive oligomers. The binding to the proteins was inhibited by other
oligodeoxynucleotides, double-stranded DNA, and RNA, but not polyanions such as
heparin, thus indicating specific receptor proteins in binding of oligomers to mammalian
cells.

A fluoroescein conjugate of the 28-mer phosphorothioate anti-*rev* sequence[23] has
been used by Egan and coworkers (private communication) in a flow cytometric study
of its fluxes into and out of cells, primarily H9, but also U937, K562, and peripheral
blood lymphocytes (PBLs). At concentrations from < 1 μM to 60 μM of this labeled
oligomer in the medium, there was rapid uptake during the first 30 min, followed by
a more gradual, sustained uptake that leveled off after 1-2 hours. Calibration against
standardized beads revealed that at 25 μM the measurable internal concentration was
0.5 μM after 1 hour at 37 °C. Following incubation in fresh medium, this internal
concentration fell to 0.25 μM, but then leveled off, thus suggesting some sequestration.
The uptake by PBLs was markedly lower (10-fold) than that exhibited by the other
cells after correction for cell volumes. Significantly, no remarkable big differences in
uptake were seen when the unmodified phosphodiester conjugate was studied. This
latter observation is in contrast to the report by Neckers and coworkers[40] that phosphorothioate oligomers were taken up by cells much more slowly than their unmodified
phosphodiester counterparts.

ONGOING ANALOGUE STUDIES

The automated solid-phase synthesis of methylphosphonate analogues is now
achieved by use of methylphosphonamidite precursors.[41-44] Purification of these compounds can be achieved by either reversed-phase HPCL[45] or ion-exchange chromatography.[42,45] A detailed study[42] of the effect of ionic strength on the hybridization of
methylphosphonate oligomers to unmodified oligodeoxynucleotides indicates that, at
high salt, the substitution of methylphosphonate linkages only affects the dissociation
rate constant. Oligomers with different arrangements of methylphosphonate linkages
have been examined for nuclease sensitivity *in vitro*, stability in tissue culture, and
ability to form RNase H-sensitive substrates with complementary RNA.[44] The latter
results indicated that a span of three internal phosphodiester linkages was necessary
and sufficient to direct cleavage of the RNA in the duplex. An earlier investigation[46]
of RNase H activity using oligomers with 2'-*O*-methylroboside residues also indicated
the necessity of internal phosphodiester linkages, whereas in the case of phosphorothio-

ates,[32] no internal phosphodiester linkages were needed. By contrast, α-anomeric oligomers bound to β-globin RNA did not lead to cleavage by *E. coli* RNase H.[32] These results agree with relative inhibitory strengths of oligodeoxynucleotides and various analogues in microinjected *Xenopus* oocytes, where the phosphorothioates were the most potent inhibitors of protein synthesis.[32] The same conclusion obtains for acellular translation of the mRNA for *ras p21*.[33] In view of the fact that relatively high concentrations (*ca* 100 μM) of methylphosphonate oligomers are needed for high levels of inhibition of protein synthesis, attention is being given to increasing their efficiency by functionalization with photoactivatable (cross-linking) psoralens[47] and free-radical generating groups.[43] A more novel approach to this end has been investigated by Bischofberger and Matteucci,[48] who incorporated an extra polycyclic base (intercalator) into oligodeoxynucleotides to achieve hybridization characterized by enhanced thermal stability.

STEREOCHEMISTRY

In an oligonucleotide analogue, the presence of asymmetric linkages, such as $O = P - S^-$ and $O = P - CH_3$, leads to the possibility of 2^n stereoisomers, where n is the number of asymmetric linkages. This can, in principle, afford a large set of stereoisomers that have different binding constants in interactions with putative receptors, polymerases, other proteins, and target RNA sequences. Investigations[9,11] aimed at elucidating the magnitude and significance of these effects have been hampered by the unavailability of convenient and, one hopes, automatable methods for synthesis of stereoisomers having either the R or S absolute configuration at each asymmetric internucleoside linkage. Progress is being made with relatively short ($\leq$ 8-mer) homopolymers, which contain either ethylphosphotriester ($O = P - OCH_2 CH_3$),[49,50] $O = P - CH_3$,[51] or $O = P - S^-$ linkages;[52] however, a considerable amount of additional work is needed for efficient practical synthesis of sufficiently long mixed-sequence oligomers for testing of their relative potency as antisense inhibitors.

Two fundamentally different approaches to bypass asymmetric linkages have been independently investigated by various laboratories. One strategy involves the use of modified nonchiral linkages, achieved in several ways: (1) isosteric substitution of the naturally occurring $O = P - O^-$ moiety with $X = Y - X$, as in phosphorodithioate[53] ($S = P - S^-$), dialkylsilyl[54] (R-Si-R), or formacetal (H-C-H) (M. Matteucci, private communication) analogues; (2) isosteric substitution of either the 3' or 5' oxygen in the phosphate moiety as in 3'S-PO_2-O5' recently reported by Cosstick and Vyle,[55] 3'O-PO_2-S5' reported earlier,[56] or 3'O-PO_2-NH5';[57,58] and (3) replacement of the entire phosphate moiety with either $CH_2C(O)$[3] or carbamate[59,60] linkages between the intact D-ribose residues (or cognates[61] thereof). The second strategy involves retention of the naturally occurring nonchiral phosphate moiety and use of either α-anomeric D-ribose or β-anomeric L-ribose[62] moieties, as the former has been bound to be relatively stable toward degradation by nucleases.[63,64]

Although not strictly apropos to the subject of oligomer stereoisomerism, it is nevertheless worthwhile to note increasing interest in acyclic oligonucleotide analogues that have either no C-3' moiety[63] or no nucleoside moiety (W. J. Stec, private communication), and cyclic oligonucleotide analogues that have no base residue (W. Egan, private communication).

ANALYTICAL METHODS

Polyacrylamide gel electrophoresis (PAGE) of unmodified oligonucleotides and their structurally modified analogues continues to be perhaps the most widely employed and most useful method for analysis and purification.[64] PAGE can be used for sequencing unmodified oligonucleotides[65] as well as methylphosphonate[66] and phosphorothioate[67] analogues. Continuous-flow electrophoresis with tube gels, multiple-mode monitoring in real time, and automated fraction collection have been recently made available, and are referred to as high-performance electrophoretic chromatography (HPEC™).[68] This new technology can lead to significant time saving in analytical and micropreparative applications because of the ability to conduct real-time quantitative measurements and use collected fractions without further processing.

Capillary electrophoresis (CE) systems,[69] a second major advance in electrophoretic separation technology, have received recent widespread attention.[70] CE can be conducted either without a sizing matrix, such as polyacrylamide or agarose, or in the presence of such matrices. The chief advantages of CE are its relatively high sensitivity, high performance with regard to separation, and speed, as runs can typically be completed in less than 10 minutes. Another useful feature is the ability to inject sample volumes in the nanoliter range, which allows direct monitoring of the usual microliter-scale *in vitro* reactions and, possibly, intracellular processes through sampling the contents of a single cell.

As more and more analogues of oligonucleotides are investigated, the need for reliable, generally useful mass spectrometric methods of analysis becomes increasingly more desirable. Most of the reports in this area have apparently dealt with fast atom bombardment (FAB) mass spectrometry;[71] however, ^{252}Cf plasma desorption mass spectra[72] may also prove to be useful, especially with the advent of relatively easy to operate and lower-cost systems (Bio Ion).[73] Polyanionic oligonucleotides with O = P − O$^-$ and O = P − S$^-$ linkages can, in principle, be peralkylated[74] to give neutral derivatives that may allow more tractable materials for these mass spectrometric analyses.

Computer-assisted analytical methods of importance to the development of antisense oligonucleotides include calculations of RNA secondary structure and comparison of sequences. These calculations need to be routinely applied by nonexperts in a user-friendly manner. Calculations of this sort are now available[75] but have been applied in only a few strategies for the selection of sequences of antisense oligonucleotides.[76,77] Much more work needs to be done before the success of this approach can be evaluated, especially in view of complications due to the unknown tertiary structure of RNA, the dynamics of its processing, and possible involvement of RNase Hs, which have undefined sequence specificities and "footprints". Regardless of the method of sequence selection, which can range from strictly empirical testing to computer-directed testing from RNA calculations, the sequences of the intended antisense oligomers should be compared with currently available sequence information in Genbank and similar data bases. Ideally, one would aim to always work with antisense oligomers that have minimum complementarity to nontarget sequences currently in Genbank, whether DNA or RNA. For interactive sequence comparisons between the target RNA, RNA calculations, and data base libraries, one can take advantage of new fast-data finder (FDF) technology.[78] This technology, which has user-transparent programmable hardware (as opposed to software), can greatly facilitate the searching speed of a conventional VAX computer. For example, in a comparison of the *ca* 10 kb HIV sequence with the 30 million bases of sequence information currently in Genbank, use of a VAX computer would take about 10 days, which can be reduced to about 24 hours with a Cray Supercomputer, and to only 10 minutes with the FDF.

SUMMARY

The use of antisense oligonucleotides for controlling genetic expression has recently received widespread attention, especially as a new class of potential chemotherapeutic agents. This coupled with the urgency of developing new effective therapies for acquired immunodeficiency syndrome (AIDS) has led to various antisense studies dealing with human immunodeficiency virus (HIV), which are briefly reviewed here. Anti-HIV and other biological activities found for oligonucleotides suggest that sequence-specific and sequence-nonspecific mechanisms of action can be found. Recent developments in oligonucleotide analogue chemistry and relevant analytical methods are also described, including fast-data finder technology.

REFERENCES

1. BELIKOVA, A. M., V. F. ZARYTOVA & N. I. GRINEVA. 1967. Synthesis of ribonucleosides and diribonucleoside phosphates containing 2-chloroethylamine and nitrogen mustard residues. Tetrahedron Lett. No. 37: 3557-3562.
2. SUMMERTON, J. 1979. Intracellular inactivation of specific nucleotide sequences: a general approach to the treatment of viral diseases and virally-mediated cancers. J. Theor. Biol. 78: 77-99.
3. HALFORD, M. H. & A. S. JONES. 1968. Synthetic analogues of polynucleotides. Nature 217: 638-640.
4. MILLER, P. S., L. T. BRAITERMAN & P. O. P. Ts'o. 1977. Effects of a trinucleotide ethyl phosphotriester, G^M p (Et) G^M p (ET) U, on mammalian cells in culture. Biochemistry 16: 1988-1996.
5. ZAMECNIK, P. C. & M. L. STEPHENSON. 1978. Inhibition of Rous Sarcoma virus replication and cell transformation by a specific oligodeoxynucleotide. Proc. Natl. Acad. Sci. USA 75: 280-284.
6. STEPHENSON, M. L. & P. C. ZAMECNIK. 1978. Inhibition of Rous Sarcoma viral RNA translation by a specific oligodeoxyribonucleotide. Proc. Natl. Acad. Sci. USA 75: 285-288.
7. CARUTHERS, M. H. 1985. Gene synthesis machines: DNA chemistry and its uses. Science 230: 281-285.
8. VAN DER KROL, A. R., J. N. M. MOL & A. R. STUITJE. 1988. Modulation of eukaryotic gene expression by complementary RNA or DNA sequences. Biotechniques 6: 958-975.
9. MILLER, P. S. & P. O. P. Ts'o. 1988. Oligonucleotide inhibitors of gene expression in living cells: new opportunities in drug design. Annu. Rep. Med. Chem. 23: 295-304.
10. STEIN, C. A. & J. S. COHEN. 1988. Oligodeoxynucleotides as inhibitors of gene expression: a review. Cancer Res. 48: 2659-2668.
11. ZON, G. 1988. Oligonucleotide analogues as potential chemotherapeutic agents. Pharmacol. Res. Commun. 5: 539-549.
12. TOULME, J.-J. & C. HELENE. 1988. Antimessenger oligodeoxyribonucleotides: an alternative to antisense RNA for artificial regulation of gene expression—a review. Gene 72: 51-58.
13. ZON, G. 1989. Oligonucleotide analogues as potential chemotherapeutic agents. In ACS Symposium Series 401. J. C. Martin, Ed.: 170-184. American Chemical Society. Washington, DC.

14. COHEN, J. S., Ed. 1989. Oligodeoxynucleotides: Antisense Inhibitors of Gene Expression. CRC Press, Inc. Boca Raton, FL.
15. ZAMECNIK, P. C., J. GOODCHILD, Y. TAGUCHI & P. S. SARIN. 1986. Inhibition of replication and expression of human T-cell lymphotropic virus type III in cultured cells by exogenous synthetic oligonucleotides complementary to viral RNA. Proc. Natl. Acad. Sci. USA **83:** 4143-4146.
16. GOODCHILD, J., S. AGRAWAL, M. P. CIVEIRA, P. S. SARIN, D. SUN & P. C. ZAMECNIK. 1988. Inhibition of human immunodeficiency virus replication by antisense oligonucleotides. Proc. Natl. Acad. Sci. USA **85:** 5507-5511.
17. AGRAWAL, S., J. GOODCHILD, M. P. CIVEIRA, A. H. THORNTON, P. S. SARIN & P. C. ZAMECNIK. 1988. Oligodeoxynucleoside phosphoramidates and phosphorothioates as inhibitors of human immunodeficiency virus. Proc. Natl. Acad. Sci. USA **85:** 7079-7083.
18. SARIN, P. S., S. AGRAWAL, M. P. CIVEIRA, J. GOODCHILD, T. IKEUCHI & P. C. ZAMECNIK. 1988. Inhibition of acquired immunodeficiency syndrome virus by oligodeoxynucleoside methylphosphonates. Proc. Natl. Acad. Sci. USA **85:** 7448-7451.
19. ZAIA, J. A., J. J. ROSSI, G. J. MURAKAWA, P. A. SPALLONE, D. A. STEPHENS, B. E. KAPLAN, R. ERITJA, R. B. WALLACE & E. M. CANTIN. 1988. Inhibition of human immunodeficiency virus by using an oligonucleoside methylphosphonate targeted to the *tat*-3 gene. J. Virol. **62:** 3914-3917.
20. MATSUKURA, M., K. SHINOZUKA, G. ZON, H. MITSUYA, M. REITZ, J. S. COHEN & S. BRODER. 1987. Phosphorothioate analogs of oligodeoxynucleotides: inhibitors of replication and cytopathic effects of human immunodeficiency virus. Proc. Natl. Acad. Sci. USA **84:** 7706-7710.
21. HAMMARSKJOLD, M.-L., J. HEIMER, B. HAMMARSKJOLD, I. SANGWAN, L. ALBERT & D. REKOSH. 1989. Regulation of human immunodeficiency virus *env* expression by the *rev* gene product. J. Virol. **63:** 1959-1966.
22. STEIN, C. A., M. MATSUKURA, C. SUBASINGHE, S. BRODER & J. S. COHEN. 1989. Phosphorothioate oligodeoxynucleotides are potent sequence non-specific inhibitors of *de novo* infection by HIV. AIDS Res. Hum. Retroviruses **5:** 639-646.
23. MATSUKURA, M., G. ZON, K. SHINOZUKA, M. ROBERT-GUROFF, T. SHIMADA, C. A. STEIN, H. MITSUYA, F. WONG-STAAL, J. S. COHEN & S. BRODER. 1989. Regulation of viral expression of human immunodeficiency virus *in vitro* by an antisense phosphorothioate oligodeoxynucleotide against *rev(art/trs)* in chronically infected cells. Proc. Natl. Acad. Sci. USA **86:** 4244-4248.
24. SHIBAHARA, S., S. MUKAI, H. MORISAWA, H. NAKASHIMA, S. KOBAYASHI & N. YAMAMOTO. 1989. Inhibition of human immunodeficiency virus (HIV-1) replication by synthetic oligo-RNA derivatives. Nucleic Acids Res. **17:** 239-252.
25. LETSINGER, R. L., G. ZHANG, D. K. SUN, T. IKEUCHI & P. S. SARIN. 1989. Cholesteryl-conjugated oligonucleotides: synthesis, properties, and activity as inhibitors of replication of human immunodeficiency virus in cell culture. Proc. Natl. Acad. Sci. USA **86:** 6553-6556.
26. CAVANAUGH, P. F., Y.-K. HO, R. G. HUGHES, JR. & T. J. BARDOS. 1982. Selectivity of antitemplates as inhibitors of deoxyribonucleic acid polymerases. Biochem. Pharmacol. **31:** 4055-4060.
27. MAJUMDAR, C., C. A. STEIN, J. S. COHEN, S. BRODER & S. H. WILSON. 1989. Stepwise mechanism of HIV reverse transcriptase: primer function of phosphorothioate oligodeoxynucleotide. Biochemistry **28:** 1340-1346.
28. GAO, W., C. A. STEIN, J. S. COHEN, G. E. DUTSCHMAN & Y.-C. CHENG. 1989. Effect of phosphorothioate homo-oligodeoxynucleotides on herpes simplex virus type 2-induced DNA polymerase. J. Biol. Chem. **264:** 11521-11526.
29. MONTEFIORI, D. C., R. W. SOBOL, JR., S. W. LI, N. L. REICHENBACH, R. J. SUHADOLNIK, R. CHARUBALA, W. PFLEIDERER, A. MODLISZEWSKI, W. E. ROBINSON, JR. & W. M. MITHCHELL. 1989. Phosphorothioate and cordycepin analogues of 2',5'-oligoadenylate: inhibition of human immunodeficiency virus 1 reverse transcriptase and infection *in vitro.* Proc. Natl. Acad. Sci USA **86:** 7191-7194.
30. LAVIGNON, M., J.-R. BETRAND, B. RAYNER, J.-L. IMACH, C. MALVY & C. PAOLETTI. 1989. Inhibition of Moloney murine leukemia virus reverse transcriptase by α-anomeric oligonucleotides. Biochem. Biophys. Res. Commun. **161:** 1184-1190.

31. THIELE, B., H. R. BRAIG, I. EHM, R. KUNZE & B. RUF. 1989. Influence of sulfated carbohydrates on the accessibility of CD4 and other CD molecules on the cell surface and implications for human immunodeficiency virus infection. Eur. J. Immunol. **19:** 1161-1164.

32. CAZENAVE, C., C. A. STEIN, N. LOREAU, N. T. THUONG, L. M. NECKERS, C. SUBASINGHE, C. HELENE, J. S. COHEN & J.-J. TOULME. 1989. Comparative inhibition of rabbit globin mRNA translation by modified antisense oligodeoxynucleotides. Nucleic Acids Res. **17:** 4255-4273.

33. CHANG, E. H., Z. YU, K. SHINOZUKA, G. ZON, W. D. WILSON & A. STREKOWSKA. 1989. Comparative inhibition of *ras* p21 protein synthesis with phosphorus-modified antisense oligonucleotides. Anti-Cancer Drug Des. **4:** 221-232.

34. SPITZER, S. & F. ECKSTEIN. 1988. Inhibition of deoxyribonculeases by phosphorothioate groups in oligodeoxyribonucleotides. Nucleic Acids Res. **16:** 11691-11704.

35. LATIMER, L. J. P., K. HAMPEL & J. S. LEE. 1989. Synthetic repeating sequence DNAs containing phosphorothioates: nuclease sensitivity and triplex formation. Nucleic Acids Res. **17:** 1549-1561.

36. MILLIGAN, J. F. & O. C. ULLENBECK. 1989. Determination of RNA-protein contacts using thiophosphate substitutions. Biochemistry **28:** 2849-2855.

37. BUZAYAN, J. M., P. A. FELDSTEIN, C. SEGRELLES & G. BRUENING. 1988. Autolytic processing of a phosphorothioate diester bond. Nucleic Acids Res. **16:** 4009-4022.

38. LOKE, S. L., C. A. STEIN, X. H. ZHANG, K. MORI, M. NAKANISHI, C. SUBASINGHE, J. S. COHEN & L. M. NECKERS. 1989. Characterization of oligonucleotide transport into living cells. Proc. Natl. Acad. Sci. USA **86:** 3474-3478.

39. YAKUBOV, L. A., E. A. DEEVA, V. F. ZARYTOVA, E. M. IVANOVA, A. S. RYTE, L. V. YURCHENKO & V. V. VLASSOV. 1989. Mechanism of oligonucleotide uptake by cells: involvement of specific receptors? Proc. Natl. Acad. Sci. USA **86:** 6454-6458.

40. LOKE, S. L., C. STIN, X. ZHANG, M. AVIGAN, J. COHEN & L. M. NECKERS. 1988. Delivery of c-*myc* antisense phosphorothioate oligodeoxynucleotides to hematopoietic cells in culture by liposome fusion: specific reduction of c-*myc* protein expression correlates with inhibition of cell growth and DNA synthesis. Curr. Top. Microbiol. Immunol. **141:** 282-289.

41. LOSCHNER, T. & J. W. ENGELS. 1988. Methylphosphonamidites: preparation and application in oligodeoxynucleoside methylphosphonate synthesis. Nucleosides & Nucleotides **7:** 729-732.

42. QUARTIN, R. S. & J. G. WETMUR. 1989. Effect of ionic strength on hybridization of oligodeoxynucleotides with reduced charge due to methylphosphonate linkages to unmodified oligodeoxynucleotides containing the complementary sequence. Biochemistry **28:** 1040-1047.

43. LIN, S.-B., K. R. BLAKE, P. S. MILLER & P. O. P. Ts'o. 1989. Use of EDTA derivatization to characterize interactions between oligodeoxyribonucleoside methylphosphonates and nucleic acids. Biochemistry **28:** 1054-1061.

44. QUARTIN, R. S., C. L. BRAKEL & J. G. WETMUR. 1989. Number and distribution of methylphosphonate linkages in oligodeoxynucleotides affect exo- and endonuclease sensitivity and ability to form RNase substrates. Nucleic Acids Res. **17:** 7253-7262.

45. EBRIGHT, Y., G. I. TOUS, J. TSAO, J. FAUSNAUGH & S. STEIN. 1988. Chromatographic purification of non-ionic methylphosphonate oligodeoxyribonucleosides. J. Liq. Chromatogr. **11:** 2005-2017.

46. INOUR, H., Y. HAYASE, S. IWAI & E. OHTSUKA. 1987. Sequence-dependent hydrolysis of RNA using modified oligonucleotide splints and RNase H. FEBS Lett. **215:** 327-330.

47. KUKLA, M., C. C. SMITH, L. AURELIAN, R. FISHELEVICH, K. MEADE, P. MILLER & P. O. P. Ts'o. 1989. Site specificity of the inhibitory effects of olig(nucleoside methylphophonates)s complementary to the acceptor splice junction of herpes simplex virus type 1 immediate early mRNA 4. Proc. Natl. Acad. Sci. USA **86:** 6868-6872.

48. BISCHOFBERGER, N. & M. D. MATTEUCCI. 1989. Synthesis of novel polycyclic nucleoside analogues, incorporation into oligodeoxynucleotides, and interaction with complementary sequences. J. Am. Chem. Soc. **111:** 3041-3046.

49. KNORRE, D. G., V. V. VLASSOV, V. F. ZARYTOVA & A. V. LEBEDER. 1988. Reactive

oligonucleotide derivatives as tools for site specific modification of biopolymers. Sov. Sci. Rev. B Chem. **13**: 1-68.

50. DURAND, M., J. C. MAURIZOT, U. ASSELINE, C. BARBIER, N. T. THUONG & C. HELENE. 1989. Oligothymidylates covalently linked to an acridine derivative and with modified phosphodiester backbone: circular dichroism studies of their interactions with complementary sequences. Nucleic Acids Res. **17**: 1823-1837.

51. LESNIKOWSKI, Z. J., M. JAWORSKA & W. J. STEC. 1988. Stereoselective synthesis of P-homochiral oligo(thymidine methanephosphonates). Nucleic Acids Res. **16**: 11675-11689.

52. LESNIKOWSKI, Z. J. & M. M. JAWORSKA. 1989. Studies on stereospecific formation of P-chiral internucleotide linkage. Synthesis of (Rp, Rp)- and (Sp, Sp)-thymidyl (3',5') thymidyl (3',5') thymidine di(O, O-phosphorothioate) using 2 nitrobenzyl group as a new S-protection. Tetrahedron Lett. **30**: 3821-3824.

53. BRILL, W. K.-D., J.-Y. TANG, Y.-X. MA & M. H. CARUTHERS. 1989. Synthesis of oligodeoxynucleoside phosphorodithioates via thioamidites. J. Am. Chem. Soc. **111**: 2321-2322.

54. CORMIER, J. F. & K. K. OGILVIE. 1988. Synthesis of hexanucleoside analogues containing diisopropylsilyl internucleotide linkages. Nucleic Acids Res. **16**: 4583-4594.

55. COSSTICK, R. & J. S. VYLE. 1988. Synthesis and phosphorus-sulfur bond cleavage of 3'-thiothymidylyl (3'-5') thymidine. J. Chem. Soc. Chem. Commun. 992-993.

56. RYBAKOV, V. N., M. I. RIVKIN & V. P. KUMAREV. 1981. Some substrate properties of analogues of oligothymidylates with p-s-C^5 bonds. Nucleic Acids Res. **9**: 189-201.

57. BANNWARTH, W. 1988. Solid-phase synthesis of oligodeoxynucleotides containing phosphoramidate internucleotide linkages and their specific chemical cleavage. Helv. Chim. Acta **71**: 1517-1527.

58. MAG, M. & J. W. ENGELS. 1989. Synthesis and selective cleavage of oligodeoxyribonucleotides containing non-chiral internucleotide phosphoramidate linkages. Nucleic Acids Res. **17**: 5973-5988.

59. COULL, J. M., D. V. CARLSON & H. L. WEITH. 1987. Synthesis and characterization of a carbamate-linked oligonucleotide. Tetrahedron Lett. **28**: 745-748.

60. STIRCHAK, E. P., J. E. SUMMERTON & D. D. WELLER. 1987. Uncharged stereoregular nucleic acid analogs: 1. Synthesis of a cytosine-containing oligomer with carbamate intersubunit linkages. J. Org. Chem. **52**: 4202-4206.

61. STIRCHAK, E. P., J. E. SUMMERTON & D. D. WELLER. 1989. Uncharged stereoregular nucleic acid analogs: 2. Morpholino nucleoside oligomers with carbamate internucleoside linkages. Nucleic Acids Res. **17**: 6129-6141.

62. RAKACZY, P. & L. OTVOS. 1989. Synthesis of L-oligodeoxyribonucleotides. Chem. Abst. **110**: 115261t.

63. USMAN, N., C. D. JUBY & K. K. OGILVIE. 1988. Preparation of glyceronucleoside phosphoramidite synthons and their use in the solid phase synthesis of acyclic oligonucleotides. Tetrahedron Lett. **29**: 4831-4834.

64. EFCAVITCH, J. W. 1990. The electrophoresis of synthetic oligonucleotides. In Gel electrophoresis of nucleic acids. A practical approach. D. Rickwood & B. D. Hames, Eds. IRL Press. Washington, DC. In press.

65. HINDLEY, J. 1983. DNA Sequencing. Elsevier Biomedical Press. New York, NY.

66. MILLER, P. S., M. P. REDDY, A. MURAKAMI, K. R. BLAKE, D. D. LIN & C. H. AGRIS. 1986. Solid-phase synthesis of oligodeoxyribonucleoside methylphosphonates. Biochemistry **25**: 5092-5097.

67. GISH, G. & F. ECKSTEIN. 1988. DNA and RNA sequence determination based on phosphorothioate chemistry. Science **240**: 1520-1522.

68. Model 230A HPEC™ System User Bulletin. 1990. Applied Biosystems, Inc. Foster City, CA.

69. Model 270A Analytical Capillary Electrophoresis System User Bulletin. 1989. Applied Biosystems, Inc. Foster City, CA.

70. COMPTON, S. W. & R. G. BROWNLEE. 1988. Capillary electrophoresis. Biotechniques **6**: 432-440.

71. IDEN, C. R. & R. A. RIEGER. 1989. Structure analysis of modified oligodeoxyribonucleotides by negative ion fast atom bombardment mass spectrometry. Biomed. Environ. Mass Spectrom. **18**: 617-619.

72. VIARI, A., J. P. BALLINI, P. MELEARD, P. VIGNY, P. DOUSSET, C. BLONSKI & D. SHIRE. 1988. Characterization and sequencing of normal and modified oligonucleotides by ^{252}Cf plasma desorption mass spectrometry. Biomed. Environ. Mass Spectrom. **16:** 225-228.

73. SUNDQVIST, B., P. ROEPSTORFF, J. FOHLMAN, A. HEDIN, P. HAKANSSON, I. KAMENSKY, M. LINDBERG, M. SALEHPOUR & G. SAVE. 1984. Molecular weight determinations of protein by californium plasma desorption mass spectrometry. Science **226:** 696-698.

74. MOODY, H. M., M. H. P. VAN GENDEREN, L. H. KOOLE, H. J. M. KOCKEN, E. M. MEIJER & H. M. BUCK. 1989. Regiospecific inhibition of DNA duplication of antisense phosphate-methylated oligodeoxynucleotides. Nucleic Acids Res. **17:** 4769-4782.

75. JAEGER, J. A., D. H. TURNER & M. ZUKER. 1990. Predicting optimal and suboptimal secondary structure for RNA. Methods Enzymol. **183:** 281-306.

76. CAVANAUGH, P. F., JR. & W. F. PILGERMAYER, JR. 1989. Antisense DNA (ASD) mRNA primary and secondary structure. Proc. Am. Assoc. Cancer Res. **30:** 417, abstr. no. 1657.

77. WICKSTROM, E. T., A. BACON & A. GONZALEZ. 1989. Walking along human c-*myc* mRNA with antisense DNA oligomers. Proc. Am. Assoc. Cancer Res. **30:** 706a, Abstr. no. 3996.

78. ROBERTS, L. 1989. New chip may speed genome analysis. Science **244:** 655-656.

Large-Scale Economic Synthesis of Antisense Phosphorothioate Analogues of DNA for Preclinical Investigations

TIM GEISER

Applied Biosystems, Inc.
Foster City, California 94404

The use of oligonucleotide analogues as potential chemotherapeutic agents has captured widening interest over the last several years. The possibility of using modified "antisense" oligonucleotides to inhibit the expression of genomic DNA and RNA at the level of transcription or translation through sequence-specific hybridization has been convincingly demonstrated in a variety of *in vitro* systems (recently reviewed by Zon[1]).

In anticipation that biological activities in cell culture experiments will continue to improve through a combination of molecular modification and a better understanding of genetic targeting, the requirement for producing unprecedentedly large quantities of oligonucleotide analogues for biological, pharmacological, and toxicological testing will demand increasing attention. Current DNA synthesis and purification technologies provide material on the microgram to milligram scale for use in basic and applied research. The multiple grams that will be required for pharmacokinetic and toxicological studies in small animals represents roughly a 1000-fold increase in scale over current automated synthesis technologies. More importantly, the quantities required for preclinical and clinical evaluation and, eventually, commercialization will necessitate cost-effective processes for the synthesis, purification, and postchromatographic processing of oligonucleotide analogues on a scale 10^4-10^7 times greater than current technologies.

Irrespective of a growing number of promising and diverse examples of inhibition of genetic expression in cell culture, the real potential of antisense therapeutics can only be developed through extensive *in vivo* testing. Among the many substantial challenges facing the development of antisense chemotherapeutics *in vivo* are two challenges that must be met very early. First, pharmacokinetic studies will require existing chain assembly technologies to be scaled up to enable the reliable production of gram quantities of crude oligonucleotide analogues that can be purified by conventional chromatography systems; second, innovative technology must be developed that allows reliable and cost-effective production, characterization, and quality assurance of tens of grams to kilograms of test material under Good Manufacturing Practice (GMP) guidelines. The latter objective must be met in order to commence with preclinical and clinical testing.

The anticipated high cost of treatment using antisense oligomers must be modulated through a balance of pharmacological optimization and reduced cost of production. An obvious approach to reducing production costs would involve extensive scale-up of synthesis and purification processes in order to dilute the effect of high labor costs. Our experience in all aspects of oligonucleotide synthesis, however, suggests that extrapolation of current technologies to scales commensurate with the above needs would fall far short of costs that would allow even affordable clinical evaluation. One need only consider that the chain assembly of unmodified oligonucleotides in the length range of 25-30 bases would entail material costs of between $8000-12,000 per gram and that batch size will be limited by the risk exposure represented by such costs. As a corollary, the considerable processing labor costs can be only moderately reduced by upscaling, unless the basic material costs are dramatically lowered so that batch sizes can be substantially increased.

A brief discussion of practical considerations for the synthesis of a particular kind of oligonucleotide analogue can be used to illustrate a strategy for developing eventual cost-effective production technology. DNA analogues are represented by a great variety of base, sugar, and backbone modifications, but our current focus is concentrated on analogues with the phosphorothioate backbone linkage (FIG. 1, structure III). This class of analogue is of particular interest due, in part, to the recently reported antisense activity against the messenger RNA of the HIV-III gene *rev*,[2] and the following discussion largely derives from experience gained in developing gram-scale synthesis and purification methods for such oligonucleotides.

All DNA analogues incorporating this modification will derive from nucleoside precursors (FIG. 2, I) that will have their reactive functionality protected (FIG. 2, II). In solid-phase synthesis methodologies, the four types of protected nucleoside are converted to their respective generically "loaded" monomer forms (FIG. 2, III) in which X, Y, and Z enable both efficient chemical synthesis and ultimate expression of the desired modification.

Current, practical technologies for synthesizing oligonucleotide phosphorothioates use loaded monomer in the form of either a phosphoramidite[3] or a hydrogen phosphonate[4] synthon (FIG. 3). These two distinctly different building blocks can be used to assemble phosphorothioate oligonucleotides in qualitatively different ways: the phosphoramidite method involves oxidative sulfurization at each cycle of monomer incorporation, whereas the hydrogen phosphonate (H-phosphonate) route allows postponement of oxidative sulfurization until the entire oligonucleotide chain has been

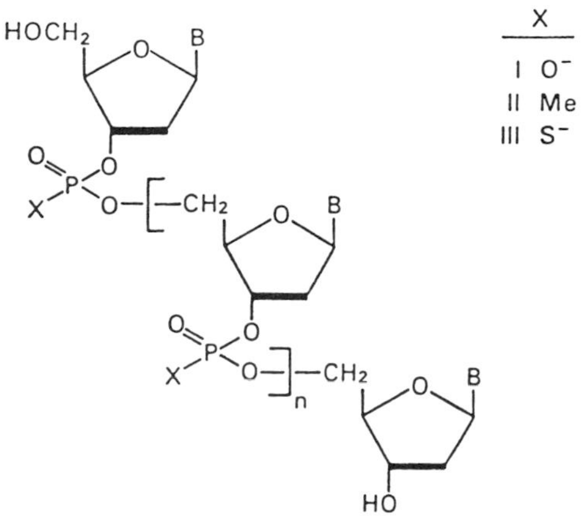

FIGURE 1. DNA analogues.

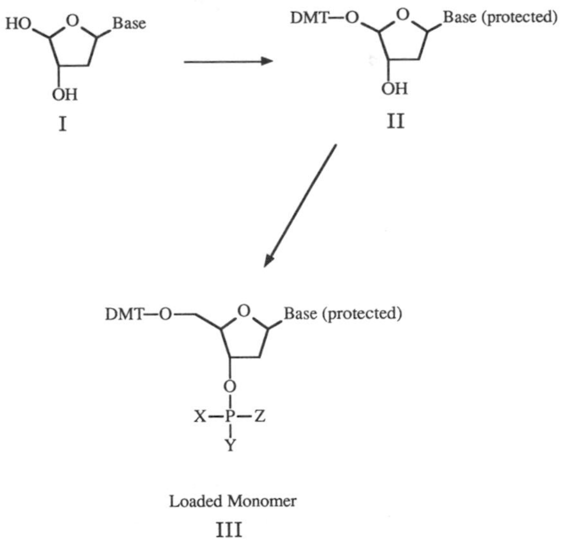

FIGURE 2.

constructed. Both of these methods use a common set of 5'-OH and base-protecting groups in their loaded monomer forms.

The efficiency of each monomer coupling step (*i.e.*, step yield) dictates the maximum yield of desired oligonucleotide in a heterogeneous mixture of all possible deletion sequences, capped failure sequences, and noncapped shorter sequences. After each cycle of monomer addition, step yields are measured by dividing the UV absorbance of trityl cation effluent resulting from 5'-hydroxyl deprotection by the trityl absorbance of the previous cycle. Such measurements hide inefficiencies in the 5'-OH deprotection step preceding monomer addition and reflect only the precision of monomer coupling. Individual measurements of trityl cation always suffer a significant degree of uncertainty, but when averaged over all monomer addition cycles of a synthesis (and over many syntheses of the same base sequence), a credible degree of precision is realized. For an oligonucleotide of length "n," there are n-1 linkages, and the maximum yield of a desired sequence is: (average step yield/100)$^{n-1}$. The consequences of 95%, 99%, and 99.5% step yields are illustrated in FIGURE 4. It is important to note that 100% minus the percentage yield of the target compound is, minimally, the aggregate yield of all possible shorter, capped sequences resulting from inefficient monomer coupling. More realistically, the failure population can also contain (n − 1) and (n + 1) sequences resulting from incomplete 5'-OH deprotection and dimer addition, respectively. In addition, a population of all possible shorter lengths of 5'-ODMT (trityl) terminal oligomers can result from inadvertent chain growth on incipient functionality that may be continually revealed on the solid controlled pore glass (CPG) support through the course of synthesis. There is, then, a potentially significant difference between real step yields and apparent step yields measured by trityl cation.

The factors affecting both apparent (by trityl measurement) and real step yields derive from the nature of the solid support, and the precise chemical means by which deprotection, monomer coupling, capping, oxidation, and washing of the support are effected. Measured step yields distinguish major differences between the use of phosphoramidite and hydrogen phosphonate methodologies in the "large scale" synthesis

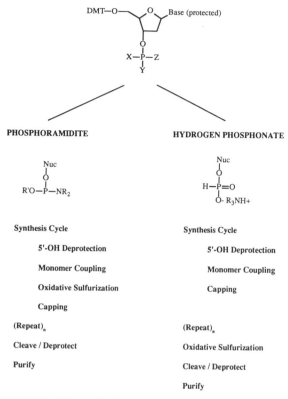

FIGURE 3. Oligonucleotide phosphorothioate synthetic routes.

of phosphorothioate analogues. In our hands, a large number of automated solid phase syntheses of an antisense phosphorothioate 28-mer complimentary to the HIV-III gene *rev*[2] revealed a consistent pattern inherent in the two methods. The average step yields in the H-phosphonate method on a 200 micromole scale were generally in the 95-97% range, irrespective of monomer stoichiometries in the range of 2-10 times substrate, whereas the step yields in the phosphoramidite method consistently averaged in the 98.5-99.5% range.

On the other hand, the H-phosphonate method has the distinct advantage of yielding oligonucleotide product with ~100% phosphorothioate linkages resulting from a single oxidative sulfurization step with elemental sulfur (S_8)/pyridine/triethylamine at the end of the chain assembly. By contrast, the relatively high yield coupling efficiency of the phosphoramidite monomers is compromised by the requirement for oxidative sulfurization at each cycle of monomer addition. The originally reported automated method for phosphorothioate synthesis[3] using S_8 suffers from 5-10% phosphodiester contamination in the phosphorothioate product. Recently, a very promising sulfurizing reagent was reported[5] that effects rapid oxidative sulfurization at ambient temperatures of the intermediate phosphite triester linkage. This reagent, 3*H*-1,2-benzodithiol-3-one-1,1-dioxide, may possess the requisite high sulfurization efficiency and other characteristics that would allow the utilization of the highly efficient phosphoramidite methodology to produce phosphorothioate analogues.

The goal of achieving the highest possible step yield in oligonucleotide synthesis is usually appreciated in terms of the simplest sense of maximizing final yield. The high-step yield goal, however, underlies the more important objective of using a blend of affinity and reverse phase chromatography to isolate the target sequence. Polymeric chromatographic supports have been developed that have a strong affinity for oligonucleotides bearing highly lipophilic 5'-ODMT protected termini. If the chain assembly conditions are sufficiently well-controlled to minimize or eliminate the (n + 1) and (n − 1) by-product populations, ignoring for the moment the possible class of 5'-ODMT shorter oligomers, then the final population of molecules will primarily consist of 5'-ODMT terminal–desired sequence and a complex mixture of shorter capped sequences. The use of such a chromatographic support is illustrated in FIGURES 5 and 6. The reverse-phase analytical profile shown in FIGURE 5 reveals 80.8% of 5'-ODMT terminal product peak and an 11.2% collection of capped failure sequences resulting from an automated 200 micromole synthesis of the anti-*rev* (HIV-III) phosphorothioate. This result correlates well with the measured trityl yields averaging 99.2% and which also predicted an 80% yield of the desired anti-*rev* phosphorothioate product. FIGURE 6 shows the analytical profile of 700 mg of the 5'-ODMT product isolated from a single injection of the entirety of crude, cleaved, base deprotected product from the same 200 micromole synthesis onto a 2.5 × 15 cm column containing a trityl affinity polymer matrix.[6] As long as the true step yields are maintained at a very high level (*e.g.*, > >99%), the trityl-bearing species will be highly homogeneous, and such trityl-specific isolation modalities may be refined to enable higher throughput and capacity for increasing scales of purification. New chromatographic matrices and new pumping/ fraction splitting systems are envisaged for the future that will enable isolation of 10-20 grams of phosphorothioate product per hour from the same size column.

The point made above about a potential by-product population of 5'-ODMT shorter oligonucleotides underscores a problem that may be most inherent in syntheses con-

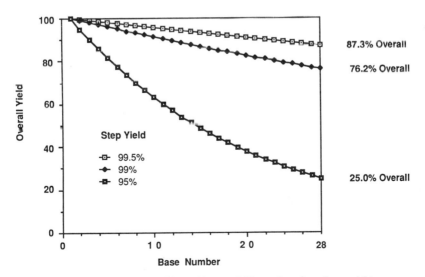

FIGURE 4. Phosphorothioate 28-mer yield as a function of step yield.

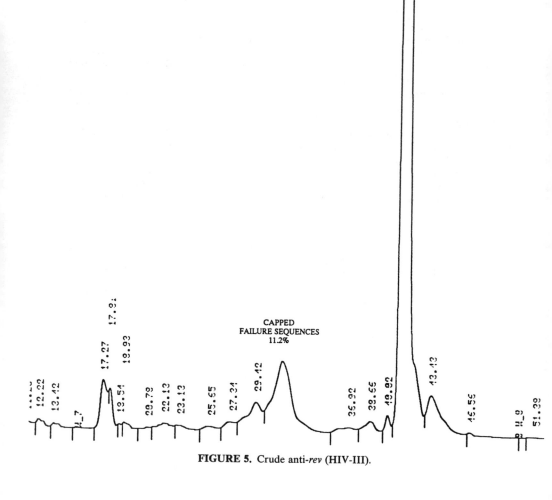

FIGURE 5. Crude anti-*rev* (HIV-III).

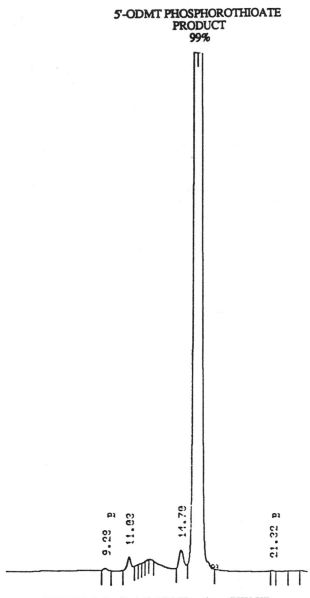

FIGURE 6. Purified 5′-ODMT anti-*rev* (HIV-III).

TABLE 1. Cost for Oligonucleotide Phosphorothioate (28-mer)[a]

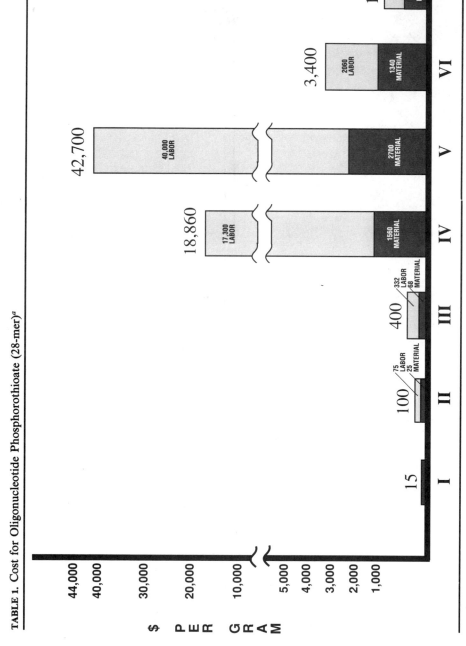

[a] I. Raw nucleosides, 100% yield. II. Protected nucleosides, 100% yield. III. "Loaded" monomer, 100% yield; + solid support. IV. "Loaded" monomer, 100% yield; + solid support; + all reagents; + labor. V. "Loaded" monomer, 26% yield; costs calculated from actual production of three grams of anti-*rev* (HIV-III); 200 micromole scale. VI. "Loaded" monomer, 60% yield; stoichiometric optimization; new catalyst; new solid support; automation; 2500 micromole scale. VII. 70% yield; fully integrated processing; 12.5 millimole scale.

ducted on glass supports where there is the possibility of continually "expressed" silanol functionality resulting from the cleavage of Si-O-Si linkages by solvolysis or other means through the course of synthesis. Such functionality would serve as unwanted sites for inadvertent chain growth, with new oligomer chains starting at each cycle of synthesis on newly expressed S-OH functionality. The problem may be exacerbated in large scale batch operations where the fragile glass beads may crack and spall when subjected to shear not common to flow processes. In addition, the low loading of 3'-terminal nucleoside necessitated by the requirements of high-yield synthesis chemistry further compromises the use of glass supports. Reactor designs for large-scale chain assembly may require strong agitation under very concentrated conditions in order to achieve adequate mixing of reactants for high synthesis efficiency. Thus, new polymer-based supports with much higher nucleoside loading must be developed that can tolerate high shear and whose bulk density and loading are such that chain assembly chemistry can be conducted at very high concentration.

Some of the foregoing considerations can now be viewed from perspectives illustrated in TABLE 1 concerning various synthesis strategies of an oligonucleotide phosphorothioate 28-mer. The costs at the top of the bars roughly approximate wholesale transfer costs that a primary producer might charge for purified, bulk oligonucleotide product. Bar I represents the minimum cost ($15) of one gram of phosphorothioate 28-mer that would somehow be miraculously assembled by coupling the appropriate nucleosides together through phosphate linkages in 100% yield, using no labor, solvents, or reagents other than the raw nucleosides. Bar II makes the same assumptions but uses a higher level monomer, namely the commonly used set of protected nucleosides: the $100/gram of 28-mer is broken down into a material and labor component, with the labor representing the cost associated with producing the protected monomer from the raw nucleoside precursor. Bar III illustrates the cost of 28-mer with similar assumptions (100% yields and 1:1 stoichiometry between monomer and support bound substrate), but it incorporates both loaded monomers and solid support (CPG): again, the labor component represents only the labor associated with producing the loaded monomer and loaded solid support. It is important to recognize that, so far, no reagents, solvents, or processing labor appear in the costs.

Bar IV assumes 100% yields, loaded monomer at 1:1 stoichiometry, solid support, all reagents, and all processing labor, including the analysis of intermediates and final products. The labor component now contains all labor costs associated with producing loaded monomer, solid support, reagent preparation, and all processing labor associated with producing the oligonucleotide phosphorothioate. It is instructive to note that the $1560 material cost is predicated on a 1X monomer stoichiometry, and 100% yields in chain assembly, purification, and postchromatography processing. Superficially, it would appear that the total cost here ($18,860) would be the lowest cost for producing a gram of phosphorothioate 28-mer, until the leveraging effect of scale on labor is considered. Before considering scale effects, it is instructive to discuss the real costs calculated from the actual synthesis of several grams of a phosphorothioate oligomer.

The costs in Bar V are calculated from the real costs of an actual large scale production of 3 grams of the above-mentioned anti-*rev* (HIV-III) phosphorothioate analogue, which is undergoing pharmacokinetic analysis and toxicological testing by the Developmental Therapeutics arm of the National Cancer Institute. The isolation of 3 grams of phosphorothioate product produced a 26% overall yield resulting from 12,600 micromoles of chain assembly at a repeated scale of ~200 micromoles, with about a 4:1 monomer to substrate stoichiometry. The relative enormity of the labor-cost component derives mostly from labor intensive postchain assembly processing. The $2700 material component appears much smaller than the usual calculation of material costs would indicate, because, as in the previous cases, the labor associated with the production of loaded monomers, loaded solid support, and all reagents is transferred to the labor cost component. Thus, when labor is properly accounted for, this analysis reveals that the upper limit of wholesale transfer cost for such an oligonucleotide phosphorothioate would be in the vicinity of $40,000/gram.

When the labor associated with producing loaded monomer, loaded support, and reagents is added back to those materials, the materials cost will be closer to $12,000/ gram of oligonucleotide. It is against this fact, which will dominate the early efforts to achieve the benefits of upscaling, that the leveraging effects of scale must be considered. The risk exposure represented by such materials costs, as mentioned earlier, will limit the degree to which batch processing can be scaled up. Thus, a number of improvements must be simultaneously developed in order to evolve processing to larger and larger scales.

Bar VI illustrates a cost objective for which a strategy is developed that we believe is achievable in a period envisaged for future clinical trials. Details cannot be given here, but the strategy assumes a 60% overall yield at a chain assembly scale of 2500 micromoles, development of a new activation catalyst that will facilitate the stoichiometric optimization of monomer coupling, the development of a new, high-loaded polymer-based synthesis support, a number of improvements to the methodology of chain assembly, and automation of postchain assembly processing. These major changes must be implemented while maintaining the integrity of the chain assembly chemistry to achieve real coupling yields > 99 percent.

Bar VII represents costs that would be attainable by combining the above developments with innovative, fully integrated processing at a 12.5 millimole chain assembly scale with overall yield in the range of 70 percent. Both in this and the previous case, the risk exposure represented by the material inputs of a single batch is minimal and allows for significant, progressive scale-up from each newly established technology base. The foregoing discussion outlining the benefits and pitfalls of chain assembly efficiency serves to underscore some of the considerations that must be given to the elaboration of innovative improvements in automated synthesis. The point is clear, however, that such cost efficiencies will never be achieved by simply scaling up the existing oligonucleotide synthesis technology.

These projected costs appear to be high in an absolute sense, but it is worth noting that some of the newer, chemically sophisticated drugs also have high wholesale transfer costs on a weight basis: tissue plasminogen activator (TPA) at ~$15,000/gram, erythropoietin at ~$1 million/gram, and salmon calcitonin at ~$160,000/gram. Data is yet to be developed for the potential dose size of an antisense oligonucleotide therapeutic, but these potentially achievable production costs may serve to better define first approximation dose objectives in specific therapeutic applications. We believe that the great potential of this new therapeutic technology justifies considerable effort to develop innovative production technology up front, so to speak, so that the probable discovery of therapeutic candidates will be coupled with the timely ability to produce quantities for clinical evaluation and, eventually, commercialization.

SUMMARY

The therapeutic potential of antisense oligonucleotides will heavily depend on a balance of two factors: pharmacologic effectiveness and cost of production. Pharmacologic optimization will be achieved to a limited degree in *in vitro* systems, but substantial progress can only be made in the context of appropriate *in vivo* models. The quantities of synthetic oligonucleotides required for modest *in vivo* testing are several thousandfold greater than can be produced by conventional DNA synthesis technology and 10^5-10^7-fold greater for preclinical and clinical evaluation. Cost-effective synthesis and purification cannot be achieved by extrapolating current technologies to scales commensurate with these quantities. Recent interest in anti-HIV (anti-*rev*) phosphorothioate analogues of DNA ($\sim$28-mers) has prompted us to develop scale-up methodology for routinely producing gram amounts of such analogues. These results and considerations given to producing clinical and commercial quantities were discussed.

REFERENCES

1. ZON, G. 1988. Oligonucleotide analogues as potential chemotherapeutic agents. Pharma. Res. Commun. **5**(9): 539-549.
2. MATSUKURA, M., G. ZON, K. SHINOZUKA, M. ROBERT-GUROFF, T. SHIMADA, C. A. STEIN, H. MITSUYA, F. WONG-STAAL, J. COHEN & S. BRODER. 1989. Proc. Natl. Acad. Sci. USA **86:** 4244-4248.
3. STEC, W. J., G. ZON, W. EGAN & B. STEC. 1984. J. Am. Chem. Soc. **106:** 6077-6079.
4. FROEHLER, B. C. 1986. Tetrahedron Lett. **27:** 5565.
5. IYER, R. P., L. R. PHILLIPS, W. EGAN, J. B. REGAN & S. L. BEAUCAGE. 1990. The automated synthesis of sulfur-containing oligodeoxyribonucleotides using 3*H*-1,2-benzodithiol-3-one-1,1-dioxide as a sulfur-transfer reagent. J. Org. Chem. **55:** 4693-4699.
6. BERGOT, J. Applied Biosystems, Inc. Unpublished results.

Ribozymes as Therapies for AIDS[a]

JOHN J. ROSSI,[b] EDOUARD M. CANTIN,[c]
JOHN A. ZAIA,[d] PAULA A. LADNE,[c] JIAN CHEN,[c]
DELILAH A. STEPHENS,[d] NAVA SARVER,[e] AND
PAIROJ S. CHANG[b,f]

[b]Department of Molecular Genetics
[c]Department of Neurology
[d]Department of Pediatrics
Beckman Research Institute of the City of Hope
Duarte, California 91010
[e]AIDS Program
National Institute of Allergy and Infectious Diseases
Rockville, Maryland 20852
[f]Department of Biochemistry
Loma Linda University
School of Medicine
Loma Linda, California 92350

INTRODUCTION

Certain RNA molecules have enzymatic activity as was first described for the autocatalytic removal of the intervening sequence from the large ribosomal RNA precursor of *Tetrahymena thermophila*.[1-5] This important discovery has changed our views of macromolecular evolution, recognizing the fact that an informational molecule can simultaneously possess enzymatic activity. Catalytic RNAs have now been described in a number of systems from bacteria through humans;[1,2,6-14] the ubiquity of catalytic RNAs has prompted intense investigation into potential applications as well as the mechanisms of catalysis.

Perhaps the simplest RNA autocleavage domain involves the formation of a catalytic active center that has been termed a "hammerhead."[8-10] This autocleavage domain is common to several plant viroids and virusoids as well as to a repetitive satellite transcript from an amphibious newt[6] and is graphically illustrated in FIGURE 1. There is a high degree of sequence homology among the selfcleavage domains of the hammerhead family of ribozymes, including 13 conserved nucleotides that form the catalytic center.[8,9,12] For the cleavage reaction to occur, only a divalent cation such as magnesium is required. The catalysis involves cleavage of a phosphodiester bond with resultant 2'-

[a]This research was supported by a PHS National Cooperative Drug Discovery Group Grant from the National Institutes of Health AI25959. J. J. Rossi, E. M. Cantin, and, J. A. Zaia are members of the Cancer Center CA34991. P. S. Chang was supported in part by a MSTP fellowship from Loma Linda University, School of Medicine.

184

3' cyclic phosphate and 5'OH groups at the termini of the cleaved fragments,[8,9,12] as is depicted in FIGURE 2.

A critical finding is that the essential constituents for the hammerhead ribozyme can be brought together in *trans*, with one molecule serving as a catalyst for the cleavage of the other in an *in vitro* reaction.[8,12,15,16] In these *trans*-cleavage reactions, the catalytic center is flanked by base-paired sequences as depicted in FIGURE 1. The inherent specificity of base pairing ensures that the cleavage takes place at a targeted site in the substrate. Because the catalytic strand is unaltered during the reaction, it can dissociate

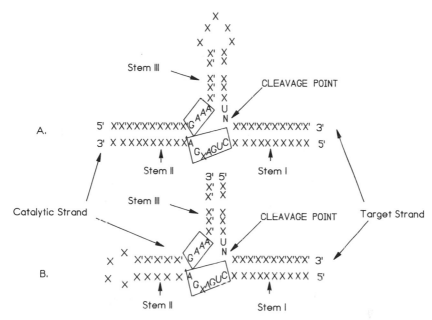

FIGURE 1. Comparison of two classes of *trans*-acting hammerhead ribozymes. The boxed-in nucleotides (nts) indicate the essential bases for formation of the catalytic center of the hammerhead ribozymes. The symbol X represents any of the four nucleotides A,C,G or U, and X' represents the complementary base-pairing partner. The symbol N represents any of the three nucleotides, A, C, or U, which can function as the cleavage site, XUN. G is a very poor cleavage site nucleotide and should be avoided in ribozyme designs. Ribozyme A requires target sequences to provide half of the catalytic center as well as stem III. In contrast to ribozyme A, ribozyme B contains all of the required nucleotides in the catalytic strand with the exception of the cleavage site. In this ribozyme, stem III is formed by intermolecular base-pairing interactions.

from the cleaved products and reanneal with another target to catalyze multiple cleavage reactions as diagrammed in FIGURE 2.

A second important finding relevant to the potential use of catalytic RNAs as antiviral or gene-inactivating agents is the development of a ribozyme in which the catalytic strand harbors 11 out of the 13 conserved catalytic center nucleotides (we will herein refer to this as a holo-ribozyme to distinguish it from the other models).[16] By incorporating all but the cleavage site nucleotides into the *trans*-acting catalyst, the potential number of cleavage sites along a target strand of RNA is greatly expanded.

It should be noted that some investigators find that a cleavage after a guanosine (G) occurs poorly, or not at all, but the cleavage site can be XUN, where X is any nucleotide and N is either C, U, or A.[12,17,18] Thus by random chance, there should be a potential hammerhead ribozyme catalyzed cleavage site found at least once every 5 or 6 nucleotides.

As an extension of antisense RNA experiments in which the target is the HIV-1 genome and transcribed mRNAs, we realized that *trans*-acting catalytic RNAs have potential as antiviral, and in particular, anti-HIV-1 therapeutic agents. Using the plant viroid and virusoid hammerhead ribozyme motif in which the catalytic domains are

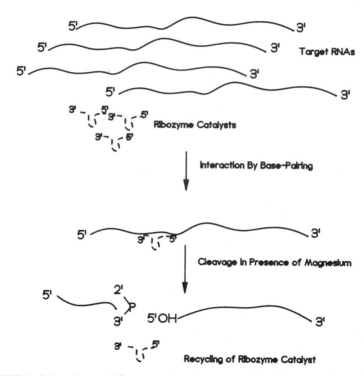

FIGURE 2. Schematic model for *trans*-acting ribozyme-mediated cleavage of target RNAs.

composed of three groups of highly conserved sequence elements, we have designed several *trans*-acting ribozymes targeted to HIV-1 RNAs. We demonstrate two modes of cleavage, one in which HIV-1 RNA sequences form part of the active site of the ribozyme and are subsequently cleaved by a *trans*-acting catalytic strand, and the other, based upon the Haseloff and Gerlach design,[16] in which only an XUN is supplied by the HIV-1 RNA. *In vitro,* these cleavage reactions are specific; multiple substrate turnover is observed, and specific cleavage reactions can take place in a mileux containing total cellular RNAs. We also demonstrate that a biologically active ribozyme is expressed in a cell culture system. These results have important implications for the potential use of ribozymes as anti-HIV-1 therapeutic agents.

RESULTS AND DISCUSSION

General Principles Behind Designs of Trans-*acting Ribozymes*

FIGURE 1 depicts two generalized designs for *trans*-acting ribozymes. In FIGURE 1A, the substrate contributes nucleotides to the active site of the ribozyme (boxed in bases). The catalytic strand supplies the remainder of active center nucleotides (boxed in bases) and is targeted to a specific site within the substrate by base-pairing. The cleavage reaction takes place between the "N" and adjoining nucleotide as indicated. The catalyst can dissociate from the cleaved target, reanneal with another intact target molecule, and effect cleavage of that molecule. The three stems indicated in this figure are crucial to the cleavage reaction. Stems I and II are supplied by the base-pairing of sequences flanking the catalytic center. Stem III, which is in the target molecule, is the most difficult to establish because it depends upon the fortuitous combination of a GAAAX followed by a region that can form a stem (see FIG. 1A), which in turn is followed by an XUN cleavage site.

FIGURE 1B depicts a generalized ribozyme structure based upon the findings of Haseloff and Gerlach.[16] The catalytic strand is designed such that stem III is supplied by the flanking base-paired regions. Because only an XUN cleavage site is required in the target, the frequency of cleavage sites using the model B ribozyme greatly exceeds that for model A.

RNA-Catalyzed Autocleavage of HIV-1 RNA

Based upon the model presented in FIGURE 1A, we reasoned that a hammerhead ribozyme could be formed by combining HIV-1 RNA and a *trans*-supplied catalyst, which would thus effect self-cleavage of the HIV-1 target. To carry this out, we searched for sequence elements in HIV-1 that conformed to the viroid and virusoid autocleavage motif and harbored the sequences GAAACX$_n$ and CUN in relatively close juxtaposition. The third required sequence block (CUGANGA) would be supplied in *trans* (as depicted in FIGURES 1A and 3A). Using this strategy, 11 possible targets were identified in HIVHXB2 proviral DNA.[19] Those regions that had the greatest potential for forming a stable stem III were examined further. The first target that met these criteria was the *gag* gene sequence illustrated in FIGURE 3. In order to incorporate this *gag* sequence into an autocleavage domain, we synthesized a 20 base long catalytic strand by *in vitro* transcription. This catalyst supplied the third block of required nucleotides and was targeted to sequences flanking the HIV-1 GAAAC—GUC block (FIG. 3). When this ribozyme was incubated in equimolar amount with a 138 base, *in vitro*-produced *gag* transcript, cleavage of the substrate into two fragments of the expected size was observed (FIG. 3). The smaller cleavage product was actually composed of several fragments of heterogenous lengths. This heterogeneity was shown by direct sequencing to be at the 3' end of the *gag* transcript, the consequence of erratic *in vitro* transcription termination, and not a variation in the cleavage site (data not presented).

The catalytic efficiency of this ribozyme was examined under several different temperatures (data not presented). Surprisingly, the cleavage efficiency was uniform

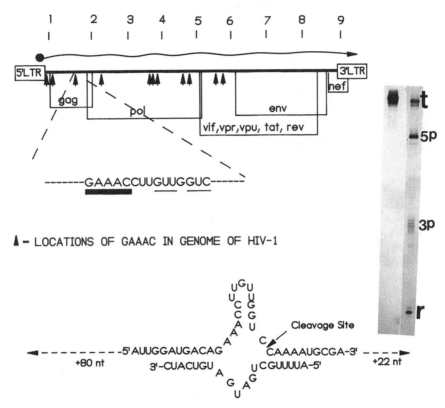

A — LOCATIONS OF GAAAC IN GENOME OF HIV-1

FIGURE 3. Ribozyme-mediated autocleavage of HIV-1 RNA. Ribozyme-mediated cleavage of *gag* gene target harboring GAAAC and GUC nucleotide blocks. The occurrences of GAAAC in HIV-1 isolate HIVXHB2 were identified by computer search and are indicated schematically in this FIGURE. The target of choice encompasses nucleotides 1743-1757. A 138 nucleotide (HIV nucleotides 1711-1789 plus 60 nucleotides of vector polylinker), *in vitro*-produced transcript was used as substrate for the cleavage reactions in both A and B. The reaction depicted was carried out for 14 hours at 37°C in 10 mM $MgCl_2$, 50 mM Tris-HCl pH7.5, and 1 mM EDTA with equimolar amounts of [^{32}P]UTP-labeled ribozyme and substrate. The reaction mixtures were electrophoresed in a denaturing acrylamide gel and autoradiographed. The left lane depicts the 138 nt uncleaved target, whereas the right lane depicts the results of a cleavage reaction. The target (t), cleavage products (5p and 3p), which are 106 and 32 nts, respectively, as well as the ribozyme (r), are indicated.

over a rather broad range of temperatures, from 37° to 55°C, with maximal activity observed between 37° and 45°C. It should be noted that in contrast to the results described below, complete cleavage of the substrate using this ribozyme has not been observed at any temperature after 14 hours incubation. We believe this to be a consequence of instability of stem III, which is crucial to formation of the hammerhead catalytic center. Nevertheless, we have clearly shown that HIV-1 RNA can participate in the formation of a hammerhead autocleavage center.

Holo-ribozyme-Mediated Cleavage of HIV-1 RNAs

Subsequent to our studies with the above-described catalytic RNA, Haseloff and Gerlach published studies of *trans*-acting ribozymes targeted to the bacterial CAT gene.[16] Their ribozyme design was based upon the structure of the catalytic center of the satellite RNA of Tobacco Ringspot Virus and harbored two of the three required catalytic center elements (FIG. 1, ribozyme B). This ribozyme design allows much greater flexibility in the choice of target sites. Using the same *gag* RNA substrate described above, we designed a catalytic RNA (FIG. 3) following the principles of Haseloff and Gerlach. When a temperature profile for this ribozyme was carried out, relatively uniform cleavage activity was also observed over a broad range of temperatures, with maximal activity also between 37°C and 45°C (data not presented). At a 1:1 ribozyme to substrate ratio, this ribozyme effected complete cleavage of the substrate at 37°C, following a 14 hour incubation (FIG. 4). As described above, the heterogeneity of the shorter 3' cleavage product is due to the erratic transcriptional termination of the *in vitro* produced transcript. Investigation of the specificity of the cleavage site by dideoxy sequencing of the cleavage reaction products demonstrated that the cleavage takes place after the predicted C nucleotide (data not presented).

Time Course of the Cleavage Event

The holo-ribozyme described in FIGURE 4 was incubated with an equimolar amount of the 138 nt long *gag* target transcript for varying amounts of time at 37°C. Under these conditions, substantial cleavage was observed after 30 minutes and progressed continually over the 4 hours of incubation at 37°C (FIG. 5). Complete cleavage of the *gag* transcript at a 1:1 substrate to ribozyme molar ratio was observed following prolonged incubation as demonstrated in FIGURE 4.

The Anti-HIV-1 Ribozymes Turnover Multiple Substrates

We have examined the substrate turnover abilities of two holo-ribozymes targeted to *gag* and to 5' long terminal repeat (LTR) sequences, respectively. In these experiments (FIG. 6), the amounts of substrate were kept constant, whereas the ribozymes were titrated to vary the substrate to ribozyme ratios from 1:1 to 50:1. In each case, incubation of the ribozymes with molar excesses of substrate resulted in catalytic turnover of molar excesses of substrate. It must be emphasized that we have made no deliberate attempts to optimize the turnover rate of these ribozymes. These data simply demonstrate that the anti-HIV-1 molecules are capable of multiple substrate cleavages.

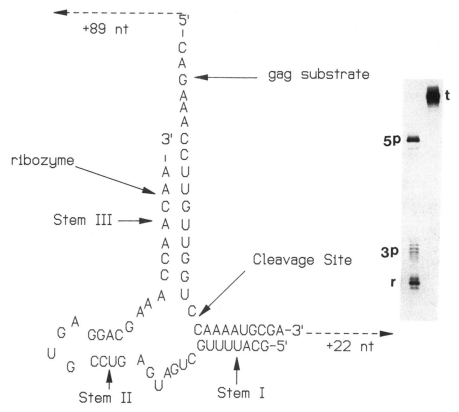

FIGURE 4. Holo-ribozyme-mediated cleavage of HIV-1 RNA. An illustration of the interaction and cleavage site of the Haseloff and Gerlach holo-ribozyme targeted to the same region of HIV-1 *gag* RNA as described in the legend to FIG. 3. The stems corresponding to those presented in FIG. 3 are also illustrated. The autoradiogram depicts an experiment in which the holo-ribozyme was incubated under cleavage conditions with the 138 nt *gag* region substrate. The left lane depicts the cleavage reaction, whereas the right lane depicts uncleaved substrate. Symbols are the same as described for FIG. 3.

Anti-HIV-1 Ribozymes Can Function in a Milieu of Total Cellular RNA

The ultimate goal of developing catalytic RNAs that cleave HIV-1 sequences is their utility as therapeutic agents in patients. Before ribozymes can be effective therapeutic agents, the many variables that could potentially influence the effective use of ribozymes in a living cell must be experimentally examined. Some of these variables can be examined using an *in vitro* cell-free system. In an attempt to begin examining some of these variables, we have synthesized a gene coding for a holo-ribozyme that is targeted to the translational initiation region of the HIV-1 *gag* gene. This ribozyme was initially cloned into a transcription vector such that the *in vitro* transcript resulted in a ribozyme with 70 non-HIV-1 complementary nucleotides. Fifty of these are appended to the 5' end of the ribozyme and 20 to the 3' end (FIG. 7). These extra nucleotides were derived from the polylinker sequences of the cloning vector. This ribozyme was tested against a 610 nucleotide long *gag* region RNA substrate in a cell-free system. In addition to the substrate, varying amounts of total RNA prepared from H9 lymphocytes either uninfected, or infected with HIV-1, were added to the ribozyme-*gag* substrate reaction. This was done to simulate a complex *in vivo* milieu. The results, depicted in FIGURE 7, clearly demonstrate that the extra flanking nucleotides did not inhibit cleavage of the target sequence. Additionally, the added total cellular RNAs

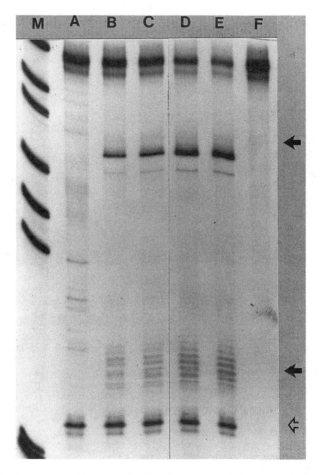

FIGURE 5. Time versus activity profiles of holo-ribozyme. Ribozyme activities were assayed under standard cleavage reaction conditions in the presence of 10 mM $MgCl_2$ and at a 1:1 substrate to ribozyme molar ratio. The substrate or target is the 138 nt *gag* transcript described in FIG. 3. The reactions were stopped after the times indicated below. Lanes: M, molecular weight marker, *Hpa*II digested pBR322 DNA; A, 4 hours incubation without $MgCl_2$ added (negative control); B, 0.5 hour reaction; C, 1 hour reaction; D, 3 hour reaction; E, 4 hour reaction; F, 4 hour incubation of substrate without ribozyme B and $MgCl_2$. The open arrow indicates the ribozyme position, and the solid arrows indicate the two cleavage products that are the same as described in the FIG. 3 legend.

from both uninfected as well as HIV-1-infected H9 cells had no marked effect on the cleavage reaction. In these experiments, the ribozyme was present in molar excess over the target substrate, and the incubations were carried out at 37°C for 14 hours, conditions that favor the complete cleavage of the target RNA. It should also be pointed out that the target itself was somewhat degraded when incubated under reaction conditions in the absence of ribozyme (2nd lane, FIG. 7B). By focusing upon the

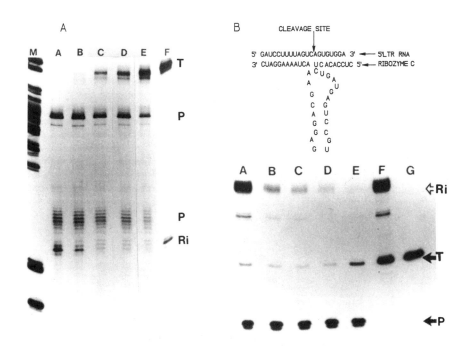

FIGURE 6. Holo-ribozyme titrations versus *gag* and 5′ LTR substrates, respectively. (A) The *gag*-targeted holo-ribozyme (FIG. 4) was titrated relative to a fixed amount of 138 nt *gag* substrate, such that substrate to ribozyme molar ratios were as follows: A, 1:1; B, 5:1; C, 10:1; D, 25:1; E, 50:1; F, 1:1 in the absence of MgCl$_2$. The target (T), ribozyme (Ri), and products (P) are the same as described in FIG. 4. Reactions were assayed under standard conditions with 20 mM MgCl$_2$. (B) The LTR-targeted holo-ribozyme (ribozyme C) depicted in this FIGURE was titrated relative to a fixed amount of 5′LTR substrate (coordinate:602–622) such that the target to ribozyme ratios were as follows: A, 1:1; B, 5:1; C, 10:1; D, 20:1; E, 50:1; F, 1:1, without MgCl$_2$ added; G, substrate alone, no ribozyme, plus MgCl$_2$. Standard reaction conditions were employed using 20 mM MgCl$_2$. Symbols: Ri indicates ribozyme C, T indicates 5′LTR substrate, and P indicates cleavage products that are 13 nts and 8 nts.

amounts of the smaller cleavage product, which does not appear to be subjected to the breakdown observed with the input transcript and larger cleavage product, it can be observed that inclusion of RNA from HIV-1-infected cells in the reaction resulted in substrate competition for ribozyme-mediated cleavage of the input labeled target. This is evidenced by reduced amounts of the smaller cleavage product in the lanes containing the HIV-1-infected, H-9 total cellular RNAs (compare the + lanes to the − lanes

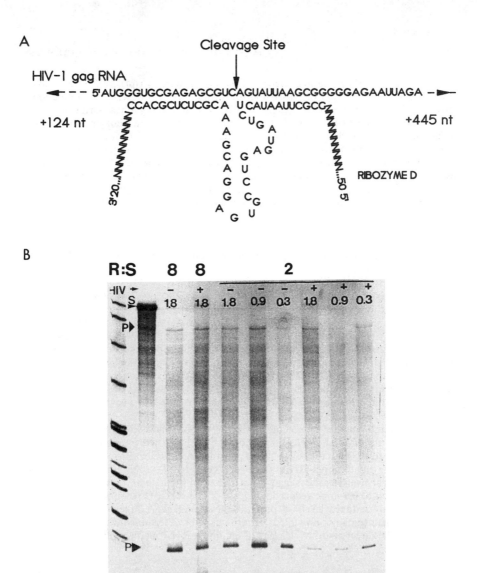

FIGURE 7. Evaluation of the catalytic activity of a holo-ribozyme harboring non-HIV-1 complementary nucleotides in a complex milieu. This holo-ribozyme is targeted to the *gag* gene between nucleotides 805 and 806, just downstream of the AUG translational initiation codon at 789-791. The ribozyme has 70 nts that are noncomplementary to HIV-1 sequences. These extra nucleotides, designated by "N", are derived from the polylinker sequence of the vector in which the ribozyme is cloned. The cleavage reaction experiments were designed to simulate an *in vivo* milieu by adding total RNA from HIV-1-infected (+) or -uninfected (−) H9 lymphocytes. Two different ratios of ribozyme to substrate (R:S) were used, 2:1 and 8:1 as indicated. The amounts of total RNA from either the HIV-1-infected or -uninfected cells are indicated and range from 0.3 through 1.8 μg as indicated above each lane. The substrate (in this case a 610 nt containing transcript) containing coordinates 675-1275 (plus 10 bases of polylinker on the 5' end) is indicated (S), as are the cleavage products (P), which are 141 (5') and 469 (3') nts, and the ribozyme (R). The reactions were performed under standard conditions with 20 mM $MgCl_2$.

under conditions of a 2:1 ratio of ribozyme to input *gag* transcript). When the ratio of ribozyme to template was increased fourfold, there was no observable competition effect (compare + and − lanes, where the ribozyme to input *gag* transcript ratio was 8:1). These results provide several important conclusions. First, a ribozyme with 5' and 3' flanking sequences noncomplementary to the target can still effect specific cleavage of the target. Second, competition by total cellular RNA does not markedly affect the specificity or efficiency of the cleavage reaction. Third, the ribozyme cleavage is affected by an input of RNA from HIV-1-infected cells, suggesting that the *gag* region transcripts from these cells were, as expected, a competitor for ribozyme cleavage. When the amount of ribozyme was increased, the competition was no longer discernible.

Expression of an Anti-gag Ribozyme in Transfected CD4⁺ HeLa Cells

Intracellular expression of the ribozyme depicted in FIGURE 7 was obtained following cloning of the ribozyme DNA into a mammalian expression vector containing the human β-actin promoter and an SV-40 late transcriptional termination and polyadenylation signals.[20] This recombinant vector was transfected into CD4⁺ HeLA cells,[21] and stably transfected clones were isolated and assayed for ribozyme expression using a polymerase chain reaction assay[22,23] (FIG. 8A). A Northern blot analysis was also performed on poly A⁺ RNA isolated from one of the expressing clones. A rather diffuse hybridizing band, centered at approximately 450 nts, was observed (FIG. 8B), suggesting that approximately 200-300 polyadenosines appended to the primary transcripts.

To determine whether or not the ribozyme transcripts were catalytically active, varying amounts of total RNA from one of the clones were tested against an *in vitro*-transcribed *gag* target RNA. At the highest RNA concentration (5 μg), detectable cleavage of the input target RNA was observed (FIG. 9). Preliminary results with pooled clones of transfectants suggest that these cells are somewhat protected from HIV-1 infection based upon reduced amounts of *gag* RNA (FIG. 10). These data are corroborated by reduced levels of proviral DNA and *gag* antigen in the ribozyme expressing clones (data not presented). It remains to be determined whether or not this reduction is the direct result of cleavage of incoming RNA mediated by the ribozyme.

CONCLUSIONS AND FUTURE PROSPECTS

We have exploited a class of selfcleaving molecules, the hammerhead ribozyme, to design and test RNAs that can specifically cleave HIV-1 genomic and messenger RNAs at predetermined sites. The cleavage reactions can take place at physiological temperatures in a complex milieu of total RNAs. Furthermore, the ribozymes act as true catalysts in that they turn over multiple substrate molecules.

As a prelude to experiments in which a ribozyme can be used therapeutically to treat HIV-1-infected cells, we have obtained expression of the anti-*gag* ribozyme in CD4⁺ HeLa cells. The ribozyme expressed in these cells is biologically active, effecting cleavage of input target RNA in an *in vitro* reaction. These results demonstrate that despite the extended length of the ribozyme transcripts (*ca* 400 extra nts), biologically

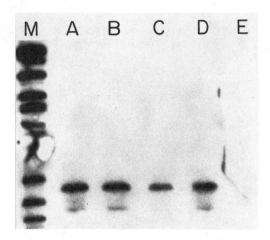

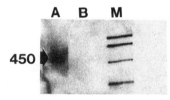

FIGURE 8. RNA analyses of HeLa CD4+ cells transfected with a *gag*-targeted holo-ribozyme. The expression of the holo ribozyme depicted in Fig. 7 from a mammalian expression vector transfected into HeLa CD4+ cells was assayed by both RNA-based PCR (**A: upper panel**) and Northern blot analysis (**B: lower panel**). (**A**) For the polymerase chain reaction (PCR) analyses, 0.5 μg of total RNAs from transfected clones or pools of clones were extracted, subjected to one round of reverse transcription using a primer complementary to transcribed vector sequences 3' of the ribozyme, followed by DNA amplification with the addition of a second primer carrying the ribozyme sense sequence. The PCR products were treated as described previously[23] and hybridized with a ^{32}P-labeled oligonucleotide complementary to the ribozyme sequences. The lanes depicted are as follows: M, *Hpa*II-digested pBR322 marker; A–D, PCR-amplified ribozyme from transfected cells; E, contamination control lacking template. Controls in which the RNA templates were present, but the reverse transcription step was omitted, gave no detectable products (not shown). (**B**) The Northern analyses were done on poly (A) + RNA from HeLa CD4+ cells expressing the holo-ribozyme of FIGURE 7 from the human β-actin promoter, (lane A). RNA from the untransformed HeLa CD4+ parent line was electrophoresed in lane B. The RNAs were electroblotted from a denaturing polyacrylamide gel onto a nylon membrane and probed with a ^{32}P-labeled oligonucleotide probe complementary to the expressed ribozyme. M is the *Hpa*II-digested pBR322 molecular weight marker.

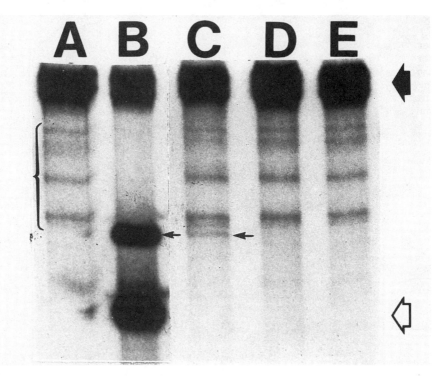

FIGURE 9. Cleavage of *in vitro*-transcribed *gag* substrate by intracellularly expressed holo-ribozyme. Total RNA from a HeLa CD4⁺ clone expressing the ribozyme of FIGURE 7 was tested for cleavage activity. A 178 nt *in vitro*-transcribed *gag* substrate (large solid arrow, coordinates 675-841 plus 10 polylinker nts) (lane A) was mixed with *in vitro*-transcribed ribozyme (lane B) or 5 μg (C), 1 μg (D), or 0.2 μg (E) of total RNA from the ribozyme-expressing HeLA clone. The *in vitro* cleavage reaction conditions were as described in the legend to FIG. 3, except that the MgCl₂ concentration was 20 mM MgCl₂. The bracketed bands are spontaneous degradation products of the ³²UTP-labeled substrate. As can be seen in lane B, these are substrates for the ribozyme, because the *in vitro* transcribed molecules completely cleave these to smaller products (not seen in this picture). The small arrow indicates the 5′ cleavage product, which is 141 nts in length. The 3′ product of 36 nts is not shown. The large open arrow indicates the electrophoretic position of the *in vitro*-produced ribozyme.

functional ribozyme molecules are produced in this system. We have also obtained preliminary data suggesting cleavage of HIV-1 *gag* region RNAs in HIV-1-infected HeLa CD4⁺ cells expressing this ribozyme.

The therapeutic use of ribozymes in treating HIV-1 infections is a goal of our research efforts. Two possible modes of treatment are envisioned. The first is exogenous delivery of preformed ribozymes targeted to highly conserved regions of the virus. The delivery to infected cells may take place through liposome carriers capable of targeting these molecules to the cytoplasm of infected cells, or simply by infusion of ribozymes into peripheral blood. In both cases, the ribozymes will need to be modified to protect them against rapid degradation by both serum and cellular nucleases. There are several possible strategies for doing this. One approach is the development of chimeric DNA-RNA molecules with nuclease-resistant DNA analogues flanking the RNA catalytic center. The flanking DNA sequences can provide the base-pairing specificity but may contain thioester bonds or methylphosphonate residues to protect the molecules from exonucleases. Another strategy is the use of modified ribose moieties such as 2'-O-methylribose, which may also resist nuclease degradation. The chemistry for these strategies is currently available and needs to be applied to ribozyme syntheses. If a simple infusion approach is used, the ribozymes may need to be complexed with some

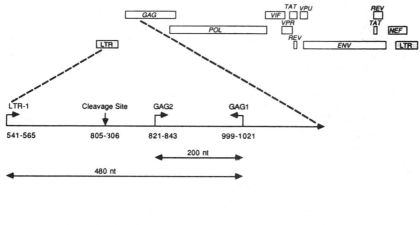

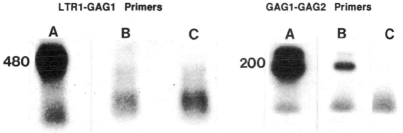

FIGURE 10. PCR analyses of HIV-1 RNAs and DNAs from HeLa CD4⁺ cells expressing a *gag*-targeted holoribozyme. HeLa CD4⁺ cells transfected with, and expressing the holo-ribozyme depicted in FIG. 7 were challenged with HIV-1, as previously described.[27] Seven days postinfection, total RNA or DNA was extracted from these and control cells and analyzed for HIV-1 LTR-*gag* RNAs (using LTR-1 and GAG-1 primers), which amplify a product that spans the cleavage site of the ribozyme, as illustrated. As a control, RNA adjacent to the cleavage site was also assayed using PCR primers that amplify a *gag* segment adjacent to the cleavage site (GAG-1 and GAG-2). In both cases the amplified products were treated as previously described[23] and probed with a ³²P-labeled oligonucleotide complementary to *gag* sequences common to both PCR products. Lane A in both cases depicts PCR-amplified product from the HeLa CD4⁺ parental cells. Lane B in both cases depicts PCR-amplified product from HeLa CD4⁺ ribozyme-expressing cells. Lane C in both cases is a contamination control in which only primers, no templates, were included in the PCR reactions. The product sizes and their derivations are diagramed in the upper panel of the FIGURE.

molecule that will facilitate intracellular transport. It should be possible to combine ribozymes with recombinant proteins that will bind to a specific cellular receptor and allow endocytosis of these molecules. Clearly, the potential for exogenous delivery exists, but a great deal of basic research is still necessary before this delivery strategy can be implemented.

The second potential method of ribozyme delivery is through gene therapy. We have already demonstrated that ribozymes can be expressed in cultured cells. Intracellular expression of these molecules could lead to either cytoplasmic or nuclear localization. It is not clear at this time where an anti-HIV-1 ribozyme will be most effective. The most effective localization is certainly going to depend on the target (*gag, rev, tat, nef,* etc.) RNA and where it is most susceptible to base-pairing and subsequent cleavage. It is now possible to use expression vectors and strategies that will allow for localization of expressed ribozymes in a particular compartment within the cell. We are currently investigating a number of parameters that will affect intracellular ribozyme expression and localization. The results obtained from these experiments should facilitate our understanding of what factors will enhance the efficacy of these molecules as anti-HIV-1 therapeutic agents.

The gene therapy approach will depend upon availability of safe and efficient vectors for delivering the constructs to pluripotent stem cells and/or other cells that are potential targets for HIV-1 infection. A great deal of progress has been made in the use of retroviral vectors for gene therapy.[24] Testing delivery methods for ribozyme gene constructs in appropriate animal models[25] is an important step in evaluating the potential efficacy of these molecules in a gene-therapy situation. Such experiments are presently underway.

As with any anti-HIV-1 therapeutic strategy, the problem of genetic variability must be addressed.[26] In the ribozyme strategy, genetic variability is critical, because a base change at the cleavage site would destroy the effectiveness of the ribozyme. A first approach to this problem is to define targets, which when mutated, destroy the biological function of the gene. Targets such as splice signals, translational initiation codons, and binding sites for RNA regulatory factors such as *tat* and *rev* are among those that should be used. Multivalent ribozymes that simultaneously target two or more sites will increase the probability that at least one site will be cleaved. As we learn more about the mechanisms of ribozyme-mediated catalysis, it is conceivable that some genetic changes will be tolerable. This is clearly an important area for future investigation.

In summary, catalytic RNAs or ribozymes represent a new class of potentially potent antiviral therapeutic agents. The field is still in its infancy and will require many hours of investigation before ribozymes can be used as therapeutic agents. It is our hope and intention that these studies will ultimately lead to a ribozyme therapy for the treatment and management of AIDS.

ACKNOWLEDGMENTS

The authors wish to acknowledge the technical assistance of Jian Chen. We thank W. Mutter for help in preparing this manuscript.

REFERENCES

1. CECH, T. R. 1988. Ribozymes and their medical implications. J. Am. Med. Assoc. **260:** 3030-3034.
2. CECH, T. R. & B. BASS. 1986. Biological catalysis by RNA. Annu. Rev. Biochem. **55:** 599-629.
3. ZAUG, A. J. & T. R. CECH. 1982. The intervening sequence excised from the ribosomal RNA precursor of *Tetrahymena* contains a 5'-terminal guanosine residue not encoded by the DNA. Nucleic Acids Res. **10:** 2823-2838.
4. ZAUG, A. J. & T. R. CECH. 1986. The intervening sequence RNA of *Tetrahymena* is an enzyme. Science **231:** 470-475.
5. ZAUG, A. J., P. J. GRABOWSKI & T. R. CECH. 1983. Autocatalytic cyclization of an excised intervening sequence is a cleavage-ligation reaction. Nature **301:** 578-583.
6. EPSTEIN, L. M. & J. G. GALL. 1987. Transcripts of newt satellite DNA self-cleave *in vitro*. Cold Spring Harbor Symp. Quant. Biol. **52:** 261-265.
7. FORSTER, A. C., C. DAVIES, C. SHELDON, A. C. JEFRIES & R. H. SYMONS. 1988. Self-cleaving viroid and newt RNAs may only be active as dimers. Nature **334:** 265-267.
8. FORSTER, A. C., A. C. JEFFRIES, C. C. SHELDON & R. H. SYMONS. 1987. Structural and ionic requirements for self-cleavage of virusoid RNAs and trans self-cleavage of viroid RNA. Cold Spring Harbor Symp. Quant. Biol. **52:** 249-259.
9. FORSTER, A. C. & R. H. SYMONS. 1987. Self-cleavage of plus and minus RNAs of a virusoid and a structural model for the active sites. Cell **49:** 211-220.
10. FORSTER, A. C. & R. H. SYMONS. 1987. Self-cleavage of virusoid RNA is performed by the proposed 55 nucleotide active site. Cell **50:** 9-16.
11. PRODY, G. A., J. T. BAKOS, J. M. BUZAYAN, I. R. SCHNEIDER & G. BRUENING. 1986. Autolytic processing of dimeric plant virus satellite RNA. Science **231:** 1577-1580.
12. UHLENBECK, O. C. 1987. A small catalytic oligoribonucleotide. Nature **328:** 596-600.
13. WU, H-N. & M. M. C. LAI. 1989. Reversible cleavage and ligation of hepatitis delta virus RNA. Science **243:** 652-654.
14. WU, H-N., Y.-J. LIN, F.-P. LIN, S. MAKINO, M.-F. CHANG & M. M. C. LAI. 1989. Human hepatitis delta virus RNA subfragments contain an autocleavage activity. Proc. Natl. Acad. Sci. USA **86:** 1831-1835.
15. JEFRIES, A. C. & R. H. SYMONS. 1989. A catalytic 13-mer ribozyme. Nucleic Acids Res. **17:** 1371-1377.
16. HASELOFF, J. & W. L. GERLACH. 1988. Simple RNA enzymes with new and highly specific endoribonuclease activities. Nature **334:** 585-591.
17. KOIZUMI, M., Y. HAYASE, S. IWAI, H. KAMIYA, H. INOUE & E. OHTSUKA. 1989. Design of RNA enzymes distinguishing a single base mutation in RNA. Nucleic Acids Res. **17:** 7059-7071.
18. SHELDON, C. C. & R. H. SYMONS. 1989. Mutagenesis analysis of a self-cleaving RNA. Nucleic Acids Res. **17:** 5679-5685.
19. RATNER, L., A. FISHER, L. L. JAGODZINSKI, H. MITSUYA, R.-S. LIOU, R. C. GALLO & F. WONG-STAAL. 1987. Complete nucleotide sequence of functional clones of the AIDS virus. AIDS Res. Hum. Retroviruses **3:** 57-69.
20. GUNNING, P., J. LEAVITT, G. MUSCAT, S.-Y. NG & L. KEDES. 1987. A human β-actin expression vector system directs high-level accumulation of antisense transcripts. Proc. Natl. Acad. Sci. USA **84:** 4831-4835.
21. MADDON, P. J., A. G. DALGLEISH, J. S. MCDOUGAL, P. R. CLAPHAM, R. A. WEISS & R. AXEL. 1986. The T4 gene encodes the AIDS virus receptor and is expressed in the immune system and the brain. Cell **47:** 333-348.
22. SAIKI, R. K., S. SCHARF, F. FALOONA, K. MULLIS, G. HORN, A. ERLICH & N. ARNHEIM. 1985. Enzymatic amplification of beta-globin genomic sequences and restriction site analysis for diagnosis of sickle cell anemia. Science **230:** 1350-1354.
23. MURAKAWA, G. J., J. A. ZAIA, P. A. SPALLONE, D. A. STEPHENS, B. E. KAPLAN, R. B. WALLACE & J. J. ROSSI. 1988. Direct detection of HIV-1 RNA from AIDS and ARC patient samples. DNA **7:** 287-295.

24. MILLER, A. D. & G. J. ROSMAN. 1989. Improved retroviral vectors for gene transfer and expression. Biotechniques **7:** 980-989.
25. NAMIKAWA, R., H. KANESHIMA, M. LIEBERMAN, I. L. WEISSMAN & J. M. McCUNE. 1988. Infection of the SCID-hu mouse by HIV-1. Science **242:** 1684-1686.
26. MEYERHANS, A., R. CHEYNIER, J. ALBERT, M. SETH, S. KWOK, J. SNINSKY, L. MOR-FELDT-MANSNON, B. ASJO & S. WAIN-HOBSON. 1989. Temporal fluctuations in HIV quasispecies *in vivo* are not reflected by sequential HIV isolations. Cell **58:** 901-910.
27. ZAIA, J. A., J. J. ROSSI, G. J. MURAKAWA, P. A. SPALLONE, D. A. STEPHENS, B. E. KAPLAN, R. ERITJA, R. B. WALLACE & E. M. CANTIN. 1988. Inhibition of human immunodeficiency virus by using an oligonucleoside methylphosphonate targeted to the *tat-3* gene. J. Virol. **62:** 3914-3917.

Antisense and Antiviral Therapy

MICHAEL I. SHERMAN[a]

Department of Cell Biology
Roche Research Center
Hoffmann-La Roche Inc.
Nutley, New Jersey 07110

HIV is a complex virus and AIDS is a difficult disease to contend with. In view of this, the speed with which basic research and clinical discoveries have contributed to our understanding of HIV and AIDS has been impressive. In considerable part, this is because AIDS has become prevalent in the midst of the biotechnology explosion. On the other hand, current therapeutic strategies for combatting AIDS are still relatively unsophisticated. It will be interesting, in retrospect, to examine how ultimate therapeutic approaches to this disease have been influenced by opportunities that our new-found technology base allows.

One of the innovative approaches being considered as an anti-AIDS therapeutic strategy is the use of antisense oligonucleotides. The concept of using antisense sequences to block gene expression dates back several years and has been used against numerous genetic targets (see ref. 1). Indeed, in 1986, Zamecnik et al.[2] first reported the feasibility of the approach for HIV, at least for infected cells in culture. As the other articles in Part III of this volume attest, we are becoming progressively more sophisticated in our ideas of how to exploit the antisense strategy effectively for therapeutic purposes. One can now imagine the use of DNA antisense oligonucleotides to block expression of viral mRNA or more complex antisense structures and strategies that would interfere with either retroviral replication or transcription of provirus. Conjugated oligonucleotides have been designed that variously lead to enhanced binding to, covalent binding to, or degradation of, the target nucleic acid sequence (reviewed by Cohen and Zon[1]). Combined ribozyme-antisense technology is another example of a more elaborate approach that has already been shown to elicit cleavage of HIV viral RNA in a catalytic manner.[3]

The antisense strategy is particularly suited to application in anti-HIV and other antiviral therapies because it should be possible to target unique viral sequences that do not have functional counterparts in the human genome. In theory, then, an antisense therapy could have exquisite specificity.

As is so often the case with new therapeutic approaches, there are significant difficulties that must be overcome before antisense therapy can become a reality. Although the strategy might be novel, the major problems are not fundamentally different from generic ones that must be addressed in the development of any therapeutic, namely how to generate an active, safe, and cost-effective drug. A number of technical issues are relevant to such concerns, including optimization of potency of antisense molecules, determination of the most effective and safest ways of getting antisense sequences into cells, evaluation of the pharmacokinetics of antisense mole-

[a] Present address: PharmaGenics, Inc., 4 Pearl Court, Allendale, NJ 07401.

cules, production of adequate amounts of antisense therapeutics to do animal and clinical testing, and generation of antisense therapeutics in a cost-effective manner.

POTENCY OF ANTISENSE SEQUENCES

Antisense sequences directed against different regions of the target nucleic acid can be differentially active; there are several possible reasons for this.[1] For example, antisense sequences that hybridize with the 5' end of mRNA are often relatively good inhibitors of translation, presumably because they block initiation.[4] On the other hand, antisense sequences that hybridize to internal regions of the mRNA molecule can also be effective, ostensibly because they serve as substrates for RNase H action;[5] unlike the former event, the latter one would irreversibly inactivate the mRNA molecule. Superimposed upon these factors must be general considerations such as base composition (which would influence strength of hybridization) and tertiary structure of the target sequence (which would determine accessibility to the target antisense molecule). Such issues will be assessed with increasing success as we generate progressively more effective models for predicting nucleic acid tertiary structure.[6] Building catalytic properties into antisense molecules through ribozyme structures could significantly contribute to their efficacy, although it will be necessary to generate such therapeutics with reaction rates that are markedly increased over existing constructs. Finally, although the technological challenge is considerable, efforts are in progress to use antisense molecules to block gene expression at the level of the genome.[7] Success in these attempts could greatly enhance the potency of antisense therapeutics because the number of target molecules would be vastly reduced relative to that of the mRNA or protein products of the target gene.

CELLULAR UPTAKE

There is much work to be done to optimize cellular uptake of antisense oligonucleotides. Oligonucleotides consisting of some types of monomers appear to be actively transported into cells, whereas others are most likely taken up by passive diffusion.[8,9] Facilitation of oligonucleotide uptake by chemical linkage to nonoligonucleotide conjugates has also been considered.[10] There are advantages and disadvantages for all of these cell uptake routes, and it is too early to predict which strategy (or combination thereof) is likely to be the most effective. In the case of ribozyme technology, the most obvious approach would be to introduce such sequences by way of viral transduction. This route carries the potential advantages of efficient cell penetration and even targeted delivery, but care will have to be taken to ensure that the viral sequences will not cause undesirable mutations (leading to malignancy), for example, by integration into the cellular genome.

PHARMACOKINETICS

In order to be maximally effective the antisense molecule must reach its intracellular target in an intact state. It is likely that in patients there will be a series of impediments to achieving this end. For example, nucleases in blood will undoubtedly reduce the circulating half-life of such molecules unless they are constructed so as to prevent this occurrence. Notwithstanding the importance of this issue, there has been a paucity of documented studies on the pharmacokinetics of antisense molecules in animal models because of production difficulties and cost considerations.

PRODUCTION

In order to carry out animal studies with antisense molecules, relatively large amounts of material are required. Generation of such amounts of material is difficult and expensive because of limitations of current technology. This will no doubt slow progress in elaboration of critical animal studies to evaluate utility, pharmacokinetics, and toxicity of antisense therapeutics. The article by Geiser[11] in this volume addresses some of the key issues regarding production of antisense therapeutics.

COST EFFECTIVENESS

Several factors will ultimately influence cost effectiveness of antisense therapeutics. In the space of just a few years, the costs of producing natural and modified oligonucleotides have dropped dramatically;[11] however, costs of labor and starting materials will probably soon prohibit further significant reductions. A more hopeful consideration for achieving competitiveness of antisense therapy will be to dramatically reduce the effective dose (currently in the micromolar range[9]) by improving a combination of properties of the molecules including potency, cellular accessibility, and pharmacokinetic profile.

In conclusion, several events are likely to be required before antisense therapy becomes an effective and competitive strategy in AIDS or any other major disease category. The requisite changes will probably occur in an incremental and step-wise fashion. Some of these future achievements are likely to have considerably more impact than others; for example, we are only beginning to evaluate feasibility of designing antisense molecules that will act upon genomic DNA rather than mRNA;[7] success in this area could dramatically increase the scope and utility of antisense therapy. It is difficult to predict when such breakthroughs will occur. Nevertheless, the concept of an antisense drug is compelling because it offers the opportunity to act pharmacologically at very early stages of gene expression; this approach could ultimately provide us with a therapeutic strategy with broad generic utility that is efficient, effective, nontoxic, and specific.

REFERENCES

1. STEIN, C. A. & G. ZON. 1988. Cancer Res. **48:** 2659-2668.
2. ROSSI, J. J., E. M. CANTIN, J. A. ZAIA, P. A. LADNE, J. CHEN, D. A. STEPHENS, N. SARVER & P. S. CHANG. 1990. Ann. N. Y. Acad. Sci. This volume.
3. ZAMECNIK, P. C., J. GOODCHILD, Y. YAGUCHI & P. SARIN. 1986. Proc. Nat. Acad. Sci. USA **75:** 285-288.
4. LIEBHABER, S. A., F. E. CASH & S. H. SHAKIN. 1984. J. Biol. Chem. **259:** 15597-15602.
5. WALDER, R. Y. & J. A. WALDER. 1988. Proc. Natl. Acad. Sci. USA **85:** 5011-5015.
6. WICKSTROM, E. L., T. A. BACON, A. GONZALEZ, D. L. FREEMAN, G. H. LYMAN & E. WICKSTROM. 1988. Proc. Natl. Acad. Sci. USA **85:** 1028-1032.
7. MOSER, H. E. & P. B. DERVAN. 1987. Science **238:** 645-650.
8. LOKE, S. J., C. A. STEIN, X. H. ZHANG, K. MORI, M. NAKANISHI, C. SUBASINGHE, J. S. COHEN & L. M. NECKERS. 1989. Proc. Natl. Acad. Sci. USA **86:** 3474-3478.
9. MARCUS-SEKURA, C. J. 1988. Anal. Biochem. **172:** 289-295.
10. LEMAITRE, M., B. BAYARD & B. LEBLEU. 1987. Proc. Natl. Acad. Sci. USA **84:** 648-652.
11. GEISER, T. 1990. Ann. N. Y. Acad. Sci. This volume.

Metabolism in Human Leukocytes of Anti-HIV Dideoxypurine Nucleosides[a]

ARNOLD FRIDLAND,[b] MARK A. JOHNSON,[b]
DAVID A. COONEY,[c] G. AHLUWALIA,[c]
VICTOR E. MARQUEZ,[c] JOHN S. DRISCOLL,[c] AND
DAVID G. JOHNS [c]

[b]*Department of Biochemical and Clinical Pharmacology*
St. Jude Children's Research Hospital
Memphis, Tennessee 38101
[c]*Developmental Therapeutics Program*
Division of Cancer Treatment
National Cancer Institute
National Institutes of Health
Bethesda, Maryland 20892

INTRODUCTION

A number of 2',3'-dideoxynucleosides inhibit the *in vitro* infectivity of human immunodeficiency virus (HIV), the etiologic agent of the acquired immunodeficiency syndrome (AIDS).[1,2] Of the dideoxynucleosides studied to date the dideoxypurine nucleoside 2,3'-dideoxyadenosine (ddA) and its deaminated derivative 2',3'-dideoxyinosine (ddI) exhibit particularly favorable therapeutic ratios and appear to be equally effective in the ATH-8 cell system.[2,3] Phase I studies also have shown that ddI produces objective responses in patients with AIDS and severe AIDS-related complex.[4]

The antiviral activity of these drugs is thought to be mediated by inhibition of reverse transcriptase (viral RNA-directed DNA polymerase) in virus-infected cells.[1] Hence phosphorylation of the nucleoside prodrug is required for activation to the putative active triphosphate. In earlier studies,[3,5] we showed that ddA could be metabolized in human lymphoid cells to its metabolite ddATP but also was rapidly converted through the ubiquitous enzyme adenosine deaminase to ddI, which was cleaved to the purine base hypoxanthine by purine nucleoside phosphorylase. Additionally, attempts were made to see if prevention of deamination of ddA by the potent inhibitor 2'-deoxycoformycin (dCF) could enhance the antiviral activity of the drug; however, this inhibitor did not greatly improve either the antiviral activity of ddA or its activation

[a]This work was generously supported in part by PHS Grants 1 R01 AI27652 and 1 R01 CA43296; by (CORE) Grant P30 CA21765 from the National Institutes of Health; and by the American Lebanese Syrian Associated Charities.

to the active metabolite ddATP. These results suggested that there might be alternate modes by which dideoxypurine nucleosides could be metabolized to the putative active inhibitor of HIV replication in human cells.

In this report, we would like to review our recent studies that deal with the enzymatic basis for, and regulation of, dideoxynucleotide accumulation from ddA, ddI, and a novel dideoxypurine nucleoside 2',3'-dideoxy-2'-fluoroarabinosyladenine (2'-F-dd-ara-A) (FIG. 1).

EXPERIMENTAL PROCEDURES

Material

Cells

Human T lymphoid cells CCRF-CEM and Molt-4 were maintained as described previously.[6] The CAR-1, Py9, and CARA mutants, defined by their deficiencies in deoxycytidine (dCyd) kinase, adenosine (Ado) kinase, and both dCyd kinase and Ado kinase, respectively, were grown as described.[6]

Radiochemicals

[2',3'-^{3}H]ddAdo, 30 Ci/mmol; [2,8-^{3} H]ddAdo and [8-^{3}H] carbocyclic 2',3'-didehydro-2',3'-dideoxyguanosine (Carbovir), both 1.3 Ci/mmol; [8-^{3}H]ddguanosine (Guo), 2-3.5 Ci/mmol; [8-^{3}H]dGuo, 16 Ci/mmol; and [2-^{3}H]inosine (Ino), 35 Ci/mmol were obtained from Moravek Biochemicals (Brea, CA). [8-^{3}H]dAdo, 20 Ci/mmol was from ICN Radiochemicals, Irvine, CA. [2,pr,3'-^{3}H]ddIno was prepared by means of enzymatic deamination of either the sugar-labeled or base-labeled ddAdo using calf intestinal adenosine deaminase (Sigma Chemical Co., St. Louis, MO). 2'-F-[^{3}H]-dd-ara-A (25 Ci/mmol) was purchased from American Radiolabeled Chemicals Inc. (St. Louis, MO).

Chemicals

ddADP and ddATP were purchased from Pharmacia (Piscataway, NJ), 2'-F-ddara-AMP was synthesized by means of the general method of Yoshikawa et al.,[7] and 2'-F-dd-ara-ATP was synthesized according to the general method of Kovacs and Otvos.[8] ddAdo (NSC98700) and 2'-F-dd-ara-A (NSC613792) were obtained from the Drug Synthesis and Chemistry Branch (NCI, NIH). Carbovir was provided by the courtesy of Dr. Charles Litterst of the Developmental Therapeutics Branch (NIAID). All other nucleoside and nucleotide standards were purchased from Sigma Chemical Co. (St.

Louis, MO).[1] Enzymes: adenosine deaminase (calf intestine) (200 U/mg) and alkaline phosphatase (*E. coli;* 45 U/mg) were purchased from Boehringer-Mannheim Biochemicals, Indianapolis, IN and Sigma Chemical Co., MO., respectively. PEI-cellulose TLC plates (20 × 20 cm) with UV_{254} fluor were from Brinkman Instruments (Westburg, NY). Dithiothreitol and ATP were from Research Organic, Cleveland, OH.

Methods

Metabolism Studies

For metabolism studies, cells (Molt-4, CEM, or ATH-8) or CEM variants deficient in either dCyd kinase, Ado kinase, or in both enzyme activities growing in log phase were incubated at a density of about 1×10^6 cells with either [³H]ddAdo, [³H]ddIno, or 2'-F-[³H]-dd-ara-A (10 µM final concentration, with 5 µCi/mL cell suspension), in the presence or absence of 5 µM dCF for 15 min prior to addition of the dideoxynucleo-

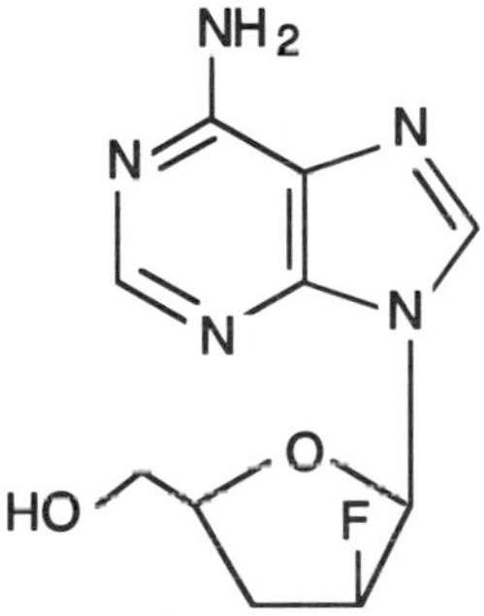

FIGURE 1. Structure of 2',3'-dideoxy-2'-fluoroarabinosyladenine.

sides. After 5 h of incubation, cells were centrifuged and pellets were washed with cold phosphate-buffered saline and extracted with 60% aqueous methanol (−20°C). After centrifugation, 200 µL of the supernatant was subjected to chromatography on an anion exchange Partisil 10 SAX column. One minute fractions were collected and radioactivity determined by liquid scintillation counting. Radioactive dideoxynucleotides in the HPLC fractions were identified by comparing their retention times with those of authentic standards.

Enzyme Assays

Ado kinase and dCyd kinase were purified from CCRF-CEM cells or from human leukemic blasts obtained by leukopheresis from patients with leukemias, as described.[5] The kinase activities were separated from nucleotidase activity and other nucleoside phosphorylating enzymes. The standard reaction mixture for the assay of dideoxy-nucleoside phosphorylation contained 10 to 25 μg protein for dideoxynucleosides and 0.1 to 2 μg protein for natural substrates in a total volume of 26 μL containing 10 mM sodium HEPES buffer, pH 7.5; 3 mM dithiothreitol; 5 mM ascorbate; 20 mM MgCl$_2$; 10 mM ATP; 15 mM phosphoenolpyruvate; 0.3 units pyruvate kinase; and 20 mM NaF. The assays were started by addition of substrate with incubation for 30 min at 37°C; the rate of phosphorylation was constant over the time period used. Reactions were terminated by addition of 75 μL of 1 mM unlabeled substrate in water. Aliquots (45 μL) were pipetted onto DEAE cellulose discs (2.4 cm Whatman DE81); the discs were dried at 75°C, washed three times with water, and counted. Background controls (zero time) were determined as above and subtracted from each test assay.

Nucleoside phosphorylation by 5'-nucleotidase was done with 2.4 mM ^{3}H-labeled nucleoside (0.5 μCi) in a volume of 15 μL buffer containing 100 mM HEPES pH 7.4, 50 mM MgCl$_2$, 500 mM KCl, 5 mM IMP, 3 mM dithiotreitol, 5 mM ATP, and 15 μg protein from the fast-flow Q/Blue Sepharose-purified nucleotidase(s). After 30 min at 37°C, reactions were terminated; 20-25% hydrolysis of the substrate IMP occurred during such incubations. Products from these reactions were measured by using poly-ethyleneimine (PEI)-cellulose thin layer chromatography. The thin layer plates were prespotted with carriers (10 nmol) and developed in water. Products and substrates were located visually by UV absorption, cut out, and quantitated by liquid scintillation counting as described.

Purification of Human Leukemic Cells 5'-Nucleotidase

The cytoplasmic 5'-nucleotidase was purified from fresh leukemic blasts obtained by leukopheresis from patients. Briefly, a suspension of white cells freed of erythrocytes was homogenized in Tris HCl buffer, pH 7.4, containing 3 mM dithiothreitol, 10% (v/v) glycerol, 0.5 mM phenylmethylsulfonyl fluoride (PMSF), 0.5 mM O-phenanthroline, 5 mM benzamidine, and 0.5 mg soybean trypsin inhibitor. After centrifugation at 105,000 g, the supernatant was stirred with 200 mL ion exchange resin (fast-flow Q-Sepharose that had previously been equilibrated with homogenization buffer). 5'-Nucleotidase activity was eluted from the Q-Sepharose using a linear gradient buffer of 0-0.6 M KCl in homogenation buffer after packing the resin in a 2.5 × 30 cm column (Pharmacia XK-26). 5'-Nucleotidase activity was then further purified on a Blue Sepharose affinity gel (Reactive Blue 2 Sepharose CL-6B, Sigma), which previously had equilibrated with 50 mM Tris buffer, pH 7.5, containing 3 mM dithiothreitol and 10% glycerol. The final 5'-nucleotidase activity was free of the major cellular nucleoside kinase activities and non-specific alkaline or acid-phosphatase and was stable, stored at −70°C for several months.

EXPERIMENTAL RESULTS AND DISCUSSION

Dideoxynucleotide Phosphorylating Activities

In extracts of human T lymphoid cells (CCRF-CEM) there are two enzyme activi-ties, dCyd kinase and Ado kinase, that can phosphorylate ddA. As shown in TABLE

1, both enzymes bind ddA with approximately the same affinity as their natural substrate 2′-deoxyadenosine (dAdo). The reaction velocity, however, is substantially slower with ddA than with dAdo, such that the maximum efficiencies are only 1 and 0.06%, respectively, of that reached with dAdo. Even at a concentration of 5 mM, no phosphorylation of ddI was detected with either dCyd kinase or Ado kinase.

The results of preliminary experiments suggested that the phosphorylation of ddI might be catalyzed in the reverse reaction of a cytoplasmic 5′-nucleotidase. TABLE 2 summarizes the procedure used to isolate this activity from CEM cells; a 24-fold purification of this enzyme was achieved. This enzyme preparation was free of detectable ATP-dependent nucleoside kinases and nonspecific phosphatases (with phenyl phosphate or ribose-5-phosphate as donors), was Mg^{2+}-dependent, and exhibited an apparent K_a of 2 mM $MgCl_2$ with 1 mM IMP (results not shown). The enzyme displayed a fairly sharp pH optimum at pH 7.4 (results not shown).

As shown in FIGURE 2, this partially purified 5′-nucleotidase activity from CEM cells, in the presence of IMP as a phosphate donor, 50 mM $MgCl_2$, 500 mM KCl, and

TABLE 1. Kinetics of Dideoxynucleoside Phosphorylation by Deoxycytidine Kinase and Adenosine Kinase[a]

Enzyme	Substrate	K_m μM	V_{max} nmol/h/mg	Relative Efficiency V/K_m
dCyd kinase	dAdo	190	340	100
	ddA	290	4	1.2
	ddI	ND[b]	<0.1	<0.001
Ado kinase	dAdo	340	160	100
	ddA	140	0.1	0.06
	ddI	ND	<0.01	<0.001

[a] The ratio V/K_m is termed catalytic efficiency, with values for dAdo set at 100 with dCyd kinase and Ado kinase, respectively. Phosphorylation kinetics were plotted using the Enzfitter computer program. Data shown represent the best fit to the Michaelis-Menten equation. Each assay was done with 10-25 μg of partially purified enzyme protein.
[b] Not determined.

5 mM ATP, catalyzed the formation of a phosphorylated product. The compound synthesized in this reaction mixture coeluted with authentic ddIMP on HPLC; after incubation with bacterial alkaline phosphatase and rechromatography on reverse-phase HPLC, ddI was generated (data not shown). The role of ATP in the stimulation of ddI phosphorylation was primarily as an activator and not a phosphate donor. For example, in a reaction mixture containing ATP without IMP, phosphorylation of ddI was not detectable (<0.5% of reaction with IMP and ATP). By contrast, phosphorylation of radiolabeled ddI was increased 3-5-fold in the presence of ATP and IMP. In addition, the phosphorylation of ddI by the 5′-nucleotidase was also stimulated 3-5-fold by GTP and endogenous compounds such as glycerate 2,3-biphosphate and diadenosine tetraphosphate (Ap4A).

The specificity of the phosphotransferase/5′-nucleotidase for ddI phosphorylation was compared to that for other dideoxypurine nucleosides. TABLE 3 indicates that several other nucleosides, including 2′,3′-dideoxyguanosine and carbocyclic 2′,3′-didehydro-2′,3′-dideoxyguanosine (Carbovir), but not ddA, served as substrate for this

TABLE 2. Purification of 5'-Nucleotidase from Human Lymphoblast Cells[a]

Step	Total protein mg	Total activity nmol/h	Specific activity nmol/h/mg	Fold purification
105,000 g supernatant	2600	260,000	100	1
Fast-flow Q-sepharose	660	174,000	290	3
Blue sepharose	30	70,000	2300	23

[a] Activities were measured with 2.4 mM Ino in the presence of 5 mM ATP and 5 mM IMP. Activity is expressed in terms of nmol/h Ino phosphorylation to IMP.

phosphorylation. Obviously much work remains to be done with this enzyme in the area of structure-function relationships; however, of the 2',3'-dideoxy compounds tested to date, ddI appears to be the best substrate for the 5'-nucleotidase.

Metabolism of ddA and ddI in Kinase-Deficient CEM Cells

We also investigated the metabolism of radioactively labeled ddA and ddI in intact human lymphoid cells and mutants of these cells deficient in deoxycytidine kinase, adenosine kinase, or in both enzyme activities in order to identify the anabolic routes

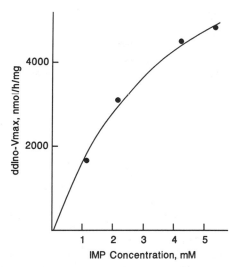

FIGURE 2. Effect of IMP concentration on V_{max} for ddIno phosphorylation by 5'-nucleotidase. Assays were performed with 400-2000 μM ddIno at variable IMP concentration and 5 mM ATP at each point. Rates are expressed as V_{max}-nmol/h/mg for ddIno phosphorylation to IMP. Rate data were fitted to the Michaelis-Menten equation using the Enzfitter computer program. Each assay was done with 18 μg protein. Analysis by the Enzfitter program showed a K_m for IMP at 4.4 mM and a V_{max} for ddIno phosphorylation at saturating IMP of 9000 nmol/h/mg.

TABLE 3. Dideoxynucleoside Phosphorylation by 5'-Nucleotidase[a]

Substrate	K_m mM	V_{max} nmol/h/mg	V_{max}/K_m	V_{max}/K_m % Ino
Ino	3.4	49000	14000	100
ddIno	0.52	870	1700	12
ddGuo	0.85	630	740	5
Carbovir	1.7	470	280	2

[a] Assays were performed with 2 mM nucleoside, 1 mM IMP, and 5 mM ATP using purified nucleotidase. Phosphorylation kinetics were plotted using the Enzfitter computer program. Data shown represents the best fit to the Michaelis-Menten equation. Each assay was done with 18 μg of protein and from 0.2 to 2 mM nucleoside.

responsible for the intracellular activation of these compounds. When ddA or ddI was incubated with wild-type CEM cells or MOLT-4 cells at concentrations of 5 to 10 μM (which represents an ED_{50} concentration for inhibition of HIV replication for these drugs), identical metabolites were generated.[9] Thus, ddI, like ddA, was metabolized to dideoxyadenosine nucleotides (ddAMP, ddADP, and ddATP) and also to the monophosphate of ddI, but not to ddIDP or ddITP. The results in TABLE 4 show that elimination of either dCyd kinase or Ado kinase or both enzyme activities had little effect on the conversion of ddA to its nucleotides unless the ADA inhibitor 2'-dCF was present. As shown in TABLE 4, 2'-dCF, at a concentration of 5 μM, blocked almost entirely the conversion of ddA to the nucleotides in the double mutant deficient in both kinase activities. By contrast, 2'-dCF had no effect on the anabolism of ddI in these mutants.

From these results, it could be proposed that ddA can be metabolized by either of two different metabolic pathways, that is, directly, by way of phosphorylation to ddAMP by either dCyd kinase or Ado kinase, or indirectly, by a route that involves its deamination to ddI followed by phosphorylation of the latter to ddIMP and reamina-

TABLE 4. Phosphorylation of Dideoxyadenosine by Kinase-Deficient CEM Cells[a]

Cell Line	2'-dCF 5 μM	ddIMP	ddADP pmol/10⁶cells	ddATP
wild type	−	1.1	0.35	0.66
	+	0.15	0.33	0.61
dCK	−	0.73	0.26	0.64
	+	0.18	0.05	0.28
AK	−	0.91	0.48	0.69
	+	0.26	0.11	0.34
dCK/AK	−	1.2	0.28	0.70
	+	0.12	<0.1	0.13

[a] Wild-type or kinase-deficient CEM mutants (1×10^7 cells) were preincubated with (+) or without (−) 5 μM 2'-dCF for 30 min, after which 10 μM [³H]ddA was added; the incubations continued for 6 h. Extracts of the cells were prepared and analyzed on Partisil-SAX (Whatman) HPLC column as described in MATERIAL AND METHODS. Each data point represents the mean of duplicate analyses.

tion to ddAMP (FIG. 3), with the latter being quantitatively the predominant route in human T lymphoid cells. To further verify this proposed route of activation, we used L-alanosine, an inhibitor of the enzymes adenylosuccinate synthetase/lyase, which converts IMP to AMP.[10] As shown in TABLE 5, pretreatment of CEM with 20 μM L-alanosine markedly decreased the accumulation of ddATP from either ddA or ddI in Molt-4 cells or kinase-deficient CEM mutants.[5]

Comparative Studies with 2′,3′-Dideoxy-2′-Fluoroarabinosyladenine

Both ddA and ddI undergo a rapid cleavage in acid to form the base and dideoxyribose.[11] This may reduce their bioavailability after oral administration and limit their efficacy. With this in mind, Marquez et al.[11] recently synthesized a series of 2′-substituted derivatives that is highly resistant to acid hydrolysis. One of these compounds is 2′,3′-dideoxy-2′-fluoroarabinosyladenine (2′-F-dd-ara-A) (FIG. 3), which has shown

TABLE 5. Effect of L-Alanosine on the Formation of Dideoxynucleotides from ddA and ddI[a]

Substrate	L-Alanosine 20 μM	ddIMP	ddADP pmol/10^6 cells	ddATP
ddA	−	0.28	0.13	0.06
	+	1.44	0.02	0.01
ddI	−	0.28	0.07	0.04
	+	1.39	0.03	<0.01

[a] [^{3}H]ddA (5 μM) or [^{3}H]ddI (5 μM) was incubated with Molt-4 cells (12 $\times$ 10^6 cells) for 4 h (ddA) or 6 h (ddI) with or without 20 μM L-alanosine. Extracts of the cells were taken and analyzed by HPLC.

interesting anti-HIV activity in ATH-8 cells and MT-4 cell systems.[11,12] These results led us to investigate whether the modification at the 2′ "up" position leads to any other changes in the biochemical properties of this analogue. 2′-F-dd-ara-A is deaminated by adenosine deaminase at only one-tenth the rate that of ddA, and the resulting deaminated derivative, 2′-F-dd-arahypoxanthine, is resistant to further cleavage by purine nucleoside phosphorylase. It is also metabolized to the triphosphate, 2′-F-dd-ara-ATP, approximately 2- and 5-fold more extensively than ddA in Molt-4 and CEM cells, respectively (TABLE 6). We also analyzed the metabolism of 2′-F-dd-ara-A in the kinase-deficient CEM cells. As shown in TABLE 7, phosphorylation of 2′-F-dd-ara-A to its nucleotides decreased about 45% in the dCyd kinase-deficient variant and in the double mutant lacking in both dCyd kinase and Ado kinase activities but was unchanged vis-a-vis wild-type CEM cells in the Ado kinase-deficient variant. The adenosine deaminase inhibitor, 2′-dCF, was found to suppress even further the capacity of either dCyd kinase or the double mutant to accumulate 2′-F-dd-ara-ATP from 2′-F-dd-ara-A.

L-Alanosine also inhibited (ca. 45%) the conversion of 2′-F-dd-ara-A to its nucleotides in CEM cells with a concomitant increase in the formation of the monophosphate,

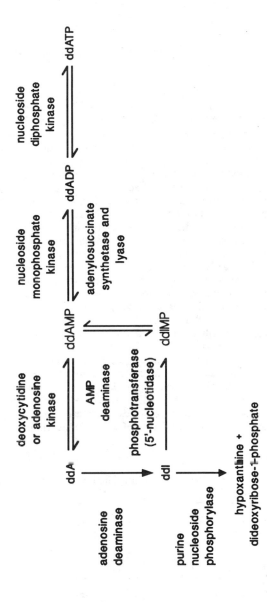

FIGURE 3. Scheme showing the metabolic pathways for anabolism of dideoxypurine nucleosides in human lymphoid cells: 2′,3′-dideoxyadenosine and 2′,3′-dideoxyinosine in human lymphoid cells.

2'-F-dd-ara-IMP. Taken together, these results indicate that unlike ddA, 2'-F-dd-ara-A is able to use both the direct and indirect route for its activation toward formation of the putative active metabolite, 2'-F-dd-ara-ATP.

SUMMARY

Of the dideoxynucleosides described to date, the purine analogues ddA and ddI have exhibited very favorable therapeutic ratios *in vitro*.[1] ddI is presently undergoing extensive phase I-II clinical trials. Whereas the action of adenosine deaminase (ADA) and purine nucleoside phosphorylase (PNP) is usually to convert a given analogue of Ado to an inactive or less active form, ddI appears to retain the same biological activity as that of the parent ddA. An explanation for these observations was possible when we found that ddI (1) underwent only a slow cleavage to hypoxanthine through the action of PNP and (2) accumulated the same active antiviral metabolite (*i.e.,* ddATP) as ddA in human lymphoid cells. The use of human lymphoid cells with deficiencies in cellular nucleoside kinases and of inhibitors of pathways of nucleotide metabolism have also revealed new aspects of dideoxypurine metabolism in human lymphoid cells, including the identification of a salvage pathway (phosphotransferase/5'-nucleotidase pathway) by which ddA/ddI may be metabolized preferentially to the active nucleotide.

The effectiveness of ddA and ddI as orally administered antiviral agents may be limited by their susceptibility to acid hydrolysis and the low efficiency for nucleotide conversion in human lymphoid cells. The presence of a fluorine atom in the arabinose configuration on C-2 confers resistance to solvolysis and renders the analogue less susceptible to enzymatic deamination and resistant to phosphorylytic cleavage by PNP. In addition, human lymphoid cells accumulated several fold higher levels of the putative active triphosphate, 2'-F-dd-ara-ATP, than those of ddA or ddI. This increased accumulation of the analogue triphosphate could be accounted for by a more direct conversion of 2'-F-dd-ara-A by a direct phosphorylation through dCyd kinase than ddA.

Thus, a single substitution with fluorine at the 2' "up" position of the sugar moiety of ddA markedly improves several biochemical properties relating to dideoxynucleotide accumulation in human lymphoid cells. Whether there are significant alterations of other biochemical properties, such as the ability of the analogue triphosphate to interact

TABLE 6. Comparison of Formation of Phosphorylated Metabolites of 2'-F-dd-ara-A and ddA in Molt-4 and CEM Cells[a]

Dideoxynucleotide	Molt-4	CEM
	pmol/10^6cells	
ddATP	0.18	0.99
2'-F-dd-ara-ATP	0.86	2.14

[a] Molt-4 cells were incubated with 5 μM [^{3}H]ddA or [^{3}H]2'-F-dd-ara-A and CEM cells with 10 μM of the same labeled dideoxynucleosides for 5 h. Extracts of the cells were taken and analyzed by Partisil-SAX (Whatman) HPLC.

TABLE 7. Phosphorylation of 2'-F-dd-ara-A by Kinase-Deficient CEM Cells[a]

Cell Line	dCF 5μM	2'-F-dd-ara-ADP pmol/10⁶ cells	2'-F-dd-ara-ATP	Total
Wild-type cells (CEM)	−	1.30	2.14	3.44
	+	1.29	2.36	3.65
Deoxycytidine kinase-	−	0.84	1.09	1.93
deficient	+	0.35	<0.10	0.35
Adenosine kinase-	−	0.59	2.48	3.07
deficient	+	0.83	2.78	3.61
Deoxycytidine kinase-	−	0.24	1.60	1.84
and adenosine kinase-deficient	+	<0.10	<0.10	<0.10

[a] Studies with kinase-deficient CEM mutants were carried out as described in TABLE 4 and MATERIAL AND METHODS section.

with the target enzyme reverse transcriptase, has not yet been determined. Thus, a definitive resolution of the relative merit of ddA/ddI and its 2'-fluoro-arabinosyl analogue is not yet possible on the basis of the studies described here.

REFERENCES

1. MITSUYA, H. & S. BRODER. 1986. Inhibition of the *in vitro* infectivity and cytopathic effect of human T-lymphotropic virus type III/lymphadenopathy-associated virus (HTLV/LAV) by 2',3'-dideoxynucleosides. Proc. Natl. Acad. Sci. USA **83:** 1911-1915.
2. YARCHOAN, R. & S. BRODER. 1987. Development of an antiretroviral therapy for the acquired immunodeficiency syndrome and related disorders. A progress report. N. Engl. J. Med. **316:** 557-564.
3. COONEY, D. A., G. AHLUWALIA, H. MITSUYA, A. FRIDLAND, M. JOHNSON, Z. HAO, M. DALAL, J. BALZARINI, S. BRODER & D. G. JOHNS. 1987. Initial studies on the cellular pharmacology of 2',3'-dideoxyadenosine, an inhibitor of HTLV-III infectivity. Biochem. Pharmacol. **36:** 1765-1768.
4. YARCHOAN, R., H. MITSUYA, R. V. THOMAS, J. M. PLUDA, N. R. HARTMAN, C. F. PERNO, K. S. MARCZYK, J.-P. ALLAIN, D. G. JOHNS & S. BRODER. 1989. *In vivo* activity against HIV and favorable toxicity profile of 2',3'-dideoxyinosine. Science **245:** 412-415.
5. JOHNSON, M. A., G. AHLUWALIA, M. C. CONNELLY, D. A. COONEY, S. BRODER, D. G. JOHNS & A. FRIDLAND. 1988. Metabolic pathways for the activation of the antiretroviral agent 2',3'-dideoxyadenosine in human lymphoid cells. J. Biol. Chem. **263:** 15354-15357.
6. VERHOEF, V., J. SARUP & A. FRIDLAND. 1981. Identification of the mechanism of activation of 9-β-D-arabinofuranosyladenine in human lymphoid cells using mutants deficient in nucleoside kinases. Cancer Res. **41:** 4478-4483.
7. YOSHIKAWA, T. K. & T. TAKENISHI. 1969. Studies of phosphorylation. III. Selective phosphorylation of unprotected nucleosides. Bull. Chem. Soc. Jpn. **42:** 3505-3508.
8. KOVACS, T. & L. OTVOS. 1988. Simple synthesis of 5-vinyl and 5-ethynyl-2'-deoxyuridine-5'-triphosphate. Tetrahedron Lett. **29:** 4525-4528.

9. AHLUWALIA, G., D. A. COONEY, H. MITSUYA, A. FRIDLAND, K. P. FLORA, Z. HAO, M. DALAL, S. BRODER & D. G. JOHNS. 1987. Initial studies on the cellular pharmacology of 2',3'-dideoxyinosine, an inhibitor of HIV infectivity. Biochem. Pharmacol. 36: 3797-3800.
10. TYAGI, A. K. & D. A. COONEY. 1980. Identification of the antimetabolite of L-alanosine L-alanosyl-5-amino-4-imidazolecarboxylic acid ribonucleotide in tumors and assessment of its inhibition of adenylosuccinate synthetase. Cancer Res. 40: 4390-4397.
11. MARQUEZ, V. E., C. K-H. TSENG, J. A. KELLEY, H. MITSUYA, S. BRODER, J. S. ROTH & J. S. DRISCOLL. 1987. 2',3'-Dideoxy-2'-fluoro-ara-A. An acid-stable purine nucleoside active against human immunodeficiency virus (HIV). Biochem. Pharmacol. 36: 2719-2722.
12. HERDEWIJN, P., R. PAUWELS, M. BABA, J. BALZARINI & E. DECLERCQ. 1987. Synthesis and anti-HIV activity of various 2'- and 3'-substituted 2',3'-dideoxyadenosine: A structure activity analysis. J. Med. Chem. 30: 2131-2137.

DNA Polymerases versus HIV Reverse Transcriptase in AIDS Therapy

YUNG-CHI CHENG, WEN-YI GAO, CHIN-HO CHEN,
MIGUEL VAZQUEZ-PADUA, AND
MILBREY C. STARNES

Department of Pharmacology
Yale University School of Medicine
New Haven, Connecticut 06510

Acquired immunodeficiency syndrome (AIDS) is one of the major health concerns around the world.[1] The key etiological agent being identified is the human immunodeficiency virus (HIV).[2] Attempts to control the replication and propagation of HIV for treatment of patients with acquired immunodeficiency syndrome are being pursued by many laboratories worldwide. One logical way to explore selective antiviral agents is to target virus-specific proteins. Such compounds could have a higher therapeutic index, although they could also have a narrower spectrum of activity.

One of the most attractive targets for developing anti-HIV agents is HIV reverse transcriptase (RT). This enzyme is essential for the early phase of viral nucleic acid replication in cells. Once the viral genome is integrated into chromosomal DNA the viral nucleic acid synthesis is no longer dependent on this enzyme.[3,4] Thus, the drug targeted at HIV-RT will be useful for preventing infection in cells and will not be useful for preventing viral production in chronically infected cells. Long-term usage of those compounds is required to control the progress of AIDS. This raises the issue of whether the compounds targeting at HIV-RT will ever be curative for patients with AIDS. It is conceivable that chronically infected cells have a defined life span. Preventing infection of cells by virus from the chronically infected cells for a period covering their life span by using drugs targeting HIV-RT should be able to cure individuals with AIDS, providing drug resistance is not an issue. At present, the turnover rate, and enhancement of turnover, of chronically infected cells is not clear.

HIV-RT is a heterodimer composed of two polypeptides with molecular masses of 66,000 and 51,000 daltons, respectively. These two polypeptides differ only in their carboxyl terminal. The 51,000 dalton polypeptide is the result of a 15,000 dalton polypeptide deletion (which has an intrinsic RNaseH activity) from the carboxyl terminal of the 66,000 dalton polypeptide.[5,6] Why the native virus prefers to have a heterodimer instead of a homodimer of 66,000 dalton polypeptides is not clear. Using activity gel analysis it was found the 66,000 dalton polypeptide has DNA polymerase, reverse transcriptase, and RNaseH activities, whereas the 51,000 dalton polypeptide has only DNA polymerase and reverse transcriptase activities.[7,8] The association of RNaseH activity domain with the carboxyl terminal of 66,000 dalton was supported by the sequence analysis.[9] As a heterodimer, HIV-RT has three intrinsic activities; these are DNA polymerase, reverse transcriptase, and RNaseH. The properties of those intrinsic activities are regulated differently in spite of their association with the same enzymes and their common ability to bind to nucleic acid. For instance, a phosphothioate oligodeoxycytidine (S-dC$_{28}$) could inhibit the intrinsic RT and RNaseH and have no effect on the intrinsic DNA polymerase (TABLE 1), whereas phosphonoformic acid (PFA) could inhibit both DNA polymerase as well as reverse transcriptase and have no effect on intrinsic RNaseH. Furthermore, the properties of this RT are quite different from that of RT associated with other viruses, such as AMV. Thus, if the goal is to develop anti-HIV RT compounds, it is essential to employ HIV-RT from virion in the studies and to examine the impact of the compounds on all three intrinsic activities, which are all critical for viral nucleic acid replication. Using HIV-RT from recombinant sources should always be done with caution despite its sharing some common properties with HIV-RT from virion.

There are two approaches that may be taken for developing anti-HIV compounds based on virus-associated RT. The first one is to look for selective HIV-RT inhibitors. These include PFA[10] and phosphothioate oligonucleotides.[11] The second approach is to look for compounds that can be preferentially used by HIV-RT as a substrate over that of host DNA polymerases such as α, β, γ, and δ. The mechanisms of a number of anti-HIV nucleoside analogues appear to fit into this category, and many of those nucleoside analogues are at different stages of clinical usage or trial for the treatment of AIDS.

AZT has been approved and widely used for the treatment of AIDS.[12] The active metabolite of AZT was suggested to be AZT triphosphate (AZTTP).[13] The interaction of AZTTP with virus RT and human DNA polymerases is shown in TABLE 2. All of those enzymes except DNA polymerase α could incorporate AZT into DNA despite different affinities for AZTTP.[14] The preferential interaction of AZTTP with HIV-RT could be responsible for the selectivity of AZT in inhibiting HIV replication. Therefore, alteration of the interaction between AZTTP and HIV-RT, induced by either a different strain of HIV from different individuals or as a mutation of HIV, could alter the sensitivity of HIV to AZT. This could be partly responsible for the drug resistance issues encountered in the clinic. Furthermore, genetic and phenotypic variations of HIV-harboring tissues could also play a role. For instance, AZT requires phosphorylation through several steps to the triphosphate level in order to exert an anti-HIV effect. Individual variations in any of these steps at targeting tissues could have an impact on the formation of AZTTP. Even if HIV-RT from different individuals has the same sensitivity to AZTTP, the target tissues of AZT of different individuals may have a different deoxythymidine 5' triphosphate content, which could compete with AZTTP for its incorporation into DNA. This could also influence the response of HIV to AZT. Thus, the variation in HIV sensitivity to AZT, the metabolism of AZT or thymidine at the HIV-harboring tissues, AZT catabolism through the courses of AZT treatment,

TABLE 1. Sensitivity of HIV-RT–Associated Activity to Phosphorothioate Oligodeoxycytidine (S-dC$_{28}$) and PFA[a]

Associate activity	Template used	S-dC$_{28}$ (100 nM)	PFA (5 μM)
		Percent Inhibition	
DNA polymerase	$(dC)_n(dG)_{12}$	12	48
Reverse transcriptase	$(rC)_n(dG)_{12}$	82	68
RNase H	$(dC)_n(rG)_n$	89	0

[a] Details will be published. The enzyme employed is the purified HIV-RT from virions.

TABLE 2. Interaction of AZTTP and ddCTP with HIV-RT and Human DNA Polymerase[a]

Enzyme	K_m (μM)		K_i (μM)	
	TTP	dCTP	AZTTP	ddCTP
HIV-RT	1.6	1.5	0.073	0.024
Human α	1.3	0.9	45	110
Human δ	2.4	—	0.36	—
Human β	4.3	4.3	0.67	2.6
Human γ	0.4	0.3	0.23	0.016

[a]Activated calf thymus DNA was used as a template for all the enzymes studied. The conditions for assays are the same except the amount of salt employed for different enzymes. See details in refs. 14, 18, 19, and 20.

and genetic variation in AZT metabolism in target tissues could play a role in clinical drug resistance. All these issues should be addressed in exploring the mechanism of drug resistance.

Regarding AZT toxicity, it is likely due to the ability of AZT to be incorporated into chromosomal DNA by host DNA polymerases. Different individuals were reported to have different tolerances to AZT. The pharmacokinetic variations among individuals could be partly responsible for this difference. The variation of AZT and thymidine metabolism in toxified tissues from different individuals could also play a key role. It was reported that at the toxic dosage of AZT, the toxicity of cells in culture is proportional to the amount of AZT incorporated into DNA.[15] Thus, it is conceivable that its metabolic variations in target tissues for AZT incorporation into DNA or its excision from DNA could also account for the differential tolerance among individuals. Recently, it was also observed in this laboratory that AZT could still be incorporated into DNA at a noncytotoxic dosage. This is unexpected inasmuch as AZT should act as a DNA chain terminator, which should stop DNA synthesis and cell growth, unless the incorporated AZT could be transferred from one segment of DNA to another through the combined actions of a DNA exonuclease and DNA polymerase in the presence of AZTTP. The presence of a unique exonuclease that is capable of removing AZT from the terminal of DNA was identified.[14] This exonuclease, which we termed DNA exonuclease VI, has properties quite different from other exonucleases. A summary of its properties in comparison to others is described in TABLE 4. The longer half-life of AZTTP over that of AZT monophosphate (AZTMP) has been demonstrated by several laboratories. A metabolic chart of AZT in target tissues is shown in FIGURE 1. It is proposed that, in addition to the possible differences in the activities of AZT metabolism, the activity of this novel exonuclease could also play an important role in AZT tolerance among different individuals.

Dideoxycytidine (ddC) was found to be a potent anti-HIV compound in cell culture and shown to be effective in the treatment of AIDS.[16,17] The antiviral specificity was also attributed to the potent interaction of its active metabolite ddCTP and HIV-RT (TABLE 2). The toxicity profiles of ddC and AZT are quite different. The limiting toxicity of ddC in the clinic is the development of peripheral neuropathy and pancreatitis after long-term usage of the compound. Due to the potent effect of ddCTP on DNA polymerase γ, which is a key enzyme for mitochondrial DNA synthesis, we suspect that the cause of peripheral neuropathy and other delayed toxicity, such as pancreatitis, could be due to the depletion of mitochondrial DNA in those tissues by ddC or other compounds that show similar limiting toxicities. In order to explore this hypothesis, the potential of ddC in causing the delayed cytotoxicity in cell growth in culture was examined. ddC, at a clinically relevant dosage of 0.2 μM, inhibited mitochondrial DNA synthesis within one day and had no impact on cell growth for the first five days. During this period, cells responding to the mitochondria depletion by ddC increased glycolysis, and there was no significant alteration of either intracellular ATP or energy charge. On the sixth day postexposure to ddC, cell growth was retarded, and mitochondrial DNA content was depleted at least 50-fold. The delayed cytotoxicity observed could be due to the minimum content of mitochondrial DNA having been reached in order for cells to have normal growth.[21]

It is conceivable that neuron tissue or some other tissues that show delayed-type toxicity, as the result of ddC or other drug treatment, may also respond to those compounds in a similar fashion as culture cells. The selective manifestation of those tissue toxicities could be that those tissues have less tolerance for change in mitochondrial DNA content than other tissues. Currently, we are examining the impact of a clinically relevant dose of ddC on mitochondrial DNA content and the neuronal

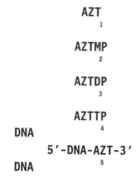

FIGURE 1. Metabolic chart of AZT. Enzyme activities responsible for each step: 1. thymidine kinase, 2. TMP kinase, 3. NDP kinase, 4. DNA polymerase or reverse transcriptase, and 5. DNA exonuclease VI.

function of well-differentiated neuron cells, such as the nerve growth factor-treated PC12 cell line in culture. Several other anti-HIV nucleosides with known clinical limiting toxicities were also examined for their effect on cell growth as well as for their effect on mitochondrial DNA content in cells during several days of treatment. These results are summarized in TABLE 3. The limiting toxicity of ddC, ddI, and D4T was suggested to cause peripheral neuropathy or pancreatitis. This occurs usually after two to three months of treatment. All three compounds could inhibit mitochondrial DNA synthesis at a dosage that does not have much impact on cell growth for the first four days after drug exposure in cell culture, whereas AZT could inhibit cell growth without much impact on the mitochondrial DNA synthesis. At high dosage, AZT can also cause mitochondrial DNA depletion. It is known that the limiting toxicity of AZT is anemia and bone marrow suppression, which can happen within a month of treatment. The lack of peripheral neuropathy and other delayed toxicities with AZT treatment could be due to the fact that the dosage used was not high enough to cause a similar effect as was caused with ddC on mitochondrial DNA synthesis in susceptible tissues.

TABLE 3. Effects of Anti-HIV Nucleosides on Mitochondrial DNA in CEM Cells after Three-Day Treatment

	Concentration (μM)	Cell growth inhibition	Inhibition of mitochondrial DNA
ddC	0.10	—	$++++$[b]
ddI[a]	200.00	—	$++$[c]
	1000.00	—	$++++$
AZT	5.00	—	—
	20.00	$+$[d]	$++$
D4T	20.00	$+$	$++++$
D4C	2.00	—	$++$
	10.00	—	$+++$
araC	0.02	$+$	—

[a] Dideoxyinosine.
[b] More than 90% decrease in mitochondrial DNA content.
[c] More than 50% inhibition. Methodologies for assessing mitochondrial DNA previously published.[21]
[d] Approximately 50% inhibition. Unpublished data.

There is a good correlation of relative sensitivity of the effect on mitochondrial DNA and cell growth to the clinical limiting toxicity, which further supports our hypothesis. This raises an interesting possibility for assessing a given compound for its delayed toxicity (similar to that of ddC), that is, to assess its impact on mitochondrial DNA content in cell culture. This could resolve the issue of the lack of an *in vitro* or animal model for this type of toxicity.

In summary, HIV-RT plays a critical role in viral nucleic acid replication in the early phase of viral cell infection. There are sufficient differences between HIV-RT and host DNA polymerases that include polymerases α, β, γ, and δ. Thus, to develop a selective anti-HIV compound that targets HIV-RT is logical. The compounds selected should be effective in preventing new cells from serving as reservoirs for virus production. It is not expected that these compounds will be able to cure HIV infection in

TABLE 4.

Enzyme	Mode of action	pH Optimum	Mg^{2+} requirement	Product nucleotides	Molecular weight
DNase I	endo	7.1	yes	5'-oligo	31,000
DNase II	endo	4.8	no	3'-oligo	38,000
DNase III	exo	8.5	yes	5'-mono/di	52,000
DNase IV	exo	8.5	yes	5'-mono	42,000
DNase V	exo	8.8	yes	5'-mono	12,000
Lysomal exonuclease	exo	5.5	no	3'-mono	70,000
DNase VI	exo	7–8	yes	5'-mono	100 to 150,000

patients with a short course of treatment. HIV-RT has high infidelity in making DNA. The alteration of RT in virion during the course of treatment or through virus propagation is also anticipated. The presence and appearance of a drug-resistant population is predictable. Thus a single drug treatment for AIDS patients is unlikely to have a high degree of success in the long run. A combination of compounds that shows no cross-resistant pattern will eventually be more successful. With regard to those nucleoside analogues that are currently used in the clinic, metabolizing and interacting with human cellular components, they should have toxicity. Their spectrum of toxicity could be quite different depending on how they are metabolized in tissues, how well their active metabolites interact with the host DNA polymerases, and how important the target molecule for cell function is. By knowing the mechanism of their toxicity, an individual's tolerance to a given drug may become predictable, based on laboratory testing. This should help in the choice of compounds for treatment. Furthermore, it could also help in selecting compounds for combination therapy.

REFERENCES

1. MANN, J. M., J. CHIN, P. PIOT & T. QUINN. 1988. The international epidemiology of AIDS. Sci. Am. **259:** 82-89.
2. GALLO, R. C. & L. MONTAGNIER. 1988. AIDS in 1988. Sci. Am. **259:** 41-48.
3. VARMUS, H. E. 1982. Form and function of retroviral proviruses. Science **216:** 812-20.
4. GERARD, G. F. & D. P. GRANDGENETT. 1980. *In* Molecular Biology of RNA Tumor Viruses. C. J. R. Stephenson, Ed.: 245-394. Academic Press Inc. New York.
5. HANSEN, J., T. SCHULZE, W. MELLERT & K. MOELLING. 1988. EMBO J. **7:** 239-243.
6. FARMERIE, W. G., D. D. LOEB, N. C. CASAVANT, C. A. HUTCHISON, III, M. H. EDGELL & R. SWANTROM. 1987. Science **236:** 305-308.
7. STARNES, M. C., W. GAO, R. C. TING & Y. C. CHENG. 1987. J. Biol. Chem. **263:** 5132-5134.
8. STARNES, M. C. & Y. C. CHENG. 1989. J. Biol. Chem. **264:** 7073-7077.
9. JOHNSON, M. S., M. A. MCCLURE, D. F. FENG, J. GRAY & R. F. DOOLITTLE. 1986. Proc. Natl. Acad. Sci. USA **83:** 7648-7652.
10. SANDSTROM, E. G., R. E. BYINGTON, J. C. KAPLAN & M. S. HIRSCH. 1985. Inhibition of human T cell lymphotropic virus type III *in vitro* by phosphonoformate. Lancet **i:** 1480-1482.
11. MATSUKURA, M., K. SINOZUKA, G. ZON, H. MITSUYA, M. REITZ, J. S. COHEN & S. BRODER. 1987. Proc. Natl. Acad. Sci. USA **84:** 7706-7710.
12. FISCHL, M. A. *et al.* 1987. The efficacy of azidothymidine (AZT) in the treatment of patients with AIDS and AIDS-related complex: A double-blind, placebo-controlled trial. N. Engl. J. Med. **317:** 185-191.
13. FURMAN, P. A. *et al.* 1986. Phosphorylatation of 3'-azido-3'-deoxythymidine and selective interaction of the 5'-triphosphate with human immunodeficiency virus reverse transcriptase. Proc. Natl. Acad. Sci. USA **83:** 8333-8337.
14. VAZQUEZ-PADUA, M. A., M. C. STARNES & Y-C. CHENG. 1990. Incorporation of 3'-azido-3'-deoxythymidine into cellular DNA and its removal in a human leukemic cell line. Cancer Comm. **2:** 55-62.
15. SOMMADOSSI, J-P., R. CARLISLE & Z. ZHOU. 1989. Cellular pharmacology of 3'-azido-3'-deoxythymidine with evidence of incorporation into DNA of human bone marrow cells. Mol. Pharmacol. **36:** 9-14.
16. MITSUYA, H. & S. BRODER. 1986. Inhibition of the *in vitro* infectivity and cytopathic effect of human T-lymphotropic virus type III/lymphadenopathy-associated virus (HTLV-III/LAV) by 2',3'-dideoxynucleosides. Proc. Natl. Acad. Sci. USA **83:** 1911-1915.
17. YARCHOAN, R., R. V. THOMAS, J-P. MCATEE *et al.* 1988. Phase I studies of 2',3'-dideoxycytidine in severe human immunodeficiency virus infection as a single agent and alternating with zidovudine (AZT). Lancet **i:** 76-80.

18. STARNES, M. C. & Y-C. CHENG. 1987. Cellular metabolism of 2',3'-dideoxycytidine, a compound active against human immunodeficiency virus *in vitro.* J. Biol. Chem. **262:** 988-991.
19. CHENG, Y-C., G. E. DUTSCHMAN, K. F. BASTOW, M. G. SARNGADHARAN & R. Y. C. TING. 1987. Human immunodeficiency virus reverse transcriptase: General properties and its interactions with nucleoside triphosphate analogs. J. Biol. Chem. **262:** 2187-2189.
20. STARNES, M. C. & Y-C. CHENG. 1989. Inhibition of human immunodeficiency virus reverse transcriptase by 2',3'-dideoxynucleoside triphosphates: Template dependence, and combination with phosphonoformate. Virus Genes **2:** 269-281.
21. CHEN, C. H. & Y-C. CHENG. 1989. Delayed cytotoxicity and selective loss of mitochondrial DNA in cells treated with the anti-human immunodeficiency virus compound 2',3'-dideoxycytidine. J. Biol. Chem. **264:** 11934-11937.

Antiviral Drug Resistance[a]

DONALD M. COEN

Department of Biological Chemistry and Molecular Pharmacology
Harvard Medical School
Boston, Massachusetts 02115

INTRODUCTION

Antiviral drugs, which were only pipe dreams not so long ago, are now successful enough that we have considerable knowledge about the ways in which viruses can become resistant to them. In the context of AIDS, there are several good reasons to start a discussion of antiviral drug resistance with agents that have been successful in treating herpesvirus infections. We know the most about resistance to these agents in part because the most widely prescribed antivirals are those against the herpesviruses, particularly herpes simplex virus (HSV). Herpesviruses are also common and dangerous opportunistic pathogens in AIDS patients and resistance to antiherpesvirus drugs has become an important clinical problem in this setting.[1-4] The lessons that we have learned in studying resistance to antiherpesvirus drugs are quite germane to the possibilities and realities[5] of resistance to anti-HIV drugs.

CLASSES OF ANTIHERPESVIRUS AND ANTI-HIV DRUGS

There are two major classes of antiherpesvirus drugs. The first class, which has had the most clinical success, comprises a wide variety of nucleoside analogues. These include idoxuridine (IUdR); vidarabine (araA); acyclovir (ACV), which is the most successful and widely used antiviral drug with indications against many herpesvirus diseases; and ganciclovir (DHPG), which is seeing considerable use against cytomegalovirus (CMV) retinitis. These nucleoside analogues are converted to mono-, di-, and triphosphorylated forms by cellular and/or viral kinases, and it is these phosphorylated forms that are active intracellularly. For example, in HSV-infected cells, araA is converted to araA-triphosphate through cellular enzymes[6] and then goes on to inhibit HSV DNA polymerase.[7] ACV, however, is converted to ACV-monophosphate almost exclusively by the HSV thymidine kinase (TK)[8] and then primarily, if not exclusively, by cellular enzymes to the triphosphate,[9,10] which is a potent inhibitor of HSV DNA polymerase.[11]

The second major class of antiherpesvirus drugs are analogues of pyrophosphate. These include phosphonoacetic acid (PAA) and phosphonoformic acid (foscarnet,

[a]Grant support from the National Institutes of Health (RO1 AI19838, RO1 AI26126, PO1 AI24010, UO1 AI26077, and SO7 RR05381) is acknowledged.

PFA). The latter is beginning to see some clinical use. These drugs do not require activation; rather they inhibit viral DNA polymerases directly, evidently by binding to the site involved in releasing the pyrophosphate product of DNA synthesis.[12]

It is not surprising that many successful and promising anti-HIV drugs are also nucleoside or pyrophosphate analogues. The one that has seen the greatest clinical use thus far, zidovudine (azidothymidine, AZT) is a nucleoside analogue. Like the antiherpesvirus nucleoside analogues, it is activated by conversion to its triphosphate and inhibits the viral DNA polymerase, retrovirus reverse transcriptase.[13] As with the herpesviruses, PFA has direct anti-DNA polymerase activity.[14] Of course, for both herpesviruses and retroviruses, other classes of drugs, some with much promise, are being developed.

WHY STUDY DRUG RESISTANCE?

There are at least three good reasons for studying drug resistance. Studies of drug resistance can shed considerable light on drug mechanism, can help enable dissection of viral proteins that serve as drug targets, and can help predict the frequency and properties of drug resistance in the clinic. All three kinds of studies can lead to improved therapies that might overcome or circumvent problems of drug resistance.

DRUG RESISTANCE AND DRUG MECHANISM

Because viruses are obligate intracellular parasites, the detection of resistance to an antiviral implies a certain level of "selectivity" in the action of the antiviral. Put another way, virus replication can be inhibited either by interfering directly with virus-specific processes or by incapacitating the host. The isolation of virus mutants resistant to a drug strongly implies that the drug acts at least in part by the former mechanism. This idea was probably first put into print by Herrmann and Herrmann.[15]

Several disclaimers must be made. For example, aphidicolin, which is an inhibitor of eukaryotic cellular replicative polymerases,[16] is surely a cytotoxic agent and not very selective against viruses. Yet, aphidicolin-resistant HSV and vaccinia-virus mutants have been isolated[17–19] (although the concentrations of aphidicolin used in such experiments are deleterious to the health of cell monolayers). Additionally, studies in cell culture cannot predict organ or whole animal toxicities. Moreover, antivirals can act selectively by modifying the host cell. Interferon operates this way. This selectivity has been built into virus hosts over millions of years of evolution, however. It will be difficult to develop selective artificial antiviral drugs with this kind of mechanism.

Selectivity by Inhibition of Viral Polymerase

In the HSV system, the use of resistance to determine the selectivity and mechanism of a drug has probably been most applicable to araA. As reviewed previously,[7] there was considerable disagreement regarding the mechanism of the antiviral activity of araA. AraA is cytotoxic and as a result it was suggested that it is not a selective antiviral agent.[20] Several investigators reported that it was difficult to isolate HSV mutants resistant to araA.[21–23] Eventually, however, it proved to be fairly easy to isolate mutants resistant to araA.[7,24] Thus, araA is indeed a selective antiviral, although some of its antiviral activity is related to its cytotoxicity.

Once a drug-resistant virus mutant is identified, a drug target can be identified by defining the gene in which mutation to drug resistance has occurred. It can be inferred that this drug target contributes to the selectivity of the antiviral. Herpesvirus drug-resistance mutations can be assigned to specific genes by genetic analyses, including complementation and recombination analyses[25,26] and more precise marker rescue methods. All HSV araA-resistance mutations studied thus far have been assigned to the gene encoding the viral DNA polymerase.[7,24,27,28] Thus, HSV DNA polymerase is a target for araA and contributes to its selectivity.

In a similar fashion, the HSV DNA polymerase has been shown to contribute to the selectivity of ACV. ACV-triphosphate inhibits viral polymerase at concentrations much lower than it does cellular polymerase.[13] Selectivity has also been demonstrated by mutations in the HSV DNA polymerase gene that confer resistance to ACV.[17] This is not a trivial point. One could imagine that the selectivity of ACV resided entirely in its activation by HSV TK; subsequent effects could be due entirely to phosphorylated derivatives incapacitating the host cell. Indeed that may be the case with some of the other anti-HSV drugs that have been developed, most of which have been more toxic than ACV.

In the HIV system, the report that virus mutants containing engineered changes in the *pol* gene were resistant to PFA[29] or AZT[30] demonstrates that these drugs inhibit HIV replication selectively through inhibition of reverse transcriptase.

Mechanism of Ganciclovir Action and Resistance in CMV

In HSV, DHPG, like ACV, is activated by conversion to its monophosphate by viral TK. CMV, however, is not known to encode or express a TK like that of HSV. Despite that, CMV induces an increase in DHPG-triphosphate upon infection.[31,32] Because CMV also induces numerous cellular nucleoside kinases, including one with weak activity towards DHPG,[32] it was widely assumed that DHPG is activated by a cellular kinase that is induced upon CMV infection.

The analysis of a CMV mutant that is resistant to DHPG, however, challenged this assumption.[33] This mutant, which was readily isolated by serial passage in increasing concentrations of DHPG, exhibited a tenfold increase in the dose that decreased virus growth 50% (ED_{50}). Strikingly, this was associated with a tenfold decrease in the level of phosphorylated DHPG. This decrease was not due to decreased stability of phosphorylated drug or to decreased induction of cellular nucleoside kinases or nucleotide pools. Moreover, the mutant is not deficient in induction of the weak cellular DHPG-kinase activity (K. Biron and J. Fyfe, personal communication).

These data demonstrated that DHPG is indeed a selective anti-CMV drug and provided substantial evidence that selectivity was due, at least in part, to specific phosphorylation of the drug. More importantly, they demonstrate that CMV encodes a gene product that contributes to DHPG phosphorylation. Although this product could induce very specifically a hitherto-unknown cellular kinase, a much simpler interpretation is that this gene product is a viral enzyme that phosphorylates DHPG or possibly its mono- or diphosphate. Thus, a genetic approach provided evidence for a unique virus drug target, which was not forthcoming from biochemical studies.

Pitfalls of Biochemical Approaches

Biochemical approaches can be limited not only in assessing mechanisms of drug action, but also in assessing how a given virus mutant becomes resistant to an antiviral agent. Such understanding is critical when dealing with issues of pathogenicity and resistance in the clinic (as will be discussed subsequently). Two examples from HSV illustrate the pitfalls of a strict biochemical approach to resistance. In the first example, there is an HSV mutant that contains a *tk* mutation leading to very low levels of TK polypeptide, which is unstable.[34] As a result, a standard TK enzyme assay on extracts of cells infected with this mutant gives the result that the mutant is TK-negative.[35] The standard interpretation would be that the mutant was drug-resistant due to a TK defect. In fact, the mutant's TK defect has little if any effect on its drug sensitivity.[36] Instead, the mutant is a recombinant virus containing a DNA polymerase mutation that confers the drug resistance (unpublished results). Sorting this out would be very difficult without genetic approaches to map the drug-resistance mutation.

In the second example, there has been a report of a mutant that specifies a DNA polymerase with an increased K_i value for bromovinyldeoxyuridine (BVdU) -triphosphate; yet, this mutant is more sensitive to BVdU than its wild-type parent.[37] Thus, the biochemical analyses did not match the situation in virus-infected cells.

These pitfalls have recurred in analysis of HIV mutants. Site-directed mutagenesis of a cloned HIV *pol* gene resulted in a reverse transcriptase that requires higher levels of AZT-triphosphate for inhibition.[38] Despite this, as in the second example provided above, viruses containing the mutant *pol* genes were more sensitive to AZT than their wild-type parent.[29] Moreover, reverse transcriptase from bona fide AZT-resistant mutants, which contain *pol* mutations, did not require higher levels of AZT-triphosphate for inhibition.[5,30] Thus, biochemical assays often do not assess resistance appropriately. By contrast, genetic approaches by definition measure resistance in the authentic context of the virus-infected cell.

ANTIVIRAL DRUG RESISTANCE AND PROTEIN STRUCTURE AND FUNCTION

General Considerations

Once drug-resistance mutations identify a gene product, they can then be used to dissect it functionally. They can be particularly useful in studies of essential gene products because the resistance mutation does not abrogate protein function, but rather alters specific functional features. A fine example of this is provided by the analysis of amantadine resistance mutations mapping to the hemagglutinin gene of influenza virus.[39]

HSV DNA Polymerase

Studies to dissect functionally the HSV DNA polymerase with the aid of drug-resistance mutations have met with some success. Mutations conferring altered sensitivity to pyrophosphate analogues are expected to alter amino acids involved in pyrophosphate recognition. Mutations conferring altered sensitivity to aphidicolin, which inhibits competitively with deoxynucleoside triphosphate (dNTP) substrates, and mutations conferring altered sensitivity to nucleoside analogues are expected to alter amino acids involved in dNTP recognition. For structure-function studies, it is important to study many different drug-resistance mutations, because any one could be due to mutations at a position removed from a substrate-binding site, exerting its effects by changing protein folding.

Sequence analyses of fourteen different polymerase mutants with altered drug sensitivity have been published. In the most extensive study,[40] nine different mutations were found in four distinct clusters within about one-quarter of the polymerase, starting from about halfway in from the N terminus. The majority of the nine mutations and four of the five others[41-43] lie in or near two regions of sequence similarity with diverse other DNA polymerases. This result led to the proposal that these two regions directly participate in substrate recognition.[40] On the other hand, there is no region that seems solely to be involved in pyrophosphate recognition or dNTP recognition. Rather, it seems likely that folding brings the various amino acids together to form substrate recognition sites.

One region, region A,[40] is found in viruses that are susceptible to certain antiviral drugs and not in viruses that are not susceptible. This raises the possibility that region A serves as a determinant of antiviral drug sensitivity.

The data argue that substrate recognition and thus polymerizing activity lie in the C-terminal half of the polymerase, consistent with the crystal structure of the large fragment of E. coli DNA polymerase I.[44] Recent work indicates that for phage $\phi29$ DNA polymerase, a member of the family of polymerases that includes HSV polymerase, amino acids required for $3'-5'$ exonuclease activity are N terminal to those involved in substrate recognition,[45] as is the case for E. coli DNA polymerase I. Remarkably, these amino acids share sequence similarity with the $3'-5'$ exonuclease domain of the otherwise unrelated E. coli DNA polymerase I.

HIV Reverse Transcriptase

Site-directed mutagenesis of certain conserved regions of the HIV reverse transcriptase resulted in altered sensitivity of reverse transcriptase in vitro to PFA and AZT.[29,38] Viruses containing mutations near certain conserved regions are resistant to AZT.[30] The results raise the possibility that the conserved regions are important for drug and substrate recognition, but as yet, too few virus mutants have been assessed to draw that conclusion.

In both the herpesvirus and retrovirus systems, these kinds of mutational analyses should complement structural studies underway. Such a combined approach should lead to detailed information about the active sites of these enzymes, which may permit the design of highly specific antiviral drugs.

STUDIES OF THE FREQUENCY AND PROPERTIES OF DRUG-RESISTANT MUTANTS

Frequency of Drug-Resistant Mutants

Drug-resistance mutations arise frequently in laboratory stocks of HSV. This is true not only for mutations in the *tk* gene, which is nonessential in cell culture, but for mutations in the polymerase. A compilation of the available data[46] gives an estimate of mutation frequency for either ACV-, araA-, or PAA-resistance of 10^{-4}-10^{-3}. One source of this high frequency of mutation to drug resistance is the HSV DNA polymerase. Mutations conferring an antimutator phenotype map to the DNA polymerase gene.[47] For one antimutator derivative, the lower mutation frequency appears to be due to improved selection of nucleotides rather than increased editing by the 3'-5' exonuclease.[48]

There have been no published reports on the frequency of CMV mutants arising in the laboratory, but they may arise at a lower frequency than do HSV mutants (unpublished data). With respect to HIV, its reverse transcriptase is highly error-prone,[49,50] and there is abundant evidence that extensive and biologically important variation is rapidly generated at other loci, resulting in clinical isolates that are heterogeneous mixtures of virus.[51-53] It is surprising that spontaneous drug-resistant mutants have not yet been isolated in the laboratory.

Are these high frequencies of mutation in the laboratory a cause for alarm regarding the use of antiviral agents in the clinic? It is still difficult to say with certainty. Two features of these mutants that can be studied in the laboratory are relevant in considering their clinical importance: sensitivity to other antiviral agents and pathogenicity in animal models.

Sensitivities to Other Antiviral Agents

Experience with bacterial pathogens has highlighted the importance of having agents that can combat organisms that are resistant to other useful drugs. TABLE 1 summarizes the results from studies too numerous to cite here that have been obtained with HSV mutants resistant to ACV. There are four classes of single mutations that confer ACV resistance. Three of these affect TK: mutations that completely abolish enzyme activity (TK-negative); mutations that decrease activity, for example by reducing the amount of activity or by decreasing affinity for substrates (TK-partial); and mutations that have little if any effect on activity towards the natural substrate, but substantial effect on the ability to phosphorylate ACV (TK-altered). The remaining class of single mutations results in altered DNA polymerase, which is less able to be inhibited by ACV-triphosphate. Double mutants with mutations in both the *tk* and DNA polymerase genes can also be found.

In general, TK mutants of all three classes remain sensitive to drugs that inhibit viral polymerase without requiring phosphorylation by TK. The TK-negative mutants are generally resistant to any drug such as DHPG that requires TK for activation, whereas TK-partial or -altered mutants are sometimes sensitive to certain of these drugs depending on their relative affinity for TK and the nature of the mutation. It is

TABLE 1. Cross-Resistance and Sensitivities of HSV ACV-Resistant Mutants

Type of Mutant	Resistant to	Sensitive to
TK-negative	DHPG	PFA, araA
TK altered or partial	depends	PFA, araA
Polymerase altered	often PFA	often DHPG
TK, polymerase double	possibly all	possibly none

much harder to generalize with polymerase mutants, which can vary widely in cross-sensitivity. Many ACV-resistant polymerase mutants, but not all, are resistant to PFA, and many, but not all, are sensitive to DHPG. One can imagine a double mutant that could be resistant to all currently available anti-HSV drugs. As will be discussed subsequently, one can also imagine a double mutant that would be highly resistant to ACV and retain considerable pathogenicity. This is an argument for continuing development of new agents. Even if such agents are too toxic for widespread systemic use, they should be kept available should life-threatening infections by drug-resistant HSV mutants occur.

Sensitivities of Drug-Resistant CMV and HIV

A DHPG-resistant CMV isolated in the laboratory proved sensitive to every other compound tested, except for a slight decrease in sensitivity to ACV.[33] Two PFA-resistant CMV mutants are sensitive to DHPG, but fairly resistant to ACV (Sullivan and Coen, manuscript in preparation), which also demonstrates that ACV is selective against CMV. The two PFA-resistant HIV mutants isolated by Larder et al.[29] were actually hypersensitive to AZT. All AZT-resistant mutants published to date have come from patients; they showed no more than two- or threefold increases in ED_{50} with PFA or dideoxycytidine, but some showed meaningful resistance to compounds more closely related to AZT.[5] More mutants from both CMV and HIV need to be studied before generalizations can be made. It seems prudent, however, to keep the issue of alternate therapies in the forefront.

Pathogenicities of HSV Drug-Resistant Mutants

Pathogenesis studies on drug-resistant CMV or HIV have not yet been performed. Such studies, just now becoming possible, should provide much interesting data, as has been obtained with HSV. TABLE 2 summarizes the results of studies, too numerous to cite here, of single ACV-resistant mutants in mouse models of HSV disease. Of course, caution must be used in extrapolating these results to humans.

All of the classes of mutants are generally capable of replication at peripheral sites of inoculation. TK-negative and TK-partial mutants are the most impaired in this category, but such mutants replicate to wild-type titers after corneal inoculation.[54,55] TK mutants are more impaired in their ability to reactivate from latent infections upon explant of ganglia, with truly TK-negative viruses being completely reactivation-incompetent.[54,55] In general, polymerase mutants have no difficulty reactivating from latency. The assay that is most sensitive to drug-resistance mutation is the ability of the virus to kill mice after intracerebral inoculation. Even in this assay, TK-altered mutants and some polymerase mutants are only modestly impaired.

Why Are Certain Drug-Resistant Mutants Altered in Pathogenicity?

This question can be rationalized for TK-deficient viruses that account for the majority of ACV-resistant mutants isolated in the laboratory. Presumably, because HSV is neurotropic and avoids immune surveillance in the nervous system, it must build up its own nucleotide pools in nonreplicating nerve cells. Thus, HSV TK becomes much more important in this setting than in cell culture. This would also explain why many ACV-resistant, TK-deficient clinical isolates have come from immunocompromised patients where the virus can replicate in nonnervous tissue.

Less understood is why polymerase mutants would be less pathogenic, as most have proven to be. One possible explanation would be that these mutants generally display lower affinities for normal dNTPs.[48,56,57] Thus, because dNTP pools may be lower in nerve cells than in cell culture, these mutants, like TK mutants, may be at a disadvantage. Nevertheless, as described above one can isolate drug-resistant mutants that exhibit substantial pathogenicity in several assays.

TK-Negative Mutants Establish Latent Infections

Even though it is not possible to recover virus upon explant of ganglia from mice infected with TK-negative mutants, recent results argue that these mutants establish latent infections. Viral DNA can be found in these ganglia (Katz, Bodin, and Coen, unpublished results), which expresses the latency-associated transcript,[55,58] and which

TABLE 2. Behavior of ACV-Resistant Mutants in Mouse Models of HSV Disease

Type of mutant	Replication at Periphery	Reactivation from Latency	Neurovirulence upon I.C. Inoculation
Wild-type	+ + + +[a]	+ + + +	+ + + +
TK-negative	+ + - + + +	0[b]	0
TK-partial	+ + - + + +	+ - + + +	+[c]
TK-altered	+ + + +	+ + - + + +	+ + +
POL-altered	+ + + +	+ + + +	0 - + + +

[a] + + + + = wild-type levels of activity.
[b] 0 = little or no activity.
[c] +, + +, + + + refer to intermediate levels of activity with + + + being nearly wild-type and + being nearly no activity.

can be rescued from ganglia upon superinfection with a TK-competent virus.[55,59] This has a number of clinical implications, assuming that the mouse studies can be extrapolated to humans. ACV-resistant, TK-negative virus would be present in ganglia of patients who have developed resistant infections. This might be reactivated by TK-positive virus present in the same neurons giving rise to mixed populations of virus that retain both pathogenicity and resistance (see below). Additionally, drugs targeted to inhibit HSV TK might be useful prophylactically during immunosuppression but would be unlikely to prevent establishment of latency during acute infection.

Behavior of Mixtures of ACV-Sensitive and -Resistant HSV in Mice

Field and Ellis and colleagues have explored how mixtures of ACV-resistant and sensitive viruses behave in infections of ACV-treated mice.[60–62] Mice infected with defined mixtures of ACV-resistant and sensitive viruses could cause disease that was less responsive to ACV therapy. Mixtures of pathogenic TK-altered and wild-type viruses were particularly more difficult to treat. After passage of either defined mixtures or wild-type virus in mice treated with ACV, highly heterogeneous mixtures of virus were derived that retained pathogenicity and were more resistant than the input virus. These viruses caused the most serious ACV-resistant disease. These results suggest that sensitive viruses can complement resistant viruses for pathogenicity, and resistant viruses can complement sensitive ones for resistance. In view of the latter idea, one can speculate that the particularly pathogenic and resistant highly heterogeneous viruses contained some DNA polymerase mutants, as these mutants are known to complement sensitive viruses for resistance.[25] Such heterogeneity may already have reared its head in resistant isolates from patients suffering from severe, progressive HSV infections that do not respond to ACV (see subsequent section).

Summary of Pathogenicity Studies in Mice

The relevance of any animal study to human disease is always in question. Nevertheless, based on these studies, among single mutants, TK-altered and DNA polymerase mutants have the greatest potential for causing dangerous drug-resistant infections. Infections caused by mixed infections may be even more worrisome, especially if they contain polymerase mutants.

DRUG-RESISTANT HSV INFECTIONS IN IMMUNOCOMPROMISED PATIENTS

The first several ACV-resistant HSV strains isolated from patients in the early 1980s were not convincingly shown to contribute to disease, as reviewed by Larder and Darby,[63] and in some cases ACV treatment did not seem to be impeded. More recently, however, there have been several reports, especially from AIDS patients, of severe, progressive disease in the face of appropriate ACV therapy.[2,3,64,65] Nevertheless in reviewing all of the cases thus far, there has been tremendous variation in the severity of disease, ranging from mere shedding, through "indolent" lesions, to life-threatening illness. The few cases of DHPG-resistant CMV infections reported thus far were associated with disease that progressed and was refractory to drug treatment.[1]

Types of Mutations Found in Clinical Isolates

As yet there have been few if any virological correlates with clinical outcome. All of the ACV-resistant clinical HSV isolates except two have exhibited TK-deficiency, mainly as assayed by *in vitro* enzyme assays. It should be stressed, however, that most of the TK-deficient isolates were not examined adequately for whether they were TK-partial as opposed to TK-negative. Neither were most of these examined for the heterogeneity of the virus population. There is nothing to rule out the presence of TK-positive, altered DNA polymerase mutants in most of the TK-deficient isolates. Two isolates have been predominantly TK-positive, altered DNA polymerase.[64,66,67] Both types of isolates—predominantly TK-deficient and predominantly TK-positive—have been associated with severe disease.

In the few cases when heterogeneity has been examined, both relatively uniform populations and highly heterogeneous mixtures have been found. Interestingly, in one case, the former was associated with an indolent infection,[67] and in a second the latter was associated with a severe, progressive infection.[64] Both populations contained DNA polymerase mutants. It may be that the polymerase mutations, combined with heterogeneity, led to severe disease in the latter case and not the former.

There is no published data yet on the nature of the alterations in the DHPG-resistant CMV isolates; however, preliminary studies indicate that these isolates, like the original laboratory isolate, are deficient in phosphorylation of drug (K. Biron, personal communication).

Pathogenicity Studies in Mice

There has been some examination of the pathogenicity of some ACV-resistant HSV isolates from patients in mouse models; however, in many cases the resistant isolates were not compared appropriately with sensitive, pretreatment isolates. There does not seem to be sufficient recognition that mouse models of pathogenicity are not absolute measures of pathogenic potential in humans. Different ACV-sensitive HSV isolates from patients with severe HSV disease require very different titers of virus to establish reactivable latent infections in mice or to kill mice after various routes of inoculation. Thus, finding that 10^5 plaque-forming units (PFU) cause 100% mortality after intranasal inoculation does not imply that this isolate is "fully neurovirulent."[2] It may well be 10^4-fold less virulent than its ACV-sensitive parent.

Only a few ACV-resistant isolates from patients have been compared appropriately with a sensitive, pretreatment isolate that can be inferred to be the parent of the resistant isolate by restriction enzyme fingerprinting.[64,67–69] Of these, some have exhibited decreased pathogenicity, and some have exhibited substantial pathogenicity in mice. As yet, no obvious correlation has emerged between behavior in mice and clinical course.

Treatment of Drug-Resistant Infections in Humans

Treatment of ACV-resistant HSV infection with PFA has been associated with clinical improvement.[3,64,70–72] Although this has been interpreted in some cases as reflecting successful treatment, it is difficult to be sure that clinical improvement was not the result of improvement in immune status, perhaps due to PFA suppression of HIV in the case of AIDS patients. There are no published reports yet on treatment of DHPG-resistant CMV; PFA would be a likely candidate for treatment in such situations, too.

DRUG RESISTANCE IN HIV: SIMILARITIES WITH HERPESVIRUSES

To coalesce points made separately above, there are many similarities between drug resistance in HIV and in herpesviruses that raise common issues. Many anti-HIV drugs are analogues of nucleosides or pyrophosphates. Many anti-HIV drugs target the viral polymerase. HIV polymerase is relatively unfaithful and is likely to be responsible for much of the genetic variation observed. Clinical isolates are often heterogeneous mixtures of virus.

Unlike the case with herpesviruses, drug-resistant HIV isolated in the clinic has preceded the spontaneous isolation of such virus in the laboratory. Nevertheless, the analysis of the clinical isolates and engineered mutants constructed in the laboratory has demonstrated that, as is true for herpesvirus mutants, biochemical assays can be misleading, and alternate drugs may be useful in treating resistant isolates.

Among the issues outstanding in considering HIV drug resistance are whether sites of mutations conferring drug resistance in the virus will reveal surprises regarding the mechanisms of these drugs; whether the frequency of mutation to drug resistance will be high; whether the initial indications that alternate drugs will be available to treat resistant HIV hold up; and probably most important, whether drug-resistance HIV will have serious pathogenic potential. In particular, will mixtures consisting of drug-resistant and -sensitive virus play a role in pathogenic, drug-resistant infections? Further results in this area are eagerly anticipated.

SUMMARY

Antiviral drug resistance is an area of increasing importance in acquired immunodeficiency syndrome (AIDS), not only in terms of the human immunodeficiency virus (HIV), but also opportunistic pathogens such as herpes simplex virus (HSV) and human cytomegalovirus (CMV). Studies of drug resistance in these and other viruses have proven valuable both for the molecular dissection of drug mechanisms and drug targets and for predicting the features of drug resistance in clinical settings: Drug-resistance mutations arise readily, due in part to a lack of fidelity of viral polymerase. Both biochemical and genetic analyses are generally required to understand the basis of drug resistance. Novel drug targets, such as a CMV gene product that contributes to ganciclovir phosphorylation, can be identified by analysis of such mutations. Regions of drug targets that are involved in drug recognition can be identified by sequencing of drug-resistance mutations. Analysis of drug-resistant viruses, obtained either in the laboratory or from patients, reveals a broad spectrum of alterations and points to the importance of heterogeneous populations of virus in resistance and pathogenesis.

ACKNOWLEDGMENTS

I thank many colleagues for helpful discussions.

REFERENCES

1. ERICE, A., S. CHOU, K. K. BIRON, S. C. STANAT, H. H. BALFOUR & M. C. JORDAN. 1989. N. Engl. J. Med. **320:** 289-293.
2. ERLICH, K. S., J. MILLS, P. CHATIS, G. J. MERTZ, D. F. BUSCH, S. E. FOLLANSBEE, R. M. GRANT & C. S. CRUMPACKER. 1989. N. Engl. J. Med. **320:** 293-296.
3. CHATIS, P. A., C. H. MILLER, L. E. SCHRAGER & C.S. CRUMPACKER. 1989. N. Engl. J. Med. **320:** 297-300.
4. HIRSCH, M. S. & R. T. SCHOOLEY. 1989. N. Engl. J. Med. **320:** 313-314.
5. LARDER, B. A., G. DARBY & D. D. RICHMAN. 1989. Science **243:** 1731-1734.
6. BENNET, L. L., W. M. SHANNON, P. W. ALLEN & G. ARNETT. 1978. Ann. N.Y. Acad. Sci. **255:** 342-352.
7. COEN, D. M., P. A. FURMAN, P. T. GELEP & P. A. SCHAFFER. 1982. J. Virol. **41:** 909-918.
8. FYFE, J. A., P. M. KELLER, P. A. FURMAN, R. L. MILLER & G. B. ELION. 1978. J. Biol. Chem. **253:** 8721-8727.
9. MILLER, W. H. & R. L. MILLER. 1980. J. Biol. Chem. **255:** 7204-7207.
10. MILLER, W. H. & R. L. MILLER. 1982. Biochem. Pharmacol. **31:** 3879-3884.
11. FURMAN, P.A., M.H. ST. CLAIR, J. A. FYFE, J. L. RIDEOUT, P. M. KELLER & G. B. ELION. 1979. J. Virol. **32:** 72-77.
12. LEINBACH, S. S., J. M. RENO, L. F. LEE, A. F. ISBELL & J. A. BOEZI. 1976. Biochemistry **15:** 426-430.
13. FURMAN, P. A., J. A. FYFE, M. H. ST. CLAIR, K. WEINHOLD, J. L. RIDEOUT, G. A. FREEMAN, S. N. LEHRMAN, D. P. BOLOGNESI, S. BRODER, H. MITSUYA & D. W. BARRY. 1986. Proc. Natl. Acad. Sci. USA **83:** 8333-8337.
14. VRANG, L. & B. OBERG. 1986. Antimicrob. Agents Chemother. **29:** 867-892.
15. HERRMANN, E. C. JR. & J. A. HERRMANN. 1977. Ann. N.Y. Acad. Sci. **284:** 632-637.
16. HUBERMAN, J. A. 1981. Cell **23:** 833-836.
17. COEN, D. M., H. E. FLEMING, JR., L. K. LESLIE & M. J. RETONDO. 1984. Drug resistant and hypersensitive herpes simplex virus mutants: isolation and application to dissection of the *pol* locus. *In* Herpesvirus. F. Rapp, Ed.: 373-385. Alan R. Liss. New York.
18. DEFILLIPPES, F. M. 1984. J. Virol. **52:** 474-482.
19. HALL, J. D. & S. WOODWARD. 1989. J. Virol. **63:** 2874-2876.
20. DE CLERCQ, E., J. DESCAMPS, G. VERHELST, R. T. WALKER, A. A. JONES, P. F. TORRENCE & D. SHUGAR. 1980. J. Infect. Dis. **141:** 563-574.
21. KLEIN, R. J. 1975. Arch. Virology **49:** 73-80.
22. SHIPMAN, C. & B. J. SLOAN. 1977. Ann. N.Y. Acad. Sci. **284:** 105.
23. BASTOW, K. F., D. D. DERSE & Y.-C. CHENG. 1983. Antimicrob. Agents Chemother. **23:** 914-917.
24. FLEMING, H. E., JR. & D. M. COEN. 1984. Antimicrob. Agents Chemother. **26:** 382-387.
25. COEN, D. M. & P. A. SCHAFFER. 1980. Proc. Natl. Acad. Sci. USA **77:** 2265-2269.

26. SANDFORD, G. R., J. W. SIMONS, J. R. WINGARD, S. P. STAAL, R. SARAL & W. H. BURNS. 1985. J. Virol. **53:** 104-113.
27. CRUMPACKER, C. S., L. E. SCHNIPPER, P. N. KOWALSKY & D. N. SHERMAN. 1982. J. Infect. Dis. **146:** 167-172.
28. CHIOU, H. C. 1988. A Combined Pharmacological and Genetic Analysis of the Herpes Simplex Virus DNA Polymerase. Ph.D. Thesis. Harvard University. Cambridge, MA.
29. LARDER, B. A., S. D. KEMP & D. J. M. PURIFOY. 1989. Proc. Natl. Acad. Sci. USA **86:** 4803-4807.
30. LARDER, B. A. & S. D. KEMP. 1989. Science **246:** 1155-1158.
31. BIRON, K. K., S. C. STANAT, J. B. SORRELL, J. A. FYFE, P. M. KELLER, C. U. LAMBE & D. J. NELSON. 1985. Proc. Natl. Acad. Sci. USA **82:** 2473-2477.
32. FREITAS, V. R., D. F. SMEE, N. CHERNOW, R. BOEHME & T. R. MATTHEWS. 1985. Antimicrob. Agents Chemother. **28:** 240-245.
33. BIRON, K. K., J. A. FYFE, S. C. STANAT, L. K. LESLIE, J. B. SORRELL, C. U. LAMBE & D. M. COEN. 1986. Proc. Natl. Acad. Sci. USA **83:** 8769-8773.
34. IRMIERE, A. F., M. M. MANOS, J. G. JACOBSON, J. S. GIBBS & D. M. COEN. 1989. Virology **168:** 210-220.
35. COEN, D. M., R. A. F. DIXON, S. W. RUBY & P. A. SCHAFFER. 1980. Genetics of acycloguanosine resistance and the thymidine kinase gene in HSV-1. *In* Animal Virus Genetics. B. N. Fields, R. Jaenisch & C. F. Fox, Eds.: 581-590. Academic Press. New York.
36. COEN, D. M., A. F. IRMIERE, J. G. JACOBSON & K. M. KERNS. 1989. Virology **168:** 221-231.
37. DARBY, G., M. J. CHURCHER & B. A. LARDER. 1984. J. Virol. **50:** 838-846.
38. LARDER, B. A., D. J. M. PURIFOY, K. L. POWELL & G. DARBY. 1987. Nature (London) **327:** 716-717.
39. DANIELS, R. S., J. C. DOWNIE, A. J. HAY, M. KNOSSOW, J. J. SKEHEL, M. L. WANG & D. C. WILEY. 1985. Cell **40:** 431-439.
40. GIBBS, J. S., H. C. CHIOU, K. F. BASTOW, Y.-C. CHENG & D. M. COEN. 1988. Proc. Natl. Acad. Sci. USA **85:** 6672-6676.
41. LARDER, B. A., S. D. KEMP & G. DARBY. 1987. EMBO J. **6:** 169-175.
42. KNOPF, C. W. 1986. Nucleic Acids Res. **14:** 8225-8226.
43. TSURUMI, T., K. MAENO & Y. NISHIYAMA. 1987. J. Virol. **61:** 388-394.
44. OLLIS, D. L., P. BRICK, R. HAMLIN, N. G. XUONG & T. A. STEITZ. 1985. Nature (London) **313:** 762-766.
45. BERNAD, A., L. BLANCO, J. M. LAZARO, G. MARTIN & M. SALAS. 1989. Cell **59:** 219-228.
46. COEN, D. M. 1986. J. Antimicrob. Chemother. **18** (Suppl.B): 1-10.
47. HALL, J. D., D. M. COEN, B. L. FISHER, M. WEISSLITZ, R. E. ALMY, P. T. GELEP & P. A. SCHAFFER. 1984. Virology **132:** 26-37.
48. HALL, J. D., P. A. FURMAN, M. H. ST. CLAIR & C. W. KNOPF. 1985. Proc. Natl. Acad. Sci. USA **82:** 3889-3893.
49. PRESTON, B. D., B. J. POIESZ & L. A. LOEB. 1988. Science **242:** 1168-1171.
50. ROBERTS, J. D., K. BEBENEK & T. A. KUNKEL. 1988. Science **242:** 1171-1173.
51. SAAG, M. S., B. H. HAHN, J. GIBBONS, Y. LI, E. S. PARKS, W. P. PARKS & G. M. SHAW. 1988. Nature (London) **334:** 440-444.
52. FISHER, A. G., B. ENSOLI, D. LOONEY, A. ROSE, R. C. GALLO, M. S. SAAG, G. M. SHAW, B. H. HAHN & F. WONG-STAAL. 1988. Nature (London) **334:** 444-447.
53. SAKAI, K., S. DEWHURST, X. MA & D. J. VOLSKY. 1988. J. Virol. **62:** 4078-4085.
54. TENSER, R. B. & M. E. DUNSTAN. 1979. Virology **99:** 417-422.
55. COEN, D. M., M. KOSZ-VNENCHAK, J. G. JACOBSON, D. A. LEIB, C. L. BOGARD, P. A. SCHAFFER, K. L. TYLER & D. M. KNIPE. 1989. Proc. Natl. Acad. Sci. USA **86:** 4736-4740.
56. DERSE, D., K. F. BASTOW & Y.-C. CHENG. 1982. J. Biol. Chem. **257:** 10251-10260.
57. ST. CLAIR, M. H., W. H. MILLER, R. L. MILLER, C. U. LAMBE & P. A. FURMAN. Antimicrob. Agents Chemother. **25:** 191-194.
58. TENSER, R. B., K. A. HAY & W. A. EDRIS. 1989. J. Virol. **63:** 2861-2865.
59. EFSTATHIOU, S., S. KEMP, G. DARBY & A. C. MINSON. 1989. J. Gen. Virol. **70:** 869-879.
60. FIELD, H. J. 1982. Antimicrob. Agents Chemother. **21:** 744-752.
61. FIELD, H. J. & E. LAY. 1984. Antiviral Res. **4:** 43-52.

62. ELLIS, M. N., R. WATERS, E. L. HILL, D. C. LOBE, D. W. SELLESETH & D. W. BARRY. 1989. Antimicrob. Agents Chemother. **33:** 304-310.
63. LARDER, B. A. & G. DARBY. 1984. Antiviral Res. **4:** 1-42.
64. SACKS, S. L., R. J. WANKLIN, D. E. REECE, K. A. HICKS, K. L. TYLER & D. M. COEN. 1989. Ann. Intern. Med. **111:** 893-899.
65. NORRIS, S. A., H. A. KESSLER & K. H. FIFE. 1988. J. Infect. Dis. **157:** 209-210.
66. PARKER, A. C., J. I. CRAIG, P. COLLINS, N. OLIVER & I. SMITH. 1987. Lancet **ii:** 1461.
67. COLLINS, P., B. A. LARDER, N. M. OLIVER, S. KEMP, I. W. SMITH & G. DARBY. 1989. J. Gen. Virol. **70:** 375-382.
68. ELLIS, M. N., P. M. KELLER, J. A. FYFE, J. L. MARTIN, J. F. ROONEY, S. E. STRAUS, S. NUSINOFF-LEHRMAN & D. W. BARRY. 1987. Antimicrob. Agents Chemother. **31:** 1117-1125.
69. OLIVER, N. M., P. COLLINS, J. VAN DER MEER & J.W. VAN' T. WOUT. 1989. Antimicrob. Agents Chemother. **33:** 635-640.
70. ERLICH, K. S., M. A. JACOBSON, J. E. KOEHLER, S. E. FOLLANSBEE, D. P. DRENNAN, L. GOOZE, S. SAFRIN & J. MILLS. 1989. Ann. Intern. Med. **110:** 710-713.
71. VINCKIER, F., M. BOOGAERTS, D. DECLERCQ & E. DECLERCQ. 1987. J. Oral Maxillofac. Surg. **45:** 723-728.
72. YOULE, M. M., D. A. HAWKINS, P. COLLINS, D. C. SHANSON, R. EVANS, N. OLIVER & A. LAWRENCE. 1988. Lancet **ii:** 341-342.

Use of a Neonatal Murine Retrovirus Model To Evaluate the Long-Term Efficacy and Toxicity of Antiviral Agents[a]

J. A. BILELLO,[b,c,e] C. MacAULEY,[b]

T. N. FREDRICKSON,[f] M. M. BELL,[c] C. McKISSICK,[b]

S. G. SHAPIRO,[c] R. PERSONETTE,[b] AND

J. L. EISEMAN [b,c,d]

[b]Research Service
Veterans Administration Medical Center
Baltimore, Maryland 21218

[c]University of Maryland Cancer Center
Departments of [d]Pathology and [e]Microbiology
University of Maryland School of Medicine
Baltimore, Maryland 21201

[f]Department of Pathobiology
University of Connecticut
Storrs, Connecticut 06269-0389

INTRODUCTION

Infants born to mothers infected with either human lentiviruses (HIV) or oncornaviruses (HTLV-I) are an expanding population who are at risk for retrovirus exposure *in utero,* during parturition, and after birth through breast milk.[1,2] Chemotherapeutic approaches directed toward reducing perinatal retrovirus infection require *in vivo* model systems to develop effective treatment regimens that minimize toxicity. Cas-Br-M MuLV infection of neonatal NFS/N mice is used to evaluate perinatal intervention with antiviral agents. Infection of neonatal mice with Cas-Br-M MuLV leads to replication of the virus in spleen with dissemination to other organs, most notably to the CNS where pathologic lesions (spongiform encephalopathy) develop in the brain stem and spinal cord. A chronic progressive neurodegenerative disease ensues that results in weakness and paralysis in susceptible mice.[3-5] Because NFS/N mice are a genetically inbred strain, the latent period for viral replication, dissemination, and the onset of disease are highly reproducible, and the effects of antiviral agents can be clearly demonstrated

[a]These studies were supported by NIAID Contract NIH-NIAID-MIDP-1-YO1-60002. Three of us (J. A. Bilello, R. Personette, and J. L. Eiseman) are partially supported by Merit Review Awards from the Department of Veterans Affairs.

using both virological and clinical end points. Viral core (p30) and envelope (gp70) proteins are detected in the spleen of infected untreated mice 2-3 weeks postinfection (p.i.), in brain at 4 weeks, and in spinal cord 5-6 weeks p.i. Neurologic symptoms can be evaluated within 5-8 weeks p.i. This well-defined pathogenesis of Cas-Br-M MuLV in NFS/N mice permitted us to document the ability of the antiviral agent 3' azidothymidine (AZT) to prevent retrovirus dissemination to the CNS and to alter the course of neurologic disease.

Although Cas-Br-M MuLV differs from HIV and HTLV-I in genetic constitution, all retroviruses are nearly identical with regard to the early replication steps: adsorption, penetration, reverse transcription, and integration of the proviral DNA. Two observations are particularly relevant to this study: MuLV reverse transcriptase is inhibited by AZTTP, the nucleoside triphosphate form of AZT;[6] and AZT inhibits *de novo* infection of murine cells with Cas-Br-M MuLV, but has no effect on viral replication once integration has occurred.[7]

Clinical efficacy of an antiviral agent is dependent upon attaining effective (inhibitory or virucidal) concentrations of the agent at sites of infection. For a nucleoside analogue such as AZT, which has as its molecular target the retroviral reverse transcriptase, it is important that an inhibitory concentration of the nucleotide triphosphate is present in target cells. In this murine model we are able to determine the pharmacokinetics and pharmacodynamics of AZT or other antivirals and the impact of the dosing regimen on drug distribution and the disease course.

METHODS

Mice

Pregnant NFS/N mice were obtained from the Animal Program administered by the Animal Genetics and Production Branch of the National Cancer Institute. To minimize exogenous infection, animals were housed singly in microisolator cages for filtration of room air. Sentinel mice are routinely monitored for infection by exogenous viruses in the environment, including mouse hepatitis, pneumonia virus of mice, minute virus of mice, reovirus type 3, lymphocytic choriomeningitis, and Sendai virus.

Inoculation and Clinical Observation

Pregnant NFS/N mice were observed daily, and their pups were inoculated with Cas-Br-M MuLV (1×10^6 plaque-forming units (PFU)/mL, 0.03 mL intracranially or intraperitoneally) 1 to 2 days after birth. Pups were weaned at 21-28 days of age and housed by sex, litter, and treatment. Observations of general health status were done daily, and symptoms of neurologic disease, including tremor, toe splay, and hind limb weakness were recorded weekly.

Preparation of Tissue Homogenates and Virus Titration

At the designated time points, mice were euthanized and bled by cardiac puncture. Spleen, brain, spinal cord, and other tissues of interest were removed and rapidly frozen on dry ice or liquid nitrogen and stored at −70°C or less. Prior to assay the tissue was weighed and homogenized at 4°C in phosphate-buffered saline. Protein content of the homogenate was determined by Coomassie blue dye binding (BioRad, Rockville Center, NY). Dilutions of the homogenates were made in duplicate in Eagles MEM tissue culture medium without serum. Virus was titered by XC assay[8] after infecting SC-1 fibroblasts in duplicate with serial dilutions of tissue homogenates.

Polyacrylamide Gel Electrophoresis and Immunoblotting

Samples (300-400 ng of protein) were analyzed on 3 mm thick, 16 cm long, 12.5% SDS-polyacrylamide slab gels.[9] Transfer of proteins to nitrocellulose was for 16 hours at 19 volts using Tris-glycine-methanol buffer as described by Burnette.[10] Viral proteins were identified after reaction with primary antisera (goat anti-Rauscher MuLV p30 or Friend MuLV gp70) and ^{125}I-labeled Protein G (Amersham, Oak Park, IL). Autoradiography was performed using Chronex 4 film and Quanta III enhancing screens at −70°C.

Assay of AZT Levels in Murine Tissues

A high-performance liquid chromatographic (HPLC) method was developed to measure the concentration of AZT in murine tissues and plasma. Briefly, tissue homogenates or heparinized plasma samples (200-500 μL) were spiked with 50 μL of the internal standard (a 200 μM solution of the beta isomer of AZT). HPLC separation was achieved with gradient flow of 1.2 mL/min from a Brownlee 22 cm Speri 5 RP-18, 5 μM column. The mobile phases were acetonitrile and 10 mM ammonium acetate, pH 4.0. Gradient was maintained at 17% acetonitrile in buffer for the first 7 minutes, increasing to 30% acetonitrile in buffer for 5 minutes, and decreasing to 17% acetonitrile by 30 minutes. All samples were analyzed by comparison to an AZT standard curve that was quantified at 267 nm and was linear from 0.1 μM to 200 μM AZT, with less than 5% interassay variation (Eiseman et al., submitted.).

RESULTS

Efficacy of AZT Administered in Drinking Water

In vitro studies showed that 0.1 μM AZT was effective in protecting cells from *de novo* infection, but concentrations of AZT up to 10 μM did not effect the release of virus from cells chronically infected with Cas-Br-M MuLV.[7,11] Cocultivation experiments, shown in FIGURE 1, demonstrate that continuous exposure to 1.0 μM AZT in tissue culture media protected uninfected cells *in vitro* from the cell to cell spread of Cas-Br-M MuLV for a period of one month.

Pharmacokinetic studies of AZT in Cas-Br-M MuLV-infected and uninfected NFS/N mice (manuscript in preparation) indicated the plasma half-life of AZT was 16 minutes in males and 18 minutes in females. Total body clearance in male and female Cas-Br-M MuLV-infected mice was 1.3 L/kg/h and 1.0 L /kg/h, respectively, after i.v. dosing. AZT was not detected in murine plasma collected beyond 4 h after dosing (lower detection limit, 0.1 μM). A comparison of AZT plasma pharmacokinetics

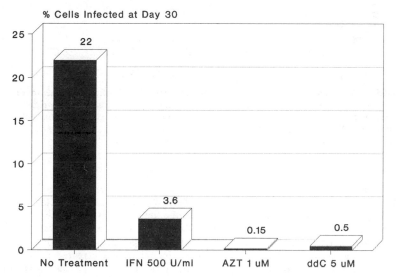

FIGURE 1. Mouse SC-1 cells chronically infected with Cas-Br-M MuLV were cocultivated with a 250-fold excess of uninfected SC-1 cells in the presence of inhibitory concentrations of AZT (1 μM), dideoxycytidine (ddC 5 μM), or murine beta interferon (IFN, 500 units/mL) in the medium for a period of one month. Cells were passaged weekly, and the media was changed (to maintain levels of IFN and AZT or ddC) every 72 hours. Virus-infected cells were measured by trypsinizing cell monolayers and plating dilutions of the cells with $10^{4.5}$ uninfected SC-1 cells. After 5 days cells were exposed to UV and overlayered with XC cells.

in mice after oral and i.v. dosing demonstrated AZT was 100% bioavailable by the oral route. FIGURE 2 shows that AZT accumulates more slowly in the brain, and peak concentrations are an order of magnitude lower than in plasma or spleen. Notably the concentration of AZT in the spleen was twofold higher than in the plasma of NFS/N mice, which indicates that AZT rapidly accumulates and may concentrate in this organ, which is the primary site of Cas-Br-M MuLV replication.

Based upon the pharmacokinetic data, pregnant NFS/N mice were treated with AZT (1 mg/mL in drinking water) beginning five days prior to parturition or when the newborns were inoculated intracranially (i.c.) with Cas-Br-M MuLV (0 to 2 days after parturition). Three weeks postinfection, 1–3 pups per litter were euthanized, and spleen and brain homogenates were analyzed for the presence of infectious virus. As seen in TABLE 1, no virus was found in the spleen and brain homogenates from a litter

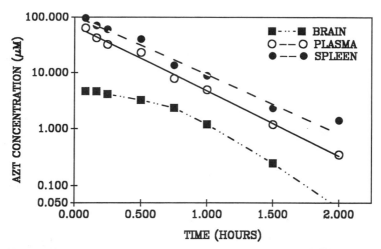

FIGURE 2. AZT pharmacokinetics in plasma and tissues of NFS/N mice. AZT was administered at a dose of 50 mg/kg (0.05 mL of a 10 mg/mL solution for 10 grams body weight). At the indicated time points after dosing, one animal of each sex was sacrificed. Plasma was obtained by centrifugation of heparinized blood at 1200 rpm for 10 minutes. Plasma, spleen, and brain were frozen for subsequent assay of AZT as described in the METHODS.

where dams were treated with AZT prior to delivery. Only one of three pups tested from a dam treated with AZT at the time of virus challenge had detectable virus in the spleen. This pup had a four log lower titer than found in Cas-Br-M MuLV-infected three-week-old mice from untreated dams (TABLE 1). At four weeks postinoculation therapy was either halted or continued at 1 mg AZT per mL in the drinking water. All animals were observed for 15 months postinoculation. Untreated infected mice were paralyzed and/or moribund and sacrificed by 18 weeks. The 16 Cas-Br-M MuLV--challenged mice who received AZT only during lactation and the 5 mice who received AZT during lactation and for an additional 4 weeks were all normal by physical diagnosis and histological examination of brain and cord. XC assay of homogenates of brain, spleen, and spinal cord from these mice were negative. No viral p30 or gp70 was detectable by Western blot of homogenates from uninfected or AZT-treated mice (FIG. 3). In another study where Cas-Br-M MuLV-infected pups received AZT only through milk from treated dams, 1 of 23 brain and 2 of 23 spleen homogenates were positive for MuLV p30.[7] By contrast, when AZT was administered to dams for the first week of lactation, all pups were virus-positive, albeit that virus titer in spleen and brain was reduced by a factor of 5 to 10.

HEMATOPOIETIC TOXICITY OF AZT

By 4 weeks of treatment with 1 mg/mL AZT, the hematocrits of treated dams fell to 9.0% ± 1.3% compared to control hematocrits of 52.7% ± 3.4% (FIG. 4). Due to a fourfold increase in water consumed by the lactating dams, the total dose of AZT per mouse per day increased from approximately 190 mg/kg at day 1 of lactation to a peak of approximately 800 mg/kg at day 24. Histological examination of bone marrow from AZT-treated dams confirmed aplasia. Further, a marked decrease in the red cell precursors in splenic red pulp was noted. Megakaryocytes and myelocytic cell types were less affected (FIG. 5). AZT-mediated depression of hematocrit was readily reversed upon the removal of the drug from the drinking water (FIG. 6).

Weanlings who had received AZT by way of maternal transfer were either continued on treatment (5 mice) with AZT at 1 mg/mL in the drinking water for an additional 4 weeks or had therapy terminated (16 mice). Those mice (12-14 g) who continued AZT therapy for 4 weeks showed signs of weakness and inactivity when compared to weanlings whose therapy had been terminated. This weakness was associated with hematocrits below 30% as compared to normal values of approximately 50 percent. As in dams, anemia and associated weakness were reversed when AZT dose was reduced or terminated.

Toxicity and Efficacy of AZT Administered by Constant Infusion

Because of the short half-life, detection of AZT in the plasma of mice drinking 1 mg/mL AZT was highly variable. In 16 dams the level of AZT varied from 21 μM to undetectable (less than 0.1 μM). Similarly plasma levels of AZT were variable and usually not detectable in pups of such AZT-treated dams at the time of euthanasia. To maintain therapeutic levels of AZT for prolonged periods, AZT was administered by constant infusion using ALZET^{tm} 2001 miniosmotic pumps implanted subcutaneously in near-term pregnant or lactating dams. Three successive implants of an ALZET^{tm} 2001 were required in order to maintain AZT levels for 21 days. Plasma AZT concentra-

TABLE 1. Virus Titer in Spleen and Brain Tissue Homogenates from Three-Week-Old Cas-Br-M MuLV-Infected NFS/N Mice

AZT treatment[a] of dam	Number/ total[b]	Tissue	Virus titer[c] PFU/0.1 g $\times$ 1000
Control (No MuLV)	3/3	Spleen Brain	<0.0005 <0.0005
none	3/3	Spleen Brain	90 6
AZT 5 days prior to birth	3/3	Spleen Brain	<0.0005 <0.0005
AZT 2 days after birth	2/3	Spleen Brain	<0.0005 <0.0005
AZT 2 days after birth	1/3	Spleen Brain	0.006 <0.0005

[a] AZT 1 mg/mL was administered in the drinking water. At 2 days after birth the newborn mice were infected with Cas-Br-M MuLV intracranially as described in the METHODS.

[b] The fraction reflects the number of pups with the indicated response/the number tested.

[c] Virus in tissue homogenates was titered using the XC plaque assay. Results are expressed as the average of each sample in duplicate at each of the three dilutions tested.

tions obtained from these dams demonstrated that ALZET^{tm} 2001 pumps loaded with 250 μL of a 25 mg/mL solution of AZT were maintained at approximately 1 μM (0.854 $\pm$ 0.145 μM) in lactating NFS/N mice. Pups from dams receiving AZT through continuous infusion were sacrificed, and the plasma from 6 pups per litter was pooled. Only one litter of 14 had a detectable plasma level (0.176 μM AZT) at the time of sacrifice.

Administration of AZT to dams by constant infusion limited virus spread and delayed the onset of symptoms in their offspring challenged with Cas-Br-M MuLV. At

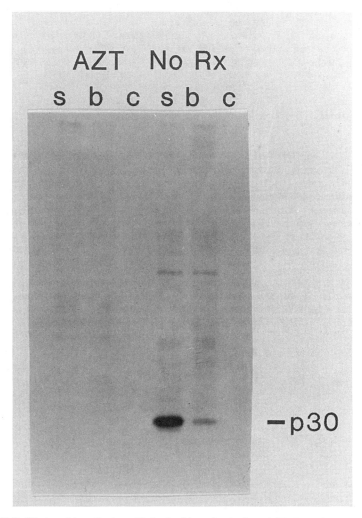

FIGURE 3. Western blot of spleen (s), brain (b), and spinal cord (c) tissue from control and AZT-treated NFS/N mice. Tissue homogenates from Cas-Br-M MuLV-infected and AZT-treated infected pups were analyzed by PAGE and immunoblotted as described in METHODS. Antiserum to Rauscher MuLV p30 was used to identify MuLV-specific proteins with p30 antigenic determinants.

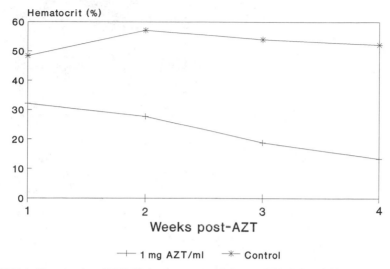

FIGURE 4. Hematocrits of NFS/N dams treated with 1 mg AZT/mL in drinking water. NFS/ N dams were permitted to drink untreated water or water containing AZT *ad libitum* for a period of three weeks. Hematocrits were measured weekly on blood obtained from the orbital sinus.

4 weeks postinoculation 2 pups per litter were sacrificed, and brain tissue homogenates were analyzed by XC assay. Four of four pups from continuously infused dams were virus-positive and had an average of 2.1×10^3 XC PFU, whereas untreated mice had an average of 5.2×10^3 XC PFU per 0.1 g of brain tissue. This difference was reproducible, and variation between animals was minimal. Consistent with other data on the drinking water regimen, brain homogenates from mice treated with AZT (1 mg/mL) in drinking water had no detectable virus (less than 1 PFU per 0.5 mL of homogenate) and were p30 negative by Western blot. At 18 weeks p.i. 16 of 16 untreated Cas-Br-M MuLV-infected NFS/N mice were in late stage of neurologic disease, whereas 3 of 7 offspring from continuously infused dams were symptomatic but with less overt disease. Splenic hyperplasia and increased numbers of erythroblasts were readily observed in dams continuously infused with AZT at 25 μg/h (FIG. 5). At necropsy dams with an AZT-releasing implant had an average spleen weight that was twofold higher than untreated mice or mice with a saline containing ALZET implant. Using standard hematopoietic colony-forming assays, we observed an increase in hematopoietic precursors (BFU-e, CFU-c) in spleen and bone marrow of mice continuously infused with AZT (data not shown).

FIGURE 5 (*See overleaf*). Histopathology of the spleen following AZT-treatment of NFS/N dams. Sections of spleen or bone marrow stained with hematoxylin eosin and magnified × 600. Panel A: Spleen from an untreated NFS/N dam; panel B: hypoplastic spleen from a dam on 0.5 mg/mL AZT; panel C: hyperplastic spleen from a dam with an ALZET miniosmotic pump maintaining plasma AZT levels of approximately 1 μM; panel D: normal bone marrow, untreated; panel E: severely hypoplastic bone marrow, 0.5 mg/mL AZT; panel F: bone marrow from continuously infused dam, showing extensive erythropoiesis.

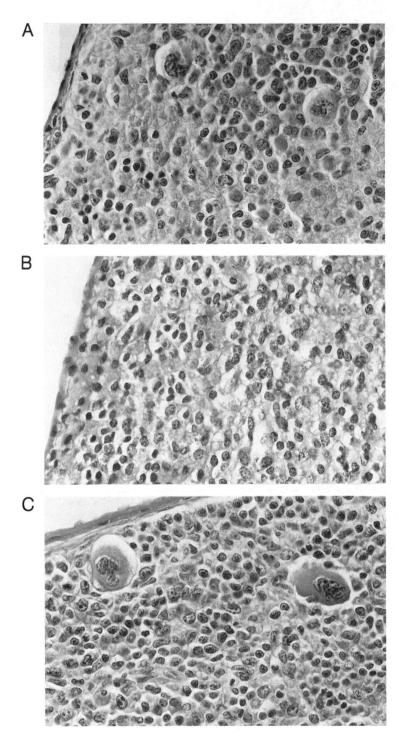

FIGURES 5A-C.

246

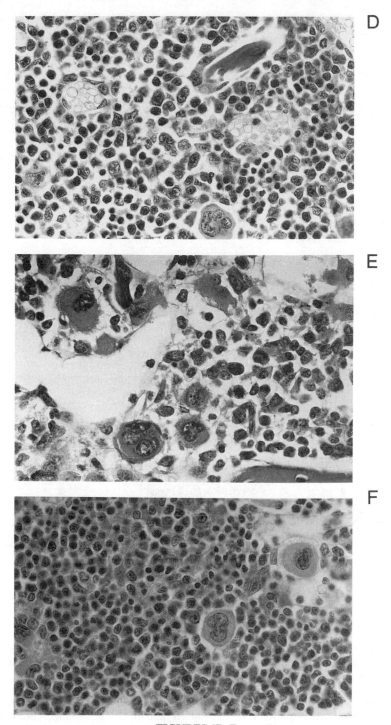

FIGURES 5D-F.

Absence of Long-Term Toxicity upon AZT Administration

We observed no differences in the weight, size, or the general health status of litters receiving AZT for three to four weeks by way of maternal transfer. Mice from AZT-treated litters were brother-sister mated to determine whether AZT had an effect on the reproductive capacity of the F_1 litters. No difference in fertility was observed. Further, no significant difference in the litter size (7.8 $\pm$ 0.91 vs 7.9 $\pm$ 1.47), weight at one week (5.21 $\pm$ 1.24 vs 5.41 $\pm$ 0.5), or general health status of the F_2 generation was apparent. During the 18 months of observation and at necropsy no neoplastic disease was documented in AZT-treated F_1 offspring.

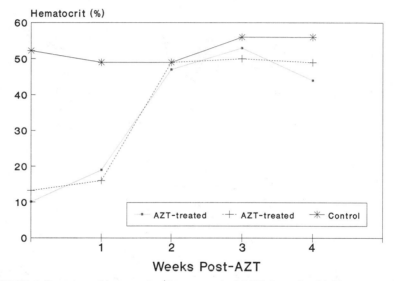

FIGURE 6. Recovery of hematocrits after removal of AZT from the drinking water of two lactating NFS/N dams. The three dams, one control and two AZT-treated (1 mg/mL in drinking water for four weeks) were all permitted to drink normal untreated water *ad libitum* for a period of three weeks. Hematocrits were measured weekly on blood obtained from the orbital sinus.

DISCUSSION

These data indicate that AZT can be administered to newborn mice by way of nursing dams to prevent both the initiation of retrovirus replication and the establishment of reservoirs of infection *in vivo*. Perinatal challenge with Cas-Br-M MuLV was chosen because natural transmission of several retroviruses occurs perinatally either during parturition or through milk-borne transmission.[1,2,13] This model may represent a situation more like pediatric AIDS in children than other murine models using other routes of infection, such as the one described by Sharpe *et al.*[12]

Ruprecht and her colleagues first reported that AZT in the drinking water was able to limit Rauscher MuLV infection of adult BALB/c mice. AZT therapy that began four hours postchallenge with 10,000 PFU of R-MuLV prevented the establishment of disease; spleen and plasma were virus-free 20 days postinoculation.[14] Our present study demonstrates that AZT administered orally to dams by way of drinking water is remarkably effective in preventing the establishment of MuLV infection in the offspring after a single injection of Cas-Br-M MuLV. Infection with Cas-Br-E MuLV, however, was not prevented by AZT therapy begun after introduction of virus-infected cells *in utero*.[12] Timing of AZT therapy is critical; increased viremia was observed in cats treated 3, 7, or 28 days after infection with feline leukemia virus[15] and in BALB/c mice inoculated with R-MuLV and treated 19 days postinfection.[14] Further, the length of the treatment period is also important. AZT administered to lactating NFS/N mice for a period of one week was not sufficient to prevent infection of their offspring challenged with Cas-Br-M MuLV.

Our results suggest that the enhanced efficacy of the drinking water regimen over continuous infusion may be directly related to AZT pharmacokinetics. Dams with implanted ALZET miniosmotic pumps loaded with 25 mg/mL AZT had plasma levels of AZT of approximately 1 μM. Levels of AZT in the spleen, the primary site of Cas-Br-M MuLV replication, were approximately twofold higher than plasma AZT levels, whereas the concentration of AZT in brain was approximately tenfold lower, presumably due to the limited penetration of AZT across the blood brain barrier. Mice drinking AZT in water, in effect, receive AZT by way of pulsed delivery with high-peak concentrations followed by low "though" levels of drug. Direct measurement of AZT levels in NFS/N plasma and tissue showed that levels of AZT above 150 μM were reached within 5 minutes after oral gavage. Other studies also suggest greater efficacy of intermittent dosing regimens. Human polymorphonuclear leukocytes pulsed with AZT in tissue culture maintained higher intracellular levels of AZT di- and triphosphates.[16] AZT is effective when administered at 250 mg/kg every four hours to patients with AIDS. Continuous administration of AZT to pediatric patients was shown to be effective in limiting and possibly reversing neurologic symptoms with minimal toxicity.[17] AZT delivered through continuous infusion to NFS/N dams was not as effective in preventing infection as intermittent dosing. This may be due to lower levels of AZT transferred to the offspring or the intermittent delivery through nursing. Other studies in adult C57BL/6 mice, however, have shown that continuous infusion of AZT for 21 days (maintaining concentrations of 1 μM) was not as effective as longer treatment with 1 mg/mL AZT in drinking water.[11] These data suggest that high-peak levels of AZT achieved on the drinking water regimen may enhance the chemotherapeutic application of AZT. Onset of neurologic disease, however, was delayed in mice nursed by NFS/N dams continuously dosed for three weeks by way of ALZET pump, and Cas-Br-M MuLV replication and/or spread was reduced. By contrast, no disease or Cas-Br-M MuLV replication was observed in Cas-Br-M MuLV-challenged offspring after receiving AZT at 1 mg/mL in drinking water for three weeks.

Lastly, anemia, bone marrow suppression, and neutropenia develop during treatment of AIDS patients with AZT.[18] Similarly, nursing NFS/N mice treated with AZT in drinking water had a marked decrease in the red cell precursors in the red pulp of the spleen. Colony-forming assays performed by Bogliolo *et al.*[19] confirm AZT-mediated toxicity for murine hematopoietic progenitor cells. Hematopoietic stem cells were capable of renewal after stopping treatment of NFS/N mice at 21 or 28 days, whereas continued treatment resulted in aplastic anemia and death. By contrast, splenic hyperplasia and an increase in spleen weight but no depression of hematocrit was observed in NFS/N dams with plasma levels of AZT maintained at nearly one micromolar, using an ALZET miniosmotic pump. These data suggest that AZT alters erythropoiesis in the absence of overt hematopoietic toxicity or anemia. Because long-term continuous infusion experiments were not performed, it is not clear whether AZT-induced hyperplasia and increased hematopoietic precursor cell proliferation/differentiation would lead to neoplastic conversion or extensive depletion of marrow precursor cells.

In conclusion, these data demonstrate the utility of this murine model in evaluating the efficacy and toxicity of therapeutic regimens and favor the chemotherapeutic use of AZT at high dose for a limited period of time. Inasmuch as we do not know whether macrophages (a primary target of HIV) are infected by Cas-Br-M MuLV and/or are involved in MuLV dissemination to the CNS, it is not clear whether this regimen will be sufficient to prevent the establishment of HIV infection. In contrast to T cells, macrophages are not readily killed by HIV and may function as a long-lived reservoir of infection. Clearly, chemoprophylactic regimens for HIV infection should be administered for a period of time long enough to permit turnover and/or elimination of potential cellular reservoirs.

ACKNOWLEDGMENTS

We acknowledge Dr. Paul Hoffman for advice and comment on this study and Melissa Smith-Meek for technical assistance.

REFERENCES

1. FALLOON, J., J. EDDY, M. ROPER & P. A. PIZZO. 1988. AIDS in the pediatric population. *In* AIDS: Etiology, diagnosis, treatment and prevention. V. T. DeVita, S. Hellman & S. A. Rosenberg, Eds.: 339-349. J. B. Lippincott. Philadelphia.
2. ZEIGLER, J. B., D. A. COOPER, R. O. JOHNSON & J. GOLD. 1985. Postnatal transmission of AIDS-associated retrovirus from mother to infant. Lancet 1: 896-898.
3. HOFFMAN, P. M., S. K. RUSCETTI & H. C. MORSE III. 1981. Pathogenesis of paralysis and lymphoma associated with retrovirus infection. I. Age and dose related effects in susceptible laboratory mice. J. Neuroimmunology 1: 272-285.
4. HOFFMAN, P. M. & H. C. MORSE III. 1985. Host genetic determinants of neurologic disease induced by Cas-Br-M murine leukemia virus infection. J. Virol. 53: 40-43.
5. OLDSTONE, M. B. A., P. W. LAMPERT, S. LEE & F. J. DIXON. 1977. Pathogenesis of the slow disease of the central nervous system associated with WM 1504E virus I. Relationship of strain susceptibility and replication to disease. Am. J. Pathol. 8: 193-206.
6. FURMAN, P. A., J. A. FYFE & M. H. ST. CLAIR *et al.* 1986. Phosphorylation of 3'-azido-3'deoxythymidine and selective interaction of the 5'-triphosphate with human immunodeficiency virus reverse transcriptase. Proc. Natl. Acad. Sci. USA 83: 8333-8337.
7. ROBBINS, D. S., J. A. BILELLO & P. M. HOFFMAN. 1989. Pathogenesis and treatment of neurotropic retrovirus infections. *In* HTLV-1 and the Nervous System. G. C. Roman, J. C. Vernant & M. Osame, Eds.: 575-587. Alan R. Liss, Inc. New York.
8. ROWE, W. P., W. E. PUGH & J. W. HARTLEY. 1970. Plaque assay techniques for murine leukemia viruses. Virology 42: 1136-1139.
9. BILELLO, J. A., O. M. PITTS & P. M. HOFFMAN. 1986. Characterization of a progressive neurodegenerative disease induced by a temperature sensitive Moloney leukemia virus infection. J. Virol. 59: 234-241.
10. BURNETTE, W. N. 1982. "Western Blotting": electrophoretic transfer of proteins from SDS-polyacrylamide gels to unmodified nitrocellulose and detection with antibody and radioiodinated protein A. Anal. Biochem. 112: 195-203.

11. BILELLO, J. A., C. MACAULEY, R. YETTER, S. G. SHAPIRO, T. FREDRICKSON, M. BELL & J. L. EISEMAN. 1989. Use of AZT as a chemotherapeutic agent: Efficacy and toxicity in murine retrovirus infections. Fifth International Conference on Acquired Immunodeficiency Syndrome. The Scientific and Social Challenge. R. A. Morisset, Ed.: p. 550. International Development Research Centre. Ottawa. Ontario. Canada.

12. SHARPE, A. H., R. JAENISCH & R. M. RUPRECHT. 1987. Retroviruses and mouse embryos: a rapid model for neurovirulence and transplacental antiviral therapy. Science **236:** 1671-1674.

13. GROSS, L. Oncogenic viruses. 2nd Edition. 1970. Pergamon Press. Oxford.

14. RUPRECHT, R. M., L. G. O'BRIEN, L. D. ROSSONI & S. NUSSINOFF-LEHRMAN. 1987. Suppression of mouse viremia and retroviral disease by 3'-azido-3'-deoxythymidine. Nature **323:** 467-469.

15. TAVARES, L., C. RONECKER, K. JOHNSTON, S. N. LEHRMAN & F. DE NORONHA. 1987. 3'Azidothymidine in feline leukemia virus infected cats: a model for therapy and prophylaxis of AIDS. Cancer Res. **47:** 3190-3194.

16. VOGT, M., H. KUSTER, V. NADAI, B. JOOS, W. SEIGENTHALER & R. LUETHY. 1989. Experimental azidothymidine (AZT) pulse therapy leads to adequate and prolonged intracellular levels of intracellular AZT-triphosphate (AZT-TP). Fifth International Conference on Acquired Immunodeficiency Syndrome. The Scientific and Social Challenge. R. A. Morisset, Ed: p. 555. International Development Research Centre. Ottawa. Ontario. Canada.

17. PIZZO, P. A., J. EDDY, J. FALLOON, F. M. BALIS, R. F. MURPHY, H. MOSS, P. WOLTERS, P. JAROSINISKI, M. RUBIN, S. BRODER, R. YARCHOAN, A. BRUNETTI, M. MAHA, S. N. LEHRMAN & D. G. POPLACK. 1988. Effect of continuous intravenous infusion of zidovudine (AZT) in children with symptomatic HIV infection. N. Engl. J. Med. **319:** 889-896.

18. RICHMAN, D. D., M. A. FISCHL, M. H. GRIECO, M. S. GOTTLIEB, P. A. VOLBERDING, O. L. LASKIN, J. M. LEEDOM, J. E. GROOPMAN, D. MILDVAN, M.S. HIRSCH, G.G. JACKSON, D.T. DURACK, S. NUSSINOFF-LEHRMAN & THE AZT COLLABORATIVE WORKING GROUP. 1987. The toxicity of azidothymidine (AZT) in the treatment of patients with AIDS and AIDS-related complex. A double-blind placebo-controlled trial. N. Engl. J. Med. **317:** 192-197.

19. BOGLIOLO, G., R. LERZA, R. MENCOBONI, A. SAVIANE & I. PANNACCIULLI. 1988. Azidothymidine-induced depression of murine hemopoietic progenitor cells. Exp. Hematol. **16:** 938-940.

Strategies to Inhibit Viral Polyprotein Cleavages

BRUCE D. KORANT

Central Research and Development Department
Du Pont Company Experimental Station E328
Wilmington, Delaware 19880-0328

INTRODUCTION

Some viruses encode their own protein-processing machinery. Following the initial reports[1-3] of this discovery, there have been numerous detailed accounts of viral proteases and their substrate preferences (for a recent review see ref. 4), as well as several approaches to inhibitors (reviewed in ref. 5).

Thus far, biochemical studies of viral protein processing have proceeded independently of any significant clinical results with virus-targeted protease inhibitors, but in light of the current AIDS epidemic, one may expect that this will change dramatically over the coming months and years.

In this paper, I will briefly give a personal view of some possible approaches to inhibiting viral proteases, using data for HIV, as well as other viruses in the assessment. Given constraints on space, much of the experimental evidence supporting one approach over another will be presented in a very abbreviated way, and for that I apologize at the outset.

Features of Viral Proteases That Make Them Attractive Chemotherapeutic Targets

Some salient characteristics of viral proteases are listed in TABLE 1. They represent an interesting class of processing enzymes because they are much more selective than standard protein-degrading enzymes, but paradoxically they are substantially ($\frac{1}{2}$-$\frac{2}{3}$) smaller (less complicated?) than cellular proteases. So far, all are synthesized as part of a much larger precursor protein and seem to be self-activating, capable of freeing themselves from their precursor by clipping away their N- and C-terminal extensions. They appear to be related to conventional active-site protease families, although this has not been proven rigorously in all cases.

In general, there is irrefutable homology among the members of a virus group regarding the protease and the cleavage sites used. Particularly at the active site, all members of a virus family are identical or show very conservative substitutions. This implies that viruses will have no easy task in escaping active-site directed inhibitors by genetic drift, particularly if elements of their cleavage sites are included in the drugs.

From studies of a variety of animal viruses, inactivation of the viral protease cannot be rescued by the host cell.

The assignment of viral proteases to a known active-site class presents the drug designer with an unwelcome potential technical hurdle. Although understanding the basis of the catalytic site is of obvious benefit, it means that certain cellular proteases may be partially sensitive to inhibitors of viral proteases. Possibly this can be overcome by incorporating features of the viral cleavage sites into the inhibitors, but this will *a priori* complicate the synthesis. Thus far, no claims of novel active-site chemistries for viral proteases have appeared, and the HIV protease structure and inhibition pattern clearly place it within the diverse and physiologically important family of aspartic proteases.[6,7]

At the present time, we have available an extensive catalog of viral cleavage sites, but these sites are known only to the extent of the amino acids present as a linear array surrounding the site. Virtually nothing is known of the folded structure of the site, whether it exists as a surface loop or in some other form. This should become a fruitful area for further detailed investigation.

TABLE 1. Characteristics of Viral Proteases

Virus-coded
Essential for replication
Smaller than cellular counterparts
High substrate specificity
Self-processing
Conserved active site; conserved cleavage sites

APPROACHES TO INHIBITORS OF VIRAL PROTEIN CLEAVAGES

Assessment of Inhibitors

There have been two distinct, but overlapping, approaches for assaying inhibitors for their ability to block viral protein cleavages. The traditional approach has been to examine the pattern of viral protein synthesis and processing in infected cells in culture.[1,8] This approach is fairly complex, usually requires several days, may involve handling of radioactive compounds, and is somewhat indirect, because inhibition of protein processing may be the result of effects other than direct inhibition of a viral protease. It offers, however, the major advantage of yielding results on intact cells, which often translates better into genuine antiviral activity than exclusively cell-free experiments.

Cell-free experiments can now be performed with semipurified or homogeneous components in several convenient formats. Often these assay systems contain a purified viral protease, which is reacted with a synthetic peptide substrate, based on the elements of a viral cleavage site, plus a reporter group.[9,10] A recent report described a convenient chromogenic substrate for the HIV protease.[11] The cell-free approach is inherently faster, less complicated, and more quantitative than experiments with intact cells, but suffers from an inability to directly predict biological availability and efficacy of a test compound. It is probably wisest to build a program seeking virus-specific protease inhibitors based on a marriage of the cell-free and cell-based approaches. A program based solely on the latter, however, is also reasonable.

Only rarely have protease inhibitors been reported in the literature to have antiviral effects *in vivo*, [12,13] and those have exclusively been carried out in model (rodent) systems with RNA viruses. In spite of these limitations, those reports do contain data showing efficacy of natural and synthetic protease inhibitors in selected viral infections in animals. The reports also support the view that such an approach could lead to useful antiviral drugs, although side effects or toxicities of the test compounds were not carefully considered in the published accounts.

New techniques for rapid assessment of cleavage inhibitors in intact cells would be of value. Our laboratory recently devised "inverted" plasmid constructions that were processed faithfully in *E. coli,* under control of a viral protease.[14] We have adapted that format to one in which the HIV protease is fused to a bacterial protein, namely beta-lactamase. The construct yields lactamase activity after autocatalytic removal of the viral protease (TABLE 2) and permits the cells to grow on penicillin-containing media. Such an assay should be useful in testing large numbers of compounds for their ability to inhibit the viral protease, scoring bacterial growth in the presence of penicillin.

Inhibitors of Viral Protein Cleavages

A multiplicity of approaches to inhibitors of viral protein cleavages have recently been reviewed.[5] They fall into two fundamentally different categories (see TABLE 3): alteration of the substrate so that it cannot be properly cleaved, and direct inactivation of viral proteases.

Alterations of the viral polyprotein to prevent its cleavage are relatively simply attained: high temperatures ($> 37°C$), incorporation of amino acid analogues during biosynthesis, exposure to certain metal ions, or denaturants, such as guanidino compounds, as well as many other physical or chemical treatments, will lead to stabilization or inappropriate cleavages of the viral polyprotein and associated loss of viral infectivity. The negative side of these approaches is fairly obvious: they cannot readily be tailored to the virus. Amino acid analogues, for example, will be incorporated equally well into cellular proteins as viral proteins, and such alterations will likely lead to undesirable effects on host metabolic regulation.

The second category is more conventional in a pharmaceutical sense, that is, the inhibition of viral proteases by natural or synthetic inhibitors. Naturally occurring

TABLE 2. Beta-Lactamase Expression in *E. coli* from a Fusion Protein Containing the HIV-1 Protease

Clone	Lactamase units/mg protein
Wild-type HIV protease-lactamase fusion	470
Inactive HIV protease (D25/G)-lactamase fusion	185
Wild-type HIV protease (no lactamase present)	< 10

TABLE 3. Classes of Inhibitors of Viral Protein Cleavages

Class	Activity range for $ED_{90}(M)$
Substrate modifiers	
Amino acid analogues	10^{-3}
Chelating agents	10^{-3}
Metal ions	10^{-3} to 10^{-5}
High temperature ($> 37°C$)	
Natural inhibitors	
Pepstatins	10^{-4} to 10^{-6}
Pancreatic trypsin inhibitor	10^{-5a}
Cystatins	10^{-5}
Macroglobulins	10^{-8b}
Synthetic inhibitors	
Affinity labels	10^{-3} to 10^{-4}
Cleavage-site mimics	10^{-5} to 10^{-7a}
Retro-inverso peptides	10^{-4} to 10^{-5}
Dimerization inhibitors	?

[a] *In vivo* experiments in mice.
[b] Microinjected into infected cells.

protease inhibitors (including derivatives of compounds found in nature) that are reported to be inhibitory to viral proteases range from small, antibiotic-like compounds, such as pepstatin A,[15] to small proteins, such as cystatins,[16] to very large, oligomeric protease inhibitors, such as alpha-2-macroglobulin, sometimes present in serum at concentrations of several milligrams per milliliter.[17] In several studies,[8,12,16] ability of such inhibitors to block virus replication was reported.

With the proteinaceous inhibitors, the one-to-one stoichiometry of the protease-protease inhibitor complex means that substantial quantities of the inhibitors are required (molecular mass of alpha-2-macroglobulin is nearly 800,000 daltons). Furthermore, they penetrate intact cells poorly, or not at all, thus making for problems in delivering them to an appropriate site of action. They are very effective inhibitors of extracellular proteolytic reactions, however, and could play a prominent role in deactivating any viral protease molecules that are released following exocytosis of virus particles or cell lysis.

By comparison, small inhibitors, such as pepstatin derivatives, are likely to become genuine leads for antiviral therapy. In one recent study,[18] the activity of pepstatin A was enhanced against HIV-1 protease up to 100-fold with a simple chemical modification. Assuming enhanced potency will translate into antiviral activity in cultured cells and animals, a structure-activity relationship should begin to elaborate improved pepstatin derivatives.

Completely synthetic protease inhibitors may offer the best opportunity to develop new antiviral drugs. The recent successful entry of synthetic-converting enzyme inhibitors as clinical antihypertensives provides an optimistic outlook for generalizing the approach to include viral proteases. It was recently shown[19,20] that peptide mimics of viral cleavage sites, containing organic blocking groups at their ends, can have substantial antiviral activity against a variety of viruses. A-peptidic analogues may be expected to have improved stability in a physiologic sense and eventually to be made highly specific for viral processing events. Finally, in the particular case of the retroviruses, inhibitors of the dimerization process, which are required to form active enzyme,[21] may provide another avenue for devising exquisitely specific inhibitors of HIV and its relatives, independent of the active-site chemistry of the aspartyl protease family.

Prospects

The study of viral protein processing events has unfolded in the past twenty years to offer many insights attractive for inhibitor design, not the least of which are the recent descriptions of the structure of the HIV-1 protease, at nearly atomic level resolution.[6,22]

A complete knowledge of the structure of a viral cleavage site undoubtedly would help in the design efforts, but sufficient information is contained in the primary sequences of the cleavage sites to allow the building of potent inhibitors that contain peptidic linkages. Future efforts must rely on further structural information and trial and error to synthesize simplified nonpeptidic compounds that retain selectivity and potency. For the retroviruses, this will include information on substrate binding sites as well as monomer-monomer docking sites.

There will still be other barriers to overcome, as with any new drugs. The distribution into infected organs as well as into cells will have to be addressed. Perhaps more formidable will be the avoidance of inhibiting cellular proteolytic enzymes that have important roles in host physiology. Inasmuch as many such enzymes have yet to be fully appreciated, it is premature to predict the eventual outcome with absolute optimism.

On the positive side of the ledger, we are rapidly reaching a status where we have a nearly complete portrait of some viral proteases, including their biological functions, mechanism, substrate specificity, structure, and genetics. No other viral functions have yet been described in such intimate and useful detail. Our obligation is to see that this strategic approach receives the best basic research support possible, and that inhibitors that arise from the research studies are expeditiously guided and promoted through thoughtful, well-designed clinical trials.

ACKNOWLEDGMENTS

Some of the studies reported here began as collaborations with James Powers of the Georgia Institute of Technology and Vito Turk of the Stefan Institute. Thanks to my colleagues at DuPont who have directly contributed to the work including Charles Kettner, Chris Rizzo, Steve Foundling, and Edmond Cheng.

REFERENCES

1. KORANT, B. 1972. J. Virol. **10:** 751.
2. SHOWE, M. & E. KELLENBERGER. 1975. *In* Control Processes in Virus Multiplication. D. Burke & W. Russell, Eds.: 407. Cambridge University Press. London.
3. VON DER HELM, K. 1977. Proc. Natl. Acad. Sci. USA **74:** 911.

4. KRAUSSLICH, H. & E. WIMMER. 1988. Annu. Rev. Biochem. **57:** 701.
5. KORANT, B. 1989. *In* Viral Proteinases. H. Krausslish, S. Oroszlan & E. Wimmer, Eds.: 277. Cold Spring Harbor Laboratory Press. Cold Spring Harbor, NY.
6. WLODOWER, A., M. MILLER, M. JASKOLSKI, B. SATHYANARAYANA, E. BALDWIN, I. WEBER, L. SELK, L. CLAWSON, J. SCHNEIDER & S. KENT. 1989. Science **245:** 616.
7. KATOH, I., T. YASUNAGA, Y. IKAWA & Y. YOSHINAKA. 1987. Nature **329:** 654.
8. SEELMEIR, S., H. SCHMIDT, V. TURK & K. VON DER HELM. 1988. Proc. Natl. Acad. Sci. USA **85:** 6612.
9. BILLICH, S., M. KNOOP, J. HANSEN, P. STROP, J. SEDLACEK, R. MERTZ & K. MOELLING. 1988. J. Biol. Chem. **263:** 17905.
10. MOORE, M., W. BRYAN, S. FAKHOWRY, V. MAGAARD, W. HUFFMAN, B. DAYTON, T. MEEK, L. HYLAND, G. DREYER, B. METCALF, J. STRICKLER, J. GORNIAK & C. DE-BOUCK. 1989. Biochem. Biophys. Res. Commun. **159:** 420.
11. NASHED, N., J. LOUIS, J. SAYER, E. WONDRAK, P. MOVA, S. OROSZLAN & D. JERINA. 1989. Biochem. Biophys. Res. Commun. **163:** 1079.
12. ZHIRNOV, O., A. OVCHARENKO & A. BUKRINSKAYA. 1985. J. Gen. Virol. **66:** 1633.
13. ZHIRNOV, O., A. OVCHARENKO, E. MELNICKOVA, A. BUKRINSKAYA & S. GAIDAMOVICH. 1986. Antiviral Res. **6:** 255.
14. KORANT, B. & A. CORDOVA. 1989 *In* Intracellular Proteolysis. N. Katunuma & E. Kominami, Eds.: 92. Japan Scientific Societies Press. Tokyo.
15. AOYAGI, T. & H. UMEZAWA. 1975. *In* Proteases and Biological Control. E. Reich, D. Rifkin & E. Shaw, Eds.: 429. Cold Spring Harbor Laboratory. Cold Spring Harbor, NY.
16. KORANT, B., T. TOWATARI, L. IVANOFF, S. PETTEWAY, J. BRZIN, B. LENARCIC & V. TURK. 1986. J. Cell Biochem. **32:** 91.
17. KORANT, B. & K. LONBERG-HOLM. 1981. Acta Biol. Med. (Gdansk) **40:** 1481.
18. RICHARDS, A., R. ROBERTS, B. DUNN, M. GRAVES & J. KAY. 1989. FEBS Lett. **247:** 113.
19. KETTNER, C. & B. KORANT. 1987. U. S. Patent 4,644,055.
20. GARTEN, W., A. STIENEKE, E. SHAW, P. WIKSTROM & H. KLENK. 1989. Virology **172:** 25.
21. MILLER, M., M. JASKOLSKI, J. RAO, J. LEIS & A. WLODOWER. 1989. Nature **337:** 576.
22. NAVIA, M., P. FITZGERALD, B. MCKEEVER, C. LEU, P. HEIMBACH, W. HERBER, I. SIGAL, P. DARKE & J. SPRINGER. 1989. Nature **337:** 615.

Therapy of Presymptomatic FeLV-Induced Immunodeficiency Syndrome with AZT in Combination with Alpha Interferon[a]

EDWARD A. HOOVER,[b] NORDIN S. ZEIDNER,[b]
AND JAMES I. MULLINS[c]

[b]Department of Pathology
Colorado State University
Fort Collins, Colorado 80523

[c]Department of Microbiology and Immunology
Stanford University
Stanford, California 94305

INTRODUCTION

Feline leukemia virus (FeLV), a contagiously transmitted feline retrovirus of the family Oncoviridae, has been recognized for over 20 years as the principal cause of lymphosarcoma, myeloproliferative diseases, aplastic anemia syndromes, and perhaps most significantly, fatal immunodeficiency syndrome in cats.[1,2] In this regard greater than 80% of FeLV-infected cats die within four years of initial diagnosis, often from opportunistic infections.[3] We have characterized and molecularly cloned a naturally occurring isolate of FeLV (FeLV-FAIDS) that induces persistent infection and fatal immunodeficiency syndrome in specific pathogen-free (SPF) cats.[4] Features of the disease include progressive depletion of total, CD4+, and colony-forming T lymphocytes, impaired T-dependent immune responses, persistent diarrhea, wasting syndrome, and terminal opportunistic infections.[4-7] Thus, FeLV-FAIDS immunodeficiency resembles symptoms associated with HIV.[8]

Studies of the pathogenesis of FeLV-FAIDS have revealed the original viral isolate to consist of a highly replication-competent common-form genome and a replication-defective but highly pathogenic major variant genome. The pathogenesis of FeLV-FAIDS infection involves viral replication in bone marrow and systemic lymphoid tissues, and onset of antigenemia and viremia by three weeks postinoculation.[4] Prefiguring the onset of immunodeficiency syndrome, high levels of the major FeLV-FAIDS pathogenic variant virus are detected in bone marrow, blood, and lymphoid tissues.[9] Transient lymphoid hyperplasia, progressive lymphoid depletion, impaired immunity, and clinical immunodeficiency disease ensue after latent periods of 80 to 311 days

[a]This work was supported by contract NO1-AI-72663 from the Developmental Therapeutics Branch, Division of AIDS, NIAID, NIH.

258

(mean 171 days), depending on age and inoculum used.[4] Studies employing viral chimeras have implicated the envelope gene of the pathogenic variant as encoding lymphocytopathic determinants of FeLV-FAIDS.[5]

Whether prophylactic chemotherapy might be effective in arresting the development of infection in individuals exposed to retroviruses, in particular HIV, is a cogent question for which there are limited data in experimental models. AZT (3'-azido-3'-deoxythymidine) (zidovudine) triphosphate has been shown to be active against a variety of mammalian and avian retroviruses, depending upon a species-specific ability to efficiently metabolize AZT to its 5'-triphosphate derivative.[10–14] AZT has also been shown to act synergistically with other antiviral agents such as IFNα, dextran sulfate, and castanospermine, which target different stages of the retrovirus life cycle.[15–17] Promising results concerning early postexposure therapy come from the studies of Ruprecht *et al.*[13] and Tavares *et al.*,[18] indicating that AZT is effective in arresting the course of Rauscher murine leukemia virus and of another strain of FeLV, FeLV-Rickard. The present study was undertaken to determine whether AZT, when administered as prophylactic therapy to animals exposed to a 100% infection-inducing dose of FeLV-FAIDS, could abort the course of progressive infection. We thus determined the capacity of AZT to inhibit *de novo* FeLV-FAIDS infectivity *in vitro* and then evaluated its capacity to abrogate a severe viral challenge *in vivo*. Our results point to the probable usefulness of oral AZT and its combination with the IFNα for prophylactic intervention in HIV infection.

MATERIAL AND METHODS

Animals

All animals were from a breeding colony of cesarean-derived SPF cats maintained at Colorado State University. These animals were age-matched, eight months of age at the time of inoculation, and free of infection and immunity to horizontally transmitted feline viruses. Cats derived from this colony have been used previously to characterize the pathogenicity of FeLV-FAIDS.[4,9,5]

Virus Inocula

The virus inoculum used consisted of the molecularly cloned pathogenic but replication-defective FeLV-FAIDS, clone 61C, rescued by its replication-competent counterpart FeLV-FAIDS, clone 61E.[5] Thus the molecular clones used represented the significant retroviral genomes contained within the infectious, pathogenic original field isolate of FeLV-FAIDS.[1] FeLV-FAIDS 61E/C was produced from AH927 feline fibroblasts cotransfected with clones 61C and 61E and expressed in approximately equal representation.[5] The inoculum for animals contained 6×10^5 focus forming units (ffu) administered intraperitoneally. The inoculum used in *in vitro* infectivity assays in Crandell feline kidney (CrFK) cells consisted of 3×10^4 ffu/mL; for neutralizing antibody assays, an inoculum containing 1×10^3 ffu per well was used.

Antiviral Compounds

3'-Azido-3'-deoxythymidine (AZT) was provided by Burroughs Wellcome Ltd., Research Triangle Park, NC, through the Developmental Therapeutics Branch, Division of AIDS, NIAID, Bethesda, MD. Human recombinant alpha-interferon 2b (IFNα) was provided by Schering Plough Research Inc., Bloomfield, NJ, by Dr. Jerome Schwartz.

In Vitro *Antiviral Assays*

The capacity of AZT and IFNα to inhibit replication of FeLV-FAIDS 61C/E was determined by FeLV p27 antigen capture ELISA of inoculated CrFK at 96 hours postinoculation (p.i.). In all cases 5×10^4 cells were seeded with antiviral compounds and Polybrene (4 μg/mL) in 1 mL of culture medium (Falcon multiwell #3047, Becton Dickinson Co., Lincoln Park, NJ) 24 hours prior to infection with FeLV-FAIDS. Media was then aspirated, and cell monolayers were exposed to FeLV-FAIDS in the absence of antiviral compounds (1 hour), washed with Dulbecco's phosphate-buffered saline (PBS) (GIBCO Laboratories, Grand Island, NY), and then replaced with 1 mL of fresh media plus antiviral agents for the duration of the assay (96 hours p.i.). Supernatants from at least three tests wells were pooled and assayed in triplicate by antigen capture ELISA. Calculations of combined drug effects of AZT and INFα *in vitro* were evaluated by the dose-effect analysis program designed by Chou and Chou.[19]

Virus-Neutralizing Antibody Assay

A microtiter assay was developed to determine serum-neutralizing antibody titers. CrFK fibroblasts (2×10^4 cells/well) were incubated with 4 μ/mL of Polybrene for 24 hours in 96-well plates (Corning #25860, Corning, NY). Monolayers were then washed with PBS before applying twofold dilutions of heat-inactivated (56°C for 30 minutes) test sera. Fifty microliters of each serum dilution was incubated with 50 μL of virus inoculum (1×10^3 ffu of FeLV-FAIDS) diluted for use in culture media. After 24 hours the inoculum was replaced with 200 μL of fresh media. At 96 hours p.i. supernatants were collected from two test wells, and pooled and assayed in triplicate by p27 capture ELISA. The virus neutralization end point was defined as the highest serum dilution that completely protected cell monolayers from infection with 1×10^3 ffu of FeLV-FAIDS.

In Vivo *Treatment Protocol*

Cats were randomized into four treatment groups. All treatment regimens were begun 24 hours prior to FeLV-FAIDS inoculation and continued for 42 days. Cats were treated with oral administration (20 mg/kg) of AZT given three times daily (TID). This dosage was reduced to 10 mg/kg TID from day 7 to 28 then increased to 20 mg/kg TID until the end of the treatment period (42 days). AZT pharmacokinetic studies were performed during the first 24 hours prior to inoculation with FeLV-FAIDS.

IFNα was administered concurrently with AZT. IFNα was injected subcutaneously once daily at 1.6×10^6 units/kg for 7 days and then reduced to 1.6×10^5 units/kg daily for the remainder of the 42 day treatment period. To determine whether a second course of AZT therapy might influence recurrent antigenemia, a second treatment period was undertaken 80 days p.i. in two cats. These animals were antigenemic at the start of the second AZT treatment regimen, and both cats received 20 mg/kg AZT administered orally three times daily for 7 weeks. FeLV status and hematologic parameters were monitored weekly in all cats (three cats per group) for the duration of the study.

Detection of Circulating FeLV p27 Antigen

FeLV p27 antigen was measured by ELISA using monoclonal antibodies (p27 A2 and B3) developed by Lutz *et al.*[20] and supplied by Dr. Niels C. Pedersen, University of California, Davis, CA. Antigen-binding antibody at 2 μg/mL was used to coat 96-well microtiter plates; 50 μL of test serum was added to each well; and 50 μL of a second horseradish peroxidase-conjugated FeLV p27 monoclonal antibody was added and incubated for 30 minutes. The plates were then rinsed and blot dried; 50 μL of 3,3', 5,5'-tetramethylbenzidine (TMB) in the presence of a peroxidase substrate solution (Kirkegaard and Perry Laboratories, Gaithersburg, MD) was added to each well. After 10 minutes absorbance was determined at 650 nm. Test well reactions were considered positive if an absorbance value of greater than 0.100 was obtained. Background readings were obtained with FeLV negative, SPF cat serum.

Statistical Analysis

Significant differences in the mean levels of p27 in serum and bone marrow reactivation cultures were determined by Student's *t* test. P values less than 0.05 were considered significant.

RESULTS

AZT Efficacy In Vitro

Anti-FeLV-FAIDS activity was evident at AZT concentrations of ≥ 0.005 μg/mL (Fig. 1); concentrations of 0.5 to 5 μg/mL completely inhibited infectivity without

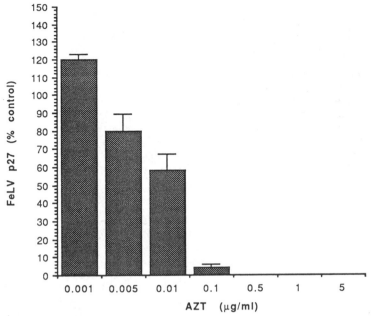

FIGURE 1. *In vitro* inhibition of FeLV-FAIDS replication by AZT. CrFK indicator cells were treated with AZT 24 h prior to inoculation with 3×10^4 ffu of FeLV-FAIDS. Supernatants from treated and nontreated wells were collected 96 h postinoculation, pooled, and assayed by ELISA for p27. Pooled samples were assayed in triplicate, and inhibition was scored as percent p27 of virus-infected control wells. Values represent the mean; bars represent the standard deviation of the mean.

producing cytotoxicity to feline fibroblasts. Antiviral activity was enhanced by the addition of IFNα at concentrations from 100-2000 units/mL (FIG. 2). IFNα at 500 and 1000 units/mL inhibited viral replication by an additional 30% at AZT concentrations of 0.01 to 0.005 μg/mL. IFNα alone inhibited viral replication by 25% at 100 units/mL and 60% at 2000 units/mL. Evaluation of this combination treatment with the combined dose-effect analysis program of Chou and Chou[19] indicated the majority of AZT/IFNα combinations (11 of 13) to be synergistic in their inhibitory activity against FeLV-FAIDS *in vitro* (FIG. 3).

AZT Efficacy In Vivo

Placebo-treated control cats challenged with FeLV-FAIDS became antigenemic by week 2 DPI; peak levels of circulating p27 were reached by week 3 (TABLE 1). The group receiving AZT alone remained negative for circulating p27 throughout the 6 week treatment period. In one of two cats, however, antigenemia developed 32 days after treatment was discontinued. At this point AZT therapy was reinstituted (TABLE 1, Rx period #2), and by week 4 of this second treatment period circulating p27 again declined below background levels. The group receiving AZT + IFNα remained negative for circulating antigen throughout the treatment period. To date (40 weeks) induction of clinical signs of FeLV-FAIDS-induced disease are delayed in all AZT-treated groups compared with those receiving either IL-2 alone or placebo controls. Thus, AZT proved able to abort the onset of persistent FeLV-FAIDS infection and to reverse the course of FeLV-FAIDS infection.

Therapy Side Effects

At 5 weeks after the start of treatment, animals receiving either AZT or IFNα developed nonregenerative anemia that was reversible when therapy was withdrawn. Blood cell numbers of animals receiving AZT alone remained within normal limits throughout the study. Both treatment groups became transiently anorexic and lost weight during the first two weeks of therapy. These symptoms dissipated thereafter.

Neutralizing Antibody Responses

Significant neutralizing antibody titers developed in all cats successfully treated with AZT by day 81 or 114 postinfection. Each of the animals that responded with

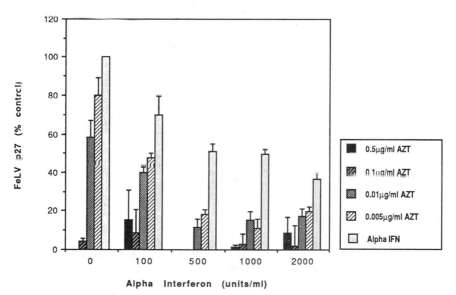

FIGURE 2. *In vitro* inhibition of FeLV-FAIDS infectivity by AZT in combination with IFNα. CrFK indicator cells were treated with AZT and IFNα 24 h prior to inoculation with 3×10^4 ffu of FeLV-FAIDS. Supernatants from treated and nontreated wells were collected 96 h postinoculation, pooled, and assayed by ELISA for p27. Inhibition was scored as percent p27 of virus-infected control wells. Values represent the mean; bars represent the standard deviation of the mean.

antibody had documented transient antigenemia after virus exposure. None of three cats treated with AZT+IFNα, in which no transient p27 antigenemia was detected, developed neutralizing antibody titers > 1:8, implying that prophylactic block of viral infection was most complete in these animals. Neutralizing antibody also was not detectable in cats that developed persistent antigenemia after virus challenge (*i.e.*, treatment failures and placebo controls).

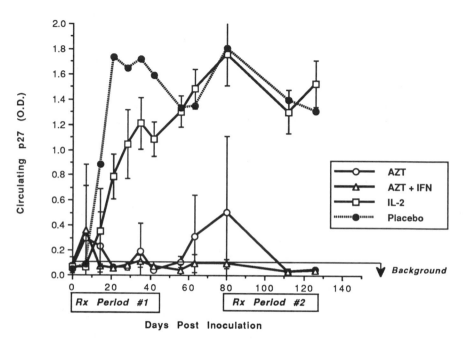

FIGURE 3. Prophylactic therapy of FeLV-FAIDS infection in cats with combined AZT/cytokine treatment. Circulating p27 antigen levels in cats treated with AZT in combination with IFNα. Lines are representative of weekly ELISA results of each treatment group. Treatment period #1 was 42 days; treatment period #2 was 44 days, as described in the MATERIALS AND METHODS section. Serum samples were assayed in triplicate; bars represent the standard deviation of the mean.

Detection of Latent FeLV

Although therapy with AZT alone was effective for blocking the development of antigenemia, latent FeLV-FAIDS could be detected in these animals by *in vitro* culture of marrow cells in the presence of hydrocortisone (TABLE 2). By contrast, no reactivatible latent virus could be detected in marrow cells cultured from cats treated with AZT+IFNα, even after culture for 5 weeks. Thus AZT+IFNα therapy appeared to confer more complete protection than AZT alone against FeLV-FAIDS infection inasmuch as viral replication appeared to be terminated prior to dissemination and integration into hemopoietic cells, an established previremic stage in the progression of FeLV infection in cats.[21]

TABLE 1. Application of the Dose-effect Analysis to Determine Combination Therapy Effects Using AZT and Alpha-Interferon in Feline Cells Infected with FeLV-FAIDS *in Vitro*

AZT (µg/mL)	IFN (units/mL)	p27 (percent virus control)	Percent affected (suppression of p27)	Fraction affected (Fa)	Combination index[a]	Diagnosis
0.005	0	79.8	20.2	0.202	ND[b]	Single agent
0.005	100	47.9	52.1	0.521	0.0238	Synergism
0.005	500	18.5	81.5	0.815	0.0006	Synergism
0.01	0	58.2	41.8	0.418	ND	Single agent
0.01	100	39.8	60.2	0.602	0.0606	Synergism
0.01	500	11.8	88.2	0.882	0.0043	Synergism
0.1	0	4.2	95.8	0.958	ND	Single agent
0.1	100	8.7	91.3	0.913	0.8388	Synergism
0.1	1000	2.8	97.2	0.972	0.0688	Synergism

[a] CI = Combination index formula. This was developed by T. C. Chou and P. Talalay (1984. Adv. Enzyme Regul. **22**: 27-55). Computer program developed by J. Chou and T. C. Chou, Elsevier-Biosoft.
[b] ND = None determined.

DISCUSSION

AZT, alone or in combination with IFNα, is the most potent nucleoside analogue we have tested to date in the FeLV-FAIDS model. Antiviral activity was attained *in vitro* at concentrations between 0.005 and 0.5 μg/mL, 10-100 times more potent than 2',3'-dideoxycytidine in this system.[22] Viral inhibition was potentiated 30% by the addition of IFNα, similar to results reported for AZT+IFNα with HIV.[15] Combined dose-effect analysis indicated these agents to be synergistic in their antiviral effect *in vitro*.

In agreement with Tavares *et al.*,[18] who conducted the only other study of AZT in cats, we found that oral administration (as opposed to subcutaneous administration) of AZT throughout a 6 week period provided protection against FeLV challenge. Moreover, we found that concomitant treatment with IFNα enhanced the antiviral activity of AZT *in vivo*. In cats treated with AZT+IFNα, FeLV p27 antigen was never

TABLE 2. Latent FeLV-FAIDS in Bone Marrow 80 Days after Inoculation

Treatment (no. of cats)	Days of marrow culture *in vitro*[a]				
	7	14	21	28	35
AZT (3)	0.0095[b]	0.154	0.163	0.275	0.386 ± .173
AZT + IFN (3)	0.011	0.076	0.133	0.123	0.110 ± .054[c]
Placebo (3)	0.318	0.788	0.838	0.959	0.913 ± .060
No Virus (1)	0.013	0	0	0	0

[a] Bone marrow mononuclear cells cultured in hydrocortisone (10^{-6} M).

[b] FeLV p27 antigen capture enzyme-linked immunosorbent assay (OD at 490 nm). Mean ± SEM. Background range extends up to 0.150.

[c] AZT + IFN group is statistically different from all treatment groups ($p < .05$).

detected in the circulation nor was latent virus reactivatible from bone marrow cells cultured *in vitro*. Our results reinforce those of Ruprecht *et al.*[23] in mice, demonstrating that IFNα and AZT synergize in their antiviral activity against retroviral infection *in vivo*.

Combined therapy with agents that act at several different stages of the virus life cycle probably will be necessary to prevent continued viral expression from integrated provirus.[24] Combined AZT/IFNα therapy proved most effective in blocking *de novo* FeLV-FAIDS infection. This is consistent with studies demonstrating that DNA chain terminators like AZT in high concentration *in vitro* greatly inhibit but do not completely thwart *de novo* HIV infection.[25] Likewise, the observed escalation in antigenemia in the face of chronic AZT therapy in AIDS patients has been observed.[26,27] Combined AZT/cytokine therapy may be an effective means of bypassing retroviral escape mechanisms and minimizing drug-induced toxicity by exploiting an additive antiviral effect while permitting lower drug dosage. AZT is toxic to normal feline erythroid precursors *in vivo* and *in vitro* (Dornsife, Zeidner, and Hoover, unpublished data), as seen in humans.[28,29] The AZT treatment regimen employed in the present study produced manageable hematological toxicity. Moreover, only maximum-tolerated dosages of all drugs were used; lower combination therapy doses may be equally efficacious in preventing viral infection. Our studies in the FeLV-FAIDS model suggest, therefore, that retroviral infection can be completely subverted through early postexposure therapy with AZT in combination with alpha-interferon.

SUMMARY

AZT inhibited replication of an immunodeficiency-inducing strain of feline leukemia virus (FeLV-FAIDS) *in vitro* at concentrations as low as 0.005 μg/mL. This antiviral activity was augmented an additional 25-30% when AZT was combined with human recombinant alpha-interferon (2b) (IFNα). Administration of AZT alone or in combination with IFNα, beginning at the time of exposure to a 100% persistent viremia-inducing dose of FeLV-FAIDS, abrogated the progression of viral infection and protected treated animals from induction of persistent antigenemia and disease. Low levels of antigenemia were detected intermittently in some AZT-treated cats throughout the 6 week treatment and 40 week observation period. Combination of AZT with IFNα appeared even more effective than AZT alone. In this treatment group even transient antigenemia was undetectable throughout the therapy and posttherapy observation periods, and latent virus could not be reactivated from bone marrow cells of protected animals. These results provide additional evidence that early treatment with AZT or AZT/IFNα therapy can be effective in completely aborting retroviral infections.

ACKNOWLEDGMENTS

We thank Matthew J. Dreitz and Susan A. Fiscus for expertise in development of the antigen capture assay, Sandra L. Quackenbush for expertise with virus infectivity and neutralization assays, and Matthew H. Myles and Candace K. Mathiason-DuBard for special assistance with the *in vivo* therapy studies. We also thank Burroughs Wellcome Inc., Research Triangle Park, NC, for providing the AZT and Schering Plough Research Inc., Kenilworth, NJ, for supplying the IFNα (2b) used in these studies.

REFERENCES

1. GILDEN, R. V. & S. OROSZLAN. 1971. Structural and immunologic relationships among mammalian C-type viruses. J. Am. Vet. Med. Assoc. **158:** 1099-1103.
2. HARDY, W. D. 1980. The virology, immunology and epidemiology of the feline leukemia virus. *In* Feline leukemia virus. Developments in cancer research. W. D. Hardy, M. Essex & A. J. McClelland, Eds.: 33-79. Elsevier. Amsterdam.
3. HARDY, W. D. & A. J. MCCLELLAND. 1977. Feline leukemia virus: Its related diseases and control. Vet. Clin. North Am. **7:** 93-103.

4. HOOVER, E. A., J. I. MULLINS, S. L. QUACKENBUSH & P. W. GASPER. 1987. Experimental transmission and pathogenesis of immunodeficiency syndrome in cats. Blood **70:** 1880-1892.

5. OVERBAUGH, J., P. R. DONAHUE, S. L. QUACKENBUSH, E. A. HOOVER & J. I. MULLINS. 1988. Molecular cloning of a feline leukemia virus that induces fatal immunodeficiency disease in cats. Science **239:** 906-10.

6. QUACKENBUSH, S. L., J. I. MULLINS & E. A. HOOVER. 1989. Colony forming T lymphocyte deficit in the development of feline retrovirus induced immunodeficiency syndrome. Blood **73:** 509-16.

7. HOOVER, E. A., S. L. QUACKENBUSH, C. D. ACKLEY, G. A. DEAN, P. R. DONAHUE, D. PARDI, G. N. CALLAHAN, J. I. MULLINS & M. D. COOPER. 1989. Lymphocyte subset alterations in cats infected with immunodeficiency disease inducing chimeras of FeLV-FAIDS. (Abstract) XIVth International Symposium for Comparative Research on Leukemia and Related Disease. p. 84.

8. CURRAN, J. W., W. M. MORGAN, A. M. HARDY, H. W. JAFFE, W. W. DARROW & W. R. DOWDLE. 1985. The epidemiology of AIDS: Current status and future prospects. Science **229:** 1352.

9. MULLINS, J. I., C. S. CHEN & E. A. HOOVER. 1986. Disease-specific and tissue-specific production of unintegrated feline leukaemia virus variant DNA in feline AIDS. Nature **319:** 333-35.

10. DAHLBERG, J. E., H. MITSUYA, S. B. BLAM, S. BRODER & S. A. AARONSON. 1987. Broad spectrum antiretroviral activity of 2′,3′-dideoxynucleosides. Proc. Natl. Acad. Sci. USA **84:** 2469-2473.

11. FRANK, K. B., P. A. MCKERNAN, R. A. SMITH & D. F. SMEE. 1987. Visna virus as an *in vitro* model for human immunodeficiency virus and inhibition by ribavirin, phosphonoformate, and 2′,3′-dideoxynucleosides. Antimicrob. Agents Chemother. **31:** 1369-1374.

12. BALZARINI, J., R. PAUWELS, B. MASANORI, P. HERDEWIJN, E. DECLERCQ, S. BRODER & D. G. JOHNS. 1988. The *in vitro* and *in vivo* anti-retrovirus activity, and intracellular metabolism of 3′-azido-2′,3′-dideoxythymidine and 2′,3′-dideoxycytidine are highly dependent on the cell species. Biochem. Pharmacol. **37:** 897-903.

13. RUPRECHT, R. M., L. G. O'BRIEN, L. D. ROSSONI & S. NUSINOFF-LEHRMAN. 1986. Suppression of mouse viraemia and retroviral disease by 3′-azido-3′-deoxythymidine. Nature **323:** 467-9.

14. OLSEN, J. C., P. FURMAN, J. A. FYFE & R. SWANSTROM. 1987. 3′-Azido-3′-deoxythymidine inhibits the replication of avian leukosis virus. J. Virol. **61:** 2800-2806.

15. HARSHORN, K. L., M. W. VOGT, T. CHOU, R. S. BLUMBERG, R. BYINGTON, R. T. SCHOOLEY & M. S. HIRSCH. 1987. Synergistic inhibition of human immunodeficiency virus *in vitro* by azidothymidine and recombinant alpha A interferon. Antimicrob. Agents Chemother. **31:** 168-172.

16. UENO, R. & S. KUNO. 1987. Dextran sulfate, a potent anti-HIV agent *in vitro* having synergism with zidovudine. Lancet **1:** 1379.

17. JOHNSON, V. A., B. D. WALKER, M. A. BARLOW, T. J. PARADIS, T. C. CHOU & M. S. HIRSCH. 1989. Synergistic inhibition of human immunodeficiency virus type 1 and type 2 replication *in vitro* by castanospermine and 3′-azido-3′-deoxythymidine. Antimicrob. Agents Chemother. **33:** 53-57.

18. TAVARES, L., C. RONEKER, K. JOHNSTON, S. NUSINOFF-LEHRMAN & F. DE NORONHA. 1987. 3′-azido-3′-deoxythymidine in feline leukemia virus-infected cats: A model for therapy and prophylaxis of AIDS. Cancer Res. **47:** 3190-3194.

19. CHOU, J. & T. C. CHOU. 1987. Dose-effect analysis with microcomputers. Quantitation of ED_{50}, LD_{50}, synergism and antagonism, low-dose risk, receptor-ligand binding and enzyme kinetics. A computer software manual. Elsevier-Biosoft. Elsevier Science Publishers. Cambridge.

20. LUTZ, H., N. C. PEDERSEN, R. DURBIN & G. H. THEILEN. 1983. Monoclonal antibodies to three epitopic regions of feline leukemia virus p27 and their use in enzyme-linked immunosorbent assay of p27. J. Immunol. Methods **56:** 209-220.

21. ROJKO, J. L., E. A. HOOVER, L. E. MATHES, R. G. OLSEN & J. P. SCHALLER. 1979. Pathogenesis of experimental feline leukemia virus infection. J. Natl. Cancer Inst. **63:** 759-768.

22. ZEIDNER, N. S., J. D. STROBEL, N. A. PERIGO, D. L. HILL, J. I. MULLINS & E. A. HOOVER. 1989. Treatment of FeLV-induced immunodeficiency syndrome (FeLV-FAIDS) with controlled release capsular implantation of 2',3'-dideoxycytidine. Antiviral Res. **11:** 147-160.

23. RUPRECHT, R. M., M. A. GAMA-SOSA & D. H. ROSAS. 1988. Combination therapy after retroviral inoculation. Lancet **1:** 239-240.

24. SARIN, P. S. 1988. Pharmacologic approaches to the treatment of AIDS. Annu. Rev. Pharmacol. Toxicol. **28:** 411-428.

25. SMITH, M. S., E. L. BRIAN & J. S. PAGANO. 1987. Resumption of virus production after human immunodeficiency virus infection of T lymphocytes in the presence of azidothymidine. J. Virol. **61:** 3769-3773.

26. REISS, R., J. LANGE, C. A. BOUCHER, S. A. DANNER & G. GOUDSMIT. 1988. Resumption of HIV antigen production during continuous zidovudine treatment. Lancet **1:** 421.

27. DOURNON, E., W. ROZENBAUM, C. MICHON, C. PERRONNE, P. DETRUCHIS, E. BOUVET, M. LEVACHER, S. MATHERON, S. GHARAKHANIAN, P. M. GIRARD, D. SALMON, C. LEPORT, M. C. DAZZA & B. REGNIER. 1988. Effects of zidovudine in 365 consecutive patients with AIDS or AIDS-related complex. Lancet **2:** 1297-1302.

28. JOHNSON, M., T. CAIAZZO, J. MOLINA, R. DONAHUE & J. GROOPMAN. 1988. Inhibition of bone marrow myelopoiesis and erythropoiesis *in vitro* by anti-retroviral nucleoside derivatives. Br. J. Haematol. **70:** 137-41.

29. GANSER, A., J. GREHER, B. VOLKERS, S. STASZEWSKI & D. HOELZER. 1989. Inhibitory effect of azidothymidine, 2'-3'-dideoxyadenosine, and 2'-3'-dideoxycytidine on *in vitro* growth of hematopoietic progenitor cells from normal persons and from patients with AIDS. Exp. Hematol. **17:** 3212-3215.

Evidence for HIV-1 Infection in Rabbits

A Possible Model for AIDS

M. R. GORDON,[b] M. E. TRUCKENMILLER,
D. P. RECKER, D. R. DICKERSON, E. KUTA,
H. KULAGA,[a] AND T. J. KINDT[c]

Laboratory of Immunogenetics
National Institute of Allergy and Infectious Diseases
National Institutes of Health
Bethesda, Maryland 20892

[a]*Neuropsychiatry Branch*
National Institute of Mental Health
St. Elizabeths Hospital
Washington, D.C. 20032

INTRODUCTION

A major obstacle in the study of acquired immunodeficiency syndrome (AIDS) has been the lack of suitable animal models for testing drugs, vaccines, and other agents directed against human immunodeficiency virus-1 (HIV-1), the causative virus of this disease. Although several animal models for AIDS have been described, all have certain shortcomings. Because of the chimpanzee's close phylogenetic relationship to humans, infection of this species with HIV-1 provides the most appropriate model for the study of AIDS.[1,2] Studies are limited, however, by the scarcity of chimpanzees and by the difficulty and expense in working with higher primates. Infection of more available primates using related viruses[2-4] has yielded valuable information involving the probable course and consequences of HIV-1 infection in humans. However, because immunodeficiency viruses, which are pathogenic in these animals, are not identical to HIV-1, results from vaccine trials and other specific therapies may not relate directly to AIDS in humans. Other animal models using HIV-1 have been proposed; these include the

[b]National Research Council Fellow.
[c]Address correspondence to T. J. Kindt, Laboratory of Immunogenetics, NIAID, NIH, Building 4, Room 213, Bethesda, MD 20892.

laboratory rabbit[5-7] and severe-combined immunodeficiency (SCID) mice reconstituted with human lymphoid cells.[8,9]

The possibility that rabbits may be infected with HIV-1 was suggested by the observation that transformed rabbit cell lines infected with HIV-1 actively produced infectious virus.[5] *In vitro* infection was verified by a number of techniques, demonstrating the production of HIV-1 protein, DNA, RNA, and mature viral particles. Based on this success, *in vivo* HIV-1 infection was attempted using a protocol similar to that described by Miyoshi and his co-workers[10] for infection of rabbits with HTLV-I. This method involves intravenous injection of human cells infected with the retrovirus. In the course of our studies,[7] another group reported that rabbits could be infected with HIV-1 using an approach different from that described here.[6] These workers showed that intraperitoneal injection of HIV-1 following injection of thioglycollate resulted in HIV-1 infection. Both routes of administration result in seroconversion and presence of virus in the rabbits. The approaches are similar in that both use New Zealand white rabbits and well-characterized HIV-1 strains. The present report details evidence for HIV-1 infection in rabbits and demonstrates that immune suppression may be a consequence of this infection.

ANTIBODY RESPONSES TO HIV-1

In these experiments, A3.01 cells[11] were infected *in vitro* with HIV-1, (strain LAV) and monitored for reverse transcriptase activity and evidence of syncytia formation. At the time of peak infection the HIV-1-infected A3.01 cells were injected i.v. into rabbits. Control animals were injected with uninfected A3.01 cells. The dose of infected cells ranged from 1×10^6 to 5×10^7 infected cells. To date, 51 rabbits have been injected with HIV-1-infected A3.01 cells, and about 90% of these developed antiviral responses. Circulating antiviral antibodies were detected by a commercial ELISA test (DuPont, Wilmington, DE) identical to that used to screen human sera, with the exception that the developing antibodies (Bethesda Research Laboratories, Gaithersburg, MD) were directed against rabbit rather than human immunoglobulins. The majority of rabbits in the study were given 5×10^6 infected A3.01 cells, and these animals produced detectable levels of antibody four weeks after a single i.v. injection. When higher doses of infected cells were given or when animals received multiple injections of infected cells, higher levels of antibodies were obtained. Sera from rabbits given control injections of A3.01 cells were uniformly negative in the ELISA test. FIGURE 1 shows antibody responses to different doses of HIV-1-infected cells for a twelve week period.

Antibodies to several different proteins, mainly those encoded in the *env* and *gag* genes of the virus, were detected by preliminary Western blot analysis.[7,12] More recently, quantitative estimations of antibodies against individual HIV-1 proteins have been determined by the use of a recombinant HIV-1 protein ELISA kit (Beckman Instruments; see FIG. 2). These data have shown that the strongest antibody responses are against gp41, p55, and p24. As was seen with the standard ELISA (FIG. 1), higher doses of HIV-1-infected cells gave stronger responses to the recombinant proteins (FIG. 2). In general, a single dose of HIV-1-infected A3.01 cells produced an antibody level that persisted above background levels for at least six months.

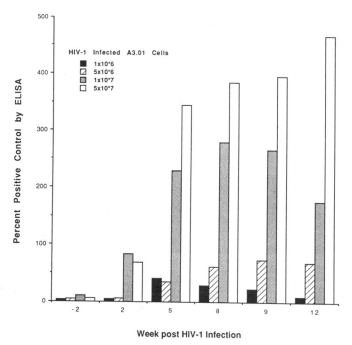

FIGURE 1. Serum antibody levels measured by HIV-1 ELISA kit for rabbits given different doses of HIV-1-infected A3.01 cells. Positive control was an anti-HIV-1 serum confirmed by recombinant protein ELISA and by Western blot analysis.

DETECTION OF VIRUS IN INFECTED ANIMALS

Experiments were carried out to determine which organ systems served as targets for HIV-1 infection in the rabbit and to follow the time course of HIV-1 infection. Rabbits were injected with either 5×10^6 HIV-1-infected A3.01 cells (low dose) or 5×10^7 infected cells (high dose), and control animals received 5×10^7 uninfected A3.01 cells. Rabbits were sacrificed at two week intervals for a ten week period; one or two from the low-dose group and one from the high-dose group were taken at each time point. Selected organs were removed from each animal, and the DNA extracted from these organs was tested for the presence of HIV-1 sequences from the *gag* region by gene amplification using the polymerase chain reaction (PCR).[13] The PCR primers were selected for sequence conservation among the published HIV-1 sequences. The analyses were carried out using a procedure reported previously;[12] a thirty-cycle PCR amplification was followed by Southern blot analysis using a probe from a portion of the amplified region lacking the primer sequences. As seen in FIGURE 2, most animals sacrificed after four weeks postinfection showed the presence of virus in lymphoid organs. Between 4 and 8 weeks the spleen appeared to be the organ in which HIV-1 proviral DNA was most commonly, but not always, found.

PCR analyses, using RNA isolated from the brain of an HIV-1-infected rabbit, demonstrated active synthesis of HIV-1 in this organ. For these studies, the brain was dissected into different regions, and RNA was individually isolated from each of these. As shown in FIGURE 3, the HIV-1 RNA was found only in frontal, occipital, temporal, and parietal lobes. Other regions of the brain were negative by this analysis.

The PCR analysis data revealed that after the second week postinfection 9 of 12 rabbits had at least one organ in which virus could be found. For the animals retained for 8-14 months, 3 of 4 were positive. The data are not yet complete, but it appears that in certain animals no organs are HIV-1 positive. It is possible that sampling methods may contribute to some of these negative results. For example, each organ taken from an animal was divided into a number of portions for DNA analysis, *in situ* hybridization, cell culture, and histologic analysis. It is possible that foci of infected cells localize within the organ and therefore virus is not uniformly present in each of the samples taken. Organs taken from control animals injected with A3.01 cells and housed with infected rabbits were consistently negative. In contrast to serologic results showing enhanced response to higher infected cell doses, the PCR data revealed no difference between high- and low-dose recipients. It should be emphasized that these gene amplifications were carried out using DNA isolated directly from rabbit organs and did not involve *in vitro* culture prior to sampling for viral DNA. Studies are currently underway to determine sequences of the viral isolates from the various animals.

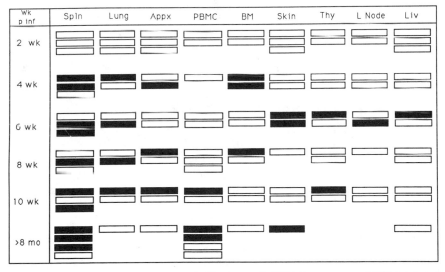

FIGURE 2. Detection of HIV-1 *gag* region sequences in DNA from organs of HIV-1-injected rabbits by PCR amplification and Southern blot analysis using procedures previously described.[12] Black boxes indicate positive detection of HIV-1 in the tissue DNA, white boxes indicate no detection, and open spaces indicate samples that were not tested. Rabbits are grouped according to the number of weeks post-HIV-1 infection that the animals were sacrificed. Organs from a given rabbit are aligned horizontally.

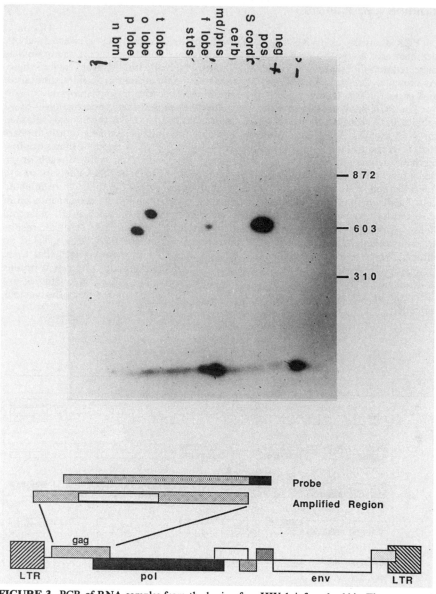

FIGURE 3. PCR of RNA samples from the brain of an HIV-1-infected rabbit. The sources of PCR samples were as follows: normal rabbit brain (n. brn); parietal lobe (p. lobe); occipital lobe (o. lobe); temporal lobe (t. lobe); blank; molecular weight standard (std); frontal lobe (f. lobe); medulla/pons (med/pons); cerebellum (cerb); spinal cord (s. cord); positive control (pos. con); negative control (neg con). Size markers were *Hae*III digests of ϕX 174. Brain regions from an HIV-1-infected rabbit were dissected and frozen immediately in liquid nitrogen. RNA from tissue samples was recovered by standard protocol.[23] First strand cDNA from the RNA samples was synthesized as previously described[24] using the HIV-1 *gag* region primer[12] G820 and M-MLV reverse transcriptase (Bethesda Research Labs, Gaithersburg, MD). PCR amplification of the cDNA was performed using the HIV-1 *gag* primers[12] G820 and GR1393. The PCR products were analyzed by Southern transfer onto nitrocellulose followed by hybridization with a ^{32}P-labeled HIV-1 probe (pBenn 3).[25]

LOCATION OF HIV-1 RNA BY *IN SITU* HYBRIDIZATION

Organs taken from infected rabbits were tested for the presence of HIV-1 RNA by *in situ* hybridization[14] using a mixture of probes from the HIV-1 genome. Spleen, lung, appendix, and other lymphoid tissues were found to contain actively reproducing virus as demonstrated by hybridization. FIGURE 4 depicts a section of a lung showing at least two major foci of HIV-1 RNA production. Correlation between PCR positive tissue and *in situ* positive tissue was not absolute, which again raises the possibility of missing infective foci due to partitioning the organs for the different tests. It must also be considered that the two techniques measure different aspects of the viral infection; *in situ* hybridization detects only actively replicating virus, whereas PCR detects the presence of proviral DNA sequences.

IMMUNE SUPPRESSION IN HIV-1-INFECTED RABBITS

The reproducible seroconversion and relative ease by which virus DNA or RNA could be detected within the infected rabbits suggested that these animals are productively infected with HIV-1. Persistence of HIV-1 in animals has been observed for more than one year after infection.[12] In spite of the ability to demonstrate the lingering presence of virus, no overt signs of illness were observed in rabbits infected with HIV-1. It should be pointed out that the rabbits used in our experiments were bred and housed under specific pathogen-free conditions and handled using biosafety level 3 practices. Consequently, there was little exposure to the diseases that commonly affect laboratory rabbits. An earlier study,[7] however, showed that animals coinfected with HTLV-I and HIV-1 were likely to show signs of illness, including weight loss, diarrhea, and evidence of neurologic dysfunction.

Consequently, the question arose as to whether the immune systems of the HIV-1-infected rabbits were altered in spite of the failure to observe signs of natural illness. To test this, the response of the HIV-1-infected animals to immunization with tetanus toxoid (TT) and a heat-killed strain of *Mycobacterium bovis* [Bacillus Calmette-Guerin (HK-BCG)] was studied. These antigens have been used for monitoring the immune responses of HIV-1-infected humans.[15] Furthermore, the use of these antigens and the resulting immune responses in the rabbit has been well characterized[16-19] The animals were immunized subcutaneously with TT and HK-BCG in oil and after one week were injected with HIV-1-infected A3.01 cells by the standard protocol. Within three weeks, control animals immunized with HK-BCG and TT, but not infected with HIV-1, developed strong serum antibody titers to TT as measured by ELISA and manifested delayed-type hypersensitivity (DTH) responses to a 10 µg intradermal injection of purified protein derivative (PPD) of *Mycobacterium tuberculosis* (Connaught Labs, Willowdale, Ontario). FIGURE 5 shows the DTH responses to PPD as monitored by skin reactivity along with the antibody responses to HIV-1 proteins. The skin test measures the thickness of skin at the test site after 48 h and is expressed in FIGURE 5 as the ratio of test site thickness to control site thickness. In HK-BCG immunized, uninfected rabbits, the normal ratio was two or above. In the HK-BCG immunized, HIV-1-infected animals, as in the nonimmunized, uninfected controls, however, the ratio was much closer to 1, indicating a lack of DTH response at the site of PPD

challenge. Note that one of the HIV-1-injected rabbits showed a positive skin test result early in the experiment, but this diminished after 10 weeks. No such loss of skin reactivity was seen in HK-BCG-immunized, A3.01-injected rabbits even after 25 weeks.

Occasionally, skin test responses to PPD in immunized rabbits may be negative for complex technical reasons;[19-21] however, in spite of this apparent state of anergy, immunized animals are always capable of mounting a DTH response in the lung to systemic HK-BCG challenge. In order to confirm that there was a true loss of immune responsiveness to BCG in the HIV-1-infected rabbits, they were given an intravenous challenge of 1 mg of HK-BCG in saline 6 months after immunization. Four days later, the animals were sacrificed, the lungs were taken intact and the reaction to BCG was evaluated. Normally the DTH response to this challenge manifests itself as a tremendous infiltration of monocytes and granulocytes into the lung interstitium. These immature cells develop rapidly, maturing into activated macrophages, giant cells, and epithelioid cells. Histologically, cells are organized into foci surrounding the HK-BCG organisms, characteristic of a granuloma response. Quantitation of this response was

TABLE 1. Lung Response to Systemic Challenge with Heat-Killed BCG

HK-BCG-immunized[a]	HIV-infected[b]	Lw/Bw $\times$ 10^{3c}	Packed cell volume[d]	n
$-$	$-$	4.0 ± 1.0^e	0.25 ± 0.07^e	$-$
$+$	$-$	8.8 ± 2.5	1.60 ± 0.05	5
$+$	$+$	4.8 ± 0.7	0.30 ± 0.1	4

[a] Immunization was by subcutaneous injection at two sites with 100 μg heat-killed BCG (HK-BCG) in 0.1 mL mineral oil each.

[b] Infection accomplished by a single intravenous injection of 1×10^6-5×10^7 HIV-1-infected A3.01 cells.

[c] The weight in grams of isolated lungs, including 3 cm of trachea, divided by the weight in grams of the whole animal. The values are multipled by 10^3 for the convenience of expression in whole numbers and are given with the standard deviation.

[d] The volume of branchial-alveolar lavage cells retrieved from 80 mL of lavage fluid and packed by centrifugation at 100 $\times$ g for 10 min.

[e] The values in this first category are based on accumulated population statistics.

accomplished by measuring lung weight normalized to body weight and determining the volume of packed cells[22] in the first 80 mL of lavage fluid (normal saline) recovered from the lungs and then centrifuged at 100 $\times$ g. TABLE 1 illustrates that HK-BCG challenge of immunized animals not infected with HIV-1 resulted in a lung weight/body weight ratio two times that of nonimmunized rabbits, and a packed cell volume six times that of nonimmunized rabbits. Both measured lung responses to HK-BCG challenge, however, were dramatically decreased in HIV-1-infected, HK-BCG-immunized animals.

After lavage, the lungs were fixed in neutral formalin and analyzed histologically. Micrographs of lungs from HK-BCG-immunized and -challenged control rabbits (including those injected with uninfected A3.01 cells) showed typical multifocal granulomas. By contrast, the lungs from BCG-immunized animals infected with HIV-1 showed little or no granulomatous response to similar challenge. Acid fast stains revealed the presence of the HK-BCG organisms in all the challenged lung tissue. Additionally, the initial positive skin-test response of one of the HIV-1-infected rabbits (see FIG. 2) verified that the immunization and challenge procedures were effectively performed. The diminution or absence of the skin test and the virtual absence of the granulomatous response to HK-BCG challenge in the BCG-immunized, HIV-1-infected rabbits suggests that an immune deficiency is present in these animals. This same pattern of depressed response in HIV-1-infected rabbits is paralleled in the studies of humoral responses to TT (data not shown).

CONCLUSIONS

Several lines of evidence show that rabbits are susceptible to infection with HIV-1. Furthermore, evidence from the present study suggests that the infection is accompanied by a striking diminution in cellular immune responses to BCG. HIV-1 infection in the rabbit appears to alter the immune system of the animal. The present data imply that the rabbit model may be useful for testing agents proposed for the prevention of HIV-1 infection or for alleviation of the immune suppression that accompanies this infection in humans.

ACKNOWLEDGMENTS

The authors thank Dr. Pete Golway and his staff for excellent care and handling of the rabbits, Dr. Alan Lock for necropsy of infected animals, Ms. Joann Bauer for help with the skin test, Ms. V. Shaw for secretarial assistance, and Dr. Tom Folks for help in all phases of the work.

REFERENCES

1. ALTER, H. J., J. W. EICHBERG, H. MASUR, W. C. SAXINGER, R. GALLO, A. M. MACHER, H. C. LANE & A. S. FAUCI. 1984. Science **226:** 549-552.
2. FULTZ, P. N., II. M. McCLURE, R. B. SWENSON, C. R. McGRATH, A. BRODIE, J. P. GETCHELL, F. C. JENSEN, D. C. ANDERSON, J. R. BRODERSON & D. P. FRANCIS. 1986. J. Virol. **58:** 116-124.
3. DESROSIERS, R. C., M. S. WYAND, T. KODAMA, D. J. RINGLER, L. O. ARTHUR, P. K. SEHGAL, N. L. LETVIN, N. W. KING & M. D. DANIEL. 1989. Proc. Natl. Acad. Sci. USA **86:** 6353-6357.
4. WATANABE, M., K. A. REIMANN, P. A. DELONG, T. LIU, R. A. FISHER & N. L. LETVIN. 1989. Nature **337:** 267-270.
5. KULAGA, H., T. M. FOLKS, R. RUTLEDGE & T. J. KINDT. 1988. Proc. Natl. Acad. Sci. USA **85:** 4455-4459.
6. FILICE, G., P. M. CEREDA & O. E. VARNIER. 1988. Nature **335:** 366-369.
7. KULAGA, H., T. FOLKS, R. RUTLEDGE, M. E. TRUCKENMILLER, E. GUGEL & T. J. KINDT. 1989. J. Exp. Med. **169:** 321-326.
8. MOSIER, D. E., R. J. GULIZIA, S. M. BAIRD & D. B. WILSON. 1988. Nature **335:** 256-259.
9. NAMIKAWA, R., H. KANESHIMA, M. LIEBERMAN, I. L. WEISSMAN & J. M. McCUNE. 1988. Science **243:** 1684-1686.

10. MIYOSHI, I., I. KUBONISHI, S. YOSHIMOT & Y. A. SHIRAISHI. 1981. GANN 72: 978-981.
11. FOLKS, T. M., A. BEEN, T. RABSON, T. THEODORE, M. D. HOGGAN, M. MARTIN, M. LIGHTFOOT & K. SELL. 1985. Proc. Natl. Acad. Sci. USA 82: 4539-4543.
12. TRUCKENMILLER, M. E., H. KULAGA, E. GUGEL, D. DICKERSON & T. J. KINDT. 1989. Res. Immunol. 140: 527-544.
13. MULLIS, K. B. & F. A. FALOONA. 1987. Methods Enzymol. 155: 335-350.
14. BRAHI, M. & A. T. HAASE. 1978. Proc. Natl. Acad. Sci. USA 75: 6125-6129.
15. CLERICI, M., N. I. STOCKS, R. A. ZAJAC, R. N. BOSWELL, D. R. LUCEY, C. S. VIA & G. M. SHEARER. 1989. J. Clin. Invest. 84: 1892-1899.
16. MYRVIK, Q. N. 1982. Adv. Exp. Med. Biol. 155: 649-57.
17. MOORE, V. L., Q. N. MYRVIK & E. S. LEAKE. 1973. Infect. Immun. 7(5): 743-746.
18. MOORE, V. L. & Q. N. MYRVIK. 1973. Infect. Immun. 7: 764-770.
19. SCHROFF, R. W., JR., E. R. HEISE, Q. N. MYRVIK & B. T. SHANNON. 1980. Infect. Immun. 28: 269-276.
20. MYRVIK, Q. N., M. R. GORDON & A. KNOX. 1982. Proc. 17th Joint U.S.-Japan Cooperative Medical Science Program. pp 51-63.
21. GORDON, M. R., I. TAKATA & Q. N. MYRVIK. 1985. Infect. Immun. 51: 134-140.
22. MCGEE, M. P. & Q. N. MYRVIK. 1981. In Manual of Macrophage Methodology. H. B. Herscowitz, H. T. Holden, J. A. Bellanti & A. Ghaffar, Eds.: 17-22. Marcel Dekker, Inc. New York.
23. CHIRGWIN, J. M., A. E. PRZYBYLA, R. J. MACDONALD & W. J. RUTTER. 1979. Biochemistry 18: 5294-5299.
24. GUBLER, A. & B. J. HOFFMAN. 1983. Gene 25: 263-269.
25. BENN, S., R. RUTLEDGE, T. M. FOLKS, J. GOLD, L. BAKER, J. MCCORMICK, P. FEORINO, P. PIOT, T. QUINN & M. MARTIN. 1985. Science 230: 949-951.

Preclinical Evaluation of Antiviral Compounds in the SCID-hu Mouse

J. M. McCUNE, H. KANESHIMA, L. RABIN,
C.-C. SHIH, AND R. NAMIKAWA

HIV Group
SyStemix, Inc.
Palo Alto, California 94303

Perhaps more is known about the human immunodeficiency virus (HIV) than about any other infectious agent that causes disease in humans. The knowledge base, though incomplete, lends confidence to the belief that the replicative cycle of this virus can eventually be suppressed *in vivo*. The scientific community has thus focused on treatments for the disease that it causes, the acquired immunodeficiency syndrome (AIDS). Systematic evaluation of the replicative cycle of HIV has identified agents that interfere at multiple steps. Most of these agents share in common a discovery process that is carefully controlled and elegant in design. Some, shown to be effective against HIV *in vitro*, are logically proposed as agents that might also be effective against HIV infection in humans and are therefore allocated to clinical trials.

Clinical testing of compounds in humans, however, necessitates a narrow focus. It is only through the careful design of such trials that meaningful statements about drug efficacy and safety can be made. The fewer the number of compounds that are chosen, the more likely it will be that they will be evaluated in a timely and meaningful manner. Today, however, focus is a problem. There is little or no rational basis by which to choose among candidate antivirals that show equivalent activity against HIV *in vitro*. Some excellent compounds will be (and perhaps have been) bypassed in favor of others that later prove useless in humans. Others may be chosen and initially dosed at a level too toxic or administered by an ineffective route.

In an effort to transform the selection process into an undertaking as rational as the design of the compounds in the first place, a number of animal models for HIV infection have been proposed. Ideally, one or several of these models might be used at a preclinical stage of drug development to ask difficult questions about bioavailability, efficacy, and toxicity that cannot be answered by experimentation *in vitro*. In this manner, the flow of novel antiviral compounds from the lab to humans might be streamlined and targeted more accurately.

Such a scenario demands a high throughput animal model, in which multiple doses of multiple congeners of a given compound might be tested, perhaps alone or in combination with other compounds. The tests should be reproducible, time-efficient, and amenable to statistical analysis. Put simply, a sufficient number of animals must be available to gather meaningful data. By these criteria, large animal models become suboptimal. Such animals are expensive, difficult to study in large numbers, and in some cases (*e.g.,* the chimpanzee) already endangered. Instead, the preferable animal model would be as small and easily bred as, for instance, the mouse.

A number of mouse models for HIV infection have been developed. Most are seriously flawed or yet unproven. Transgenic mice carrying intact copies of HIV proviral DNA, for instance, can be demonstrated in some cases to support postintegration stages of viral replication.[1] Such mice will not, however, be amenable to the evaluation of compounds that block either infection or steps that occur before integration. The system is also hampered by the fact that viral replication takes place within murine cells; certain antiviral compounds might be metabolized differently in such cells than in human cells. Another animal model is the hu-PBL-SCID mouse, made by injecting mature human peripheral blood cells into the peritoneal cavity of the congenitally immunodeficient C.B-17 scid/scid mouse (hereafter called SCID, for severe combined immunodeficiency).[2] Although very little has been published about this model, it is said to be permissive for HIV replication when virus is injected in tandem with phytohemagglutinin (PHA)-activated human T-cell blasts.[3] This is not surprising: HIV has long been (and more easily) studied *in vitro* under similar conditions. Perhaps most important to the future evaluation of this model is a resolution to the questions: Which human cells exist where and for how long after engraftment? and Does graft-versus-host (GvH) disease occur as a result of the procedure? The original authors, though not completely able to reproduce their reported findings,[4] apparently do not observe GvH. Others, following the published procedures, do see GvH disease.[5,6] A final and interesting small animal model involves the injection of adult human bone marrow cells into the beige/nude/xid stock.[7] These animals support human myelopoiesis, as least for several weeks. It has yet to be shown, however, that they can be infected with HIV.

The SCID-hu mouse[8] was constructed with the intent to avoid some of the above problems. The C.B-17 scid/scid stock[9] was chosen for several reasons. First, it has severe combined immunodeficiency (SCID), lacks murine T and B cells, and would predictably accept xenografts of human tissue. Second, in the absence of specific treatment or special handling, it is susceptible to the development of *Pneumocystis carinii* pneumonia.[10] We reasoned that the animals might be protected from this opportunistic infection, if they were implanted with a human immune system and if that system were functional. Thereafter, the transplanted human system itself might be infected with HIV.

Rather than implant mature human peripheral blood cells, we chose to transfer to the SCID mouse those cells that are most likely to be infected *in vivo* in humans, namely the cells of the hematolymphoid organs (*e.g.*, the fetal liver, bone marrow, thymus, lymph node, spleen, and skin). Because these organs are critical to the regeneration, maintenance, and coordination of hematopoietic cells, observation of infection within them may be of far greater relevance than studies using peripheral blood cells. Perhaps most importantly, most of the subpopulations of cells within these organs cannot be grown *in vitro* and cannot be transferred by injection of peripheral blood into SCID mice. They therefore cannot be studied in any other way.

To prevent the human immune system from rejecting the SCID mouse, we took advantage of a classic observation in immunology, namely, that fetal immune cells can be "taught" the difference between self and nonself major histocompatibility complex (MHC) antigens.[11] These cells, which start out as stem cells in the fetal liver or bone marrow, learn this lesson in the thymus as part of their developmental program.[12,13] Thereafter, as mature and educated cells, they circulate in the peripheral blood and live in peripheral lymphoid organs such as the lymph node. If they "see" foreign tissue after this maturation process, these lymphoid cells will engage a GvH reaction. Therefore, to reconstitute the SCID mouse with a self-regenerating and educable human immune system, we provided to the mouse both the progenitor cells (in the way of the hematopoietic fraction of human fetal liver or bone marrow) as well as the microenvironments through which these cells self-renew and/or differentiate (by surgical implantation of the fetal liver, marrow, and/or thymus organ structures themselves). Finally, to permit functional immune interactions to occur later, the microenvironments of the peripheral lymphoid system (lymph node, spleen, and skin) were surgically implanted. These organs contain subanatomic structures (*e.g.*, primary follicles) without which primary and secondary immune responses do not occur. Most obviously, such three-dimensional structures are also not normally found in the peripheral blood stream and therefore cannot be provided using such a source of cells for reconstitution of SCID mice.

Over the course of the past three years, we have established the validity of the basic concept as outlined above. It is possible to implant and to maintain stromal microenvironments for fetal liver, bone marrow, thymus, lymph node, and skin. These organs are vascularized within the SCID mouse and are, in certain circumstances, permissive to the influx of hematopoietic cell fractions. Certain of these fractions (for instance, from fetal liver) can then be shown to differentiate into numerous and more mature cell subpopulations (for instance, into myelomonocytic and T-cell subsets after movement through the cortex and medulla of the engrafted human thymus). Thereafter, mature cell subpopulations are found in the peripheral blood of the SCID-hu mouse. Importantly, no GvH disease is initiated by these human T cells against the SCID host. On the contrary, the engrafted animals appear to be more immunocompetent than their untreated littermates and, as predicted, SCID-hu mice are relatively resistant to the acquisition of *Pneumocystis carinii* pneumonia.

More precise descriptors of human T- and B-cell function in the SCID-hu mouse have been gathered on a number of levels. First, it has been observed that human B cells will differentiate into human plasma cells that secrete human IgG and IgM after human fetal lymph nodes are implanted into the SCID-hu mouse. The immunoglobulin is polyclonal, secreted to high levels in the peripheral blood, and maintained for long periods of time. Because differentiation and class-switching results as a function of interaction between B cells, T cells, and antigen-presenting cells, these interactions must occur in a functional manner in the SCID-hu. Likewise, the human T cells in the SCID-hu are both phenotypically and functionally similar to normal human T cells (John Krowka, SyStemix, unpublished observations). They express CD4 and CD8 in the appropriate ratio as well as the CD3 marker and the α/β T-cell receptor. They can be stimulated to divide by mitogens such as ConA or PHA, by antibodies against CD3, and by alloantigens. As mentioned above, even though they are functional by these assays, they do not engage in GvH disease against the SCID host. At this stage, it is not clear if the human T and/or B cells within the SCID-hu mouse can be induced to make a primary immune response against a specific antigen introduced at will. Ongoing studies should soon determine whether or not this important event can be observed. If it is, the SCID-hu should find multiple applications in the development of human monoclonal antibodies as well as in the development of vaccines against infectious agents.

In the design of the SCID-hu mouse, we wished to be able to experimentally observe and to manipulate acute and chronic infection with HIV. On one level, features related to viral replication within different cells of the hematolymphoid system might be explored. On another, it might be possible to dissect the interplay between the human immune system of the SCID-hu mouse and HIV. To accomplish these goals, it was critical to establish a reproducible and practical system for infection with HIV.

We first established that the SCID-hu mouse is permissive for HIV infection.[14] The HIV isolate used for infection was specifically chosen to be as similar as possible to that found in human patients. Reciprocally, we avoided those isolates that had been adapted to growth conditions *in vitro* (*e.g.*, HTLV-IIIB). The isolate JR-CSF was derived after short-term culture in PHA-blasts and then directly cloned into phage λ.[15] JR-CSF is preferentially tropic for normal activated human T cells, uses a CD4-dependent pathway for entry, and is nonlytic; it will not grow in continuous human T-cell lines. It has been fully sequenced and is homologous to all other isolates of HIV-1, with all known open reading frames intact.[16] In initial experiments, JR-CSF was introduced by direct intrathymic or intranodal injection. Viral replication was thereafter assayed by in situ hybridization, the polymerase chain reaction (PCR), and immunohistochemistry. Two weeks after the injection of 400-4000 infectious units of virus, 100% of animals were positive for HIV. Using a combination of immunohisto-chemistry and flow cytometry, it was shown that the infected cell subpopulations were inclusive of both T and myelomonocytic cell lineages.

To test the possibility that intrathymic infection of SCID-hu mice might represent a suitable assay for antiviral efficacy, 3'-azido-3'-deoxythymidine (AZT; 1 mg/mL in the drinking water, a dose that corresponds to 250 mg/kg/day) was administered to animals 24 hours prior to infection and continued for the next 14 days.[17] At that time, none (0/17) of the treated animals showed evidence of HIV infection by PCR analysis; 40/40 untreated animals in the experiment were positive for HIV by this assay. The protective effect of AZT was manifest against both T-tropic and monocytotropic isolates of HIV. It was not, however, complete: four weeks after cessation of AZT therapy, HIV-infected animals were once again positive by PCR. This reappearance of HIV is related to a rare population of cells in the thymus that is infected even in the presence of AZT.

These data represent the first demonstration that the efficacy of an antiviral compound against HIV can be tested directly on HIV in a small animal model. The design of the experiments (intrathymic injection, assay by biopsy, in situ hybridization) is not, however, consistent with large scale screening of such compounds, in different doses, by varying routes, or in combinations.

This problem has been solved by empiric analysis of HIV infection in the SCID-hu mouse. We have now found that if SCID-hu mice are implanted with human fetal lymph node and then infected with HIV by the intravenous route, signs of viremia may be observed in the peripheral circulation later.[18] By 10-14 days postinfection, greater than 95% of the animals are viremic (as measured by qualitative or quantitative PCR assays for virion RNA). One hundred percent of the animals show signs of HIV infection in the engrafted human lymph node. Among animals that are viremic for HIV, it is only the engrafted human lymph node that is infected. The engrafted human thymus is not infected by the intravenous route; engrafted human connective tissue as well as the endogenous murine lymphoid organs are also spared (as measured by RNA PCR, DNA PCR, in situ hybridization, immunohistochemistry, and direct viral isolation). Therefore, HIV does not acquire an altered host range under these conditions.[19] If pseudotypes do form between HIV and endogenous murine amphotropic or xenotropic viruses in the SCID-hu mouse, they do not arise with a frequency high enough to detect with the most sensitive of assays currently available.[20]

The response to intravenous injection is dependent upon the dose as well as the derivation of the input virus. For most assays, a minimum of 120,000 TCID$_{50}$s (tissue culture infectious dose) of JR-CSF are injected intravenously to result in 100% infection rates at two weeks. The SCID-hu[21] is also permissive for other isolates (JR-FL, SM) that have been isolated directly from patients and that have not been propagated in vitro. By contrast, isolates of HIV that have been maintained in CD4+ human lymphoid cell lines in vitro (e.g., HTLV-IIIB, MN, RF) have not been observed to replicate in the human organs of the SCID-hu.[21] We infer that there is a fundamental difference between these two groups of isolates; those taken directly from patients would presumably bear a closer proximity to reality.

Intravenous infection of SCID-hu mice implanted with human lymph node thus represents a simple, reproducible, time-efficient, and safe method by which to observe the events associated with acute HIV infection *in vivo*.

To test the possibility that this assay might be useful in studying the efficacy of antiviral compounds, we have studied several that have been previously used in humans and other animal models: AZT and 2',3'-dideoxyinosine (ddI).[18] Both drugs are able to suppress infection with HIV when given prior to and maintained for two weeks after infection. This effect is dose-dependent. When administered at 250 mg/kg/day, both drugs result in 100% protection of animals at the two week end point. The dose of AZT that protects 50% of the animals is approximately 66 mg/kg/day; the "protective dose 50" for ddI is 13 mg/kg/day. These doses may be compared to those currently being used in humans: 5-10 mg/kg/day for AZT and 10 mg/kg/day for ddI. Given the fact that the mouse usually requires approximately 12 times more drug (on a mg/kg basis),[22] it is apparent that the dose-response curves in the HIV-infected SCID-hu mouse generate reasonable dose ranges for humans. The critical difference between studies in humans and those in the SCID-hu are underlined, however, by the results with AZT: it took 3-4 years of empiric experimentation in human trials to determine a dose that was both efficacious and nontoxic; it took 3-4 weeks to determine a minimal efficacious dose in the SCID-hu.

In conclusion, it is now clear that the SCID-hu mouse can be implanted in a stable fashion with human hematolymphoid organs, that human cells can be observed to differentiate through these organs, that human T and B cells thereafter are functional, and that the model can be streamlined into a high throughput, reproducible system for the analysis of antiviral compounds against HIV. It is hoped that this approach will offer helpful information in the efficient transfer of promising antiviral compounds from the lab bench to the clinic.

REFERENCES

1. LEONARD, J. M., J. W. ABRAMCZUK, D. S. PEZEN, R. RUTLEDGE, J. H. BELCHER, F. HAKIM, G. SHEARER, L. LAMPERTH, W. TRAVIS, T. FREDRICKSON, A. L. NOTKINS & M. A. MARTIN. 1988. Science **242:** 1665-1670.
2. MOSIER, D. E., R. J. GULIZIA, S. BAIRD & D. B. WILSON. 1988. Nature **355:** 256-259.
3. MOSIER, D. E., R. J. GULIZIA, S. BAIRD, S. SPECTOR, D. SPECTOR, T. J. KIPPS, R. I. FOX, D. A. CARSON, N. COOPER, D. D. RICHMAN & D. B. WILSON. 1989. Studies of HIV infection and the development of Epstein-Barr virus-related B cell lymphomas following transfer of human lymphocytes to mice with severe combined immunodeficiency. *In* The Scid Mouse. Characterization and Potential Uses. M. J. Bosma, R. A. Phillips & W. Schuler, Eds.: 195-199. Springer-Verlag. Berlin.
4. MOSIER, D. E., R. J. GULIZIA, S. BAIRD & D. B. WILSON. 1989. Nature **338:** 211.
5. BANKERT, R. B., T. UMEMOTO, Y. SUGIYAMA, F. A. CHEN, E. REPASKY & S. YOKOTA. 1989. Human lung tumors, patients' peripheral blood lymphocytes and tumor infiltrating lymphocytes propagated in Scid mice. *In* The Scid Mouse. Characterization and Potential Uses. M. J. Bosma, R. A. Phillips & W. Schuler, Eds.: 201-210. Springer-Verlag. Berlin.
6. KRAMS, S. M., K. DORSHKIND & M. E. GERSHWIN. 1989. J. Exp. Med. **170:** 1919-1930.
7. KAMEL-REID, S. & J. E. DICK. 1988. Science **242:** 1706-1709.
8. McCUNE, J. M., R. NAMIKAWA, H. KANESHIMA, L. D. SHULTZ, M. LIEBERMAN & I. L. WEISSMAN. 1988. Science **241:** 1632-1639.
9. BOSMA, G. C., R. P. CUSTER & M. J. BOSMA. 1983. Nature **301:** 527-530.
10. SHULTZ, L. D., P. A. SCHWEITZER, E. J. HALL, J. P. SUNDBERG, S. TAYLOR & P. D. WALZER. 1989. *Pneumocystis carinii* pneumonia in scid/scid mice. *In* The Scid Mouse.

Characterization and Potential Uses. M. J. Bosma, R. A. Phillips & W. Schuler, Eds.: 243-249. Springer-Verlag. Berlin.

11. BILLINGHAM, R. E., L. BRENT & P. B. MEDAWAR. 1953. Nature 172: 603-605.
12. ZINKERNAGEL, R. M., G. N. CALLAHAN, A. ALTHAGE, S. COOPER, P. A. KLEIN & J. KLEIN. 1978. J. Exp. Med. 147: 882-896.
13. ZINKERNAGEL, R. M., G. N. CALLAHAN, A. ALTHAGE, S. COOPER, J. W. STREILEIN & J. KLEIN. 1978. J. Exp. Med. 147: 897-911.
14. NAMIKAWA, R., H. KANESHIMA, M. LIEBERMAN, I. L. WEISSMAN & J. M. MCCUNE. 1988. Science 242: 1684-1686.
15. KOYANAGI, Y., S. MILES, R. T. MITSUYASU, J. E. MERRILL, H. V. VINTERS & I. S. Y. CHEN. 1987. Science 236: 819-822.
16. CHEN, I. S. Y. Personal communication.
17. MCCUNE, J. M., R. NAMIKAWA, C.-C. SHIH, L. RABIN & H. KANESHIMA. 1990. Science 247: 564-566.
18. KANESHIMA, H., C.-C. SHIH, R. NAMIKAWA, L. RABIN & J. M. MCCUNE. 1990. Submitted.
19. LUSSO, P., F. DI MARZO VERONESE, B. ENSOLI, G. FRANCHINI, C. JEMMA, S. E. DEROCCO, V. S. KALYANARAMAN & R. C. GALLO. 1990. Science 247: 848-852.
20. MCCUNE, J. M., R. NAMIKAWA, C.-C. SHIH, L. RABIN & H. KANESHIMA. 1990. Pseudotypes in HIV-infected mice. Science 250: 1152-1153.
21. RABIN, L., H. KANESHIMA, C.-C. SHIH, & J. M. MCCUNE. 1990. 6th Intl. Conf. AIDS. 3: 113.
22. FREIREICH, E. J., E. A. GEHAN, D. P. RALL, L. H. SCHMIT & H. E. SKIPPER. 1966. Cancer Chemother. Rep. 50: 219-244.

Nonhuman Primate Models for Evaluation of AIDS Therapy[a]

HAROLD M. McCLURE,[b,c,f] DANIEL C. ANDERSON,[b]
AFTAB A. ANSARI,[b,c] PATRICIA N. FULTZ,[b,c]
SHERRY A. KLUMPP,[b] AND
RAYMOND F. SCHINAZI[b,d,e]

[b]Yerkes Regional Primate Research Center
Departments of [c]Pathology and [d]Pediatrics
School of Medicine
Emory University
Atlanta, Georgia 30322

and

[e]Veterans Affairs Medical Center
Decatur, Georgia 30033

INTRODUCTION

The magnitude and continuing growth of the current worldwide AIDS pandemic make the development of effective vaccines and antiviral drugs of utmost urgency.[1-5] These efforts, especially studies of the pathogenesis of retroviral infections and testing of antiretroviral drugs, immune system modulators, and vaccines will be greatly facilitated by access to appropriate animal models. The SIV-infected nonhuman primate has been established as an excellent animal model system for conducting such studies.[6-12]

The simian immunodeficiency viruses (SIVs) are a group of related lentiviruses that have been isolated from a variety of nonhuman primate species. The first isolate, SIVmac (initially designated STLV III), was reported in 1985 from rhesus macaques that were immunodeficient or had lymphoma.[13] Similar isolates were subsequently reported in 1986 from mangabey monkeys[14-16] and pigtailed macaques,[17,18] and from African green monkeys[19-21] and mandrills[22,23] in 1988. More recently, isolates have been obtained from stumptail macaques[24,25] and Sykes monkeys.[26] Based on their

[a]These investigations were supported in part by NIH Grant RR00165 from the Division of Research Resources to the Yerkes Regional Primate Research Center, Emory University Research Committee Grant No. 2-50103, NIAID Grant No. AI26055, Burroughs Wellcome Company, and by the U.S. Army Medical Research and Development Command under Project No. 87-PP-7863. Opinions, interpretations, conclusions, and recommendations are those of the authors and are not necessarily endorsed by the U.S. Army. The Yerkes Center is fully accredited by the American Association for Accreditation of Laboratory Animal Care.
[f]Address correspondence to H. M. McClure at Yerkes Regional Primate Research Center, 954 Gatewood Rd. NE, Emory University, Atlanta, Georgia 30322.

genetic, antigenic, and biologic properties, the SIVs are the closest known relatives of the human AIDS viruses (HIV-1 and HIV-2).[27-31] The mangabey (SIVsmm), macaque (SIVmac), and HIV-2 isolates are very closely related, suggesting that SIVsmm was the source of infection for macaques in captivity and humans (HIV-2) in West Africa.[31] More recently, an SIV (SIVcpz) has been isolated from a feral chimpanzee in Gabon; this isolate is reported to be more closely related to HIV-1 than to HIV-2.[32,33]

Although natural SIV infection in African species of nonhuman primates (African green monkeys, mangabeys, mandrills, Sykes monkeys) does not usually result in disease, we have noted occasional disease problems in mangabeys that appear to be related to SIV infection; increased numbers of lymphocytes in the peripheral blood, mild anemia, and lymphoid hepatitis have been reported in African green monkeys seropositive for SIV antibodies.[34] Nevertheless, SIV isolates from mangabey monkeys, when inoculated into rhesus, pig-tailed, and cynomolgus macaque monkeys results in a high incidence of a disease syndrome that is remarkably similar to human AIDS.[7,10,11] Experimental infection of macaque monkeys with SIV isolates from naturally infected rhesus (SIVmac) or pigtailed macaques (SIVmne) also results in the development of an AIDS-like disease.[6,18,35] Experimental infection of SIV-seronegative African green monkeys, cynomolgus, or rhesus macaques with SIVagm, however, usually results in seroconversion but no clinical disease; 1 of 4 pig-tailed macaques was noted to die from the infection.[36,37]

In this paper, we summarize studies done at the Yerkes Regional Primate Research Center to characterize the SIV-infected mangabey and macaque models and to provide preliminary data on drug trials using the SIV-infected macaque model.

NATURAL SIV INFECTION IN MANGABEYS

T-lymphotropic lentiviruses have been isolated from a high percentage of mangabeys in the Yerkes mangabey breeding colony.[14] This mangabey colony was established with wild-born animals in 1968, and since then has continued to reproduce well and has not shown any obvious increased incidence of disease associated with the widespread retrovirus infection. The mangabey isolate, designated SIVsmm, is morphologically identical to HIV by electron microscopy; serologically related to HIV by enzyme immunoassay, Western blot, and radioimmunoprecipitation; and is cytopathic for human CD4+ cells *in vitro*. Of 118 mangabeys tested, 73 (62%) were found to be seropositive and virus-positive for SIVsmm; 45 of 104 (43%) of the animals were also seropositive for antibodies to STLV-1. The frequency of SIVsmm infection increases with age of the animal; infection has been documented in 94% (34 of 36) of mangabeys 9 years of age or older, in 83% (5 of 6) of animals 7-8 years of age, in 73% (11 of 15) of 5-6-year-old animals, in 49% (17 of 35) of 3-4-year-old animals, and in 23% (6 of 26) of animals 1-2 years of age. Studies are currently underway to document the virus status of mangabeys less than one year of age. Observations in this naturally infected colony indicate that transmission within the colony is primarily by sexual activity and occasionally perinatally. Studies are currently underway to determine if perinatal transmission occurs *in utero* or during birth, or by ingestion of milk from SIV-infected mothers. Naturally infected, generally asymptomatic mangabeys are comparable to HIV-infected but asymptomatic humans and should prove to be an important model system for evaluation of immunologic parameters that maintain the asymptomatic state in persistently infected animals, as well as evaluation of possible cofactors associated with the induction of an AIDS-like disease.

CHRONIC SIVsmm INFECTION IN MACAQUES

In initial studies to evaluate the pathogenicity of SIVsmm for macaque monkeys, 12 rhesus and 1 pigtailed macaque were inoculated intravenously with approximately 10^4 $TCID_{50}$ of SIVsmm; the animals ranged from 1 to 15 months of age at the time of inoculation. Twelve of the 13 macaques seroconverted and became virus-positive within 3 to 6 weeks of inoculation; the remaining animal seroconverted at 6 months postinoculation, but has remained virus-negative. These SIVsmm-infected macaques developed variable degrees of lymphadenopathy, splenomegaly, diarrhea, weight loss, and hematologic abnormalities, including lymphopenia, neutropenia, and thrombocytopenia. Eight of these 13 chronically infected macaques (61.5%) died from an AIDS-like disease between 14 and 43 months postinfection. One additional animal currently has an AIDS-like disease and is showing gradual deterioration of its clinical condition. All clinically ill animals showed a progressive decrease in CD4+ T cells and in their CD4+/CD8+ cell ratios. Sentinel animals housed in the same room (3 rhesus and 2 pigtailed macaques) or same cage (4 rhesus) with macaques chronically infected with SIVsmm have remained seronegative and virus-negative for up to 52 months; animals housed together in the same cage (1 infected and 1 noninfected) were all sexually immature.[10]

Histologic findings in animals dying from an AIDS-like disease ranged from prominent follicular hyperplasia to severe lymphoid depletion, with lymphoid tissues often showing an infiltrate of syncytial giant cells. One animal had intestinal cryptosporidiosis, one had disseminated mycobacteriosis, and two had brain lesions comparable to those seen in AIDS encephalopathy in humans. These observations indicate that the disease induced by SIVsmm infection in macaque monkeys is remarkably similar to human AIDS, and that SIVsmm, like HIV, is not transmitted by casual contact.

To determine the minimal infectious dose of SIVsmm for use in vaccine or drug trials, eight juvenile rhesus macaques were divided into four groups of two animals each and inoculated intravenously with 1 log dilutions of the standard SIVsmm inoculum (10^4 $TCID_{50}$), with the experimental groups receiving 0.2 to 200 $TCID_{50}$. All animals receiving 10^{-2} or 10^{-3} dilutions (200 or 20 $TCID_{50}$) seroconverted and became virus-positive within 3 to 6 weeks of challenge; one of two animals receiving the 10^{-4} dilution (2 $TCID_{50}$) was virus-positive at 3 weeks after challenge and seroconverted at 6 weeks postchallenge. Both animals receiving the 10^{-5} dilution (0.2 $TCID_{50}$) remained seronegative and virus-negative. Results of this minimal infectious dose study are summarized in TABLE 1. Because the $TCID_{50}$ of this virus stock is about 2×10^4/mL, the above data indicate that one 50% animal infectious dose (ID_{50}) is approximately 2 $TCID_{50}$.

ACUTE SIVsmm INFECTION IN MACAQUES

A variant of SIVsmm, designated SIVsmmPBj14, that was isolated from a pigtailed macaque chronically infected with SIVsmm was found to induce acute clinical disease and death within 15 days when inoculated into other pigtailed macaques.[38] Infection with this variant SIV was fatal in 100% of pigtailed macaques receiving a dose of 10^4 $TCID_{50}$, caused death within less than 2 weeks in one of three experimentally infected rhesus monkeys, and induced acute lethal disease in SIVsmm-seronegative mangabeys but not in SIVsmm-seropositive mangabeys. Recent studies have also shown that prior infection with SIVsmm affords complete protection to challenge with SIVsmmPBj14

TABLE 1. SIVsmm Minimal Infectious Dose in Rhesus Macaques

Virus Dilution (TCID$_{50}$)	Animal	Antibody		Virus isolation	
		3 weeks	6 weeks	3 weeks	6 weeks
10^{-2} (200)	RNy	+	+	+	+
	RQq	±	+	+	+
10^{-3} (20)	RIz	±	+	+	+
	RCv	+	+	+	+
10^{-4} (2)	RKt	−	+	+	+
	REr	−	−	−	−
10^{-5} (0.2)	ROr	−	−	−	−
	RVr	−	−	−	−

in pigtailed macaques (manuscript in preparation). The results of animal inoculations with SIVsmmPBj14 are summarized in TABLE 2.

When challenged with SIVsmmPBj14, pigtailed macaques develop an acute clinical disease characterized by profuse, often bloody diarrhea, pronounced lethargy, essentially total anorexia, lymphopenia, and a marked left shift in polymorphonuclear cell counts within 4 to 5 days of challenge; infected macaques die within 7 to 12 days. Pathologic findings in these animals include severe generalized lymphadenopathy, splenomegaly, and marked hyperplasia of lymphoid tissues in the intestinal mucosa. Syncytial giant cells are often present in multiple tissues, and large numbers of mature and budding lentivirus particles are easily demonstrated by electron microscopy in mesenteric lymph nodes and intestinal lymphoid tissues; virus particles are often present in intracellular vacuoles in macrophages.

To determine the minimal infectious dose of SIVsmmPBj14 for use in vaccine or drug trials, 12 juvenile pigtailed macaques were divided into six groups of two animals each and inoculated intravenously with decreasing doses of the PBj isolate. Group 1 animals received the standard inoculum of 10^4 TCID$_{50}$, with groups 2-6 receiving 1 log dilutions of the standard inoculum (10^3 TCID$_{50}$ to 0.1 TCID$_{50}$). All animals given 10 TCID$_{50}$ or greater became infected and developed acute clinical disease. Although there was no evidence that the two recipients of 1 TCID$_{50}$ became infected, one animal that received 0.1 TCID$_{50}$ was infected and at 6 weeks postinfection had reduced numbers of CD4$^+$ cells; these decreased progressively until death nine months postinfection. In the other infected animals, disease onset ranged from day 7 (10^4 TCID$_{50}$) to day 12 (10 TCID$_{50}$) postinfection, with death occurring from day 8 to day 16 postinfection. One animal (recipient of 10^2 TCID$_{50}$) survived the acute disease but showed a progressive decrease in CD4$^+$ cells and died 7 months postinfection with emaciation, oroesophageal candidiasis, lymphadenopathy, splenomegaly, lymphopenia, and a CD4$^+$/CD8$^+$ cell ratio of 0.16. The results of this minimal infectious dose determination are summarized in TABLE 3.

PROPHYLACTIC EFFECTS OF AZT FOLLOWING EXPOSURE TO THE ACUTELY LETHAL SIV VARIANT (SIVsmmPBj14)

The prophylactic efficacy of AZT was determined in pigtailed macaques exposed to the acutely lethal variant of SIVsmm (SIVsmmPBj14). In this study, 12 juvenile pigtailed macaques were inoculated intravenously with approximately 20 $TCID_{50}$ of SIVsmmPBj14. AZT was given subcutaneously at a dose of 100 mg/kg/day, divided into three doses and administered at 8:00 A.M., 1:00 P.M., and 6:00 P.M. each day. The AZT treatment was continued for a period of 14 days in all animals that survived for that period of time. The 12 pigtailed macaques were divided into four groups of three animals each, with AZT administration initiated at 1 (group 1), 24 (group 2), and 72 (group 3) hours after virus exposure; group 4 animals did not receive any drug treatment.

Following virus exposure and the initiation of AZT treatment, the clinical condition of the experimental animals was monitored daily, and the animals were anesthetized for physical examination and blood collection at 4, 10, 15, 21, and 35 days and at 3-6-week intervals thereafter for the first year postexposure. Blood samples were used for CBC determinations, virus culture, and serology.

Results of this study are summarized in TABLES 4 and 5. All animals except one in group 1 were virus-positive at 10 days postinoculation. Three animals in groups 1 and 2 did not develop the characteristic acute clinical disease following exposure to SIVsmm PBj14 and remained clinically normal; all other animals developed clinical disease within 10-17 days of virus exposure. One death occurred in group 1, two deaths occurred in group 2, and each of the three animals in groups 3 and 4 died. In groups 3 and 4, two animals in each group died acutely, and one animal in each group survived for 13 and 14 months, respectively. One animal in group 1 continues to be virus-negative, and all 3 survivors in groups 1 and 2 continue to appear clinically normal and to have normal immunologic parameters two years postexposure. Animals in groups 3 and 4 had 30-fold higher antibody titers than animals in groups 1 and 2, suggesting that the former had more antigenic stimulation due to increased virus replication.

TABLE 2. Susceptibility of Monkeys to SIVsmmPBj14 Infection

Species	Inoculum	Number of animals	Time of death	Percent mortality
Macaca nemestrina (SIV negative)	Blood (IV)[a]	3	8 days, 9 days 10 weeks	100
M. nemestrina (SIV negative)	Virus (IV)	6	7 days (3 animals) 8 days (3 animals)	100
M. mulatta (SIV negative)	Virus (IV)	3	9 days	33
Cercocebus atys (SIV negative)	Virus (IV)	4	10 days, 11 days, 13 days	75
C. atys (SIV positive)	Virus (IV)	2	—	0
M. nemestrina (SIV negative)	Feces (oral)[b]	3	12 days	33
M. nemestrina (SIV positive)	Virus (IV)	9	—	0
M. nemestrina (SIV negative)	Virus (IV)	3	10 days, 11 days, 12 days	100

[a] 10 mL blood transfusion from a pigtailed macaque chronically infected with SIVsmm.
[b] Diarrheal material from pigtailed macaque with acute SIVsmmPBj infection administered by gastric intubation.

TABLE 3. SIVsmmPBj14 Minimal Infectious Dose Study

Group and animal designation	Day of onset of blood in stool	Time of death
Group 1 (10^4 TCID)		
PPh	Day 7 p.i.	Day 8 p.i.
PFf	Day 7 p.i.	Day 9 p.i.
Group 2 (10^3 TCID)		
PGg	Day 8 p.i.	Day 10 p.i.
PUc	Day 10 p.i.	Day 11 p.i.
Group 3 (100 TCID)		
PEf	Day 10 p.i.[a]	7 Months p.i.
PDg	Day 11 p.i.	Day 13 p.i.
Group 4 (10 TCID)		
POg	Day 12 p.i.	Day 15 p.i.
PSf	Day 12 p.i.	Day 16 p.i.
Group 5 (1 TCID)		
PSe	No Disease[b]	Alive 2 yr p.i.
PEc	No Disease[b]	Alive 2 yr p.i.
Group 6 (0.1 TCID)		
PYg	No Disease[b]	Alive 2 yr p.i.
PHb	No Acute Disease[c]	9 Months p.i.

[a] Recovered from acute clinical disease but developed severe immunosuppression and died 7 months postinoculation (p.i.).

[b] Animals did not become virus-infected and did not develop clinical disease.

[c] Animal did not develop acute clinical disease but became virus-infected and showed immunosuppression at 6 weeks postinoculation. Immunosuppression became progressively more severe, and animal died at 9 months postinoculation.

Data derived from this study indicate that some protection is provided by AZT when treatment is initiated within 24 hours of exposure to an acutely lethal simian HIV-like virus. One of three animals treated with AZT within 1 hour of exposure apparently did not become virus-infected, and 3 of 6 animals treated within 24 hours of exposure failed to develop the characteristic acute clinical disease and continued to be clinically normal two years postexposure. These data suggest that AZT treatment inhibits virus replication in animals treated within 24 hours of exposure. In previous SIVsmmPBj14 infection studies, all animals exposed to a dose of 10 $TCID_{50}$ or higher became infected and subsequently died.

TABLE 4. AZT Prophylaxis following SIVsmmPBj14 Exposure

	Treatment Time Postexposure			
	Group 1 (1 hour)	Group 2 (24 hours)	Group 3 (72 hours)	Group 4 (No Rx)
Virus-negative	1/3	0/3	0/3	0/3
Clinical disease	1/3	2/3	3/3	3/3
Death	1/3	2/3	3/3	3/3
Day of death postexposure	12	14,19	12,14, 13 mo.	12,14, 14 mo.
Normal survivors at 2 yr postexposure	2	1	0	0

PROPHYLACTIC EFFECTS OF CS-87, AZT, D4T, AND FDT IN THE SIVsmm MACAQUE MODEL

The SIVsmm-infected rhesus macaque model was used to evaluate and compare the prophylactic effects of 3'-azido-2',3'-dideoxyuridine (CS-87/AzddU), 3'-azido-3'-deoxythymidine (AZT), 2',3'-didehydro-3'-deoxythymidine (D4T), and 3'-fluoro-3'-deoxythymidine (FDT/FLT). Our objective was to determine whether the drugs tested could prevent infection when animals were treated shortly before and for a short period after exposure to SIVsmm.

In this study, 25 juvenile rhesus monkeys were placed into five groups of five animals each and treated with either CS-87, AZT, D4T, FDT, or phosphate-buffered saline (PBS). All 25 animals were inoculated intravenously with 150 TCID$_{50}$ of SIVsmm 24 hours after drug treatment was initiated. Each drug was administered subcutane-

TABLE 5. AZT Prophylaxis following SIVsmmPBj14 Exposure

AZT Treatment	Animal	EIA[a] antibody titers Weeks postexposure			
		8	18	35	42
Group 1	F86235	3,200	3,200	6,400	6,400
(1 hour)	M86338	Dead			
	F86342	< 100	< 100	< 100	< 100
Group 2	F86367	Dead			
(24 hours)	J86092	3,200	6,400	3,200	6,400
	F86386	Dead			
Group 3	J86078	Dead			
(72 hours)	T86308	Dead			
	F86387	51,200	204,800	204,800	102,400
Group 4	J86015	Dead			
(No Rx)	F86188	Dead			
	T86310	51,200	204,800	102,400	204,800

[a] Enzyme immunoassay.

ously at a dose of 100 mg/kg/day, divided into three doses, and given at 8:00 A.M., 4:00 P.M., and 12:00 A.M. Drug treatment was initiated 24 hours prior to virus exposure and continued for a period of 14 days following virus exposure. At the time of SIVsmm inoculation, the scheduled drug dosage was administered intravenously shortly before the virus inoculum was given.

Following the initiation of drug treatment and virus exposure, the animals were monitored by daily observations, and each animal was anesthetized for physical examinations and blood collection at 2, 4, 6, and 8 weeks postexposure. Blood samples were used for complete blood counts (CBC) and serum chemistry determinations, immunologic evaluations (CD4$^+$ and CD8$^+$ cells), and for virus culture and serology. Unfortunately, due to contamination of the human peripheral blood mononuclear cells used for the cocultures, virus isolation attempts were not valid until much later in the study. Nevertheless, the prophylactic effects (or lack thereof) of the drugs being tested were determined by seroconversion for antibodies to SIVsmm. These seroconversion results are summarized in TABLE 6 and clearly show that none of the drugs being tested were effective in preventing infection in animals exposed to SIVsmm by the intravenous route. All animals except two in the FDT treatment group had seroconverted by 6 weeks postexposure; one additional animal in the FDT group had seroconverted by 8 weeks postexposure. This seroconversion, and therefore lack of prophylactic efficacy, occurred despite the fact the drug treatment was initiated 24 hours prior to virus exposure.

There was a general lack of significant adverse effects on the animals with respect to clinical appearance, or hemogram or blood chemistry parameters following a two week course of treatment with CS-87, AZT, or D4T. Animals in the FDT treatment group, however, developed diarrhea shortly after initiation of treatment, which persisted throughout the treatment period and was associated with weight loss. Animals in the FDT treatment group also showed evidence of significant bone marrow toxicity, with marked decreases noted in RBC and WBC counts, hemoglobin and hematocrit values, and in reticulocyte and platelet counts. These values all returned to normal levels within two to four weeks after drug treatment was terminated. More details of this study will be provided in a separate publication (manuscript in preparation).

TABLE 6. Seroconversion in Animals Exposed to SIVsmm and Treated with Antivirals

Drug Rx Group	Time of Seroconversion Postexposure			
	2 weeks	4 weeks	6 weeks	8 weeks
PBS	0/5	4/5	5/5	5/5
CS-87	0/5	5/5	5/5	5/5
AZT	0/5	5/5	5/5	5/5
D4T	0/5	3/5	5/5	5/5
FDT	0/5	3/5	3/5	4/5

DISCUSSION

Although a number of newly developed antiretroviral drugs are presently in early phases of human clinical trials, AZT is currently the only drug approved for treatment of HIV infection.[39-41] AZT has been shown to prolong the life of AIDS patients, to decrease the incidence of opportunistic infections, and to relieve or improve the CNS problems associated with HIV infection.[42-45] AZT, however, does not cure an individual of HIV infection and often has severe toxic effects that prevent treatment or continued treatment in a significant number of AIDS patients.[46-48] These shortcomings of AZT and the growing magnitude of worldwide HIV infection make the continued search for, and development of, new more efficacious and less toxic drugs of paramount importance.

The development, testing, and eventual clinical use of new antiretroviral agents will be greatly facilitated by the availability and adequate use of appropriate animal model systems. The importance of animal models is emphasized by the fact that only about 1% of compounds that have *in vitro* antiviral activity are also active in animal systems.[49] The SIV-infected macaque provides a model for evaluating the safety and efficacy of newly developed AIDS drugs because the SIVs are serologically related to the human AIDS viruses, and we and others have documented the marked clinical, pathologic, virologic, and immunologic similarities between human AIDS and SIV infection in macaques.[6-12] This is an excellent animal model system for study of the pathogenesis of an HIV-like virus and for evaluation of vaccines and newly developed antiretroviral drugs. In addition, the acutely lethal SIV variant should prove to be extremely useful for the rapid screening and evaluation of antiretroviral agents.

Data are provided in this report that indicate that some protection is provided by AZT when treatment is initiated within 24 hours of exposure to the acutely lethal variant of SIV. Another study, however, using the more chronic SIVsmm infection model failed to show any prophylactic efficacy of CS-87, AZT, D4T, or FDT, even when drug treatment was initiated 24 hours prior to virus exposure. This study also revealed that, at the dosage used, FDT had unacceptable levels of toxicity.

Appropriate animal model systems are available for evaluating the efficacy of newly developed antiretroviral agents, and based on various factors, the SIV-infected macaque can be considered the best model currently available. These animal model systems should be used more extensively prior to initiating large scale human clinical trials. Drug evaluations can be done under more controlled conditions, in a more timely manner, and at less cost in the animal model system than in the human population. It should also be pointed out that prophylactic drug trials can be done in a timely manner only in an animal model system. Although a trial to evaluate the prophylactic effects of AZT in health care workers accidentally exposed to HIV was initiated,[50] it was later noted that the low risk for infection following occupational exposure and the difficulty in obtaining an adequate number of subjects for inclusion in the trial have impeded progress and made completion of the study unlikely.[51]

SUMMARY

Infection of macaque monkeys with simian immunodeficiency virus (SIV) has been established as an excellent animal model system for studying the pathogenesis of an HIV-like virus and for evaluating newly developed antiretroviral drugs and vaccines. Based on their genetic, antigenic, and biologic properties, the simian immunodeficiency viruses are the closest known relatives of the human AIDS viruses, and experimental infection of macaque monkeys results in a disease that is remarkably similar to human AIDS. Infected macaques show diarrhea, weight loss, hematologic abnormalities including lymphopenia and thrombocytopenia, lymphadenopathy/lymphoid hyperplasia that progresses to lymphoid depletion, immunosuppression with marked reduction in $CD4^+$ cells and in the $CD4^+/CD8^+$ cell ratio, and opportunistic infections. A majority of such macaques die from an AIDS-like disease within one to three years of infection. An acutely lethal variant of SIV has been identified that results in death in susceptible macaques within 7-12 days of infection.

Preliminary prophylactic treatment trials with AZT in macaque monkeys exposed to the acutely lethal SIV variant indicate that some protection is provided when AZT treatment is initiated within 24 hours of virus exposure. Other studies with the more chronic SIV infection model, however, failed to show any prophylactic efficacy of CS-87, AZT, D4T, or FDT.

ACKNOWLEDGMENTS

The authors acknowledge the excellent technical assistance of numerous technicians in the Division of Pathobiology and Immunobiology at the Yerkes Center, the daily care provided to the experimental animals by the primate care technicians, and the assistance of Elizabeth White in preparation of the manuscript.

REFERENCES

1. McGowan, J. & D. Hoth. 1989. AIDS drug discovery and development. J. AIDS **2:** 335-343.
2. Merigan, T. C. 1989. A personal view of efforts in treatment of human immunodeficiency virus infection in 1988. J. Infect. Dis. **159:** 390-399.
3. Mitsuya, H. & S. Broder. 1987. Strategies for antiviral therapy in AIDS. Nature **325:** 773-778.
4. Vogt, M. & M. S. Hirsch. 1986. Prospects for the prevention and therapy of infections with the human immunodeficiency virus. Rev. Infect. Dis. **8:** 991-1000.
5. Polsky, B. 1989. Antiviral chemotherapy for infection with human immunodeficiency virus. Rev. Infect. Dis. **11** (Suppl. 7): S1648-S1663.
6. Letvin, N. L., M. D. Daniel, P. K. Sehgal, R. C. Desrosiers, R. D. Hunt, L. M. Waldron, J. J. Mackey, D. K. Schmidt, L. V. Chalifoux & N. W. King. 1985. Induction of AIDS-like disease in macaque monkeys with T-cell tropic retrovirus STLV-III. Science **230:** 71-73.
7. Baskin, G. B., M. Murphey-Corb, E. A. Watson & L. N. Martin. 1988. Necropsy findings in rhesus monkeys experimentally infected with cultured simian immunodeficiency virus (SIV)/Delta. Vet. Pathol. **25:** 456-467.
8. Gardner, M. B. & P. A. Luciw. 1988. Simian immunodeficiency viruses and their relationship to the human immunodeficiency viruses. AIDS **2** (Suppl. 1): S3-S10.
9. Desrosiers, R. C., M. D. Daniel & Y. Li. 1989. Minireview: HIV-related lentiviruses of nonhuman primates. AIDS Res. Hum. Retroviruses **5:** 465-473.
10. McClure, H. M., D. C. Anderson, P. N. Fultz, A. A. Ansari, E. Lockwood & A. Brodie. 1989. Spectrum of disease in macaque monkeys chronically infected with SIV/SMM. Vet. Immunol. Immunopathol. **21:** 13-24.
11. Putkonen, P., K. Warstedt, R. Thorstensson, R. Benthin, J. Albert, B. Lundgren, B. Oberg, E. Norrby & G. Biberfeld. 1989. Experimental infection of cynomolgus monkeys (*Macaca fascicularis*) with simian immunodeficiency virus (SIVsm). J. AIDS **2:** 359-365.
12. Schneider, J. & G. Hunsman. 1988. Simian lentiviruses—the SIV group. AIDS **2:** 1-9.
13. Daniel, M. D., N. L. Letvin, N. W. King, M. Kannagi, P. K. Sehgal, R. D. Hunt, P. J. Kanki, M. Essex & R. C. Desrosiers. 1985. Isolation of T-cell tropic HTLV-III-like retrovirus from macaques. Science **228:** 1201-1204.
14. Fultz, P. N., H. M. McClure, D. C. Anderson, R. B. Swenson, A. Anand & A. Srinivasan. 1986. Isolation of a T-lymphotropic retrovirus from naturally infected sooty mangabey monkeys (*Cercocebus atys*). Proc. Natl. Acad. Sci. USA **83:** 5286-5290.
15. Murphey-Corb, M., L. N. Martin, S. R. S. Rangan, G. B. Baskin, B. J. Gormus, R. H. Wolf, W. A. Andes, M. West & R. C. Montelaro. 1986. Isolation of an HTLV-III-related retrovirus from macaques with simian AIDS and its possible origin in asymptomatic mangabeys. Nature **321:** 435-437.
16. Lowenstine, L. J., N. C. Pederson, J. Higgins, K. C. Pallis, A. Uyeda, P. Marx, N. W. Lerche, R. J. Munn & M. B. Gardner. 1986. Seroepidemiologic survey of captive old-world primates for antibodies to human and simian retroviruses, and isolation of a lentivirus from sooty mangabeys (*Cercocebus atys*). Int. J. Cancer **38:** 563-574.
17. Benveniste, R. E., L. O. Arthur, C.-C. Tsai, R. Sowder, T. D. Copeland, L. E.

HENDERSON & S. OROSZLAN. 1986. Isolation of a lentivirus from a macaque with lymphoma: comparison with HTLV-III/LAV and other lentiviruses. J. Virol. **60:** 483-490.

18. BENVENISTE, R. E., W. R. MORTON, E. A. CLARK, C.-C. TSAI, H. D. OCHS, J. M. WARD, L. KULLER, W. B. KNOTT, R. W. HILL, M. J. GALE & M. E. THOULESS. 1988. Inoculation of baboons and macaques with simian immunodeficiency virus/Mne, a primate lentivirus closely related to human immunodeficiency virus type 2. J. Viral **62:** 2091-2101.

19. OHTA, Y., T. MASUDA, H. TSUJIMOTO, K.-I. ISHIKAWA, T. KODAMA, S. MORIKAWA, M. NAKAI, S. HONJO & M. HAYAMI. 1988. Isolation of simian immunodeficiency virus from African green monkeys and seroepidemiologic survey of the virus in various nonhuman primates. Int. J. Cancer **41:** 115-122.

20. DANIEL, M. D., Y. LI, Y. M. NAIDU, P. J. DURDA, D. K. SCHMIDT, C. D. TROUP, D. P. SILVA, J. J. MACKEY, H. W. KESTLER, III, P. K. SEHGAL, N. W. KING, Y. OHTA, M. HAYAMI & R. C. DESROSIERS. 1988. Simian immunodeficiency virus from African green monkeys. J. Virol. **62:** 4123-4128.

21. KRAUS, G., A. WERNER, M. BAIER, D. BINNIGER, F. J. FERDINAND, S. NORLEY & R. KURTH. 1989. Isolation of human immunodeficiency virus-related simian immunodeficiency viruses from African green monkeys. Proc. Natl. Acad. Sci. USA **86:** 2892-2896.

22. TSUJIMOTO, H., R. W. COOPER, T. KODAMA, M. FUKASAWA, T. MIURA, Y. OHTA, K.-I. ISHIKAWA, M. NAKAI, E. FROST, G. E. ROELANTS, J. ROFFI & M. HAYAMI. 1988. Isolation and characterization of simian immunodeficiency virus from mandrills in Africa and its relationship to other human and simian immunodeficiency viruses. J. Virol. **62:** 4044-4050.

23. TSUJIMOTO, H., A. HASEGAWA, N. MAKI, M. FUKASAWA, T. MIURA, S. SPEIDEL, R. W. COOPER, E. N. MORIYAMA, T. GOJOBORI & M. HAYAMI. 1989. Sequence of a novel simian immunodeficiency virus from a wild-caught African mandrill. Nature **341:** 539-541.

24. LOWENSTINE, L. J., N. W. LERCHE, J. A. YEE, A. UYEDA, M. B. JENNINGS, R. J. MUNN, H. M. MCCLURE, P. N. FULTZ, D. C. ANDERSON & M. B. GARDNER. 1990. Evidence for a lentiviral etiology in an epizootic of lymphoma and immunodeficiency in stumptailed macaques (*Macaca arctoides*). Submitted.

25. ANDERSON, D. C., S. A. KLUMPP, A. A. ANSARI, P. N. FULTZ & H. M. MCCLURE. 1990. Naturally occurring SIV infection in a domestic breeding colony of stumptail macaques (*Macaca arctoides*). Manuscript in preparation.

26. EMAU, P., H. M. MCCLURE, M. ISAHAKIA, J. ELSE & P. N. FULTZ. 1990. Isolation from African Sykes monkeys (*Cercopithecus mitis*) of a lentivirus related to human and simian immunodeficiency viruses. Submitted.

27. FRANCHINI, G., C. GURGO, H.-G. GUO, R. C. GALLO, E. COLLALTI, K. A. FARGNOLI, L. F. HALL, F. WONG-STAAL & M. S. REITZ, JR. 1987. Sequence of simian immunodeficiency virus and its relationship to the human immunodeficiency viruses. Nature **328:** 539-543.

28. CHAKRABARTI, L., M. GUYADER, M. ALIZON, M. D. DANIEL, R. C. DESROSIERS, P. TIOLLAIS & P. SONIGO. 1987. Sequence of simian immunodeficiency virus from macaque and its relationship to other human and simian retroviruses. Nature **328:** 543-547.

29. SCHNEIDER, J., E. JURKIEWICZ, M. HAYAMI, R. DESROSIERS, P. MARX & G. HUNSMANN. 1987. Serological and structural comparison of HIV, SIVmac, SIVagm and SIVsm, four primate lentiviruses. Ann. Inst. Pasteur Virol. **138:** 93-99.

30. KESTLER, H. W., III, Y. LI, Y. M. NAIDU, C. V. BUTLER, M. F. OCHS, G. JAENEL, N. W. KING, M. D. DANIEL & R. C. DESROSIERS. 1988. Comparison of simian immunodeficiency virus isolates. Nature **331:** 619-621.

31. HIRSCH, V. M., R. A. OLMSTED, M. MURPHEY-CORB, R. H. PURCELL & P. R. JOHNSON. 1989. An African primate lentivirus (SIVsm) closely related to HIV-2. Nature **339:** 389-392.

32. PEETERS, M., C. HONORE, T. HUET, L. BEDJABAGA, S. OSSARI, P. BUSSI, R. W. COOPER & E. DELAPORTE. 1989. Isolation and partial characterization of an HIV-related virus occurring naturally in chimpanzees in Gabon. AIDS **3:** 625-630.

33. HUET, T., R. CHEYNIER, A. MEYERHANS, G. ROELANTS & S. WAIN-HOBSON. 1990. Genetic organization of a chimpanzee lentivirus related to HIV-1. Nature **345:** 356-359.

34. FINCHAM, J. E., F. VAN DER RIET, J. G. STEYTLER, M. T. L. TUNG, R. COOPER, J. V. SEIER, D. L. MADDEN, P. KANKI, J. A. H. CAMPBELL, J. J. F. TALJAARD & C. W.

WOODROOF. 1989. Increased peripheral lymphocytes, lymphoid hepatitis and anaemia in African vervet monkeys seropositive to retroviruses. J. Comp. Pathol. **101:** 53-68.

35. KING, N. W., L. V. CHALIFOUX, D. J. RINGLER, M. S. WYAND, P. K. SEHGAL, M. D. DANIEL, N. L. LETVIN, R. C. DESROSIERS, B. J. BLAKE & R. D. HUNT. 1990. Comparative biology of natural and experimental SIVmac infection in macaque monkeys: a review. J. Med. Primatol. **19:** 109-118.

36. HONJO, S., T. NARITA, R. KOBAYASHI, A. HIYAOKA, K. FUJIMOTO, M. TAKASAKA, I. SAKAKIBARA, R. MUKAI, K. ISHIKAWA, Y. OHTA & M. HAYAMI. 1990. Experimental infection of African green monkeys and cynomolgus monkeys with a SIVagm strain isolated from a healthy African green monkey. J. Med. Primatol. **19:** 9-20.

37. GRAVELL, M., W. T. LONDON, R. S. HAMILTON, G. STONE & M. MONZON. 1989. Infection of macaque monkeys with simian immunodeficiency virus from African green monkeys: virulence and activation of latent infection. J. Med. Primatol. **18:** 247-254.

38. FULTZ, P. N., H. M. MCCLURE, D. C. ANDERSON & W. M. SWITZER. 1989. Identification and biologic characterization of an acutely lethal variant of simian immunodeficiency virus from sooty mangabeys (SIV/SMM). AIDS Res. Human Retroviruses **5:** 397-409.

39. RICHMAN, D. D. 1988. The treatment of HIV infection. AIDS **2** (Suppl. 1): S137-S142.

40. YARCHOAN, R., R. V. THOMAS, J.-P. ALLAIN, N. MCATEE, R. DUBINSKY, H. MITSUYA, T. J. LAWLEY, B. SAFAI, C. E. MYERS, C. F. PERNO, R. W. KLECKER, R. J. WILLS, M. A. FISCHL, M. C. MCNEELY, J. M. PLUDA, M. LEUTHER, J. M. COLLINS & S. BRODER. 1988. Phase I studies of 2', 3'-dideoxycytidine in severe human immunodeficiency virus infection as a single agent and alternating with zidovudine (AZT). Lancet **1:** 76-81.

41. JOHNSON, R. P. & R. T. SCHOOLEY. 1989. Update on antiretroviral agents other than zidovudine. AIDS **3** (Suppl. 1): S145-S151.

42. FISCHL, M. A., D. D. RICHMAN, M. H. GRIECO, M. S. GOTTLIEB, P. A. VOLBERDING, O. L. LASKIN, J. M. LEEDOM, J. E. GROOPMAN, D. MILDVAN, R. T. SCHOOLEY, G. G. JACKSON, D. T. DURACK, D. KING AND THE AZT COLLABORATIVE WORKING GROUP. 1987. The efficacy of azidothymidine (AZT) in the treatment of patients with AIDS and AIDS-related complex. N. Engl. J. Med. **317:** 185-191.

43. CREAGH-KIRK, T., P. DOI, E. ANDREWS, S. NUSINOFF-LEHRMAN, H. TILSON, D. HOTH & D. W. BARRY. 1988. Survival experience among patients with AIDS receiving zidovudine. J. Am. Med. Assoc. **260:** 3009-3015.

44. HIRSCH, M. S. 1988. Azidothymidine. J. Infect. Dis. **157:** 427-431.

45. FISCHL, M. A. 1989. State of antiretroviral therapy with zidovudine. AIDS **3** (Suppl. 1): S137-S143.

46. RICHMAN, D. D., M. A. FISCHL, M. H. GRIECO, M. S. GOTTLIEB, P. A. VOLBERDING, O. L. LASKIN, J. M. LEEDOM, J. E. GROOPMAN, D. MILDVAN, M. S. HIRSCH, G. G. JACKSON, D. T. DURACK, S. NUSINOFF-LEIIRMAN, AND THE AZT COLLABORATIVE WORKING GROUP. 1987. The toxicity of azidothymidine (AZT) in the treatment of patients with AIDS and AIDS-related complex. N. Engl. J. Med. **317:** 192-197.

47. FISCHL, M. A., D. D. RICHMAN, D. M. CAUSEY, M. H. GRIECO, Y. BRYSON, D. MILDVAN, O. L. LASKIN, J. E. GROOPMAN, P. A. VOLBERDING, R. T. SCHOOLEY, G. G. JACKSON, D. T. DURACK, J. C. ANDREWS, S. NUSINOFF-LEHRMAN, D. W. BARRY, AND THE AZT COLLABORATIVE WORKING GROUP. 1989. Prolonged zidovudine therapy in patients with AIDS and advanced AIDS-related complex. J. Am. Med. Assoc. **262:** 2405-2410.

48. GELMON, K., J. S. G. MONTANER, M. FANNING, J. R. M. SMITH, J. FALUTZ, C. TSOUKAS, J. GILL, G. WELLS, M. O'SHAUGHNESSY, M. WAINBERG & J. RUEDY. 1989. Nature, time course and dose dependence of zidovudine-related side effects: results from the multicenter Canadian azidothymidine trial. AIDS **3:** 555-561.

49. PRUSOFF, W. H., T.-S. LIN, E. M. AUGUST, T. G. WOOD & M. E. MARONGIU. 1989. Approaches to antiviral drug development. Yale J. Biol. Med. **62:** 215-225.

50. LAFON, S. W., S. NUSINOFF LEHRMAN & D. W. BARRY. 1988. Prophylactically administered Retrovir in health care workers potentially exposed to the human immunodeficiency virus. J. Infect. Dis. **158:** 503.

51. HENDERSON, D. K. & J. L. GERBERDING. 1989. Prophylactic zidovudine after occupational exposure to the human immunodeficiency virus: an interim analysis. J. Infect. Dis. **160:** 321-327.

Pharmacology of Antiretroviral Drugs

Lessons Learned to Date

PAUL S. LIETMAN [a]

Division of Clinical Pharmacology
The Johns Hopkins University School of Medicine
Baltimore, Maryland 21205

The successful development of a drug for AIDS begins with drug discovery and ends with our use of the drug in patients with an optimized dose and dosing regimen that maximizes the beneficial clinical response and minimizes the toxicities. Drug discovery in the field of anti-HIV drugs is occurring at an unprecedentedly rapid pace that is already crying out for efficient means of evaluating the numerous discoveries in humans. The pressures for successes in drug development offer enormous challenges and enormous opportunities for clinical investigations. It is imperative that these clinical investigations take cognizance of the pharmacologic aspects of the drugs in order to correctly assess their efficacy and toxicity and in order to optimize doses and dosing regimens.

Optimization of the use of an antiviral agent will depend upon some understanding of the pharmacodynamics of the drug, the pharmacokinetics of the drug, and the interaction between these two, that is, the time-dependent pharmacodynamics. Three axioms underlie these pharmacologic principles.

First, for all drugs there is a relationship between the concentration of the drug at its site of action and its effect, that is, the *pharmacodynamics* of the drug. Second, for all drugs there are time-dependent effects of the host (humans) on the drug, that is, the *pharmacokinetics* of the drug. Third, for all drugs there is an important time dependency of the effects of the drug. This is often referred to as the pharmacokinetic/pharmacodynamic interactions or the time-dependent pharmacodynamics of a drug.

PHARMACODYNAMICS

The pharmacodynamics of an antiviral drug must be considered from both the standpoint of beneficial or wanted effects and toxic or unwanted effects. In each case,

[a] Address for correspondence: Osler 527, The Johns Hopkins Hospital, 600 North Wolfe Street, Baltimore, Maryland 21205.

there is a definable relationship between the concentration of the drug at the site of the desired or undesired effect and the magnitude of the effect. Two drugs that we have studied, namely, zidovudine (Z) and dextran sulfate (DS), serve to illustrate some of the facets of the pharmacodynamics of antiviral drugs.

It is generally believed that Z exerts its proven clinical efficacy by some combination of its ultimate inhibition of the retroviral reverse transcriptase and/or its chain-terminating potential following its insertion into a growing DNA chain. Each of these effects is believed to be a direct effect of an anabolite of Z, namely, zidovudine triphosphate (ZTP). The pharmacodynamics of Z, therefore, will address the relationship between the concentration of ZTP at the intracellular site of the retroviral reverse transcriptase and either the degree of inhibition of reverse transcriptase or the efficiency with which a fraudulent nucleoside analogue is inserted into the growing DNA chain with subsequent chain termination. Several important lessons have been learned.

The relationship between the concentration of ZTP and the inhibition of the retroviral reverse transcriptase can be defined in terms of the usual enzymologic parameters using isolated and purified HIV reverse transcriptase. From *in vitro* studies of the enzyme, the K_i (the concentration necessary for 50% inhibition of enzymologic activity) for ZTP may be between 0.002 and 0.04 micromolar.[1-4] As a rule of thumb, nearly complete inhibition of an enzyme is achieved at about five times the K_i or about 0.2 micromolar. Thus, as a starting point, it might be assumed that optimal Z dosing would require a concentration of ZTP at the site of the retroviral reverse transcriptase of at least 0.2 micromolar throughout all of every dosing interval. This requirement would appear to be met only with doses of greater than 5 mg/kg given every 4 hours.[5] Although effectiveness may be optimal at such doses, toxicity is unacceptably high. Currently, doses of less than 1 mg/kg every 4 hours are being recommended, and clearly, the optimal theoretical level is not being achieved. The kinetics of the chain-terminating effect of ZTP are more complex and have, in fact, not been fully developed. As food for thought, it would seem reasonable to expect that at each site on the growing DNA chain into which a deoxythymidine should be positioned, the fraudulent nucleoside triphosphate analogue (zidovudine triphosphate) would be inserted with a likelihood that bears some relationship to the K_i for the enzyme. Assuming that the chance of inserting the correct nucleoside analogue is 95% and the chance of inserting the fraudulent ZTP is 5%, then there would be a 5% chance that the chain could not continue beyond that point and a 95% chance that it would continue. At the next site of insertion of a deoxythymidine, the chances should be exactly the same. The chances of inserting a correct deoxythymidine at both of the first two sites, however, should be 95% of 95% or 90.25 percent. Similarly, at the third deoxythymidine site, the chances of inserting all three deoxythymidines correctly should be 95% of 95% of 95% or 85.74 percent. Extending this series allows one to see that the statistical chance of producing a complete DNA copy of the HIV RNA would be virtually impossible statistically, even at a relatively low degree of inhibition and a relatively low chance of inserting the fraudulent nucleoside analogue at each individual site. It would seem that the results of this type of analysis would suggest that Z would be effective at exquisitely low concentrations, probably lower than those currently known to be effective. This hypothetical model could be amended by the additional consideration of repair enzymes that might excise fraudulent nucleoside analogues in order to maintain the integrity of the proviral DNA. Thus, it might be possible to correlate the proven biologic effects with the very low plasma zidovudine levels realized from current dosing schemes.

From an enzymologic standpoint it is also apparent that both the degree of inhibition of the HIV reverse transcriptase and the statistical chance of completing a faithful proviral DNA copy are influenced by the concentration of the endogenous and correct nucleoside triphosphate (deoxythymidine triphosphate) at the site of the reverse transcriptase as well as the concentration of the ZTP at the same site. Thus, the provision of higher levels of deoxythymidine triphosphate will successfully overcome the inhibition of the HIV reverse transcriptase by ZTP. It follows, then, that the effectiveness of Z will be a function of the intracellular deoxythymidine triphosphate level as well as the intracellular ZTP level over time. It also follows that if one were to be able to deplete the intracellular deoxythymidine triphosphate concentration, Z's effectiveness should be increased at any given ZTP level. Interestingly, Z itself appears to be effective in depleting intracellular deoxythymidine triphosphate levels.[1,6] This is believed to be due to the effect of intracellular zidovudine monophosphate (ZMP) as an inhibitor of thymidine kinase. Thus, the high intracellular levels of zidovudine monophosphate that are found in Z-treated cells lead to the concurrent depletion of intracellular deoxythymidine triphosphate. Several other drugs are capable of reducing intracellular deoxythymidine triphosphate levels. Dipyridamole blocks the transport of deoxythymidine across cell membranes while not effecting the transport of Z across cell membranes. Thus, dipyridamole should, in principle, be synergistic with zidovudine, and it appears that this is the case.[7,8]

As another example of the lessons learned to date with respect to pharmacodynamics, dextran sulfate is believed to act by inhibiting the binding of the human immunodeficiency virus to the CD4-containing cells. *In vitro* data suggests that this inhibition is nearly complete at a concentration of 2 μg/mL of dextran sulfate.[9] Thus, for this inhibition to be continuously effective, one would presume that it would be necessary to maintain levels of dextran sulfate of at least 2 μg/mL throughout all of every dosing interval. As discussed below, the oral administration of dextran sulfate will not produce these levels.[10]

There will also, of course, be some relationship between that concentration of a drug and its toxicologic effects. If the exact biochemical mechanism of the toxicity is known, then the relationship between the concentration of drug (or active metabolite) can be assessed *in vitro*. Unfortunately, the exact biochemical mechanism of the toxicity is seldom known. Nevertheless, the relationship between the concentration of drug and a biologic effect may be quantifiable, *in vitro* or *in vivo*.

Dextran sulfate serves as an excellent example. The major dose-limiting toxicity of dextran sulfate is its anticoagulant effect, and this can be conveniently and appropriately measured *in vitro* using the activated partial thromboplastin time (APTT) as the assay. Using this system, it becomes clear that unacceptable prolongation of the APTT (> 55 s) occurs at dextran sulfate levels above 8 μg/mL.[10]

The relationships of drug concentration to both anemia and neutropenia with Z, to peripheral neuropathy with dideoxycytidine, and to pancreatitis with dideoxyinosine are far less clear. The hematologic toxicity of zidovudine has been addressed by assessing the relationship between Z concentrations and the growth of bone marrow-derived hematologic precursor cells in culture. The value of these systems as predictive models for the relationships between Z levels and hematologic toxicity in humans remains to be defined.

A major lesson from the pharmacodynamics of anti-HIV drug toxicity is that assessing the toxicity of an anti-HIV drug and the relationship between drug concentrations and toxicity in the same cells in culture that are used to assess antiviral efficacy is, at best, of extremely limited value because this simple assessment fails to take cognizance of the multitude of possibilities for drug toxicity that have nothing whatsoever to do with any single cell type in culture. To phrase it more simply, cells in culture do not have livers, kidneys, brains, pancreases, or peripheral nerves that can all be sites of toxicity.

PHARMACOKINETICS

The effects of the host (humans) on the drug as a function of time as the drug passes through the body constitutes the pharmacokinetics of the drug. Antiviral chemotherapy differs from most other antimicrobial chemotherapy in that the site of viral replication is always intracellular and, therefore, it will usually be the intracellular level of an active drug in infected cells over time that will be critically important. We have clearly learned, at least for some nucleoside analogues that are currently being investigated, that it is not the drug as administered that is the active drug, but instead it is a metabolite of the administered drug that is the ultimate antiviral entity. Zidovudine, dideoxycytidine, and dideoxyinosine are examples of this phenomenon. Thus, for drugs such as these, the pharmacokinetics may be considered in two interrelated parts, that is, the intracellular pharmacokinetics and the more traditional extracellular pharmacokinetics.

Intracellular Pharmacokinetics

Using Z as an example, it is the intracellular ZTP that is the ultimate antiviral agent and the time course of its intracellular concentration that really matters. Unfortunately, the quantification of intracellular ZTP concentrations over time in infected cells, after zidovudine administration to humans, has proven intractable, because accessible infected cells are few in number and the ZTP concentrations are below the detection limits of currently available analytical technology. Clearly, the ability to measure intracellular ZTP levels in infected cells over time after *in vivo* administration of zidovudine to humans remains an important challenge.

In the absence of such direct measurements of intracellular ZTP, however, much has been learned that is relevant. It has been learned that Z is handled by infected cells similarly to the way it is handled in uninfected cells.[1] Thus, one may not have to be quite so handicapped in having to measure ZTP only in infected cells. It has also been learned, however, that different cell types and even different phases of the cell cycle in the same cell type handle Z differently.[11] Thus, we will have to focus our attention on lymphocytes and cells of the monocyte-macrophage lineage inasmuch as these are believed to be the major and possibly only cell types infected with the HIV. A considerable amount of information does exist for intracellular Z kinetics in these types of cells. Zidovudine appears to enter cells by simple diffusion,[12] thus differing from nucleobases and nucleosides that have transport systems facilitating intracellular transport. Nevertheless, Z diffuses into cells quite readily. Once inside the cell, Z is phosphorylated to ZMP by a cellular "thymidine kinase."[1,4] ZMP is further phosphorylated to zidovudine diphosphate (ZDP) by a cellular thymidylate kinase,[1,4] and ZDP is further phosphorylated to ZTP by a cellular deoxynucleoside diphosphate kinase.[4] At a biochemical level, the intracellular pharmacokinetics of ZTP will be dependent on the enzymologic characteristics of each of these enzymes. In addition, the intracellular enzymes that can use or break down each of the phosphorylated metabolites, including ZTP, will influence the intracellular pharmacokinetics of ZTP. These latter enzymes remain poorly defined. Overall, the relationship between extracellular Z and intracellular ZTP has been addressed *in vitro,* and some lessons have been learned. The intracellular ZTP levels are generally very low compared to extracellular Z levels.[4] Considerably higher intracellular ZMP levels exist than ZTP levels,[4] and ZDP levels are intermediary.[4] Most of the existing data are derived by incubating cells with a constant concentration of extracellular Z. As a result, we know little about the fluctuations over time of intracellular Z, ZMP, ZDP, and ZTP with the fluctuating extracellular Z levels that occur in humans when the drug is administered intermittently. There remains another interesting challenge. It is known that abrupt removal of extracellular Z leads to a rapid dissipation of intracellular ZTP levels, with a half-life that is only marginally longer than the half-life of Z itself in humans, that is, about one hour.[1] Thus, we may assume that intracellular ZTP levels will fluctuate in some rather close relationship with the fluctuating extracellular Z levels, albeit at a considerably lower concentration.

Extracellular Pharmacokinetics

Traditionally, pharmacokinetics has been divided into the absorption, distribution, metabolism, and excretion of drugs as well as overall descriptive parameters such as half-life, volume of distribution, and clearance.

Absorption

The most dramatic lesson focuses on dextran sulfate. Oral dextran sulfate was widely used, even though unapproved, and reasonably large controlled and uncontrolled clinical trials were instituted without knowing whether or not the drug was absorbed. When examined, it became clear that dextran sulfate was not absorbed to any significant extent, and its use and study has all but ceased.[10] Clearly, a drug with a purported site of action in the interior of the body must be absorbed. This is, fortunately, an unusual example with a complete lack of attention to the most basic of clinical pharmacologic principles. More commonly, less consequential but, nevertheless, important issues revolve around defining an extent of absorption that lies between 10% and 90% and whether the extent found is or is not sufficient to provide adequate plasma and tissues to be effective. Alternatively, the issues may revolve around defining the constancy or variability in absorption. Variable absorption may well contribute to the variable responses seen with each of the anti-HIV nucleoside analogues.

Distribution

In order to be effective any drug must have access to its site of action. Thus, a drug that acts inside cells must be distributed intracellularly as well as extracellularly, and if the drug must act in certain specific tissues, then it must be distributed to those tissues. Z illustrates this point. Z acts intracellularly and enters cells easily; thus, its ability to get to the site of action is excellent as long as it can get to the extracellular fluid surrounding the infected cell. In general, Z also appears to distribute throughout the body rather well, thus getting to the extracellular fluid surrounding most infected cells. The brain, however, appears to provide a sanctuary for HIV-infected cells.

Although some data exist with respect to cerebrospinal fluid concentrations in humans,[13] few data exist for brain concentrations, and it is the brain that is the usual CNS site of HIV infection rather than the meninges, that is, there is an encephalitis rather than a meningitis.[14] Within the brain, HIV may infect neural cells or may be confined to resident cells of the monocyte-macrophage lineage. In either case, the distribution of Z to the brain is important and incompletely understood.

Metabolism

Using Z as an example, its metabolism includes not only the intracellular anabolism to the active ZTP and the dissipation of ZTP as discussed above, but also the metabolism of Z to other products that do not lie on the pathway to ZTP. The major metabolic pathway, from a quantitative perspective, is the formation of the more water soluble zidovudine glucuronide (ZG) by the liver and possibly other tissues as well.[15] An understanding of the metabolic pathways followed for Z or any other drug allows one to predict clinical situations where dosing may need to be altered. For example, one could predict that newborns, who in general, cannot glucuronidate many drugs, would eliminate Z less rapidly than other children who, in turn, might eliminate Z more rapidly than do adults. Furthermore, one could intentionally or inadvertently lengthen or shorten the half-life of Z by inhibiting or inducing the glucuronyltransferase responsible for ZG formation. An example of the intentional inhibition of Z glucuronidization, that has been investigated as a potential means of prolonging the half-life of Z in order to reduce its cost as well as to provide a more convenient dosing interval, is the concurrent administration of probenecid.[16] Although probenecid clearly does lengthen the half-life of Z by about twofold, it may carry with it unacceptable toxicities.[17] Other possibilities remain to be tested. From a drug interaction perspective, one must be on guard for both the effects of other drugs that might inhibit or induce glucuronyltransferases as well as other drugs whose glucuronidization may be induced or inhibited by Z.

Excretion

Again, using Z as an example, its excretion is known to occur both as the parent unmetabolized drug and as the glucuronide. Diminished renal glomerular function might then be expected to have relatively little effect on the half-life of Z itself but to markedly prolong the half-life of ZG. Other drugs that are primarily excreted by glomerular filtration, should be more affected by impaired renal function.

Overall Pharmacokinetics

The overall pharmacokinetics of an anti-HIV agent, as with all drugs, can usually be summarized in terms of a few parameters such as half-life, volume of distribution, clearance, and sometimes a maximal velocity and concentration that provides half-maximal metabolism. Knowing these parameters, for any given drug, allows one to manipulate the doses and dosing regimens in numerous permutations in order to produce an array of patterns of drug concentrations versus time. The more enigmatic and ultimately more important questions, however, are What drug concentrations over time do we wish to achieve? Do we wish to attain plasma levels that correspond to an ED_{50}, ED_{90}, or ED_{99} in cells in culture? Do we wish to maintain levels above one of these values over every entire dosing interval? At the present time, we simply cannot choose our goals with any degree of confidence.

TIME-DEPENDENT PHARMACODYNAMICS

The biologic effects of some drugs correlate in a timely fashion with plasma drug levels. On the other hand, some drugs produce biologic effects that appear to have no relationship with plasma drug levels or, at best, an exceedingly complex relationship. Lessons have been learned from studies of drugs that have anti-HIV activity that are applicable to these situations as well.

As discussed above, the intracellular ZTP levels probably fluctuate over time in some relationship with simultaneously measured plasma Z levels. Dideoxycytidine (ddC) and dideoxyinosine (ddI), however, both behave differently in that the intracellular levels of dideoxycytidine triphosphate and dideoxyadenosine triphosphate, the active metabolites of ddC and ddI, respectively, appear to be maintained within cells longer than is ZTP after abrupt withdrawal of the extracellular drug.[18,19] Thus, it may be rational to dose ddC and ddI at less frequent dosing intervals than are necessary for Z because the pharmacokinetics of the active metabolites differ.

A more remarkable example of time-dependent pharmacodynamics is alpha interferon. Alpha interferon, when administered to humans either intravenously or intramuscularly, rapidly achieves peak plasma concentrations with a subsequent relatively rapid disappearance of the drug from the plasma, with a half-life of about five hours.[20] The biologic effect of interferon, however, as measured by its induction of the enzyme 2'-5'oligoadenylate synthetase and its production of an antiviral state, peaks later (6-24 hours) and persists considerably longer (2-3 days).[21,22] This is compatible with the fact that alpha interferon interacts with a receptor on the cell surface and initiates a cascade of events that continues within the target cell for some prolonged period of time even in the absence of the continued presence of alpha interferon at the cell surface. This type of relationship between the pharmacodynamics of a drug and time may be relevant to other biologic response modifiers or drugs that act by binding to a cell surface receptor and inducing a subsequent cascade of events that persists in the absence of the stimulus itself.

CONCLUSIONS

It is clear that many lessons have already been learned or relearned as the field of antiviral chemotherapy has emerged from its childhood into a vigorous adolescence. As the field matures, numerous new lessons will surely be learned that will be of enormous value for the study of AIDS as well as for the study of many other viral illnesses.

REFERENCES

1. FURMAN, P. A., J A. FYFE, M. H. ST. CLAIR, K. WEINHOLD, J. L. RIDEOUT, G. A. FREEMAN, S. N. LEHRMAN, D. P. BOLOGNESI, S. BRODER, H. MITSUYA & D. W. BARRY. 1986. Proc. Natl. Acad. Sci. USA **83:** 8333-8337.
2. VRANG, L., H. BAZIN, G. REMAUD, J. CHATTOPADHYAYA & B. OBERG. 1987. Antiviral Res. **7:** 139-149.
3. ST. CLAIR, M. H., C. A. RICHARDS, T. SPECTOR, K. J. WEINHOLD, W. H. MILLER, A. J. LANGLOIS & P. A. FURMAN. 1987. Antimicrob. Agents Chemother. **31:** 1972-1977.
4. FURMAN, P. A. & D. W. BARRY. 1988. Am. J. Med. **85:** 176-181.
5. CLOAD, P. A. 1989. J. Infect. Dis. **18:** 15-21.
6. FRICK, L. W., D. J. NELSON, M. H. ST. CLAIR, P. A. FURMAN & T. A. KRENITSKY. 1988. Biochem. Biophys. Res. Comm. **154:** 124-129.
7. SZEBENI, J., S. M. WAHL, M. POPOVIC, L. M. WAHL, S. GARTNER, R. L. FINE, U. SKALERIC, R. M. FRIEDMAN & J. N. WEINSTEIN. 1989. Proc. Natl. Acad. USA **86:** 3842-3846.
8. BETAGERI, G. V., J. SZEBENI, K. HUNG, S. S. PATEL, L. M. WAHL, M. CORCORAN & J. N. WEINSTEIN. 1990. Biochem. Pharmacol. **40:** 867-870.
9. MITSUYA, H., D. J. LOONEY, S. KUNO, R. UENO, F. WONG-STAAL & S. BRODER. 1988. Science **240:** 646-649.
10. LORENTSEN, K. J., C. W. HENDRIX, J. M. COLLINS, D. M. KORNHAUSER, B. G. PETTY, R. W. KLECKER, C. FLEXNER, R. H. ECKEL & P. S. LIETMAN. 1989. Ann. Intern. Med. **111:** 561-566.
11. RICHMAN, D. D., R. S. KORNBLUTH & D. A. CARSON. 1987. J. Exp. Med. **166:** 1144-1149.
12. ZIMMERMAN, T. P., W. B. MAHONY & K. L. PRUS. 1987. J. Biol. Chem. **262:** 5748-5754.
13. KLECKER, R. W., J. M. COLLINS, R. YARCHOAN, R. THOMAS, J. F. JENKINS, S. BRODER & C. E. MYERS. 1987. Clin. Pharmacol. Ther. **41:** 407-412.
14. TERASAKI, T. & W. M. PARDRIDGE. 1988. J. Infect. Dis. **158:** 630-632.
15. BLUM, M. R., S. H. T. LIAO, S. S. GOOD & P. DE MIRANDA. 1988. Am. J. Med. **85**(Suppl 2A): 189-194.
16. KORNHAUSER, D. M., B. G. PETTY, C. W. HENDRIX, A. S. WOODS, L. J. NERHOOD, J. G. BARTLETT & P. S. LIETMAN. 1989. Lancet ii: 473-475.
17. PETTY, B. G., D. M. KORNHAUSER & P. S. LIETMAN. LANCET i: 1044-1045.
18. STARNES, M. C. & Y.-C. CHENG. 1987. J. Biol. Chem. **262:** 988-991.
19. AHLUWALIA, G., M. A. JOHNSON, A. FRIDLAND, D. A. COONEY, S. BRODER & D. G. JOHNS. 1988. Am. Assoc. Cancer Res. **29:** 349.
20. WILLS, R. J., S. DENNIS, H. E. SPIEGEL, D. M. GIBSON & P. L. NADLER. 1984. Clin. Pharmacol. Ther. **35:** 722-727.
21. BAROUKI, F. M., F. R. WITTER, D. E. GRIFFIN *et al.* 1987. J. Interferon Res. **7:** 206-211.
22. WITTER, F., F. BAROUKI, D. GRIFFIN, P. NADLER, A. WOODS, D. WOOD & P. LIETMAN. 1987. Clin. Pharmacol. Ther. **42:** 567-575.

Impaired Immunity in AIDS

The Mechanisms Responsible and Their Potential Reversal by Antiviral Therapy[a]

CURTIS L. RUEGG AND EDGAR G. ENGLEMAN

Department of Pathology, L235
Stanford University School of Medicine
Stanford, California 94305

INTRODUCTION

The acquired immunodeficiency syndrome (AIDS) is the end stage of a progressive clinical disorder that is caused by the human immunodeficiency virus type 1 (HIV-1).[1] Since the discovery of HIV-1, much has been learned about its genetic makeup, its life cycle, and the mechanism by which it seeks out and infects a few selected cell types. Indeed, despite extensive sequence variation between different HIV-1 isolates[2] (due to an extremely high rate of mutation during replication of the viral genome in infected cells), HIV-1 appears to use a single protein as its obligate cell-surface receptor. This protein, called CD4 (or T4 or Leu 3), is expressed on the surface of certain mononuclear cells and serves as a beacon for HIV-1, which attaches to it through the virally encoded envelope glycoprotein (outer coat) gp120.[3–6] Shortly after HIV-1 attaches to CD4, its envelope fuses with the plasma membrane of the CD4-expressing cells,[7] enabling the viral capsid (consisting of viral genomic RNA and the enzyme reverse transcriptase that converts RNA to DNA) to enter the cytoplasm where the viral RNA is replicated as DNA that eventually makes its way to the nucleus and inserts ("integrates") itself into the host cell genome. Thus, cells that express the CD4 molecule (CD4+ cells) are susceptible to HIV-1 infection, whereas cells that lack CD4 (CD4− cells) are resistant.[4] There is evidence that some CD4− cells can be infected *in vitro*,[8–11] however, proof of productive HIV-1 infection of CD4− cells, *in vivo*, is still lacking. By contrast, infection of CD4+ cells is not only routinely detectable but, as described below, an obligate step in disease pathogenesis.

Because CD4 serves as an important cell-surface receptor for HIV-1, knowledge of the types and functions of cells that express CD4 should provide us with information about where HIV-1 can be found in infected persons as well as the likely consequences of infection. The CD4 protein is expressed almost exclusively by mononuclear leukocytes,[4] which are bone marrow-derived cells that participate in the body's defense against infections. Although not every mononuclear cell expresses CD4, those that do so play critical roles in the immune response. These cells include a subpopulation of lympho-

[a]This work was supported by Grants AI72657 and AI25922 from the National Institutes of Health.

307

cytes that undergo maturation in the thymus (T cells) and two other bone marrow-derived cell types, the major function of which is to present foreign antigens to T cells: the monocyte/macrophage and lymphoid dendritic cell. The latter cell type, which includes Langerhans' cells of the skin as well as dendritic cells found in the thymus, lymph nodes, and peripheral blood, should not be confused with follicular dendritic cells, which are not derived from bone marrow.

As a result of HIV-1 infection, one of these cell types, the CD4+ T cell, becomes functionally impaired, gradually decreases in number, and in late stages of disease virtually disappears.[1,12] Inasmuch as CD4+ T cells are responsible for initiating an immune response to many types of foreign antigens, including infectious pathogens, it is not surprising that HIV-1-infected patients tend to be particularly susceptible to infections. Indeed, most of the clinical manifestations resulting from HIV-1 infection are felt to be consequences of either impaired function or depletion of CD4+ T cells. On this basis, there is great interest in deciphering the mechanisms used by the virus to paralyze and ultimately destroy CD4+ T cells. The nature of these mechanisms and their potential for reversal through antiviral therapy are the subjects of this report.

MECHANISMS RESPONSIBLE FOR QUALITATIVE CD4+ T-CELL DYSFUNCTION

In addition to whatever disruption of immune function results from direct infection of CD4+ T cells by HIV-1, a number of studies have shown that noninfectious HIV-1 inhibits lymphoproliferation, *in vitro,* in response to T-cell mitogens and recall antigens independent of infection.[13] This immunosuppressive activity has been shown to reside within structural determinants of the HIV-1 envelope proteins gp120 and gp41 as well as the viral regulatory protein tat. Using recombinant forms of gp120, investigators have demonstrated that this component of HIV-1 inhibits T-cell proliferation in response to both recall antigens[14,15] and mitogens.[16] Chirmule and colleagues further characterized this effect of gp120 and showed that T-cell activation mediated by way of the CD3/T-cell receptor complex (CD3/TCR) was specifically inhibited, but gp120 had no effect on activation mediated by way of other T-cell activation pathways, such as CD2, CD28, and direct activation by costimulation with phorbol 12-myristate 13-acetate (PMA) and the Ca^{2+} ionophore ionomycin.[17] Recent data from Mittler and co-workers have extended these findings to demonstrate that gp120 and anti-gp120 antibodies from HIV-1-infected individuals synergize to inhibit CD3/TCR signal transduction at lower concentrations than that required for gp120 alone.[18] In general, it is presumed that the mechanism by which gp120 inhibits CD4+ T-cell function involves the binding of gp120 to CD4, which disrupts interactions between CD4 and MHC class II proteins as well as immune functions dependent upon those interactions.[19]

As an extension of earlier studies involving the immunosuppressive properties of the transmembrane protein p15E of animal retroviruses, we[20] and others[21] have identified a short envelope amino acid (aa) sequence, 581-597, from the HIV-1 transmembrane protein gp41 that is homologous to the suppressive sequence of p15E, is highly conserved across distinct HIV-1 isolates, and inhibits T-cell activation *in vitro* when presented to cells in the form of a synthetic peptide. We have gone on to characterize the molecular mechanism of this immunosuppressive aa581-597 peptide and demonstrated that it inhibits both protein kinase C (PKC) and intracellular Ca^{2+} influx, the two arms of the phosphoinositide hydrolysis pathway used by CD3/TCR to transduce T-cell activation.[22] In contrast to the restriction of gp120-mediated inhibition to CD3/TCR signals described above, the gp41-derived aa581-597 peptide inhibits activation mediated by CD2, CD28, and PMA/ionomycin stimulation as well as by CD3/TCR (Ruegg and Strand, submitted). This paralysis of immune activation at the level of the second messengers PKC and Ca^{2+} is similar to that observed for lymphocytes from AIDS patients.[23]

Two additional regions near the carboxy terminal end of gp41 have also been shown to contain suppressive amino acid sequences (aa735-752, aa846-860) that inhibit mitogenic T-cell stimulation[24] and natural killer cell function.[25] Neither of these sequences exhibits any homology to the aa581-597 sequence described above, and therefore they presumably inhibit immune function by way of a distinct mechanism.

Finally, gp41 has been shown to induce autoreactive antibodies in HIV-1-infected individuals due to sequence similarity of the aa837-844 region of gp41 with MHC class II antigen.[26] These autoantibodies were shown to block antigen- and allo-stimulated $CD4^+$ T-cell proliferation and thus mark uninfected $CD4^+$ MHC class II-positive T cells as targets for antibody-dependent cellular cytotoxicity (ADCC).

Direct immunosuppressive activity of HIV-1 proteins is not limited to the envelope polypeptides but has also been shown for another HIV-1 product known as tat.[27] These investigators carried out antigen- and mitogen-driven T-cell proliferation assays in the presence of tat and found that this HIV-1 protein blocked activation of T cells stimulated by way of antigen but not mitogen. A potential mechanism for this suppressive activity of tat has been supplied in a preliminary communication by Lotz et al.[28] who have reported that tat can transactivate the transcriptional promoter element of transforming growth factor-beta (TGF-beta), a cytokine with potent immunosuppressive activity. They related this finding to that observed in vivo by showing that both mRNA and protein expression for TGF-beta are upregulated in lymphocyte cultures from HIV-1-infected individuals as compared to normal lymphocytes and that the impaired proliferation of these cultures can be restored by neutralizing TGF-beta activity with specific anti-TGF-beta antibody.

Impaired antigen presentation by monocytes and dendritic cells may also contribute to $CD4^+$ T-cell dysfunction in HIV-1-infected individuals. Monocytes isolated from AIDS patients have been observed to exhibit reduced phagocytic[29] and chemotactic[30] activities as well as reduced expression of HLA class II antigens[31] and accessory function in anti-CD3-induced T-cell activation.[32] Many if not all of these defects, however, appear to be reversible by the addition of exogenous interferon-gamma[33,34] and thus may result from defective stimulation by $CD4^+$ T cells. Direct infection of monocytes with HIV-1 in vitro or treatment with purified gp120 elicits a somewhat mixed response involving both down-modulation of chemotactic function and enhanced expression of HLA class II.[35] The relevance of these in vitro observations to clinical disease is unresolved in light of the low incidence of infection of monocytes in vivo.

MECHANISMS RESPONSIBLE FOR DEPLETION OF CD4+ T CELLS

Although $CD4^+$ T-cell dysfunction is an early and prevailing symptom of HIV-1-infected individuals, there is a strong correlation between the onset of advanced and severe symptoms of AIDS, such as opportunistic infection, with dramatic reduction in the number of circulating $CD4^+$ T cells.[36] Early explanations for this quantitative depletion of CD4$^+$ T cells consisted of the direct destruction of infected cells due to the cytopathic effects of HIV-1 and the recruitment of uninfected CD4$^+$ T cells into multinucleated syncytia following interaction of gp120 expressed on the surface of HIV-1-infected cells with CD4 on the surface of uninfected cells.[6,37,38] The characteristic process of HIV-1-induced syncytium formation can be readily observed in HIV-1-infected cultures consisting of immunologically stimulated CD4$^+$ T cells or T-cell lines and has been shown conclusively to result from cell-to-cell fusion dependent upon interactions between viral envelope components and CD4.[6,37,38] In many, although certainly not all, *in vitro* assay systems, the cytopathic process of CD4-dependent HIV-1 envelope-mediated cell fusion appears to be the major mechanism by which HIV-1 infection leads to cell death.[6,37,38] A prominent feature of this process is the ability of HIV-1 envelope-expressing infected cells or syncytia to "recruit" uninfected CD4-expressing cells into increasingly large syncytia, which go on to die. Even in assay systems in which cell fusion is not a prominent feature, but in which HIV-1 infection-associated death of single cells occurs, interactions between HIV-1 envelope components and CD4 have been postulated to result in localized membrane perturbations leading eventually to metabolic disruption and osmotic death.[39] Other factors, ranging from accumulation of unintegrated viral DNA[40] to "terminal" differentiative events linked to immunologic activation of infected cells,[41,42] have been proposed to contribute to HIV-induced cell death; however, CD4-dependent cell fusion appears to be the major mechanism of HIV-1-mediated cell death in those *in vitro* assay systems characterized by prominent viral cytopathology. The CD4 molecule may also play a role in receptor-mediated superinfection, a process that has been postulated to be a cause of cytopathology in other retroviral systems[40] and recently in HIV-1 as well.[43]

In addition to the mechanisms proposed above to explain HIV-1-mediated cell killing *in vitro,* additional mechanisms have been hypothesized to explain how HIV-1 infection, *in vivo,* leads to a progressive decrease in the number of CD4$^+$ cells and resulting immunocompromise. Various autoimmune phenomena, in which uninfected CD4$^+$ cells may be destroyed in the course of immune responses triggered by HIV-1 infection, have been suggested. For example, cytotoxic autoantibodies reactive with an antigen expressed on activated or HIV-1-infected CD4$^+$ cells have been proposed to contribute to depletion of such cells *in vivo.*[44] In another suggested mechanism, free HIV-1 gp120 may be selectively adsorbed to uninfected CD4-expressing cells through gp120/CD4 interactions. This gp120, in either native or processed forms, is postulated to render CD4$^+$ cells expressing viral envelope determinants susceptible to lysis by gp120-specific cytotoxic T lymphocytes[45,46] or to render gp120-coated cells susceptible to killing through ADCC mechanisms.[47] Independent of any direct or indirect cytotoxic effects, free gp120 may also contribute to depletion of CD4-expressing cells by triggering cellular activation, potentially rendering cells more susceptible to HIV-1 infection or more permissive for viral replication.[48] Finally, recent studies by Zarling *et al.* have suggested that circulating CD8$^+$ T cells in HIV-1-infected patients are capable of selectively lysing CD4$^+$ cells in a non-MHC restricted manner (personal communication).

CAN CD4$^+$ T-CELL DEPLETION BE EXPLAINED BY THE DIRECT CYTOPATHIC EFFECT OF HIV-1 INFECTION?

Perhaps the simplest proposed explanation for CD4$^+$ T-cell depletion in HIV-1-infected patients is that these cells die as a direct consequence of infection due to viral envelope mediated events. In support of this concept is the recent report of Schnittman et al. indicating that as many as 1 in 100 CD4$^+$ T cells are HIV-1 infected in late-stage patients.[49] Although this number may seem too low to account for the massive T-cell depletion observed in such patients, if 1% of the CD4$^+$ cells are continuously being infected, dying, and disappearing, such a process could eventually result in substantial cell loss. If the cytopathic effects of CD4$^+$ T-cell infection with HIV-1 is a major cause of CD4$^+$ T-cell depletion in HIV-1-infected patients, then the total viral load would be expected to increase prior to or in parallel with reduction in the number of CD4$^+$ cells. In early-stage patients, however, with normal CD4$^+$ T-cell counts, the percentage of HIV-1-infected CD4$^+$ cells is low (estimated to be less than 1 in 1,000) compared to the percentage in late-stage (AIDS) patients (estimated to be 1 in 100).[49] Furthermore, the available data would suggest that in symptomatic as well as asymptomatic HIV-1-infected patients at least 90% of CD4$^+$ T cells containing HIV-1 DNA are in a latent stage of infection,[49] which does not, by definition, affect cell viability. Thus, higher titers of HIV-1 in blood as well as higher frequencies of HIV-1 infected cells are found after CD4$^+$ T-cell depletion, not before. The possibility exists that longitudinal, serial studies of HIV-1 DNA levels in individual patients might reveal a sudden increase in the frequency of virally infected cells or viral burden just prior to dramatic declines of CD4$^+$ T cells. In many patients, however, the decline of the CD4$^+$ T-cell count occurs gradually over a period of months or years.

It can be argued that one reason for the failure to detect a higher frequency of productively infected T cells, in vivo, is that the switch from latency to active viral replication occurs in lymphoid organs (rather than peripheral blood) where T-cell activation takes place, and that such productively infected cells do not circulate but rather die in situ shortly after the onset of viral replication. If so, examination of the lymph nodes of HIV-1-infected patients should reveal a veritable graveyard of CD4$^+$ T cells. This does not appear to be the case, however, based on available data. Therefore, whereas HIV-1 infection of CD4$^+$ T cells with cell death resulting from viral envelope-mediated events contributes to CD4$^+$ T-cell depletion, this mechanism alone probably does not account for the massive depletion of T cells observed in end-stage disease.

THE ROLE OF CD4$^+$ T-CELL DEPLETION IN THE CLINICAL MANIFESTATION OF AIDS

Despite a strong inverse correlation between the number of circulating CD4$^+$ T cells and the likelihood of opportunistic infection in HIV-1-infected patients,[36] a direct cause and effect relationship between CD4$^+$ T-cell counts and clinical outcome has not yet been proved. Indeed, mice rendered completely depleted of T cells by x-irradiation apparently survive quite well if they are reconstituted with normal T cells to a level of only 1-2% of that of untreated control animals. Moreover, humans treated with fractionated total lymphoid irradiation (TLI), the treatment of choice for early-stage Hodgkin's lymphoma and an experimental therapy for certain autoimmune diseases as well as a treatment to prevent rejection of transplant organs, tolerate this treatment well and experience no increase in the incidence of life-threatening infections despite the fact that their levels of CD4$^+$ T cells are profoundly reduced.[50,51] On the other hand, whereas abnormally low CD4$^+$ T-cell counts (200-500) persist for periods of one year and longer in such patients, levels of less than 200 are rarely seen for more than a few months following completion of TLI.[52] Therefore, it can be argued that partial depletion of CD4+ T cells can be well-tolerated for prolonged periods (greater than one year), and more profound depletion can be tolerated for at least several months in the absence of HIV-1 infection. It is possible that more prolonged CD4+ T-cell depletion (in the absence of HIV-1 infection) would increase the risk of opportunistic infections. The possibility must be considered, however, that factors in addition to CD4+ T-cell depletion play a critical role in rendering late-stage patients increasingly susceptible to the clinical manifestations of AIDS. The nature of such factors has yet to be defined.

DOES A DEFECT IN T-CELL REGENERATION PLAY A SIGNIFICANT ROLE IN THE DEPLETION OF CD4+ T CELLS?

Finally, in potential collaboration with the mechanisms listed above for the active destruction of CD4+ T cells, HIV-1 infection may also adversely affect replenishment of the CD4+ T-cell pool *in vivo*. Although the extent and role of T-cell regeneration in adults is unknown, there is indirect evidence that HIV-1 infection adversely affects the maturation of CD4+ T cells and that a failure to regenerate CD4+ T cells contributes to the overall depletion of these cells in late-stage patients. Thus, HIV-1-uninfected patients, whose CD4+ T-cell compartment is nearly ablated as a consequence of treatment with TLI, regain normal responses to alloantigen within 3-5 years.[53] By contrast, the loss of the CD4+ T-cell compartment in patients with late-stage HIV-1 infection is rarely reversed, even in the presence of antiviral therapy, suggesting that the capacity to regenerate T cells in these patients is severely compromised.

What can be said regarding the role of thymic defects in HIV-1-associated CD4+ T-cell dysfunction? Clearly, the thymus of end-stage AIDS patients is virtually destroyed.[54-56] The possibility also exists that the thymus is affected early in the course of HIV-1 infection, inasmuch as most immature thymocytes are CD4+ and presumably susceptible to HIV-1 penetration. If, however, a high proportion of T-cell precursors in the thymus or bone marrow were infected and later released into the periphery as mature T cells, a much higher proportion of circulating T cells would demonstrate the presence of HIV-1 DNA than has been observed. In addition, it is widely held that thymic precursors of CD8+ T cells express CD4 as well as CD8 molecules and, therefore, HIV-1-infected CD8+ T cells should be readily detectable in AIDS patients and/or CD8+ T cells should be depleted in parallel with CD4+ T cells. Because this is not the case, it is necessary to hypothesize that HIV-1 infection of the thymus or bone marrow results in defective T-cell maturation and/or the failure to release mature T cells into the periphery, and that precursors of CD4+ cells are more susceptible to these effects than precursors of CD8+ cells. Such effects might occur as a consequence of HIV-1 infection of cell types other than maturing T cells, such as macrophages, dendritic cells, or epithelial cells, all of which play essential roles in the maturation of T cells.

In summary, we suggest that the thymus is profoundly affected by HIV-1 infection, because destruction of peripheral T cells appears insufficient to account for the massive T-cell depletion observed in late-stage disease. Of course this assumes that in healthy, uninfected adults the thymus retains some T-cell regenerating capacity. This would seem to be the case inasmuch as adult patients rendered profoundly T lymphopenic from therapy, such as TLI, eventually regain normal or nearly normal T-cell counts and immune function. Although the hypothesized thymic defects in HIV-1-infected patients may or may not be reversible (see below), such defects may nonetheless be critical to the ultimate disappearance of CD4+ T cells in these patients. Remarkably, no direct evidence to support this hypothesis has yet emerged.

ARE CD4+ T-CELL DYSFUNCTION AND DEPLETION REVERSIBLE IN AIDS PATIENTS?

Despite the large number and diversity of the putative mechanisms responsible for CD4+ T-cell dysfunction and depletion in HIV-1-infected patients, most have in common a critical role for the HIV-1 envelope glycoproteins, gp120 and/or gp41. For example, transfection or infection with the HIV-1 envelope gene alone is sufficient for syncytia formation or single cell death,[37,38] and no other HIV-1 gene or gene product has yet been shown to contribute to these phenomena. Similarly, most of the nonlytic mechanisms proposed to explain T-cell dysfunction in early-stage disease are mediated by envelope gene products. On this basis, one might predict that suppression of HIV-1 replication, *in vivo*, would be followed by a reversal of immune suppression; that is, virtually all of the mechanisms reviewed in this report are potentially reversible. This prediction is consistent with our recent observation that incubation of T cells from HIV-1 infected patients for 1-2 days, *in vitro*, reversed defective immune responses (D. Ritter and E. Engleman, manuscript in preparation). Moreover, some azidothymidine (AZT, zidovudine)-treated HIV-1-infected patients reportedly recover delayed-type hypersensitivity responses as measured by skin-test reactivity to tuberculin and other recall antigens, and some patients show rises in the number of circulating CD4+ T cells. The fact that such "immune recovery" is transient can be ascribed to the eventual failure of AZT treatment to control viral replication, *in vivo*, due to the selection for AZT-resistant strains of HIV-1.

Can we infer from the above that more prolonged suppression of HIV-1 replication, as might be anticipated with newer anti-HIV-1 drugs or combinations of drugs, would result in prolonged recovery of the immune system? Based on the information reviewed here, the answer is yes, provided that the capacity to regenerate T cells has not been irrevocably lost as a consequence of HIV-1 infection. On an optimistic note, the fact that relatively few T cells appear to be required for maintenance of seemingly normal immune function suggests that a return to normal numbers of mature T cells may not be essential for resistance to opportunistic infections. Even if the thymus is completely or nearly completely destroyed, immunologic "recovery" may be possible if the remaining T cells are not irreversibly damaged. Of particular importance in this regard is the fate of long-lived memory T cells, which are thought to be responsible for maintaining immune responses to ubiquitous, opportunistic organisms of the types known to cause life-threatening infections in AIDS patients. As discussed previously, memory CD4+ T-cell function tends to be lost early in the course of HIV-1 infection. Whether the T cells mediating this function have been destroyed or, alternatively, "paralyzed" is unknown, but the answer to this question takes on paramount importance to the consideration of possible immunologic recovery. Clearly, if memory T cells are irreversibly damaged or deleted, then an intact thymus would be essential to reconstitute essential immune responses. In the event that the thymus is destroyed and memory T cells are deleted, then the only recourse would be that of thymic transplantation.

SUMMARY

The inability of CD4$^+$ T cells of HIV-1-infected patients to mount an effective immune response is widely believed to explain the increased susceptibility of these patients to opportunistic infections. Although the full explanation for T-cell dysfunction in HIV-1 infection is not yet understood, at least two fundamentally distinct mechanisms are thought to contribute: depletion of CD4$^+$ T cells and qualitative CD4$^+$ T-cell dysfunction independent of T-cell depletion. Many HIV-1-infected patients manifest reduced T-cell responses to recall antigens prior to measurable CD4$^+$ T-cell depletion, and among the proposed explanations for this phenomenon are gp120-mediated interference with T-cell activation by way of inhibition of CD4-class II major histocompatibility complex (MHC) determinant interactions, gp41-mediated inhibition of protein kinase C-dependent T-cell activation, formation of gp41 cross-reactive antibodies that react with MHC class II determinants, transforming growth factor-beta (TGF-beta)-mediated immunosuppression, and decreased functions of antigen-presenting and antigen-processing cells (macrophages and bone marrow-derived dendritic cells). Despite their detection in most HIV-1-infected patients, these qualitative T-cell defects do not herald the onset of life-threatening disease. The appearance of severe clinical manifestations of AIDS, particularly opportunistic infections, occurs primarily in patients whose CD4$^+$ T-cell count is significantly reduced. Depletion of CD4$^+$ T cells may be a direct consequence of HIV-1 infection that occurs as a result of syncytia formation, autoantibody-mediated cytolysis, gp120-specific antibody-dependent cytolysis, and/or gp120-specific T-cell mediated cytolysis. The thymus is severely affected in patients with late-stage disease, and although there is no proof that the failure of the thymus to regenerate new T cells contributes to T-cell depletion in patients with AIDS, the likelihood seems high that this is the case. Indeed, if prolonged suppression of HIV-1 replication can be achieved with newer anti-HIV drugs or combinations of drugs, reconstitution of a normal immune system seems likely, provided that the capacity to regenerate T cells has not been irrevocably lost as a consequence of viral infection. In summary, available evidence indicates that HIV-1 uses a complex array of mechanisms to disrupt T-cell mediated immunity, but because most of these involve a direct role for HIV-1 proteins, such mechanisms are likely to be reversible if suppression of HIV-1 replication can be achieved.

REFERENCES

1. FAUCI, A. S. 1988. The human immunodeficiency virus: infectivity and mechanisms of pathogenesis. Science **239:** 617-622.
2. STARCICH, B. R., B. H. HAHN, G. M. SHAW, P. D. MCNEELY, S. MODROW, H. WOLF, E. S. PARKS, W. P. PARKS, S. F. JOSEPHS, R. C. GALLO & F. WONG-STAAL. 1986. Identification and characterization of conserved and variable regions in the envelope gene of HTLV-III/LAV, the retrovirus of AIDS. Cell **45:** 637-648.
3. DALGLEISH, A. G., P. C. L. BEVERLEY, P. R. CLAPHAM, D. H. CRAWFORD, M. F. GREAVES & R. A. WEISS. 1984. The CD4 (T4) antigen is an essential component of the receptor for the AIDS retrovirus. Nature **312:** 763-767.
4. MADDON, P. J., A. G. DALGLEISH, J. S. MCDOUGAL, P. R. CLAPHAM, R. A. WEISS & R. AXEL. 1986. The T4 gene encodes the AIDS virus receptor and is expressed in the immune system and the brain. Cell **47:** 333-348.

5. SATTENTAU, Q. J. & R. A. WEISS. 1988. The CD4 antigen: physiological ligand and HIV receptor. Cell **52**: 631-633.
6. LIFSON, J. D., G. R. REYES, M. S. MCGRATH, B. S. STEIN & E. G. ENGLEMAN. 1986. AIDS retrovirus induced cytopathology: giant cell formation and involvement of CD4 antigen. Science **232**: 1123-1127.
7. STEIN, B. S., S. D. GOWDA, J. D. LIFSON, R. C. PENHALLOW, K. G. BENSCH & E. G. ENGLEMAN. 1987. pH-Independent HIV entry into CD4-positive T cells via virus envelope fusion to the plasma membrane. Cell **49**: 659-668.
8. TATENO, M., F. GONZALEZ-SCARANO & J. A. LEVY. 1989. Human immunodeficiency virus can infect CD4-negative human fibroblastoid cells. Proc. Natl. Acad. Sci. USA **86**: 4287-4290.
9. CHESEBRO, B., R. BULLER, J. PORTIS & K. WEHRLY. 1990. Failure of human immunodeficiency virus entry and infection in CD4-positive human brain and skin cells. J. Virol. **64**: 215-221.
10. HAROUSE, J. M., C. KUNSCH, H. T. HARTLE, M. A. LAUGHLIN, J. A. HOXIE, B. WIGDAHL & F. GONZALEZ-SCARANO. 1989. CD4-independent infection of human neural cells by human immunodeficiency virus type 1. J. Virol. **63**: 2527-2533.
11. CLAPHAM, P. R., J. N. WEBER, D. WHITBY, K. MCINTOSH, A. G. DALGLEISH, P. J. MADDON, K. C. DEEN, R. W. SWEET & R. A. WEISS. 1989. Soluble CD4 blocks the infectivity of diverse strains of HIV and SIV for T cells and monocytes but not for brain and muscle cells. Nature **337**: 368-370.
12. EDELMAN, A. S. & S. ZOLLA-PAZNER. 1989. AIDS: a syndrome of immune dysregulation, dysfunction, and deficiency. FASEB J. **3**: 22-30.
13. PAHWA, S., R. PAHWA, C. SAXINGER, R. C. GALLO & R. A. GOOD. 1985. Influence of the human T-lymphotropic virus/lymphadenopathy-associated virus on functions of human lymphocytes: Evidence for immunosuppressive effects and polyclonal B-cell activation by banded viral preparations. Proc. Natl. Acad. Sci. USA **82**: 8198-8202.
14. SHALABY, M. R., J. F. KROWKA, T. J. GREGORY, S. E. HIRABYASHI, S. M. MCCABE, D. S. KAUFMAN, D. P. STITES & A. J. AMMANN. 1987. The effects of human immunodeficiency virus recombinant envelope glycoprotein on immune cell functions *in vitro*. Cell. Immunol. **110**: 140-148.
15. MANN, D. L., F. LASANE, M. POPOVIC, L. O. ARTHER, W. G. ROBEY, W. A. BLATTNER & M. J. NEWMAN. 1987. HTLV-III large envelope protein (gp120) suppresses PHA-induced lymphocyte blastogenesis. J. Immunol. **138**: 2640-2644.
16. DIAMOND, D. C., B. P. SLECKMAN, T. GREGORY, L. A. LASKY, J. L. GREENSTEIN & S. J. BURAKOFF. 1988. Inhibition of CD4+ T cell function by the HIV envelope protein p120. J. Immunol. **141**: 3715-3717.
17. CHIRMULE, N., V. S. KALYANARAMAN, N. OYAIZU, H. B. SLADE & S. PAHWA. 1990. Inhibition of functional properties of tetanus antigen-specific T-cell clones by envelope glycoprotein gp120 of human immunodeficiency virus. Blood **75**: 152-159.
18. MITTLER, R. S. & M. K. HOFFMAN. 1989. Synergism between HIV gp120 and gp120-specific antibody in blocking human T cell activation. Science **245**: 1380-1382.
19. CHIRMULE, N., V. KALYANARAMAN, N. OYAIZU & S. PAHWA. 1988. Inhibitory influences of envelope glycoproteins of HIV-1 on normal immune responses. J. AIDS **1**: 425-430.
20. RUEGG, C. L., C. R. MONELL & M. STRAND. 1989. Inhibition of lymphoproliferation by a synthetic peptide with sequence identity to gp41 of human immunodeficiency virus type 1. J. Virol. **63**: 3257-3260.
21. CIANCIOLO, G. J., H. BOGERD & R. SNYDERMAN. 1988. Human retrovirus-related synthetic peptides inhibit T lymphocyte proliferation. Immunology Letters **19**: 7-13.
22. RUEGG, C. L. & M. STRAND. 1990. Inhibition of protein kinase C and anti-CD3-induced Ca^{2+} influx in Jurkat T cells by a synthetic peptide with sequence identity to HIV-1 gp41. J. Immunol. **144**: 3928-3935.
23. HOFMANN, B., J. MOLLER, E. LANGHOFF, K. D. JAKOBSEN, N. ODUM, E. DICKMEISS, L. P. RYDER, O. THASTRUP, O. SCHARFF, B. FODER, P. PLATZ, C. S. PETERSEN, L. MATHIESEN, T. HARTVIG-JENSEN, P. SKINHOJ & A. SVEJGAARD. 1989. Stimulation of AIDS lymphocytes with calcium ionophore (A23187) and phorbol ester (PMA): Studies of cytoplasmic free Ca, IL-2 receptor expression, IL-2 production, and proliferation. Cell. Immunol. **119**: 14-21.

24. CHANH, T. C., R. C. KENNEDY & P. KANDA. 1988. Synthetic peptides homologous to HIV transmembrane glycoprotein suppress normal human lymphocyte blastogenic response. Cell. Immunol. 111: 77-86.

25. CAUDA, R., M. TUMBARELLO, L. ORTONA, P. KANDA, R. C. KENNEDY & T. C. CHANH. 1988. Inhibition of normal human natural killer cell activity by human immunodeficiency virus synthetic transmembrane peptides. Cell. Immunol. 115: 57-65.

26. GOLDING, H., G. M. SHEARER, K. HILLMAN, P. LUCAS, J. MANISCHEWITZ, R. A. ZAJAC, M. CLERICI, R. E. GRESS, R. N. BOSWELL & B. GOLDING. 1989. Common epitope in human immunodeficiency virus (HIV) I-gp41 and HLA class II elicits immunosuppressive autoantibodies capable of contributing to immune dysfunction in HIV I-infected individuals. J. Clin. Invest. 83: 1430-1435.

27. VISCIDI, R. P., K. MAYUR, H. M. LEDERMAN & A. D. FRANKEL. 1989. Inhibition of antigen-induced lymphocyte proliferation by tat protein from HIV-1. Science 246: 1606-1608.

28. LOTZ, M., J. KEKOW, M. T. CRONIN, J. A. MCCUTCHAN, I. CLARK-LEWIS, D. A. CARSON & W. WACHSMAN. 1990. Induction of transforming growth factor-beta (TGF-beta) by HIV-1 tat; a noncytopathic pathway of immunodeficiency in HIV infection. FASEB J. 4: A2014.

29. ESTEVEZ, M. E., I. G. BALLARD, R. A. DIEZ, N. PLANES, C. SCAGLIONE & L. SIN. 1986. Early defect of phagocytic cell function in subjects at risk for acquired immunodeficiency syndrome. Scand. J. Immunol. 24: 215-221.

30. SMITH, P. D., K. CHURA, H. MASUR, H. C. LANE, A. S. FAUCI & S. M. WAHL. 1984. Monocyte function in the acquired immunodeficiency syndrome defective chemotaxis. J. Clin. Invest. 74: 2121-2124.

31. HEAGY, W., V. E. KELLEY, J. B. STROM & K. MAYER. 1984. Decreased expression of human class II antigens on monocytes from patients with acquired immune deficiency syndrome increased expression with interferon-gamma. J. Clin. Invest. 74: 2089-2096.

32. GARTNER, S., P. MARKOVITS, D. M. MARKOVITZ, M. H. KAPLAN, R. C. GALLO & M. POPOVIC. 1986. The role of mononuclear phagocytes in HTLV-III infection. Science 233: 215-219.

33. MURRAY, H. W., R. A. GELLENE, D. M. LIBBY, C. D. ROTHERMEL & B. Y. RUBIN. 1985. Activation of tissue macrophages from AIDS patients: in vitro response of AIDS alveolar macrophages to lymphokines and interferon-gamma. J. Immunol. 135: 2374-2377.

34. MURRAY, H. W., D. SCAVUZZO, J. L. JACOBS, M. H. KAPLAN, D. M. LIBBY, J. SCHINDLER & R. B. ROBERTS. 1987. In vitro and in vivo activation of human mononuclear phagocytes by interferon-gamma. Studies with normal and AIDS monocytes. J. Immunol. 138: 2457-2462.

35. WAHL, S. M., J. B. ALLEN, S. GARTNER, J. M. ORENSTEIN, M. POPOVIC, D. E. CHENOWETH, L. O. ARTHUR, W. L. FARRAR & L. M. WAHL. 1989. HIV-1 and its envelope glycoprotein down-regulate chemotactic ligand receptors and chemotactic function of peripheral blood monocytes. J. Immunol. 142: 3553-3559.

36. LIFSON, A. R., G. W. RUTHERFORD & H. W. JAFFE. 1988. The natural history of human immunodeficiency virus infection. J. Infect. Dis. 158: 1360-1367.

37. SODROSKI, J., W. C. GOH, C. ROSEN, K. CAMPBELL & W. A. HASELTINE. Role of the HTLV-III/LAV envelope in syncytium formation and cytopathology. Nature 322: 470-474.

38. LIFSON, J. D., M. B. FEINBERG, G. R. REYES, L. RABIN, B. BANAPOUR, S. CHAKRABARTI, B. MOSS, F. WONG-STAAL, K. S. STEIMER & E. G. ENGLEMAN. 1986. Induction of CD4-dependent cell fusion by the HTLV-III/LAV envelope glycoprotein. Nature 323: 725-728.

39. HASELTINE, W. A. 1988. Replication and pathogenesis of the AIDS virus. J. AIDS 1: 217.

40. TEMIN, H. M. 1988. Mechanisms of cell killing/cytopathic effects by nonhuman retroviruses. Rev. Infect. Dis. 10: 399.

41. ZAGURY, D., J. BERNARD, R. LEONARD, R. CHEYNIER, M. FELDMAN, P. S. SARIN & R. C. GALLO. 1986. Long-term cultures of HTLV-III-infected T cells: a model of T cell depletion in AIDS. Science 231: 850-853.

42. LEONARD, R., D. ZAGURY, I. DESPORTES, J. BERNARD, J.-F. ZAGURY & R. C. GALLO. 1988. Cytopathic effect of human immunodeficiency virus in T4 cells is linked to the last stage of virus infection. Proc. Natl. Acad. Sci. USA 85: 3570-3574.

43. STEVENSON, M., C. MEIER, A. M. MANN, N. CHAPMAN & A. WASIAK. 1988. Envelope glycoprotein of HIV induces interference and cytolysis resistance in CD4⁺ cells: mechanism for persistence in AIDS. Cell **53**: 483-496.
44. STRICKER, R. B., T. M. McHUGH, D. J. MOODY, W. J. W. MORROW, D. P. STITES, M. A. SHUMAN & J. A. LEVY. 1987. An AIDS-related cytotoxic autoantibody reacts with a specific antigen on stimulated CD4⁺ T cells. Nature **327**: 710-713.
45. SILICIANO, R. F., T. LAWTON, C. KNALL, R. W. KARR, P. BERMAN, T. GREGORY & E. L. REINHERZ. 1988. Analysis of host-virus interactions in AIDS with anti-gp120 T-cell clones: effect of HIV sequence variation and a mechanism for CD4⁺ cell depletion. Cell **54**: 561-575.
46. ORENTAS, R. J., J. E. K. HILDRETH, E. OBAH, M. POLYDEFKIS, G. E. SMITH, M. L. CLEMENTS & R. F. SILICIANO. 1990. Induction of CD4⁺ human cytolytic T cells specific for HIV-infected cells by a gp160 subunit vaccine. Science **248**: 1234-1237.
47. WEINHOLD, K. J., H. K. LYERLY, S. D. STANLEY, A. A. AUSTIN, T. J. MATTHEWS & D. P. BOLOGNESI. 1989. HIV-1 gp120-mediated immune suppression and lymphocyte destruction in the absence of viral infection. J. Immunol. **142**: 3091-3097.
48. KORNFELD, H., W. W. CRUIKSHANK, S. W. PYLE, J. BERMAN & D. M. CENTER. 1988. Lymphocyte activation by HIV-1 envelope glycoprotein. Nature **335**: 445-448.
49. SCHNITTMAN, S. M., M. C. PSALLIDOPOULOS, H. C. LANE, L. THOMPSON, M. BASELER, F. MASSARI, C. H. FOX, N. P. SALZMAN & A. S. FAUCI. 1989. The reservoir for HIV-1 in human peripheral blood is a T cell that maintains expression of CD4. Science **245**: 305-308.
50. KOTZIN, B. L., G. S. KANSAS, E. G. ENGLEMAN, R. T. HOPPE, H. S. KAPLAN & S. STROBER. 1983. Changes in T-cell subsets in patients with rheumatoid arthritis treated with total lymphoid irradiation. Clin. Immunol. Immunopathol. **27**: 250-260.
51. KOTZIN, B. L., S. STROBER, E. G. ENGLEMAN, A. CALIN, R. T. HOPPE, G. S. KANSAS, C. P. TERRELL & H. S. KAPLAN. 1981. Treatment of intractable rheumatoid arthritis with total lymphoid irradiation. N. Engl. J. Med. **305**: 969-976.
52. STROBER, S., E. FIELD, R. T. HOPPE, B. L. KOTZIN, O. SHEMESH, E. ENGLEMAN, J. C. ROSS & B. D. MYERS. 1985. Treatment of intractable lupus nephritis with total lymphoid irradiation. Ann. Intern. Med. **102**: 450-458.
53. FUKS, Z., S. STROBER, A. M. BOBROVE, T. SASAZUKI, A. McMICHAEL & H. S. KAPLAN. 1976. Long term effects of radiation on T and B lymphocytes in peripheral blood of patients with Hodgkin's disease. J. Clin. Invest. **58**: 803-814.
54. DAVIS, JR., A. E. 1984. The histopathological changes in the thymus gland in the acquired immune deficiency syndrome. Ann. N.Y. Acad. Sci. **437**: 493-502.
55. GRODY, W. W., S. FLIGIEL & F. NAEIM. 1985. Thymus involution in the acquired immunodeficiency syndrome. Am. J. Clin. Pathol. **84**: 85-95.
56. JOSHI, V. V., J. M. OLESKE, S. SAAD, C. GADOL, E. CONNOR, R. BOBILA & A. B. MINNEFOR. 1986. Thymus biopsy in children with acquired immunodeficiency syndrome. Arch. Pathol. Lab. Med. **110**: 837-842.

New Developments in Combination Chemotherapy of Anti-Human Immunodeficiency Virus Drugs

VICTORIA A. JOHNSON AND MARTIN S. HIRSCH

Infectious Disease Unit
Department of Medicine
Massachusetts General Hospital
Harvard Medical School
Boston, Massachusetts 02114

INTRODUCTION

Although HIV-1 continues to cause major worldwide devastation, marked progress has occurred in the development of antiviral agents to attack this virus. Advances include the demonstration of zidovudine efficacy at various stages of infection (M. Fischl, *et al.,*[1] P. Volberding, *et al.,*[2]), the early evaluation of other HIV reverse transcriptase inhibitors that may improve therapeutic indices over zidovudine, and the study of newer agents with novel mechanisms of antiretroviral action[3-7] (TABLE 1). Several of these promising agents are undergoing clinical evaluation[7] (FIG. 1). Despite these advances, the frequent dose-limiting toxicity of drugs as single agents at higher doses,[8,9] as well as the reports of emergence of zidovudine-resistant HIV variants during prolonged monotherapy,[10] have signaled the need for improved strategies. In this review, we will focus on one promising approach to this problem, that is, the development of combination therapy for HIV infection.

THE DEVELOPMENT OF COMBINATION THERAPY FOR HIV INFECTION

There is ample precedent for the use of combination therapy for HIV-1 infection in the demonstrated efficacy of multidrug treatment for many bacterial and fungal infections, as well as in cancer chemotherapy. Ideally, the major goal of this therapeutic strategy for HIV-infected individuals should be the ability to achieve increased efficacy and/or reduced toxicity. It is likely that combinations of agents that target different sites in the HIV-1 replicative cycle will afford prolonged effective therapy. When two agents are combined, they may interact in one of three ways[11]: (1) Additive effect: Two drugs are said to be additive when the activity of the drugs in combination is equal to the sum (or a partial sum) of their independent activities when studied separately. (2)

Synergism: The combined effect of a synergistic pair of agents is greater than the sum of their independent activities when measured separately (*i.e.*, greater than the expected additive effect). (3) Antagonism: If two drugs are antagonistic, the activity of the combination is less than the sum of their independent effects when measured alone (*i.e.*, less than the expected additive effect).

To assess drug interactions, a mathematical analysis of the data is preferable given the complexities of dose-effect relationships in biologic assays. We evaluate our drug interactions by the median-effect principle and the isobologram technique.[12-14] A review of the methods available, and their mathematical limitations, are described elsewhere.[12-14]

TABLE 1. Targets for Anti-HIV Agents[a]

Target in Viral Replicative Cycle	Agents
Viral adsorption or entry	Recombinant soluble CD4 or its analogues
	Neutralizing antibodies
	Inhibitors of viral uncoating
Reverse transcriptase inhibitors	Zidovudine
	Dideoxycytidine
	Dideoxyinosine
	Other nucleoside analogues
	Inhibitors of RNase H activity
Integration of DNA into host genetic material	Inhibitors of integrase function
Viral gene expression	Anti-tat agents
	Antisense oligodeoxynucleotides
Posttranscriptional or posttranslational processing, assembly, or release	Glycoprotein processing inhibitors
	castanospermine
	deoxynojirimycin derivatives
	Myristylation inhibitors
	Protease inhibitors
	Interferons

[a] The antiviral effect of some of these agents has not been firmly established; for some there may be more than one mode of action, and for others the mechanism is unclear. Some of these listings are theoretical interventions and not currently available for testing.

Anti-HIV drug combination therapies offer several potential advantages over single drug therapy, especially if antiviral synergistic interactions occur leading to more complete virus suppression. Such an approach may allow the reduction of component agents below their toxic concentrations and may reduce the opportunity for the emergence of drug-resistant HIV mutants. An optimal combination regimen should affect virus replication in a broad range of cell types and should not display overlapping (*i.e.*, additive or synergistic) toxicity. Drugs should generally not be used in combination in patients until they have been studied thoroughly as single agents to avoid incorrect conclusions concerning combined benefit or toxicity. The steps involved in the development of combination therapy for HIV infection are similar to those involved in single agent therapy.

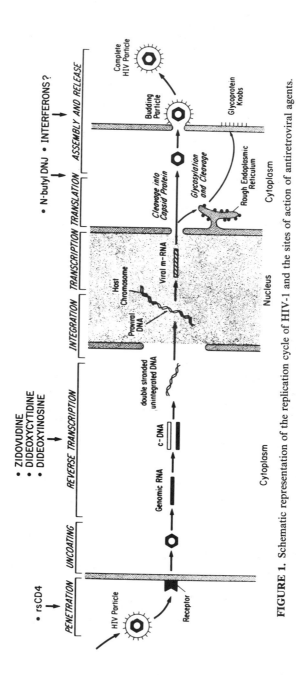

FIGURE 1. Schematic representation of the replication cycle of HIV-1 and the sites of action of antiretroviral agents.

DRUG COMBINATIONS TESTED AGAINST
HIV REPLICATION *IN VITRO*

Drug Combinations with Synergistic Activity against HIV Replication in Vitro

Combination therapies that have been found to have synergistic interactions *in vitro* in our laboratory are outlined in TABLE 2.[15-23] We will highlight recent work on several combinations: (a) zidovudine (AZT) and recombinant soluble CD4 (rsCD4), (b) zidovudine plus either castanospermine (CAS) or *N*-butyl 1-deoxynojirimycin (*N*-butyl DNJ), and (c) the three-drug regimen of zidovudine, rsCD4, and recombinant interferon-alpha-A (rIFN-α-A).

TABLE 2. *In Vitro* Interactions of Drug Combinations for HIV Infection

Combination	Interaction[a]	Reference Number
Zidovudine plus:		
Recombinant soluble CD4 (rsCD4)	Synergism	15
Interferon-alpha (rIFN-α-A)	Synergism	16
Castanospermine (CAS)	Synergism	17
N-butyl 1-deoxynojirimycin (*N*-butyl DNJ)	Synergism	18
Ribavirin	Antagonism	19
Zidovudine plus rsCD4 plus rIFN-α-A	Synergism	20
2′,3′-dideoxycytidine (ddC) plus interferon-alpha (rIFN-α-A)	Synergism	21
Foscarnet plus interferon-alpha (rIFN-α-A)	Synergism	22
Castanospermine plus recombinant soluble CD4 (rsCD4)	Synergism	23

[a] See text for definitions.

Zidovudine and rsCD4

Earlier studies in our laboratory[25] and others[24,26-28] demonstrated that rsCD4, as a single agent, is a potent inhibitor of HIV-1 in CD4-positive lymphoid cells. In our combination studies, synergism was seen with multiple drug concentrations in diverse cell types without cytotoxicity.[15] In H9 cells (a CD4$^+$ T-cell line) acutely infected with HIV-1 (500 TCID$_{50}$ of strain HTLV-IIIB/10^6 cells), combinations of rsCD4 (≥ 0.02 μg/mL) and zidovudine (≥ 0.16 μM) inhibited HIV-1 synergistically on day 10, as measured by p24 antigen production, reverse transcriptase activity, yield of infectious virus, and HIV-1 antigen expression by immunofluorescence. In acutely infected peripheral blood mononuclear cells (PBMC), a dose-dependent inhibition of HIV-1 replication was observed throughout ten days in culture with rsCD4 (0.02-0.32 μg/mL) and zidovudine (0.003-0.040 μM) when each was tested as a single agent. Combinations of rsCD4 at concentrations of ≥ 0.08 μg/mL and zidovudine at concentrations of

≥ 0.01 μM inhibited HIV-1 synergistically on day 10. Even though rsCD4 (0.02-0.32 μg/ mL) and zidovudine (0.003-0.040 μM) as single agents were less effective against HIV-1 replication by day 14 in PBMC, combinations of rsCD4 at concentrations of ≥ 0.16 μg/mL and zidovudine at concentrations of ≥ 0.02 μM demonstrated synergistic interactions that both increased over time and persisted through day 14. In an acutely HIV-1-infected CD4$^+$ monocytic cell line (the HLA-DR$^+$ clone of the BT4 cell line), synergistic interactions were seen with rsCD4 (0.001-0.080 μg/mL) and zidovudine (0.01-0.64 μM) at multiple drug concentrations over the twelve day course of the experiment. In all of these experiments, the combination index values were <1. Clinical trials of AZT and recombinant soluble CD4 are planned or underway.

Zidovudine and either CAS or N-butyl DNJ

The glycosylation inhibitors CAS and *N*-butyl DNJ have been shown by our group[29] and others[30–32] to be inhibitors of HIV-1 replication. The use of these agents as monotherapy at higher doses, however, may be limited by toxic effects on normal cellular metabolism[33] and altered glycogen distribution.[34]

We have studied both CAS and *N*-butyl DNJ in combination with AZT.[17,18] In acutely infected H9 cells, the combinations of CAS (21-339 μM) and zidovudine (0.04-0.64 μM) inhibited HIV-1 synergistically, as measured by p24 antigen production, RT activity, and infectious virus yield. In acutely infected PBMC, combinations of CAS (42-339 μM) and zidovudine (0.02-0.16 μM) synergistically inhibited both HIV-1 and HIV-2 on day 7.[17] Concentrations of CAS as low as 21-42 μM resulted in synergistic interactions with zidovudine *in vitro,* without apparent cellular toxicity.

We also evaluated *N*-butyl DNJ in combination with AZT.[18] Cultures of H9 cells were exposed simultaneously to HIV-1 and various concentrations of each agent. *N*-butyl DNJ (0.156-40 μM) and AZT (0.01-2.56 μM) were added either alone or in combined regimens. Representative data regarding the inhibition of HIV-1 p24 antigen production (ng/10^6 cells) on day 11 in culture are shown in TABLE 3. In acutely infected H9 cells, the combination of *N*-butyl DNJ (≥ 10 μg/mL) and AZT (≥ 0.64 μM) inhibited HIV-1 synergistically without additive toxicity. This combination may deserve consideration for future clinical trials.

The Three-Drug Regimen of Zidovudine, rsCD4, and rIFN-α-A

We have recently completed the first three-drug combination study in HIV-1 infection *in vitro.* We evaluated whether more complete virus suppression could be attained with three anti-HIV agents in combination, using agents that each attack different targets in the HIV-1 replicative cycle *in vitro,* when compared to one- or two-drug regimens. We found that zidovudine, rsCD4, and rIFN-α-A inhibited HIV-1 synergistically in two- and three-drug regimens using PBMC and a CD4-positive T-cell line (H9).[20] The three-drug regimen provided more complete virus suppression than the two-drug regimens. In acutely infected H9 cells, single drug regimens lost effectiveness at 10-14 days, and two-drug regimens lost effectiveness at 14-18 days with zidovudine at 2.56 μM, rsCD4 at 0.32 μg/mL, and rIFN-α-A at 128 U/mL. In contrast, the three-drug regimen showed nearly complete suppression over 28 days in culture without toxicity. Clinical trials of these three drugs in combination are planned.

Antagonistic Combination—Zidovudine plus Ribavirin in Vitro

Not all drugs have favorable interactions against HIV-1 replication when combined. As seen in TABLE 2, the combination of zidovudine plus ribavirin was found to be antagonistic.[19] The mechanism of this antagonism appears to be the ribavirin-induced elevations of deoxythymidine triphosphate levels that feed back negatively to inhibit the host cell cytosolic thymidine kinase required for phosphorylation of zidovudine to its active triphosphate form.[19,35] Thus, combination regimens should be tested *in vitro* prior to testing in clinical trials, particularly agents that may share common metabolic pathways.

Drug Combinations Tested in Vitro *Elsewhere*

Reports of anti-HIV combination testing in other laboratories are summarized in TABLE 4. Many of these studies provide insufficient data regarding the analysis of their drug interactions to assess synergistic, additive, or antagonistic effects *in vitro*.

TABLE 3. Inhibition of HIV-1 p24 Antigen Production by *N*-Butyl DNJ and AZT[a]

Experiment No.	Infected Control	*N*-butyl DNJ (10 µg/mL)	AZT (0.64 µM)	*N*-butyl DNJ and AZT
1	5423	4011	3075	73
2	4837	3694	2478	495

[a]HIV-1 p24 antigen production is expressed as ng/10^6 cells using H9 cells on day 11 in culture.

CLINICAL TRIALS OF COMBINATION THERAPY FOR HIV INFECTION

Many potential problems arise when clinical trials of combinations are considered, which represent an amplification of the problems one encounters conducting trials of single agents. These difficulties include patient heterogeneity, controversial study end points, and optimal sample sizes to achieve statistical significance. The distinction between additive and synergistic effects (for both toxicity and benefit) is often impossible due to confounding variables such as compliance, concurrent medications, and dose reductions of component drugs. Rather than be dissuaded from a combination therapy approach, however, ample insight into these potential pitfalls should help guide the proper design of clinical studies that will provide meaningful results.

Several clinical trials, planned or in progress, involve combination therapy for HIV-1 infection (see TABLE 5). These trials include combinations of antiretroviral agents, as well as combinations of antiretroviral agents with immunomodulators and/

TABLE 4. Antiretroviral Combinations Tested *in Vitro* Elsewhere

Combination
Zidovudine and acyclovir
Zidovudine and GM-CSF[a]
Zidovudine and dextran sulfate
Zidovudine and ampligen
Zidovudine and amphotericin B
Zidovudine and dipyridamole
Ribavirin and dideoxycytidine
Purine nucleoside analogue NSC-614846 and either ribavirin or zidovudine
Zidovudine and an acyclic adenosine analogue (PMEA)
Zidovudine and foscarnet
Zidovudine and interferon-beta
Zidovudine and isoprinosine
Zidovudine alternating with 2′,3′-dideoxycytidine
2′,3′-dideoxycytidine and recombinant soluble CD4
2′,3′-dideoxyinosine and recombinant soluble CD4
2′,3′-dideoxycytidine and dextran sulfate
2′,3′-dideoxyinosine and dextran sulfate
Recombinant soluble CD4 and dextran sulfate

[a] Granulocyte-macrophage colony-stimulating factor.

TABLE 5. Clinical Trials of Combination Therapies for HIV Infection

Combination
Zidovudine in combination with the following agent:
IFN-alpha
IFN-beta
acyclovir
erythropoietin (EPO)
foscarnet
interleukin-2
recombinant soluble CD4 (rsCD4)
2′,3′-dideoxycytidine
GM-CSF
Three-drug regimens:
Zidovudine plus GM-CSF plus IFN-alpha
Zidovudine plus G-CSF[a] plus EPO
Zidovudine plus IFN-alpha plus rsCD4
Zidovudine alternating with the following agent:
2′,3′-dideoxycytidine
GM-CSF

[a] Granulocyte colony-stimulating factor.

or biologic response modifiers. These two- and three-drug regimens are administered either in combination or in sequence.

CONCLUSIONS

Many anti-HIV combination therapies are undergoing evaluation in clinical trials, and preliminary results with several of these regimens look promising. Combination regimens should be evaluated *in vitro* initially, prior to the careful design of clinical trials, in order to evaluate both beneficial and toxic drug interactions. Not all combination regimens can be assumed to have favorable interactions, as noted by the demonstration of antagonistic anti-HIV effects between zidovudine and ribavirin. This may be particularly important for agents that share common intracellular metabolic pathways. Certain two- or three-drug combination regimens, however, may provide enhanced virus suppression, allowing component dose reduction below toxic concentrations. In addition, combination therapy may prevent or reduce the emergence of drug-resistant HIV-1 variants.

REFERENCES

1. FISCHL, M.A., D. D. RICHMAN, N. HANSEN, A. C. COLLIER, J. T. CAREY, M. F. PARA, W. D. HARDY, R. DOLIN, W. G. POWDERLY, J. D. ALLAN, B. WONG, T. C. MERIGAN, V. J. MCAULIFFE, N. E. HYSLOP, F. S. RHAME, H. H. BALFOUR, S. A. SPECTOR, P. VOLBERDING, C. PETTINELLI, J. ANDERSON & THE AIDS CLINICAL TRIALS GROUP. 1990. The safety and efficacy of zidovudine (AZT) in the treatment of subjects with mildly symptomatic human immunodeficiency virus type 1 (HIV) infection. A double-blind, placebo-controlled trial. Ann. Intern. Med. 112: 727-737.
2. VOLBERDING, P. A., S. W. LAGAKOS, M. A. KOCH, C. PETTINELLI, M. W. MYERS, D. K. BOOTH, H. H. BALFOUR, R. C. REICHMAN, J. A. BARTLETT, M. S. HIRSCH, R. L. MURPHY, W. D. HARDY, R. SOEIRO, M. A. FISCHL, J. G. BARTLETT, T. C. MERIGAN, N. E. HYSLOP, D. D. RICHMAN, F. T. VALENTINE, L. COREY & THE AIDS CLINICAL TRIALS GROUP OF THE NATIONAL INSTITUTE OF ALLERGY AND INFECTIOUS DISEASES. 1990. Zidovudine in asymptomatic human immunodeficiency virus infection. A controlled trial in persons with fewer than 500 CD4-positive cells per cubic millimeter. N. Engl. J. Med. 322: 941-949.
3. YARCHOAN, R., H. MITSUYA, R. V. THOMAS, J. M. PLUDA, N. R. HARTMAN, C. F. PERNO, K. S. MARCZYK, J.-P. ALLAIN, D. G. JOHNS & S. BRODER. 1989. *In vivo* activity against HIV and favorable toxicity profile of 2',3'-dideoxyinosine. Science 245: 412-415.
4. YARCHOAN, R., H. MITSUYA & S. BRODER. 1989. Clinical and basic advances in the antiretroviral therapy of human immunodeficiency virus infection. Am. J. Med. 87: 191-200.
5. YARCHOAN, R., H. MITSUYA, C. E. MYERS & S. BRODER. 1989. Clinical pharmacology of 3'-azido-2',3'-dideoxythymidine (zidovudine) and related dideoxynucleosides. N. Engl. J. Med. 321: 726-738.
6. SANDSTROM, E. 1989. Antiviral therapy in human immunodeficiency virus infection. Drugs 38: 417-450.
7. HIRSCH, M. S. 1990. Chemotherapy of human immunodeficiency virus infections: current practice and future prospects. J. Infect. Dis. 161: 845-857.
8. RICHMAN, D. D., M. A. FISCHL, M. H. GRIECO, M. S. GOTTLIEB, P. A. VOLBERDING, O. L. LASKIN, J. M. LEEDOM, J. E. GROOPMAN, D. MILDVAN, M. S. HIRSCH, G. G.

JACKSON, D. T. DURACK, S. NUSINOFF-LEHRMAN & THE AZT COLLABORATIVE WORKING GROUP. 1987. The toxicity of azidothymidine (AZT) in the treatment of patients with AIDS and AIDS-related complex. A double-blind, placebo-controlled trial. N. Engl. J. Med. **317**: 192-197.

9. MERIGAN, T. C., G. SKOWRON, S. A. BOZZETTE, D. RICHMAN, R. UTTAMCHANDANI, M. FISCHL, R. SCHOOLEY, M. HIRSCH, W. SOO, C. PETTINELLI, H. SCHAUMBURG & THE ddC STUDY GROUP OF THE AIDS CLINICAL TRIALS GROUP. 1989. Circulating p24 antigen levels and responses to dideoxycytidine in human immunodeficiency virus (HIV) infections. A phase I and II study. Ann. Intern. Med. **110**: 189-194.

10. LARDER, B. A., G. DARBY & D. D. RICHMAN. 1989. HIV with reduced sensitivity to zidovudine (AZT) isolated during prolonged therapy. Science **243**: 1731-1734.

11. MOELLERING, R. C. 1990. Principles of anti-infective therapy. *In* Principles and Practice of Infectious Diseases. G. L. Mandell, R. G. Douglas & J. E. Bennett, Eds. Third Edition: 212-3. Churchill Livingstone Inc. New York.

12. CHOU, T.-C. & P. TALALAY. 1984. Quantitative analysis of dose-effect relationships: the combined effects of multiple drugs or enzyme inhibitors. Adv. Enzyme Regul. **22**: 27-55.

13. CHOU, T.-C. & P. TALALAY. 1987. Applications of the median-effect principle for the assessment of low-dose risk of carcinogens and for the quantitation of synergism and antagonism of chemotherapeutic agents. *In* New Avenues in Developmental Cancer Chemotherapy. Bristol-Myers Cancer Symposia Series. K. R. Harrap & T. A. Connors, Eds.: 37-64. Academic Press. Orlando, FL.

14. CHOU, J. & T.-C. CHOU. 1987. Dose-effect analysis with microcomputers: quantitation of ED_{50}, LD_{50}, synergism, antagonism, low-dose risk, receptor-ligand binding and enzyme kinetics. *In* A computer software for IBM-PC and manual. Elsevier-Biosoft. Cambridge, UK.

15. JOHNSON, V. A., M. A. BARLOW, T.-C. CHOU, R. A. FISHER, B. D. WALKER, M. S. HIRSCH & R. T. SCHOOLEY. 1989. Synergistic inhibition of human immunodeficiency virus type 1 (HIV-1) replication *in vitro* by recombinant soluble CD4 and 3'-azido-3'-deoxythymidine. J. Infect. Dis. **159**: 837-844.

16. HARTSHORN, K. L., M. W. VOGT, T.-C. CHOU, R. S. BLUMBERG, R. BYINGTON, R. T. SCHOOLEY & M. S. HIRSCH. 1987. Synergistic inhibition of human immunodeficiency virus *in vitro* by azidothymidine and recombinant alpha A interferon. Antimicrob. Agents Chemother. **31**: 168-172.

17. JOHNSON, V. A., B. D. WALKER, M. A. BARLOW, T. J. PARADIS, T.-C. CHOU & M. S. HIRSCH. 1989. Synergistic inhibition of human immunodeficiency virus type 1 and type 2 replication *in vitro* by castanospermine and 3'-azido-3'-deoxythymidine. Antimicrob. Agents Chemother. **33**: 53-57.

18. JOHNSON, V. A., D. P. MERRILL, T.-C. CHOU & M. S. HIRSCH. 1989. Synergistic inhibition of HIV-1 replication by *N*-butyl deoxynojirimycin (*N*-butyl DNJ) and zidovudine (AZT) (abstr. #504). *In* Proceedings of the Twenty-ninth Interscience Conference on Antimicrobial Agents and Chemotherapy. Houston, Texas. September 17-20: 185.

19. VOGT, M. W., K. L. HARTSHORN, P. A. FURMAN, T.-C. CHOU, J. A. FYFE, L. A. COLEMAN, C. CRUMPACKER, R. T. SCHOOLEY & M. S. HIRSCH. 1987. Ribavirin antagonizes the effect of azidothymidine on HIV replication. Science **235**: 1376-1379.

20. JOHNSON, V. A., M. A. BARLOW, D. P. MERRILL, T.-C. CHOU & M. S. HIRSCH. 1990. Three-drug synergistic inhibition of HIV-1 replication *in vitro* by zidovudine, recombinant soluble CD4, and recombinant interferon-alpha A. J. Infect. Dis. **161**: 1059-1067.

21. VOGT, M. W., A. G. DURNO, T.-C. CHOU, L. A. COLEMAN, T. J. PARADIS, R. T. SCHOOLEY, J. C. KAPLAN & M. S. HIRSCH. 1988. Synergistic interaction of 2',3'-dideoxycytidine and recombinant interferon-α-A on replication of human immunodeficiency virus type I. J. Infect. Dis. **158**: 378-385.

22. HARTSHORN, K. L., E. G. SANDSTROM, D. NEUMEYER, T. J. PARADIS, T.-C. CHOU, R. T. SCHOOLEY & M. S. HIRSCH. 1986. Synergistic inhibition of human T-cell lymphotropic virus type III replication *in vitro* by phosphonoformate and recombinant alpha-A interferon. Antimicrob. Agents Chemother. **30**: 189-191.

23. JOHNSON, V. A., B. D. WALKER, T. J. PARADIS, P. A. BARLOW, J. SODROSKI, T.-C. CHOU, R. T. SCHOOLEY & M. S. HIRSCH. 1988. Synergistic inhibition of HIV-1 replication by castanospermine (CAS) and either zidovudine (AZT) or recombinant soluble CD4 (rsT4).

(Abstr. #3618). *In* Programs and Abstracts of the IV International Conference on AIDS, Stockholm, Sweden, June 12-16: Vol. 2: 171.

24. SMITH, D. H., R. A. BYRN, S. A. MARSTERS, T. GREGORY, J. E. GROOPMAN & D. J. CAPON. 1987. Blocking of HIV-1 infectivity by a soluble, secreted form of the CD4 antigen. Science **238:** 1704-1707.

25. FISHER, R. A., J. M. BERTONIS, W. MEIER, V. A. JOHNSON, D. S. COSTOPOULOS, T. LIU, R. TIZARD, B. D. WALKER, M. S. HIRSCH, R. T. SCHOOLEY & R. T. FLAVELL. 1988. HIV infection is blocked *in vitro* by recombinant soluble CD4. Nature **331:** 76-78.

26. HUSSEY, R. E., N. E. RICHARDSON, M. KOWALSKI, N. R. BROWN, H.-C. CHANG, R. F. SILICIANO, T. DORFMAN, B. WALKER, J. SODROSKI & E. L. REINHERZ. 1988. A soluble CD4 protein selectively inhibits HIV replication and syncytium formation. Nature **331:** 78-81.

27. DEEN, K. C., J. S. MCDOUGAL, R. INACKER, G. FOLENA-WASSERMAN, J. ARTHOS, J. ROSENBERG, P. J. MADDON, R. AXEL & R. W. SWEET. 1988. A soluble form of CD4 (T4) protein inhibits AIDS virus infection. Nature **331:** 82-84.

28. TRAUNECKER, A., W. LUKE & K. KARJALAINEN. 1988. Soluble CD4 molecules neutralize human immunodeficiency virus type 1. Nature **331:** 84-86.

29. WALKER, B. D., M. KOWALSKI, W. C. GOH, K. KOZARSKY, M. KRIEGER, C. ROSEN, L. ROHRSCHNEIDER, W. A. HASELTINE & J. SODROSKI. 1987. Inhibition of human immunodeficiency virus syncytium formation and virus replication by castanospermine. Proc. Natl. Acad. Sci. USA **84:** 8120-8124.

30. TYMS, A. S., E. M. BERRIE, T. A. RYDER, R. J. NASH, M. P. HEGARTY, D. L. TAYLOR, M. A. MOBBERLEY, J. M. DAVIS, E. A. BELL, D. J. JEFFRIES, D. TAYLOR-ROBINSON & L. E. FELLOWS. 1987. Castanospermine and other plant alkaloid inhibitors of glucosidase activity block the growth of HIV. Lancet **2:** 1025-1026.

31. GRUTERS, R. A., J. J. NEEFJES, M. TERSMETTE, R. E. Y. DE GOEDE, A. TULP, H. G. HUISMAN, F. MIEDEMA & H. L. PLOEGH. 1987. Interference with HIV-induced syncytium formation and viral infectivity by inhibitors of trimming glucosidase. Nature **330:** 74-77.

32. KARPAS, A., G. W. J. FLEET, R. A. DWEK, S. PETURSSON, S. K. NAMGOONG, N. G. RAMSDEN, G. S. JACOB & T. W. RADEMACHER. 1988. Aminosugar derivatives as potential anti-human immunodeficiency virus agents. Proc. Natl. Acad. Sci. USA **85:** 9229-9233.

33. ARAKAKI, R. F., J. A. HEDO, E. COLLIER & P. GORDEN. 1987. Effects of castanospermine and 1-deoxynojirimycin on insulin receptor biogenesis. J. Biol. Chem. **262:** 11886-11892.

34. SAUL, R., J. J. GHIDONI, R. J. MOLYNEUX & A. D. ELBEIN. 1985. Castanospermine inhibits α-glucosidase activities and alters glycogen distribution in animals. Proc. Natl. Acad. Sci. USA **82:** 93-97.

35. FYFE, J. A., P. FURMAN, M. VOGT & P. SHERMAN. 1988. Mechanism of ribavirin antagonism of anti-HIV activity of azidothymidine (abstr. #3617). *In* Programs and Abstracts of the IV International Conference on AIDS. Stockholm, Sweden. June 12-16. Vol 2: 170.

Initial Clinical Experience with Dideoxynucleosides as Single Agents and in Combination Therapy

ROBERT YARCHOAN, JAMES M. PLUDA,
CARLO FEDERICO PERNO, HIROAKI MITSUYA,
ROSE V. THOMAS, KATHY M. WYVILL, AND
SAMUEL BRODER

Clinical Oncology Program
National Cancer Institute
Bethesda, Maryland 20892

INTRODUCTION

The past several years have brought about a dramatic change in thinking about the therapy of AIDS and related disorders caused by infection by human immunodeficiency virus (HIV). The discovery that AIDS results from infection with a pathogenic retrovirus has enabled consideration of therapy aimed at the causative agent of this disease, and at least one antiviral agent, 3'-azido-2',3'-dideoxythymidine (AZT, zidovudine), has been shown to reduce morbidity and mortality in patients with AIDS.[1-4] Since the end of 1986, when AZT was first made widely available, the overall survival of patients diagnosed with AIDS has increased substantially.[5] Such an effect can be seen over and beyond the contribution of other treatment advances such as the institution of aerosolized pentamidine.[6] AZT can also partially reverse the dementia associated with HIV infection,[4,7,8] and, in fact, its use has been shown to be associated with a decreased incidence of AIDS dementia in patients with AIDS.[9] It is worth remembering, however, that the finding that AIDS was caused by a retrovirus was initially greeted with a certain amount of therapeutic pessimism: only a handful of antiviral drugs had been found to be clinically useful in any setting, and retroviral infections were viewed by some as inherently untreatable because of the ability of the viral genome to integrate into the DNA of host cells.

The development of AZT has done much to dispel some of that pessimism. At the same time, however, this must be viewed as only a first step. Long-term therapy with AZT is associated with a substantial amount of toxicity, particularly bone marrow suppression and myositis.[2,10-13] This toxicity is most frequent in patients with established AIDS or with underlying bone-marrow suppression, and it necessitates stopping therapy in a high percentage of such patients.[11,12] Although toxicity can be reduced with lower doses of the drug, it can still pose a problem for long-term use in certain patients.[12] In addition, it has been reported that HIV isolates from patients receiving AZT therapy for more than one year frequently have reduced *in vitro* sensitivity to AZT.[14,15] Finally, AZT is not a cure, and patients frequently have progression in their disease in spite of receiving this drug. For these reasons, there is an urgent need for new and more effective therapies for HIV infection.

Since the original discovery that HIV was the cause of AIDS, we have learned much about the life cycle of this virus and have pinpointed a number of steps of replication that may be potential targets for antiretroviral therapy (TABLE 1). In addition, we have identified a number of agents that can inhibit HIV replication *in vitro*. Whereas several years ago the question was whether any agent would be effective in this disease, we now have multiple candidate drugs for clinical testing, and an important consideration is how to best prioritize these drugs so as to use the available clinical resources most effectively. In this article, we will review some of the recent progress in moving drugs from the bench to the clinic with an eye to learning how this transition can best be effected.

TABLE 1. Stages in the Life Cycle of HIV Replication That May Be Targets for Anti-HIV Therapy

Stage	Possible therapeutic approach
Binding	Antibodies; CD4 analogues; sulfated polysaccharides
Fusion (involves *env* gp41)	Antibodies to gp41
Entry into target cell	Inhibitors can possibly be found
Uncoating of RNA	Inhibitors can possibly be found
Reverse transcription (RNA → DNA, then DNA → DNA)	Dideoxynucleosides and related nucleoside analogues; phosphonoformate; TIBO compounds
Degradation of RNaseH activity	Inhibitors being sought
Integration of viral DNA into host genome (by *pol*-encoded integrase)	Possibly inhibitors can be found
Efficient translation and transcription of RNA	Antisense constructs (may also have nonspecific activity); inhibitors of *tat* or *rev* can possibly be found
Ribosomal frameshifting	Inhibitors can possibly be found
Polyprotein cleavage and other protein modifications	Protease inhibitors, trimming glucosidase inhibitors (*e.g.* castanospermine), and possibly myristylation inhibitors
Viral component assembly and budding	Interferons may act in part at this step
Infection by cell-free virus	Possibly *vif* gene inhibitors
Selective killing of HIV infected cells	CD4-toxin constructs, possibly CD4-IgG hybrid proteins, antibodies, and possibly immunoenhancing agents
Other mechanism or not known	GLQ223; ribavirin

DIDEOXYNUCLEOSIDES AS ANTI-HIV AGENTS

The development of a rapid assay system for the testing of compounds for anti-HIV activity by Mitsuya and Broder in 1984 enabled the establishment of a rational basis for selecting candidate drugs for clinical trials.[1,16,17] Using this system, it was found that a number of deoxynucleoside analogues in which the 3'-hydroxyl group was replaced by a hydrogen group, an azido group, or another group that did not form phosphodiester linkages were potent inhibitors of HIV replication *in vitro.*[1,16] (FIG. 1). These compounds, called dideoxynucleosides, are phosphorylated by enzymes in mammalian cells to 5'-triphosphate moieties (for a review, see reference 18). These dideoxynucleoside-5'-triphosphates, in turn, are believed to inhibit the activity of reverse transcriptase, both by acting as chain terminators and as competitive inhibitors of the physiologic deoxynucleoside-5'-triphosphates.[16,19–21] They are active against HIV in human monocyte/macrophages as well as in T cells.[22,23] In addition to these true dideoxynucleosides, a number of other nucleoside analogues have been found to have anti-HIV activity. Several acyclic compounds, for example, may structurally resemble dideoxynucleosides, when viewed three-dimensionally, and act in a similar manner.[24–26]

The first dideoxynucleoside to undergo clinical testing was AZT.[27,28] This drug was selected because it already had a corporate sponsor and because animal toxicology had already been completed (it had previously been considered for development as a veterinary antibiotic). As noted above, this compound was found to benefit patients with advanced HIV infection[2–4,7,8] and is now approved for treatment of severe HIV infection. At the same time, several other dideoxynucleosides were considered for entry into clinical trials. The next dideoxynucleoside selected for phase 1 testing was 2',3'-dideoxycytidine (ddC). Upon entering cells, ddC is metabolized to the active moiety 2',3'-dideoxycytidine-5'-triphosphate (FIG. 2). This compound was chosen because of its potency against HIV *in vitro,*[16] because it was resistant to degradation by cytidine deaminase, and because animal studies suggested that it would be excreted by the kidneys with straightforward pharmacokinetics.[29]

CLINICAL EVALUATION OF 2',3'-DIDEOXYCYTIDINE (ddC)

Phase 1 studies demonstrated that ddC was well-absorbed when administered by the oral route, and that it penetrated into the cerebrospinal fluid[27,28] (TABLE 2). These studies also revealed that administration of even low doses of ddC was associated with virologic and immunologic improvement in patients with HIV infection.[27,30] At high doses, the dose-limiting toxicity was found to be a painful peripheral neuropathy primarily involving the feet. This neuropathy gradually subsided upon withdrawal of the ddC, particularly if the drug was given in doses of 0.09 mg/kg/day or less and was stopped soon after the development of symptoms.[27,30,31] The development of ddC neuropathy was found to be related both to the cumulative dose and the dose intensity; we will return to this point in discussing another dideoxynucleoside, ddI. Interestingly, ddC proved to be more potent *in vivo,* both in terms of activity and toxicity, than was predicted from *in vitro* and animal studies. Indeed, the drug proved to be active (and toxic for extended therapy) even at the lowest dosing regimen used in the initial phase 1 trials (0.06 to 0.09 mg/kg/day). Subsequent studies have explored lower doses. In particular, studies by Merigan *et al.* and Gottlieb *et al.* have shown evidence of anti-HIV activity (particularly decreased serum p24 antigen) in patients receiving 0.03 mg/kg/day of ddC.[30,32] This dose was associated with markedly reduced toxicity, and far fewer patients developed neuropathy over six months. A multicenter phase 2 trial comparing low dose ddC with AZT is presently enrolling patients.

It was also noteworthy that the toxicity profile of ddC was substantially different from that of AZT: ddC caused peripheral neuropathy as the dose-limiting toxicity, whereas AZT caused bone marrow suppression. This suggested that therapy combining

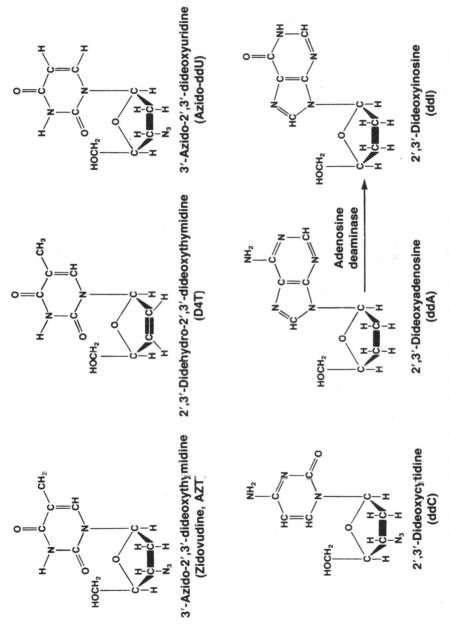

FIGURE 1. Structure of dideoxynucleosides that are in clinical trial as of the fall of 1989. 2′,3′-Dideoxyadenosine (ddA) is rapidly metabolized to 2′,3′-dideoxyinosine (ddI) by the ubiquitous enzyme adenosine deaminase.

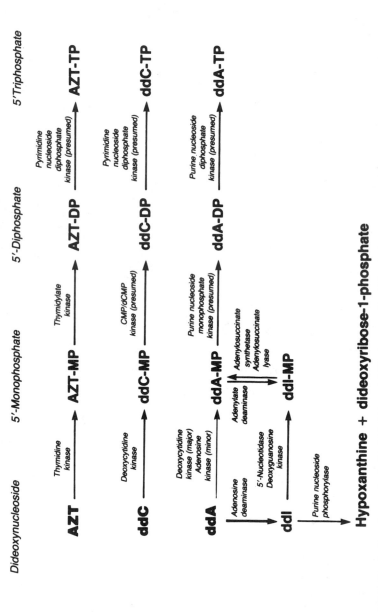

FIGURE 2. Metabolic pathways for AZT, ddC, ddA, and ddI in human cells. Abbreviations used are as follows: MP, monophosphate, DP, diphosphate, TP, triphosphate. (Yarchoan *et al.*[18] With permission from the *New England Journal of Medicine.*)

TABLE 2. Selected Pharmacokinetic Parameters for AZT, ddC, and ddI[2,7,18,20,21,27,28,34,41,43,44]

Drug	Typical dose	Peak plasma level after dose	Oral bioavailability	Terminal plasma half-life	Approximate intracellular half-life of triphosphate	CSF: plasma ratio	Chief clearance route
	mg	μM	Percent	Hours	Hours		
AZT	200	4	63	1.1	1.3	0.60	liver, kidney
ddC	2	0.1–0.2	87	1.2	2.6	0.2	kidney
ddI	250	8–10	40	0.5	12–24	0.2	probably metabolized to uric acid, kidney

these two agents might enable an anti-HIV effect to be maintained with reduced toxicity compared to each agent used alone. To this end, we have initiated an alternating trial with a week on AZT followed by a week on ddC, and so on; this regimen was designed to permit rest periods from each drug. Preliminary results from this trial indicate that an anti-HIV effect is attained, that the cumulative tolerated dose of ddC can be markedly increased when it is given under these conditions, and that there is decreased toxicity from AZT on this regimen compared to that seen on the standard dose.[27,33] Laboratory studies are now underway to determine whether the development of HIV resistance to AZT will be delayed by this regimen and whether ddC resistance will develop. Also, two larger studies comparing different regimens of AZT alternating with ddC are being conducted by the AIDS Clinical Trials Group of the National Institute of Allergy and Infectious Diseases.

RATIONALE FOR THE CLINICAL TESTING OF 2',3'-DIDEOXYINOSINE (ddI)

The next compounds that we chose for clinical testing were 2',3'-dideoxyadenosine (ddA) and the related compound 2',3'-dideoxyinosine (ddI).[16] Unlike AZT and ddC, which are dideoxypyrimidines, these compounds are dideoxypurines. Upon exposure to the ubiquitous enzyme adenosine deaminase, ddA is rapidly converted to ddI[34] (FIG. 1), so that for many purposes, these can be considered alternate forms of the same drug. (Indeed, this conversion occurs rapidly in fetal calf serum, so that even *in vitro,* the two may act similarly.) Upon entering cells, either compound is eventually metabolized to form 2',3'-dideoxyadenosine-5'-triphosphate, which is active at the level of reverse transcriptase[19,21,34–36] (FIG. 2).

Several features of ddA and ddI suggested that they might be potentially useful in patients with HIV infection. One was that they had a higher *in vitro* therapeutic index in human T cells than most other agents that had been tested; anti-HIV activity (using a high multiplicity of infection of HIV) was detectable at 2 to 10 μM, whereas T-cell toxicity did not appear at concentrations up to 200 μM.[16,17] These compounds also could completely inhibit de novo HIV infection of human peripheral blood monocyte/macrophages at concentrations down to 1 μM (FIG. 3).[22,23] Also, in contrast to AZT, ddA and ddI were relatively nontoxic for hematopoietic precursor cells when tested *in vitro.*[37–39] Finally, in contrast to AZT, the anti-HIV activity of ddA or ddI was not reversed by addition of the physiologic deoxynucleoside (*e.g.* deoxyadenosine).[40]

Animal toxicology and pharmacology studies suggested that ddA would be almost instantly converted to ddI in plasma and that ddI would have a relatively short half-life. Studies of the intracellular pharmacology of these compounds, however, indicated that once converted to ddA-5'-triphosphate, these agents would remain in cells with a half-life of over 12 hours;[34] by contrast, the triphosphates of AZT or ddC remained in cells with a half-life of only 2 to 3 hours.[20,41] This suggested that a sustained anti-HIV effect from ddA or ddI might be attained even with infrequent dosing (one to three times daily).

Both ddA and ddI are unstable at low pH (such as is found in the stomach), dissociating into 2',3'-dideoxyribose and the free base (adenine and hypoxanthine, respectively). Adenine is subsequently metabolized to 2,8-dihydroxyadenine, which is insoluble and can cause renal failure.[42] By contrast, hypoxanthine is handled better by the body; it is catabolized to uric acid and subsequently excreted (FIG. 2). (Indeed, we have observed 0.5 to 4 mg/dI rises in uric acid in patients receiving high doses of ddI[43]). Because of the toxicity of adenine, ddI is the preferred form for oral administration. Even with ddI, the issue of acid instability must be addressed when this drug is given by the oral route, for example, by administering the drug with antacids or buffers.

INITIAL CLINICAL EXPERIENCE WITH ddI

Our group at the National Cancer Institute initiated a small intravenous phase 1 study of ddA in February of 1988.[44] This study showed that ddA was instantly metabolized to ddI in the blood stream, that it was well-tolerated for short-term administration, and that patients receiving this drug had evidence of immunologic and virologic im-

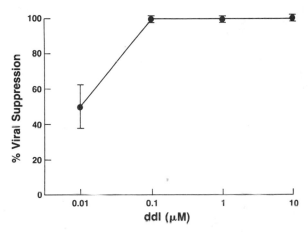

FIGURE 3. Activity of ddI in preventing *de novo* infection of fresh elutriated monocyte/macrophages by the monocytotropic strain of HIV-1, HTLV-III$_{Ba-L}$. Viral replication was assessed by measurement of HIV p24 antigen production into the supernatant at day 21 after exposure to virus.[23]

provement. In July of that same year, permission was obtained to administer ddI (both intravenously and orally) to patients, and we refocused our efforts on that form of the drug. Over the next year, we tested 11 dosing schedules of ddI in 37 patients in an ascending phase 1 study, ranging from daily oral doses of 0.8 mg/kg to 51.2 mg/kg.[43,45] Because of the long intracellular half-life of the triphosphate moiety, we administered ddI two or three times daily.

When given with antacids to fasting patients, ddI was found to be well-absorbed (average bioavailability 35 to 40%), and it penetrated into the cerebrospinal fluid (TABLE 2). In addition, patients receiving ddI had immunologic improvement over a 6 week period of time: the mean number of CD4 cells increased from 114 ± 15 cells/mm^3 at entry (mean $\pm$ SEM) to 161 ± 22 cells/mm^3 at week 6 (p = 0.00004), the mean total lymphocytes increased from 1162 ± 64 cells/mm^3 at entry to 1414 ± 106 cells at week 6 (p = 0.0008), and the CD4/CD8 ratio increased from 0.13 ± 1.18 at entry to 0.16 ± 1.18 at week 6 (p $= 0.0056$).[43,45] In some patients, these changes have been sustained for more than 18 months (Yarchoan *et al.,* unpublished observation). In addition, 7 of 23 evaluable anergic patients developed a cutaneous delayed-type hypersensitivity response when retested after 6 weeks of therapy.

Along with the evidence of immunologic reconstitution, the patients had a fall in their serum HIV p24 antigen from a mean to 234 ± 1.25 at entry to 86 ± 1.30 at week 6 (p $= 0.0034$). Of 18 patients who had detectable serum p24 antigen at entry, it became undetectable by week 6 in 7 of these patients. Finally, many of the patients reported feeling better, increased energy and appetite, upon receiving ddI, and the patients gained an average of 1.5 kg during the first 6 weeks of therapy. This weight gain was not associated with evidence of fluid retention.[43,45] These changes refer to the group as a whole, including patients who received both very low and very high doses. In general, patients receiving the lowest four doses of ddI had less pronounced evidence of improvement than those receiving 6.4 mg/kg/day of more drug. Some patients in every dose group, however, except the lowest, had some evidence of immunologic and/ or virologic improvement.

In general, patients receiving up to 9.6 mg/kg/day of ddI orally have tolerated the drug well; this includes several patients who have received ddI for over two years.[43,45] One of the purposes of a phase 1 trial was to define the dose-limiting toxicities of a drug, and to this end we continued to escalate up to 51.2 mg/kg/day. At these very high doses, the limiting toxicities were reversible painful peripheral neuropathy and, in occasional patients, pancreatitis or hepatitis.[43,45] In addition, some patients receiving ddI complained of headaches, nausea, irritability, or insomnia. Finally, we have observed asymptomatic amylase and triglyceride elevations in patients receiving ddI, and occasional patients have developed neutropenia, seizures, or a skin rash. The relationship of these latter reactions to the drug is unclear at this time. Other phase 1 trials of ddI in adults have been carried out at the University of Rochester, New York University, Boston City Hospital, and New England Deaconess Hospital. Preliminary results reported from these other trials are substantially similar to those observed in the National Cancer Institute adult study.[46,47] In addition, a trial of ddI in children, conducted at the National Cancer Institute, has shown that this drug is well-tolerated and is associated with anti-HIV activity in this population.[48] What we can say now is that ddI therapy may be associated with peripheral neuropathy and pancreatitis. How to predict, reduce, and manage these side effects is an important goal for future research.

DOSE INTENSITY AS A DETERMINANT OF ddI TOXICITY

It is worth stressing that the toxicities seen with ddI are primarily seen at the higher doses of the drug (particularly doses above 9.6 mg/kg/day orally).[43,45] By contrast, doses of 3.2 to 9.6 mg/kg/day (corresponding to daily doses of 224 to 672 mg for a 70 kg man) have been well-tolerated in our study for over 20 months in most evaluable patients. As noted above, these doses are associated with anti-HIV activity. Thus, there is a dose range for ddI that is associated with an anti-HIV effect but little toxicity in the phase 1 studies. These doses are being studied further in three multicenter phase 2 studies organized by the National Institute of Allergy and Infectious Diseases and the Bristol Myers Company. (In addition, ddI is being made available to patients with severe HIV infection who cannot tolerate AZT or who are progressing in spite of AZT therapy under the mechanisms of a Treatment IND and open label protocol).

We are presently attempting to learn how to best prevent and manage the toxicities associated with ddI. The neuropathy associated with this drug manifests itself as a sense of burning, aching, or numbness in the feet. This can be difficult to distinguish from the sensory neuropathy that is commonly seen in advanced HIV infection and that may be caused by cytomegalovirus infection.[49] In patients receiving high daily doses of ddI, this neuropathy often develops after a cumulative dose of 1.5 g/kg.[45] Patients receiving lower daily doses of ddI (up to 9.6 mg/kg/day), however, have received cumulative doses of up to 2.5 g/kg, and none of these patients have yet developed neuropathy. Based on our experience, we recommend stopping ddI when the neuropathy is mild to moderate in intensity and lasts for more than several hours; in such patients, the neuropathy generally subsides within several weeks. In certain patients, we have then been able to reinstitute therapy at a lower dose without recurrence of the neuropathy.

Two of the original 37 patients receiving ddI developed pancreatitis (both were receiving more than 15 mg/kg/day), and a third patient had an episode of nausea and vomiting associated with a rise in amylase two weeks later. In each case, the pancreatitis has resolved rapidly. One patient had an elevated triglyceride level of over 500 mg/dL for several weeks prior to the development of frank pancreatitis. In patients with triglycerides over 500 mg/dL, it may be worthwhile to temporarily discontinue use of the ddI until the triglycerides become lower. We are also exploring whether stopping the ddI for one week in patients with serum amylase levels greater than 1.5 times the upper limit of normal can prevent development of pancreatitis. We do not score asymptomatic elevations of serum amylase as pancreatitis, because transient elevations of this enzyme can occur in this setting without further sequelae. Also, some patients receiving ddI have been observed to develop isolated elevations of salivary amylase, and this bears further study. It is worth noting that a number of drugs in clinical use are also associated with the development of pancreatitis, and such drugs should probably be avoided in patients receiving ddI[50–53] (TABLE 3). Also, HIV infection itself, as well as complications of this infection, can cause pancreatic abnormalities.[54–56] Finally, it should be recalled that alcohol is most frequently a cause of pancreatitis, and patients using ddI should probably be cautioned not to ingest alcohol until more is known about the possible cumulative effect of these two agents.

COMBINATION THERAPY

It is likely that anti-HIV therapy will have to be maintained for a long time, perhaps for the life of the infected patient. Given the problems of resistance and cumulative toxicity, it is unlikely that a single agent will be able to provide optimal therapy for this disorder. Taking a cue from the development of effective therapies for certain cancers or tuberculosis, however, it is reasonable to expect that combinations of drugs might provide more effective therapy than any single drug used alone.

As mentioned above, a combination of AZT and ddC has already been found to cause reduced toxicity compared to either drug used alone;[27,33] such a regimen may also be found to reduce the development of resistance. In certain cases, anti-HIV agents may be found to be synergistic, particularly if they act at different steps of the HIV life cycle.[17,57] Also, certain opportunistic infections (e.g. herpes viruses) may activate HIV replication, and suppression of such infections may in turn reduce HIV replication. Both synergy and suppression of herpes viruses have provided a rationale for studying the simultaneous administration of AZT and acyclovir.[58] Taking another approach, certain agents such as erythropoietin or granulocyte-macrophage colony-stimulating factor (GM-CSF), which stimulates the bone marrow, might ameliorate the toxicity associated with AZT;[59] GM-CSF may also act to enhance the activity of AZT in monocyte/macrophages.[23] Finally, there is renewed interest in studying the effects of immunostimulation in combination with antiretroviral therapy.

CONCLUSION

During the past several years, much progress has been made. Scientists have dissected out the salient steps in the HIV life cycle and have pinpointed a number of

TABLE 3. Selected Drugs Whose Use Is Associated with Pancreatitis

Ethanol
Pentamidine
Sulfonamides
Azathioprine
Furosemide
Thiazide diuretics
Cimetidine, ranitidine
Corticosteroids
Methyldopa
Nitrofurantoin

potential targets for therapy. Many compounds have been identified as having some anti-HIV activity *in vitro,* and several of these have been shown to have activity when tested in patients. One of these agents, AZT, has been shown to reduce the morbidity and mortality of patients with severe HIV infection and, at least over the short term, reduce the incidence of progression to AIDS in patients with early HIV infection (less than 500 CD4 cells/mm^3). Several other of these compounds, including ddC and ddI, are now being tested in large multicenter phase 2 trials. Finally, we are beginning to make progress in the development of combination therapy for this disorder.

The genome of HIV can integrate into that of the cells of an infected individual, and no therapy, either being developed or on the drawing board, is envisioned as completely eradicating the virus from an infected individual. It is quite possible that in the future, however, therapies may be found that will be able to prolong the life expectancy of HIV-infected patients or even AIDS patients to approach that of uninfected age-matched controls. This is a feasible goal for investigators. In the quest for this goal, we should not lose sight of the importance of conducting controlled trials, for only in this manner can we progressively move towards the development of curative therapies for this disorder.

SUMMARY

Several dideoxynucleosides, including 3'-azido-2',3'-dideoxythymidine (zidovudine, azidothymidine, AZT), 2',3'-dideoxycytidine (ddC), and 2',3'-dideoxyinosine (ddI), have been shown to be potent inhibitors of human immunodeficiency virus (HIV) replication in human T cells and macrophages. These compounds undergo anabolic phosphorylation within target cells to a 3'-triphosphate moiety; as triphosphates, they act at the level of HIV DNA polymerase (reverse transcriptase). AZT has been shown to reduce the morbidity and mortality of patients with severe HIV infection and to at least temporarily ameliorate certain cases of HIV-induced dementia. In phase 1 studies, ddC and ddI have been shown to induce immunologic and virologic improvements in patients with AIDS or related disorders; phase 2 studies of ddC and ddI are underway. The use of these drugs can be associated with toxicity. AZT can cause bone marrow toxicity or myositis with prolonged use, ddC can cause peripheral neuropathy at high doses, and ddI can cause sporadic pancreatitis and peripheral neuropathy at high doses. For each compound, however, a therapeutic window exists in which an anti-HIV effect can be attained without short-term toxicity in most patients. Dose-intensity appears to be an important determinant of the toxicity of dideoxynucleosides. Studies are underway to explore how the therapeutic profiles of these compounds may be enhanced by attention to scheduling or through the use of combination therapy.

REFERENCES

1. MITSUYA, H., K. J. WEINHOLD, P. A. FURMAN, M. H. ST. CLAIR, S. NUSINOFF LEHRMAN, R. C. GALLO, D. BOLOGNESI, D. W. BARRY & S. BRODER. 1985. 3'-Azido-3'-deoxythymidine (BW A509U): an antiviral agent that inhibits the infectivity and cytopathic effect of human T-lymphotropic virus type III/lymphadenopathy-associated virus *in vitro*. Proc. Natl. Acad. Sci. USA **82:** 7096-7100.

2. YARCHOAN, R., R. W. KLECKER, K. J. WEINHOLD, P. D. MARKHAM, H. K. LYERLY, D. T. DURACK, E. GELMANN, S. N. LEHRMAN, R. M. BLUM, D. W. BARRY, G. M. SHEARER, M. A. FISCHL, H. MITSUYA, R. C. GALLO, J. M. COLLINS, D. P. BOLOGNESI, C. E. MYERS & S. BRODER. 1986. Administration of 3'-azido-3'-deoxythymidine, an inhibitor of HTLV-III/LAV replication, to patients with AIDS or AIDS-related complex. Lancet **1:** 575-580.

3. FISCHL, M. A., D. D. RICHMAN, M. H. GRIECO, M. S. GOTTLIEB, P. A. VOLBERDING, O. L. LASKIN, J. M. LEEDON, J. E. GROOPMAN, D. MILDVAN, R. T. SCHOOLEY, G. G. JACKSON, D. T. DURACK, D. KING & THE AZT COLLABORATIVE WORKING GROUP. 1987. The efficacy of azidothymidine (AZT) in the treatment of patients with AIDS and AIDS-related complex: a double-blind, placebo-controlled trial. N. Engl. J. Med. **317:** 185-191.

4. PIZZO, P. A., J. EDDY, J. FALLOON, F. M. BALIS, R. F. MURPHY, H. MOSS, P. WOLTERS, P. BROUWERS, P. JAROSINSKI, M. RUBIN, S. BRODER, R. YARCHOAN, A. BRUNETTI, M. MAHA, S. NUSINOFF-LEHRMAN & D. G. POPLACK. 1988. Effect of continuous intravenous infusion zidovudine (AZT) in children with symptomatic HIV infection. N. Engl. J. Med. **319:** 889-896.

5. NEW YORK STATE DEPARTMENT OF HEALTH. 1989. AIDS in New York State through 1988. New York State Department of Health. 78-79. Albany, New York.

6. MONTGOMERY, A. B., G. S. LEOUNG, L. A. WARDLAW, K. J. CORKERY, M. ADAMS, D. ABRAHMS & D. W. FEIGAL. 1989. Effect of zidovudine on mortality rates and *Pneumo-*

cystis carinii (PCP) incidence in AIDS and ARC patients on aerosol pentamidine. Am. Rev. Respir. Dis. **139:** A250.

7. YARCHOAN, R., G. BERG, P. BROUWERS, M. A. FISCHL, A. R. SPITZER, A. WICHMAN, J. GRAFMAN, R. V. THOMAS, B. SAFAI, A. BRUNETTI, C. F. PERNO, P. J. SCHMIDT, S. M. LARSON, C. E. MYERS & S. BRODER. 1987. Response of human-immunodeficiency-virus-associated neurological disease to 3'-azido-3'-deoxythymidine. Lancet **1:** 132-135.

8. SCHMITT, F. A., J. W. BIGLEY, R. MCKINNIS, P. E. LOGUE, R. W. EVANS, J. L. DRUCKER & THE AZT COLLABORATIVE WORKING GROUP. 1988. Neuropsychological outcome of zidovudine (AZT) treatment of patients with AIDS and AIDS-related complex. N. Engl. J. Med. **319:** 1573-1578.

9. PORTEGIES, P., J. DE GANS, J. M. A. LANGE, M. M. A. DERIX, H. SPEELMAN, M. BAKKER, S. A. DANNER & J. GOUDSMIT. 1989. Declining incidence of AIDS dementia complex after introduction of zidovudine treatment. Br. Med. J. **299:** 819-821.

10. YARCHOAN, R. & S. BRODER. 1987. Development of antiretroviral therapy for the acquired immunodeficiency syndrome and related disorders. A progress report. N. Engl. J. Med. **316:** 557-564.

11. RICHMAN, D. D., M. A. FISCHL, M. H. GRIECO, M. S. GOTTLIEB, P. A. VOLBERDING, O. L. LASKIN, J. M. LEEDOM, J. E. GROOPMAN, D. MILDVAN, M. S. HIRSCH, G. G. JACKSON, D. T. DURACK, S. NUSINOFF-LEHRMAN & T. A. C. W. GROUP. 1987. The toxicity of azidothymidine (AZT) in the treatment of patients with AIDS and AIDS-related complex: a double-blind, placebo-controlled trial. N. Engl. J. Med. **317:** 192-197.

12. DOURNON, E., S. MATHERON, W. ROZENBAUM, S. GHARAKHANIAN, C. MICHON, P. M. GIRARD, C. PERRONNE, D. SALMON, P. DE TRUCHIS, C. LEPORT, E. BOUVET, M. C. DAZZA, M. LAVACHER, B. REGNIER & THE CLAUDE BERNARD HOSPITAL AZT STUDY GROUP. 1988. Effects of zidovudine in 365 consecutive patients with AIDS or AIDS-related complex. Lancet **2:** 1297-1302.

13. BESSEN, L. J., J. B. GREENE, E. LOUIE, P. SEITZMAN & H. WEINBERG. 1988. Severe polymyositis-like syndrome associated with zidovudine therapy of AIDS and ARC. N. Engl. J. Med. **318:** 708.

14. LARDER, B. A., G. DARBY & D. D. RICHMAN. 1989. HIV with reduced sensitivity to zidovudine (AZT) isolated during prolonged therapy. Science **243:** 1731-1734.

15. LARDER, B. A. & S. D. KEMP. 1989. Multiple mutations in HIV-1 reverse transcriptase confer high-level resistance to zidovudine (AZT). Science **246:** 1155-1158.

16. MITSUYA, H. & S. BRODER. 1986. Inhibition of the in vitro infectivity and cytopathic effect of human T-lymphotropic virus type III/lymphadenopathy virus-associated virus (HTLV-III/LAV) by 2',3'-dideoxynucleosides. Proc. Natl. Acad. Sci. USA **83:** 1911-1915.

17. MITSUYA, H. & S. BRODER. 1987. Strategies for antiviral therapy in AIDS. Nature **325:** 773-778.

18. YARCHOAN, R., H. MITSUYA, C. E. MYERS & S. BRODER. 1989. Clinical pharmacology of 3'-azido-2',3'-dideoxythymidine (zidovudine) and related dideoxynucleosides. N. Engl. J. Med. **321:** 726-738.

19. WAQAR, M. A., M. J. EVANS, K. F. MANLY, R. G. HUGHES & J. A. HUBERMAN. 1984. Effects of 2',3'-dideoxynucleosides on mammalian cells and viruses. J. Cell. Physiol. **121:** 402-8.

20. STARNES, M. C. & Y.-C. CHENG. 1987. Cellular metabolism of 2',3'-dideoxycytidine, a compound active against human immunodeficiency virus in vitro. J. Biol. Chem. **262:** 988-991.

21. HAO, Z., D. A. COONEY, N. R. HARTMEN, C. F. PERNO, A. FRIDLAND, A. DEVICO, M. G. SARNGADHARAN, S. BRODER & D. G. JOHNS. 1988. Factors determining the activity of 2',3'-dideoxynucleosides in suppressing human immunodeficiency virus in vitro. Mol. Pharmacol. **34:** 431-435.

22. PERNO, C. F., R. YARCHOAN, D. A. COONEY, N. R. HARTMAN, S. GARTNER, M. POPOVIC, Z. HAO, T. L. GERRARD, Y. A. WILSON, D. G. JOHNS & S. BRODER. 1988. Inhibition of human immunodeficiency virus (HIV-1/HTLV-III$_{Ba-L}$) replication in fresh and cultured human peripheral blood monocytes/macrophages by azidothymidine and related 2',3'-dideoxynucleosides. J. Exp. Med. **168:** 1111-1125.

23. PERNO, C.-F., R. YARCHOAN, D. A. COONEY, N. R. HARTMAN, D. S. A. WEBB, Z. HAO, H. MITSUYA, D. G. JOHNS & S. BRODER. 1989. Replication of human immunodeficiency

virus in monocytes. Granulocyte/macrophage colony-stimulating factor (GM-CSF) potentiates viral production yet enhances the antiviral effect mediated by 3'-azido-2'3'-dideoxythymidine (AZT) and other dideoxynucleoside congeners of thymidine. J. Exp. Med. **169**: 933-951.

24. HAYASHI, S., S. PHADTARE, J. ZEMLICKA, M. MATSUKURA, H. MITSUYA & S. BRODER. 1988. Adenallene and cytallene: acyclic nucleoside analogues that inhibit replication and cytopathic effect of human immunodefiency virus *in vitro*. Proc. Natl. Acad. Sci. USA **85**: 6127-6131.

25. HAYASHI, S., D. W. NORBECK, J. PLATTNER, S. BRODER & H. MITSUYA. 1989. Carbocyclic oxetanocin analogues that inhibit *de novo* replication of human immunodeficiency virus in T-cells and monocyte/macrophages *in vitro*. In Abstracts of the V International Conference on AIDS. (Montreal, Canada): June 4-9, 1989. 564.

26. PAUWELS, R., J. BALZARINI, D. SCHOLS & E. DE CLERCQ. 1988. Phosphonylmethoxyethyl purine derivatives, a new class of anti-human immunodeficiency virus (HIV) *in vitro*. Antimicrob. Agents Chemother. **32**: 1025-30.

27. YARCHOAN, R., C. F. PERNO, R. V. THOMAS, R. W. KLECKER, J.-P. ALLAIN, R. J. WILLS, N. MCATEE, M. A. FISCHL, R. DUBINSKY, M. C. MCNEELY, H. MITSUYA, J. M. PLUDA, T. J. LAWLEY, M. LEUTHER, B. SAFAI, J. M. COLLINS, C. E. MYERS & S. BRODER. 1988. Phase 1 studies of 2',3'-dideoxycytidine in severe human immunodeficiency virus infection as a single agent and alternating with zidovudine (AZT). Lancet **1**: 76-81.

28. KLECKER, R. W., JR., J. M. COLLINS, R. YARCHOAN, R. THOMAS, N. MCATEE, S. BRODER & S. MYERS. 1988. Pharmacokinetics of 2',3'-dideoxycytidine in patients with AIDS and related disorders. J. Clin. Pharm. **28**: 837-842.

29. KELLY, J. A., C. L. LITTERST, J. S. ROTH, D. T. VISTICA, D. G. POPLACK, M. NADKARNI, F. M. BALIS, S. BRODER & D. G. JOHNS. 1987. The disposition and metabolism of 2',3'-dideoxycytidine, an *in vitro* inhibitor of human T-lymphotropic virus type III infectivity, in mice and monkeys. Drug Metab. Dispos. **15**: 595-601.

30. MERIGAN, T. C., G. SKOWRON, S. A. BOZZETTE, D. RICHMAN, R. UTTAMCHANDANI, M. FISCHL, R. SCHOOLEY, M. HIRSCH, W. SOO, C. PETTINELLI, H. SCHAUMBURG & the ddC Study Group of the AIDS Clinical Trials Group. 1989. Circulating p24 antigen levels and responses to dideoxycytidine in human immunodeficiency virus (HIV) infections. Ann. Int. Med. **110**: 189-194.

31. DUBINSKY, R. M., R. YARCHOAN, M. DALAKAS & S. BRODER. 1989. Reversible axonal neuropathy from the treatment of AIDS and related disorders with 2',3'-dideoxycytidine (ddC). Muscle & Nerve **12**: 856-860.

32. GOTTLIEB, M., J. GALPIN, J. THOMPKINS, D. WILSON, L. DONATACCI & W. SOO. 1989. 2',3'-Dideoxycytidine in the treatment of patients with AIDS and ARC. In Abstracts of the V International Conference on AIDS (Montreal, Canada): June 4-9, 1989. 212.

33. YARCHOAN, R., J. M. PLUDA, R. V. THOMAS, C. F. PERNO, N. MCATEE & S BRODER. 1989. Long-term (18 month) treatment of severe HIV infection with an alternating regimen of AZT and 2',3'-dideoxycytidine (ddC). In Abstracts of the V International Conference on AIDS. (Montreal, Canada): June 4-9, 1989. 406.

34. AHLUWALIA, G., M. A. JOHNSON, A. FRIDLAND, D. A. COONEY, S. BRODER & D. G. JOHNS. 1988. Cellular pharmacology of the anti-HIV agent 2',3'-dideoxyadenosine. Proc. Am. Assoc. Cancer Res. **29**: 349.

35. AHLUWALIA, G., D. A. COONEY, H. MITSUYA, A. FRIDLAND, K. P. FLORA, Z. HAO, M. DALAL, S. BRODER & D. G. JOHNS. 1987. Initial studies on the cellular pharmacology of 2',3'-dideoxyinosine, an inhibitor of HIV infectivity. Biochem. Pharmacol. **36**: 3797-3800.

36. MITSUYA, H., R. F. JARRETT, M. MATSUKURA, F. DI MARZO VERONESE, A. L. DEVICO, M. G. SARNGADHARAN, D. G. JOHNS, M. S. REITZ & S. BRODER. 1987. Long-term inhibition of human T-lymphotropic virus type III/lymphadenopathy-associated virus (human immunodeficiency virus), DNA synthesis, and RNA expression in T cells protected by 2',3'-dideoxynucleosides *in vitro*. Proc. Natl. Acad. Sci. USA **84**: 2033-2037.

37. GANSER, A., J. GREHER, B. VOLKERS, A. STASZEWSKI & D. HOELZER. 1988. Azidothymidine in the treatment of AIDS. N. Engl. J. Med. **318**: 250-251.

38. DU, D. L., D. A. VOLPE, M. J. MURPHY, JR. & C. K. GRIESHABER. 1989. Myelotoxicity of new anti-HIV drugs (2',3'-dideoxynucleosides) on human hematopoetic progenitor cells *in vitro*. Exp. Hematol. **17**: 519.

39. MOLINA, J.-M. & J. E. GROOPMAN. 1989. Bone marrow toxicity of dideoxyinosine. N. Engl.
    J. Med. **321:** 1478.
40. MITSUYA, H., M. MATSUKURA & S. BRODER. 1987. Rapid *in vitro* systems for assessing
    activity of agents against HTLV-III/LAV. *In* Rapid *in vitro* systems for assessing activity
    of agents against HTLV-III/LAV. S. Broder, Eds.: 303-333. Marcel Dekker. New York.
41. FURMAN, P. A., J. A. FYFE, M. ST. CLAIR, K. WEINHOLD, J. L. RIDEOUT, G. A. FREEMAN,
    S. NUSINOFF LEHRMAN, D. P. BOLOGNESI, S. BRODER, H. MITSUYA & D. W. BARRY.
    1986. Phosphorylation of 3'-azido-3'-deoxythymidine and selective interaction of the 5'-
    triphosphate with human immunodeficiency virus reverse transcriptase. Proc. Natl. Acad.
    Sci. USA **83:** 8333-8337.
42. LINBLAD, G., G. JOHNSSON & J. FALK. 1973. Adenine toxicity; a three week intravenous
    study in dogs. Acta Pharmacol. Toxicol. **32:** 246-256.
43. YARCHOAN, R., H. MITSUYA, R. V. THOMAS, J. M. PLUDA, N. R. HARTMAN, C.-F. PERNO,
    K. S. MARCZYK, J.-P. ALLAIN, D. G. JOHNS & S. BRODER. 1989. *In vivo* activity against
    HIV and favorable toxicity profile of 2',3'-dideoxyinosine. Science **245:** 412-415.
44. YARCHOAN, R., R. V. THOMAS, H. MITSUYA, C.-F. PERNO, J. M. PLUDA, N. R. HARTMAN,
    D. G. JOHNS & S. BRODER. 1989. Initial clinical studies of 2',3'-dideoxyadenosine (ddA)
    and 2',3'-dideoxyinosine (ddI) in patients with AIDS or AIDS-related complex (ARC).
    J. Cell Biochem. Supplement **13B:** 313.
45. YARCHOAN, R., H. MITSUYA, J. PLUDA, K. S. MARCZYK, R. V. THOMAS, N. R. HARTMAN,
    P. BROUWERS, C.-F. PERNO, J.-P. ALLAIN, D. G. JOHNS & S. BRODER. 1990. The
    National Cancer Institute phase 1 study of ddI administration in adults with AIDS or
    AIDS -related complex: analysis of activity and toxicity profiles. Rev. Infect. Dis.
    12(Suppl.5): S522-S533.
46. LAMBERT, J. S., R. DOLIN, M. SEIDLIN, C. KNUPP, G. MORSE, C. MCLAREN, C. PLANK
    & R. C. REICHMAN. 1989. 2',3'-Dideoxyinosine (ddI) administered twice daily to patients
    with AIDS/ARC. *In* Program and Abstracts of the Twenty-Ninth Interscience Confer-
    ence on Antimicrobial Agents and Chemotherapy. (Houston, Texas): September 17-20,
    1989. 105.
47. COOLEY, T., C. A. SAUNDERS, C. J. PERKINS, R. P. MCCAFFERY, C. MCLAREN & H. A.
    LIEBMAN. 1989. Phase 1 study of 2',3'-dideoxyinosine (ddI) given once daily to patients
    with AIDS or ARC. *In* V International Conference on AIDS: The Scientific and Social
    Challenge. R. A. Morisset, Ed.: 336. International Development Research Centre. Ottawa,
    Ontario, Canada.
48. BUTLER, K., J. EDDY, M. EINLOTH, P. JAROSINSKI, H. MOSS, P. WOLTERS, P. BROUWERS,
    L. WEINER, F. M. BALIS, D. G. POPLACK & P. A. PIZZO. 1989. Dideoxyinosine (ddI) in
    children with symptomatic HIV infection. A Phase I-II study. *In* Program and Abstracts
    of the Twenty-Ninth Interscience Conference on Antimicrobial Agents and Chemother-
    apy. (Houston, Texas): September 17-20, 1989. 106.
49. FULLER, G. N., J. M. JACOBS & R. J. GUILOFF. 1989. Association of painful peripheral
    neuropathy in AIDS with cytomegalovirus infection. Lancet **2:** 937-941.
50. HERER, B., T. CHINET, S. LABRUNE, M. A. COLLIGNON, J. CHRETIEN & G. HUCHON.
    1989. Pancreatitis associated with pentamidine by aerosol. Br. Med. J. **298:** 605.
51. MALLORY, A. & F. KERN, JR. 1980. Drug-induced pancreatitis: a critical review. Gastroen-
    terology **78:** 813-820.
52. PRESENT, D. H., S. J. MELTZER, M. P. KRUMHOLZ, A. WOLKE & B. I. KORELITZ. 1989.
    6-Mercaptopurine in the management of inflammatory bowel disease: short and long-term
    toxicity. Ann. Intern. Med. **111:** 641-649.
53. THOMAS, F. B. 1982. Drug-induced pancreatitis: fact vs. fiction. Drug Therapy 229-240.
54. CLAS, D., J. FALUTZ & L. ROSENBERG. 1989. Acute pancreatitis associated with HIV
    infection. Can. Med. Assoc. J. **140:** 823.
55. GRUNFELD, C., D. P. KOTLER, R. HAMADEH, A. TIERNEY & R. N. PIERSON, JR. 1989.
    Hypertriglyceridemia in the acquired immunodeficiency syndrome. Am. J. Med. **86:**
    27-31.
56. SCHWARTZ, M. S. & L. J. BRANDT. 1989. The spectrum of pancreatic disorders in patients
    with acquired immunodeficiency syndrome. Am. J. Gastroenterol. **84:** 459-462.
57. HARTSHORN, K. L., M. W. VOGT, T.-C. CHOU, R. S. BLUMBERG, R. BYINGTON, R. T.
    SCHOOLEY & M. S. HIRSCH. 1987. Synergistic inhibition of human immunodeficiency

virus *in vitro* by azidothymidine and recombinant alpha A interferon. Antimicrob. Agents Chemother. **31:** 168-172.

58. SURBONE, A., R. YARCHOAN, N. MCATEE, R. BLUM, J.-P. ALLAIN, R. V. THOMAS, H. MITSUYA, S. N. LEHRMAN, M. LEUTHER, J. M. PLUDA, F. K. JACOBSEN, H. A. KESSLER, C. E. MYERS & S. BRODER. 1988. Treatment of acquired immunodeficiency syndrome (AIDS) and AIDS-related complex with a regimen of 3'-azido-2',3'-dideoxythymidine (azidothymidine or zidovudine) and acyclovir. Ann. Intern. Med. **108:** 534-540.

59. GROOPMAN, J. E., R. T. MITSUYASU, M. J. DELEO, D. H. OETTE & D. W. GOLDE. 1987. Effect of human granulocyte-macrophage colony-stimulating factor on myelopoiesis in the acquired immunodeficiency syndrome. N. Engl. J. Med. **317:** 593-598.

Summary of Part VI

Clinical Evaluation of Anti-HIV Drugs

CARLOS LOPEZ

Eli Lilly and Company
Lilly Corporate Center
Indianapolis, Indiana 46285-0438

The very rapid development and clinical evaluation of AZT set an example that will be difficult to match anytime in the near future. This drug has clearly been shown to reduce the opportunistic infections in patients with AIDS and to prolong the life span of patients with this disease.[1] Nevertheless, AZT leaves much to be desired, and new and better therapies are required to control HIV infections. The clinical evaluation of promising new compounds or combinations of drugs in an efficient and effective manner will be necessary to introduce the required new therapies in a timely fashion.

There are several challenges to the clinical evaluation of anti-HIV drugs, not the least of which is the prioritization of the therapies to be tested in human trials. One of the problems with drug development in AIDS is that there is no one animal model of this disease that is universally accepted as an appropriate model of human disease. Much research is going into the evaluation of the simian immunodeficiency virus (SIV) model in monkeys, the SCID-hu mouse infected with HIV, and the feline immunodeficiency virus (FIV) infection of cats as models for the evaluation of antiviral drugs.[2] At present, however, there is insufficient data to conclude that one is better than the others for all candidate compounds. Far more experience will have to be obtained with each of these models before one can conclude that one is better than the others. Because it will not be possible to take every candidate compound to the clinic for evaluation, it will be important to have animal data with which to select the most meritorious compounds.

The clinical evaluation of AZT used the incidence of opportunistic infections as an indicator of efficacy of the drug, and treated individuals developed significantly fewer infections than did controls.[1] More recent studies have attempted to use surrogate markers of disease rather than opportunistic infections in order to reduce the length of time required for these studies. Although surrogate markers such as p24 antigenemia and the number of CD4 positive cells in peripheral blood have been shown to be good indicators of disease progression in groups of patients, they may not be as reliable in determining the progression of individual patients. Thus, these surrogate markers must be validated as predictive markers of effective antivirals prior to their use in clinical evaluation of antiviral agents in AIDS.

Probably the greatest challenge facing the development of chemotherapeutic agents for AIDS is the development of mutant viruses resistant to those antivirals. Resistance has been demonstrated in viruses isolated from AIDS patients treated with AZT for more than six months.[3] At present it is difficult to determine whether this resistance is clinically important, but there is an indication that patients begin to deteriorate after resistant mutants can be detected in such individuals.

In the preceding chapter, Yarchoan *et al.* present evidence of efficacy for a new series of reverse transcriptase inhibitors. Because there is no cross-resistance between the dideoxynucleosides and AZT, their use as single agents or in combination reduces the chances of resistance developing. These new agents clearly add new weapons in our armamentarium against this disease. The chapter by Johnson and Hirsch summarizes a number of studies that attempt to evaluate the potential for combination therapy for AIDS. Both offer hope for more effective therapy in the future.

REFERENCES

1. YARCHOAN, R., H. MITSUYA & S. BRODER. 1989. Clinical and basic advances in the antiretroviral therapy of human immunodeficiency virus infection. Am. J. Med. **87:** 191-200.
2. GARDNER, M. B. & P. A. LUCIW. 1989. Animal models of AIDS. FASEB J. **3:** 2593-606.
3. LARDER, B. A., G. DARBY & D. D. RICHMAN. 1989. HIV with reduced sensitivity to zidovudine (AZT) isolated during prolonged therapy. Science **243:** 1731-34.

Characterization of Reverse Transcriptase Activity and Susceptibility to Other Nucleosides of AZT-Resistant Variants of HIV-1

Results from the Canadian AZT Multicentre Study[a]

MARK A. WAINBERG,[b,c,i] MICHEL TREMBLAY,[b]
RONALD ROOKE,[b] NORMAND BLAIN,[b]
HUGO SOUDEYNS,[b] MICHAEL A. PARNIAK,[b]
X-J YAO,[b] X-G LI,[b] MARY FANNING,[d]
JULIO S. G. MONTANER,[e]
MICHAEL O'SHAUGHNESSY,[f]
CHRISTOS TSOUKAS,[c,g] JULIAN FALUTZ,[c,g]
GERVAIS DIONNE,[h] BERNARD BELLEAU,[h,j] AND
JOHN RUEDY[e]

INTRODUCTION

Several studies have shown that patients who receive 3'-azido-3'-deoxythymidine (AZT, zidovudine) for long periods are likely to develop drug-resistant strains of

[a] This research was supported by Grants from Health and Welfare Canada.
[b] Jewish General Hospital.
[c] McGill AIDS Centre, McGill University, Montreal, Canada.
[d] Toronto General Hospital, University of Toronto, Toronto, Canada.
[e] St. Paul's Hospital, University of British Columbia, Vancouver, Canada.
[f] Federal Centre for AIDS, Ottawa, Canada.
[g] Montreal General Hospital, Montreal, Canada.
[h] IAF Biochem, Montreal, Canada.
[i] Address correspondence to Dr. Mark A. Wainberg, Jewish General Hospital, 3755 Cote Ste-Catherine Road, Montreal, Canada H3T 1E2.
[j] This paper is dedicated to the memory of Dr. Bernard Belleau, Emeritus Professor of Chemistry, McGill University, who synthesized certain of the novel nucleoside structures described in this paper. Dr. Belleau died suddenly on July 2, 1989 and will be remembered by all who worked with him as a colleague and friend.

HIV-1 in their circulation.[1,2] The occurrence of such resistance is probably the result of selection by drug pressure of variants that will have developed, as a consequence of mutations within the HIV-1 genome, during the course of viral replication. It is conceivable that the responsible mutations may develop at any of a number of loci within the viral genome, although the most likely site is the *pol* gene.[3] Mutations within *pol* could give rise to changes in the structure of viral RNA-dependent RNA polymerase (reverse transcriptase, RT) which could, in turn, become insensitive to the effect of AZT.

Our laboratory has been concerned with the development of such drug resistance in patients, as a consequence of our participation in a Canada-wide clinical trial in which each of 72 patients have been treated with AZT for periods of three years or more.[4] Initially, all members of this group were relatively asymptomatic and fell within CDC groups II and III.

AZT is considered to be the treatment of choice for patients suffering from infections caused by HIV-1. Several studies have shown that treatment with AZT can both improve the quality of life and prolong survival for people suffering from HIV-1 infections, including patients with AIDS.[5,6] The drug is thought to act by interfering with viral RT activity by blocking the formation of proviral DNA from viral parental RNA.[7] This results in chain termination, after viral penetration into the cytoplasm of the infected cell has taken place. Because AZT does not apparently act at times after integration of proviral DNA into the nucleus has taken place, it cannot cure people of infection by this virus; nonetheless, it does seem to inhibit viral replication in seropositive individuals.[8]

Results of tissue culture studies have shown that AZT exerts an incomplete effect on viral RT activity. Indeed, the formation of some proviral DNA and infectious progeny virus can take place at a reduced rate, even under circumstances in which AZT treatment of susceptible cell cultures is performed continuously, from times preceding viral inoculation over periods as long as three months after infection.[9]

This paper confirms that drug-resistant viruses may be isolated from patients who have been treated with AZT for periods of 36 weeks or greater. We further report that AZT-resistant virus has now been isolated from one patient who had never received drug therapy; this was demonstrated by a modification of the technique routinely used to identify drug-resistant viruses in our laboratory. We have shown that replication of these variants can be inhibited by a number of other nucleoside analogues, including dideoxyinosine (ddI), dideoxycytidine (ddC), and a novel compound, deoxythiacytidine (dTC) (BCH-189, IAF Biochem, Montreal, Canada). Moreover, our data show that extensive cross-resistance may be present between AZT and another nucleoside analogue, 3'-didehydro, 2'3'-dideoxythymidine(d4T), widely considered for the treatment of AIDS patients. Finally, we present results on the kinetics and stoichiometry of viral RT and p51/66 of some of the AZT-resistant viruses described in this paper, in comparison with the control parental viruses from which they were derived.

METHODS AND RESULTS

Isolation of Drug-Resistant Variants of HIV-1

Viruses resistant to AZT were isolated from the peripheral blood mononuclear cells (PBMC) of 5 of 20 individuals who had received this drug for periods greater than 36 weeks. Isolation of such drug-resistant variants was demonstrated using each of two procedures. In one instance, we attempted to demonstrate the presence of these viruses by inclusion of a variety of concentrations of AZT (0.5-20 μM) directly in the primary tissue culture medium used for viral isolation. We found that 2 μM AZT worked best toward this end. In a second protocol, we thawed frozen isolates of HIV-1 obtained from individuals on long-term drug therapy and asked whether these isolates might contain variants able to grow in tissue culture in the presence of 1 μM AZT. This latter procedure has afforded us the opportunity to compare drug-resistant variants of HIV-1 with wild-type parental strains derived from the same patients at times prior to AZT therapy. In fact, it was possible to demonstrate the presence of HIV-1 variants possessing a AZT-resistant phenotype by both of these procedures.

The results of TABLE 1 show that 5 of 20 individuals studied in these ways possessed drug-resistant viruses in their circulation. This is about the same percentage isolation of drug-resistant viruses that we previously reported.[2] It is relevant that, in instances in which we successfully identified AZT-resistant viruses in the circulation of individuals on long-term drug therapy, we were also able to isolate such virus at later time points during the course of therapy.[2] We have not yet had the opportunity to study individuals from whom drug-resistant virus will have been isolated and who have subsequently been removed from AZT therapy. It is conceivable that virus possessing a wild-type phenotype may again become predominant in such individuals.

Using these procedures, we have never demonstrated the presence of drug-resistant viruses in infected individuals prior to commencement of AZT therapy. It is likely that the drug-resistant isolates thus far obtained consist of mixtures of both wild-type and resistant particles. This notion is strengthened by the fact that resistance to AZT was relative and not absolute, as indicated in TABLE 1. Virus possessing an AZT-resistant phenotype was detected more rapidly in the absence than the presence of this drug. Thus, virus that was able to replicate in the presence of AZT was nonetheless inhibited in terms of the rapidity of such growth, relative to the rate at which replication occurred in the absence of drug pressure.

Further evidence of the relative nature of drug resistance is that the AZT-resistant isolates were, in fact, sensitive to very high concentrations of this drug, that is, 10-20 μM (TABLE 2). These studies were performed using the HTLV-I-carrying MT-4 line of lymphocytes; these cells are highly susceptible to HIV-1-induced cytopathicity and produce progeny virus efficiently, as measured by production of viral p24 antigen and viral reverse transcriptase activity. Hence, it follows that the viral populations studied are heterogeneous mixtures of large numbers of viral types with a variety of different

TABLE 1. Isolation of AZT-Resistant HIV-1 from Subjects on Drug Therapy

Subjects	Weeks of treatment	Days to culture positivity[a]	
		No AZT	AZT (2 μM)
15 subjects	27-96	7-15	—
Subject A	36	9	14
Subject B	42	11	16
Subject C	51	7	11
Subject D	51	10	15
Subject E	51	11	16

[a] Cultures were considered positive when they contained p24 antigen levels greater than 1 ng/mL and reverse transcriptase activity in excess of 20,000 cpm/mL.

TABLE 2. Concentration-Dependence of Inhibition by AZT of HIV-1 Replication for both Wild-Type and Drug-Resistant Variants

Strain of HIV-1	Reverse transcriptase activity (cpm/mL)[a] when concentration of AZT was:					
	0	0.01 μM	0.1 μM	1 μM	10 μM	20 μM
Wild-type isolate	426,319	274,319	52,355	1,276	1,463	738
Wild-type isolate	372,058	346,017	26,490	842	1,601	1,152
AZT-resistant isolate	350,774	392,564	316,921	263,714	49,847	1,782
AZT-resistant isolate	414,965	406,991	361,729	312,568	21,369	1,346

[a] Cultures of MT-4 cells were assayed for presence of reverse transcriptase activity after 4 days. No cellular toxicity was observed at any of the drug concentrations employed.

genomic structures. It will probably be necessary to employ plaque-purified virus for studies that will assess mechanisms of drug resistance in a definitive way.

Cross-Resistance and Sensitivity of AZT-Resistant Variants to Other Drugs

It was, of course, important to assess whether or not these AZT-resistant isolates of HIV-1 were resistant or susceptible to other nucleosides currently proposed for therapy of HIV-1-infected individuals. We have employed five such drugs in this study: they are ddC; ddI; phosphonoformic acid (PFA; Foscarnet, Astra Pharmaceuticals, Toronto, Canada); BCH-189, in which the 3' carbon of the nucleoside pentose ring has been replaced by a sulfur atom (IAF Biochem, Montreal, Canada); and d4T, (Bristol-Myers Laboratories, New York, NY). The data of TABLE 3 indicate that each of these compounds was able to inhibit the replication of almost all the variants of AZT-resistant HIV-1 described. The inhibition effected by these nucleosides against HIV-1 replication was equivalent to that manifested by AZT against wild-type HIV-1 isolates. The one exception was that extensive cross-resistance was seen with one isolate and d4T. Furthermore, this d4T cross-resistance was demonstrable at a wide variety of drug concentrations (TABLE 4). The data of TABLE 4 also indicate that virus that was harvested from this same patient was sensitive to both AZT and d4T.

Isolation of AZT-Resistant Viruses at Times prior to Drug Therapy

We were also interested in assessing whether the emergence of drug resistance might in some cases precede drug therapy. Accordingly, we have attempted to isolate such virus by a procedure that differs from that described above. Virus that was initially propagated on cord blood lymphocytes by standard procedure was subsequently replicated in MT-4 cells in the absence of drug. Following initial amplification, this clinical isolate was replicated on MT-4 cells in the presence of very low concentrations of AZT for two weeks (.01 μM.) After this time, virus that was present in culture fluids was replicated in the presence of increasing concentrations of AZT. We found that each

TABLE 3. Sensitivity of AZT-Resistant Isolates of HIV-1 to Other Drugs

		Reverse transcriptase activity (cpm/mL)[a] when viral replication occurred in presence of:					
Phenotype of HIV-1	No drug	AZT (2 μM)	ddC (2 μM)	BCH-189 (1 μM)	ddI (1 μM)	d4T (1 μM)	PFA (40 μM)
AZT-sensitive	395,574	1,689	1,085	1,898	1,382	979	1,642
AZT-sensitive	226,890	1,842	1,696	1,853	1,603	1,401	1,681
AZT-resistant	198,968	208,921	1,842	1,604	1,138	1,644	1,276
AZT-resistant	273,504	183,576	1,055	1,478	1,657	1,436	1,485
AZT-resistant	342,092	251,493	1,462	1,511	1,511	1,682	1,081
AZT-resistant	250,735	165,840	1,890	957	1,895	1,712	699
AZT-resistant	281,417	193,718	351	814	1,014	167,912	1,204

[a] Cultures were assessed for reverse transcriptase activity 4 days after viral inoculation of MT-4 cells in the presence of drug.

cycle of viral replication yielded progeny; after two months, virus was able to grow in the presence of concentrations of drug as high as 1-2 μM. Thus, through the use of drug pressure and *in vitro* selection procedures, it was possible to demonstrate the presence of virus possessing an AZT-resistant phenotype from a clinical isolate obtained prior to initiation of drug therapy. Of course, this does not mean that such a variant was present in the patient before treatment. Rather, our selection procedure may have yielded AZT-resistant viruses that mutated during the *in vitro* replication process, but not within the infected individual. This is, nonetheless, the first demonstration that drug pressure may successfully be used to derive AZT-resistant variants of HIV-1 from viral populations that appeared initially to be universally drug-sensitive.

Kinetics and Stoichiometry of Viral Reverse Transcriptase and p51/66 in AZT-Resistant Variants of HIV-1 and Wild-Type Parental Viruses

We were interested in assessing whether the stoichiometry of our AZT-resistant variants might differ from parental types with regard to amount of p51/66 protein per pg p24 antigen. We have used a quantitative ELISA assay for this purpose, in which

TABLE 4. Cross-Resistance of AZT-Resistant HIV-1 to d4T

	Reverse transcriptase activity (percent of control)									
	AZT					d4T				
Strain of HIV-1	.001 μM	.01 μM	.1 μM	1 μM	5 μM	.05 μM	.2 μM	.5 μM	2 μM	5 μM
Parental AZT-sensitive isolate	100	100	0	0	0	78	66	58	0	0
AZT-resistant isolate[a]	100	100	22	12	2	100	100	100	100	84

[a] AZT-resistant variant of HIV-1 employed was isolated after 52 weeks of drug therapy.

monoclonal antibodies against p51/66 have been used to determine levels of this protein. Amounts of viral p24 were also established by a enzyme-linked immunosorption assay (ELISA) commercially available for this purpose (Abbott Labs, North Chicago, IL). The data of TABLE 5 reveal that both the AZT-resistant and the wild-type viruses from which they were derived contained similar levels of p51/66 protein per 2000 pg p24. This suggests that resistance to AZT is not associated with increased levels of viral p51/66 protein per virion. The HIV-III$_B$ laboratory strain of HIV-1, grown in H-9 cells, served as a control in these studies.

In addition, we have studied the ability of the various RT enzymes of our AZT-resistant and wild-type viruses to catalyse the incorporation of [³H]deoxythymidine triphosphate (dTTP) and [³H]deoxyguanosine triphosphate (dGTP) into poly(rA)-oligo(dT)$_{12-18}$ and poly(rC)-oligo(dG)$_{12-18}$, respectively.[10,11] The results of TABLE 6 show that the RTs of the AZT-resistant variants were far more efficient than their parental counterparts in this regard. We also determined kinetic parameters for each of these RTs and were unable to detect significant differences in affinity for dTTP substrate among the different parental isolates studied. By contrast, two of the AZT-resistant viral isolates possessed increased RT catalytic efficiency (V/K), when compared with the parental strains (TABLE 7). The catalytic efficiency of these enzymes,

TABLE 5. Levels of p51/66 Protein per ng p24 Antigen for each of AZT-Resistant and Parental Isolates of HIV-1[a]

Isolates of HIV-1	p51/66 (ng) per 2000 ng p24	
	Parental strains	AZT-resistant strains
Clinical isolate A	154	142
Clinical isolate B	524	564
Clinical isolate C	115	183
HIV-III$_B$	579	

[a] Determinations of p51/66 (ng) were by ELISA, as described in the text.

however, did not differ appreciably from that of the drug-sensitive HIV-III$_B$ laboratory strain of HIV-1.

We also examined the RTs of these various strains of AZT-resistant and -sensitive viruses for inhibition by each of two antagonists of enzyme activity. These were dideoxy-thymidine triphosphate (ddTTP) and the triphosphate derivative of AZT (N$_3$dTTP) (TABLE 8). No significant differences were seen in this regard between the resistant and wild-type isolates of HIV-1, using analytical procedures previously described for this purpose.[12,13]

DISCUSSION

Treatment of HIV-1-infected individuals and AIDS patients with AZT has been shown to both diminish the severity of symptoms and prolong life.[5,6] HIV-1 can continue to be isolated from patients who receive AZT therapy,[10] however, and it is

TABLE 6. Incorporation Rates (pmol/30 min) of dTTP and dGTP by RT Enzymes of Clinical and Laboratory Strains of HIV-1[a]

	dTTP		dGTP	
Strain of HIV-1	Parental strain	AZT-resistant strain	Parental strain	AZT-resistant strain
Clinical isolate A	0.50	9.39	0.06	2.05
Clinical isolate B	0.65	10.37	0.12	1.85
Clinical isolate C	3.29	10.48	0.35	2.15
HIV-III$_B$	0.97		0.19	

[a] RT activity was evaluated by measuring incorporation of [³H]dTTP (specific activity = 225.2 × 10¹⁸ dpm/pmol) into poly(rA)-oligo(dT)$_{12-18}$ and of [³H]dGTP (specific activity = 31.2 × 10¹⁸ dpm/pmol) into poly(rc)-oligo(dG)$_{12-18}$. The same quantity of viral p24 antigen (i.e. 2000 ng) was used in each case.

apparent that treatment with this nucleoside does not lead to restoration of normal levels of T-helper lymphocytes. For these reasons, it had been anticipated that AZT-resistant variants of HIV-1 would be isolated, well in advance of the initial demonstrations of this phenomenon.[1,2]

The results of this chapter confirm that resistance to AZT is likely to develop in a proportion of individuals exposed to this drug during long-term therapy. We have demonstrated that isolation of resistant viruses may be manifested in two ways. First, we have grown drug-resistant variants directly from the circulation of patients, by inclusion of AZT in the tissue culture medium used for this purpose. Second, we have thawed viruses that had previously been frozen and shown that they had the potential

TABLE 7. Kinetics of RT Activity for Each of AZT-Resistant and Drug-Sensitive Strains of HIV-1 Using dTTP as Substrate[a]

	Parental strains			AZT-resistant strains		
Strain of HIV-1	K_m (μM)	V_{max} (pmol/30'/ pg p51/66)	V/K	K_m (μM)	V_{max} (pmol/30'/ pg p51/66)	V/K
Clinical isolate A	5.4	1.3	0.24	4.2	3.5	0.83
Clinical isolate B	4.1	0.4	0.0	3.4	0.9	0.26
Clinical isolate C	4.1	7.8	1.9	3.9	6.6	1.7
HIV-III$_B$	4.4	0.7	0.16			

[a] RT was measured by the incorporation of [³H]dTTP (specific activity = 225.2 × 10¹⁸ dpm/pmol) into poly(rA)-oligo(dT)$_{12-18}$ as described in METHODS AND RESULTS. Kinetic parameters were calculated using a computer program based on a direct linear plot, as previously described.[12] Curve-fitting analyses were performed with ASYSTANT Scientific Software (MacMillan Software, New York, NY).

to replicate in the presence of AZT. This latter procedure has given us further opportunity to compare drug-resistant isolates of HIV-1 with wild-type parental strains obtained from the same patients at times prior to initiation of AZT therapy. More recently, we have been able to derive an AZT-resistant variant of HIV-1 by selective replication of a clinical strain, isolated prior to commencement of AZT therapy, in the presence of increasing concentrations of AZT. In the latter instance, we do not know whether AZT-resistance preceded drug therapy or developed as a consequence of mutations during *in vitro* replication.

The results of this study further show that a variety of other nucleosides may be used successfully to antagonize replication of AZT-resistant strains of HIV-1. These drugs include ddI and ddC[14] as well as a novel compound, deoxythiacytidine BCH-189. In addition, we have shown that cross-resistance may exist against other drugs, most notably d4T.

We have attempted to define the kinetics of the RT enzymes of the AZT-resistant variants of HIV-1 that have been isolated thus far. The data indicate that the V_{max} of

TABLE 8. Inhibition of RT from AZT-Resistant and Drug-Sensitive Strains of HIV-1 by Deoxythymidine Analogues

	K_i (nM)[a]			
	ddTTP		N_3dTTP	
	Parental strain	AZT-resistant strain	Parental strain	AZT-resistant strain
Clinical isolate A	6.6 ± 2.8	3.7 ± 1.2	20.1 ± 7.2	6.5 ± 1.3
Clinical isolate B	4.0 ± 1.5	2.4 ± 1.0	5.8 ± 0.9	3.8 ± 1.4
Clinical isolate C	3.5 ± 1.1	2.8 ± 0.5	6.4 ± 1.7	5.7 ± 1.6
HIV-III$_B$	5.1 ± 2.2		6.1 ± 1.4	

[a] Data were obtained over a range of inhibitor concentrations (0, 5, 10, 20, 50, 100, and 200 nM) using 5 μM [^{3}H]dTTP as substrate. All experiments were performed in duplicate. K_i values were calculated using an equation for competitive inhibition[13] and are reported as means ± standard deviations from each of the six different inhibitor concentrations employed.

certain of these enzymes may be higher than those of parental strains isolated from the same patients who yielded drug-resistant variants. This does not necessarily mean that the relevant mutations, which account for drug resistance, are present in the *pol* region of the viral genome, although this is a likely scenario. It is possible, for example, that mutations in regulatory genes may play a role in drug resistance. Current efforts to further define the genetic and biochemical basis for reduced AZT sensitivity are now ongoing in our laboratory. It is noteworthy that we and others have shown that interactions between the RTs of AZT-resistant and wild-type variants with the triphosphate derivative of AZT (N_3dTTP) are nearly identical.[1,12] This argues against the notion that changes in RT structure are solely responsible for the observed resistance to AZT.

We are now trying to plaque-purify individual viral isolates, so as to be able to work with material as homogeneous as possible. This is important for attempts to clone individual viral genes and for ultimate sequence analysis of genomic sites at which relevant mutations might have occurred. Efforts to date have used clinical isolates of

HIV-1 that contain heterogeneous populations of both AZT-resistant as well as sensitive viral particles, making definitive analysis impossible.

ACKNOWLEDGMENT

We thank Mrs. Suzanne Rouleau-Martinez for the preparation of the manuscript.

REFERENCES

1. LARDER, B. A., G. DARBY & D. D. RICHMAN. 1989. HIV with reduced sensitivity to zidovudine (AZT) isolated during prolonged therapy. Science **243:** 1731-1734.
2. ROOKE, R., M. TREMBLAY, H. SOUDEYNS, L. DeSTEPHANO, X. J. YAO, M. FANNING, J. S. G. MONTANER, M. O'SHAUGHNESSY, K. GELMON, C. TSOUKAS, J. GILL, J. RUEDY, M. A. WAINBERG, AND THE CANADIAN ZIDOVUDINE MULTI-CENTRE STUDY GROUP. 1989. Isolation of drug-resistant variants of HIV-1 from patients on long-term zidovudine therapy. AIDS **3:** 411-415.
3. FURMAN, P. A., J. A. FYFE, M. H. ST. CLAIR, K. WEINHOLD, J. L. RIDEOUT, G. A. FREEMAN, S. N. LEHRMAN, D. P. BOLOGNESI, S. BRODER, H. MITSUYA & D. W. BARRY. 1986. Phosphorylation of 3'-azido-3'-deoxythymidine and selective interaction of the 5'-triphosphate with human immunodeficiency virus reverse transcriptase. Proc. Natl. Acad. Sci. USA **83:** 8333-8337.
4. GELMON, K., J. S. G. MONTANER, M. FANNING, J. R. M. SMITH, J. FALUTZ, C. TSOUKAS, J. GILL, G. WELLS, M. O'SHAUGHNESSY, M. A. WAINBERG & J. RUEDY. 1989. Nature, time course and dose dependence of zidovudine-related side effects: results from the multicenter Canadian azidothymidine trial. AIDS **3:** 555-561.
5. FISCHL, M. A., D. D. RICHMAN, M. M. GRIECO, M. S. GOTTLIEB, P. A. VOLBERDING, O. L. LASKIN, J. M. LEEDOM, J. E. GROOPMAN, D. MILDVAN, R. T. SCHOOLEY, G. G. JACKSON, D. T. DURECK, D. PHIL, D. KING, AND THE AZT COLLABORATIVE WORKING GROUP. 1987. The efficacy of azidothymidine (AZT) in the treatment of patients with AIDS and AIDS-related complex. A double-blind placebo-controlled trial. N. Engl. J. Med. **317:** 185-191.
6. YARCHOAN, R., R. W. KLECKER, K. J. WEINHOLD, P. D. MARKHAM, H. K. LYERLY, D. T. DURACK, E. GELMANN, S. LEHRMAN, R. M. BLUM, D. W. BARRY, G. M. SHEARER, M. A. FISCHL, H. MITSUYA, R. C. GALLO, J. M. COLLINS, D. P. BOLOGNESI, C. M. MYERS & S. BRODER. 1986. Administration of 3'-azido-3'deoxythymidine, an inhibitor of HTLV-III/LAV replication, to patients with AIDS or AIDS-related complex. Lancet **1:** 575-580.
7. MITSUYA, H., R. F. JARRETT, M. MATSUKURA, F. D. M. VERONESE, A. L. DeVICO, M. G. SARNGADHARAN, D. G. JOHNS, M. S. REITZ & S. BRODER. 1987. Long-term inhibition of human T-lymphotropic virus type III/lymphadenopathy-associated virus (human immunodeficiency virus) DNA synthesis and RNA expression in T cells protected by 2',3'-dideoxynucleosides *in vitro.* Proc. Natl. Acad. Sci. USA **84:** 2033-2037.
8. REISS, P., J. M. A. LANGE, C. A. BOUCHER, S. A. DANNER & J. GOUDSMIT. 1988. Resumption of HIV antigen production during continuous zidovudine treatment (letter). Lancet **1:** 421.
9. TREMBLAY, M. & M. A. WAINBERG. 1989. Susceptibility to AZT of HIV-1 variants grown in Epstein-Barr virus-transformed B cell lines. J. Infect. Dis. **160:** 31-36.
10. WAINBERG, M. A., J. FALUTZ, M. FANNING, J. GILL, K. GELMON, J. S. G. MONTANER, M. O'SHAUGHNESSY, C. TSOUKAS & J. RUEDY. 1989. Cessation of zidovudine therapy may lead to increased replication of HIV-1 (letter). J. Am. Med. Assoc. **261:** 865-866.

11. LARDER, B. A., S. D. KEMP & D. J. M. PURIFOY. 1989. Infectious potential of human immunodeficiency virus type 1 reverse transcriptase mutants with altered sensitivity. Proc. Natl. Acad. Sci. USA **86:** 4803-4807.
12. EISENTHAL, R. & A. CORNISH-BOWDEN. 1974. The direct linear plot: a new graphical procedure for estimating enzyme kinetic parameters. Biochem. J. **139:** 715-720.
13. SEGEL, I. H. 1975. Enzyme kinetics: behavior and analysis of rapid equilibrium and steady-state systems. Wiley and Sons. New York.
14. STARNES, M. C. & Y. C. CHENG. 1987. Cellular metabolism of 2',3'-dideoxycytidine, a compound active against human immunodeficiency virus *in vitro.* J. Biol. Chem. **262:** 988-991.

Pharmacologic Studies of Nucleosides Active against the Human Immunodeficiency Virus[a]

JEAN-PIERRE SOMMADOSSI, ZHOU ZHU,
RICARDA CARLISLE, MENG-YU XIE, AND
DOUGLAS A. WEIDNER

Department of Pharmacology
Comprehensive Cancer Center and Center for AIDS Research
Division of Clinical Pharmacology
University of Alabama at Birmingham
Birmingham, Alabama 35294

INTRODUCTION

Since the first reports of acquired immune deficiency syndrome (AIDS) in 1981, when it was characterized by unexplained opportunistic infections and aggressive Kaposi's sarcoma in young males, AIDS has reached epidemic proportions within the homosexual community and among intravenous drug users. By June 1989, over 94,000 cases of AIDS had been reported in the United States and more than 48,000 of these patients have died. This disease has a 5- to 10-year fatality rate of almost 100 percent. There are as many as 1.5 million carriers of the AIDS virus in the United States that are currently asymptomatic, and the Center for Disease Control anticipates that by the end of 1992, the number of AIDS cases will surpass 365,000, with approximately 263,000 deaths. AIDS has already caused enormous suffering throughout the world, and even if a vaccine was available today, the World Health Organization has estimated that the over 5,000,000 people that are now infected with the virus will develop AIDS in the next 10 to 20 years. Because probability for the development and implementation of a safe, effective vaccine within the next 5 to 10 years seems unlikely, only two major approaches are currently possible in fighting the HIV epidemic: stopping the spread of the disease to noninfected individuals by public health and education and developing effective treatment for the people that are already infected with HIV.

[a] This work was supported by Public Health Service Grants HL 42125, AI 25784, and NO 1 RR 00032. J.-P. Sommadossi is a recipient of a Junior Faculty Research Award from the American Cancer Society.

CHEMOTHERAPY OF AIDS

Regarding treatment for the millions of individuals who are already infected with HIV, the tremendous efforts of scientists in academia, pharmaceutical companies, and governmental agencies have led to the discovery of several compounds that have been demonstrated to interfere with HIV replication in cell culture systems. These compounds have essentially been discovered through large screening programs and/or chemical synthesis of known active entities, including inhibitors of the absorption or penetration of HIV into a cell, such as recombinant soluble CD4, AL721, peptide T, or dextran sulphate; inhibitors of virus-encoded enzymatic activities (reverse transcriptase, RNase H, integrase, protease) with suramin, HPA23, Foscarnet, and nucleoside derivatives (including 3'-azido-3'-deoxythymidine); inhibitors of posttranscriptional processing, assembly, or release with ribavirin, interferon, ampligen, or castanospermine; and other glycosylation inhibitors, as well as various peptides. The list of agents with *in vitro* activity against HIV is growing daily, but several agents that have been brought quickly into AIDS clinical trials because of the emergency of the situation have had limited clinical benefit and/or unacceptable toxicities resulting in the discontinuation of the trials.

Among the steps in the lifecycle of HIV that are potential targets for antiviral chemotherapy, the viral DNA polymerase or reverse transcriptase has been the target of choice for the development of anti-HIV drugs, probably due to the documented clinical effectiveness of AZT. Historically, nucleoside derivatives have been among the best drugs for treating DNA and RNA viral infections, and AZT is still the only clinically approved drug in the treatment of AIDS.

TOXICITY AGAINST BONE MARROW

Among all human host tissues, bone marrow is probably one of the most crucial sites for studying potential side effects of antiretroviral compounds. Specifically, purine and pyrimidine derivatives, which are active *in vitro* against HIV, should be tested for their effects on human hemopoiesis. Indeed, AZT reduced the risk of mortality from opportunistic infections associated with AIDS, increased the number of CD4 cells, and decreased AIDS dementia effects. Unfortunately, an unacceptably high number of AZT-treated patients have developed quite severe side effects. Indeed, about 40 to 50% of the patients have been shown to develop hematologic side effects, including anemia and neutropenia, that require dosage reduction or discontinuation after 6 months of therapy.[1-3] The importance of evaluating this toxicity and elucidation of the cellular and molecular mechanisms underlying these side effects is emphasized by the fact that long-term chemotherapy will be required in using anti-HIV drugs in the treatment of AIDS. Moreover, additional depletion of hematopoietic cells in patients who already have a collapse of their immune system may actually lead to an increased risk for associated opportunistic infections.

TESTING FOR BONE MARROW TOXICITY

Our laboratory has been at the forefront for such studies and was the first to demonstrate that AZT had a direct inhibitory effect on human granulocyte-macrophage colony-forming units (CFU-GM) and erythroid burst-forming units (BFU-E) at clinically achievable concentrations of 1 to 2 μM.[4] For this purpose, clonogenic techniques were developed, as illustrated in FIGURE 1. Direct extrapolation of *in vitro* data to the clinical situation should nevertheless always be made with caution. Our preliminary clinical studies, however, indicate a good correlation between the 50% inhibitory concentration (IC_{50}) values obtained in these clonogenic assays and drug plasma levels at which cytotoxic effects are observed on human myeloid cells *in vivo*,[5] corroborating the importance of these assays as a prognostic test of toxicity in patients.

Since then, these assays have been particularly useful in the investigation of the potential toxicity of anti-HIV agents for bone marrow cells (TABLE 1). All tested compounds had previously shown some protection against HIV by using *in vitro* assays,[6–12] and some are currently in clinical trials. Inhibition of human bone marrow clonal growth varied substantially according to the compounds under study. 3′-Azido-2′,3′-dideoxy-5-ethyluridine (CS-85) and 3′-fluoro-2′,3′-dideoxythymidine (FddT) were the most toxic, with IC_{50} values in the same order of magnitude as AZT for both cell populations. The purine analogues, 2′,3′-dideoxyadenosine and 2′,3′-dideoxyinosine, were the least toxic. Previous *in vitro* studies have shown, however, that the concentrations required to inhibit HIV replication by these purine analogues are several orders of magnitude higher than that of AZT.[7] 2′,3′-Dideoxycytidine (ddC) was particularly toxic for human BFU-E, in agreement with published data.[13] 3′-Azido-2′,3′-dideoxyuridine (CS-87, AzdU) and 2′,3′-didehydro-2′,3′-dideoxythymidine (D_4T) were among the most selective compounds in our system. Phase I clinical trials were recently initiated with both compounds. The continuing evaluation of the effects of nucleosides towards these cells will permit us to ascertain a structure-toxicity profile for these drugs that will help in the development of novel entities. Of special note is the fact that all nucleoside analogues tested were substantially more toxic toward human BFU-E than CFU-GM. It is probable that the drug-induced toxicity may vary with the degree of maturation (or cell proliferation pattern): thus the observed higher toxicity for BFU-E, which are earlier progenitors than the CFU-GM. Recent studies from our laboratory, however, using a K-562 human erythroleukemia model, which can be induced to synthesize hemoglobin, indicate that AZT inhibits, in a dose-dependent manner, hemoglobin synthesis as measured by a benzidine staining method[14] (TABLE 2).

Hemoglobin is the predominant gene product of erythroid progenitor cells, and its synthesis is conducted only upon full maturation of reticulocytes. The synthesis of hemoglobin involves the collaboration between two very different metabolic pathways. One, globin synthesis through the regulation of different genes, is carried out by cytoplasmic ribosomes. The other, heme synthesis, involves extensive participation by mitochondria (FIG. 2). Inhibition of globin gene expression by AZT, associated to a decreased globin polypeptide chain synthesis in these human K-562 leukemia cells induced to synthesized hemoglobin, suggests that these mechanisms may play a role in the quantitative differences in toxicity of the various anti-HIV nucleoside analogues towards human erythroid and myeloid cells and, in particular, may explain the AZT-induced anemia observed in patients.

MECHANISMS OF TOXICITY

Elucidation of the cellular and molecular mechanism(s) of toxicity of these potential anti-HIV drugs is an important element in developing strategies for the treatment of AIDS. For example, several hypotheses have been suggested for the biochemical

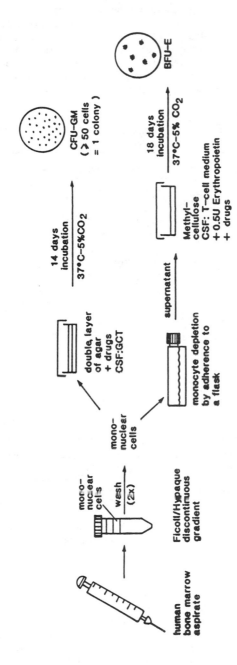

FIGURE 1. Schematic representation of culture assays for human granulocyte-macrophage CFU (CFU-GM) and human erythroid burst-forming units (BFU-E).

mechanism(s) responsible for the cytotoxic effects of AZT to human host cells. One hypothesis is that thymidylate kinase is inhibited by 3'-azido-3'-deoxythymidine-5'-monophosphate (AZT-MP), resulting in decreased formation of deoxythymidine triphosphate (dTTP) pools needed for DNA synthesis.[15] Significant variations in the degree of AZT-induced perturbations of deoxyribonucleotide pools have been reported.[15-19] These variations may reflect differences among cell populations or use of methodologies with limited sensitivity[19] and suggest that adequate studies will require use of cells representative of the toxicity site, as bone marrow cells concomitant with

TABLE 1. Effects of Anti-HIV Nucleoside Analogues on Human CFU-GM and BFU-E Clonal Growth[a]

Compound	Clonogenic assay	IC$_{50}$ (μM)
AZT	CFU-GM	1
AZT	BFU-E	1-5
CS-85	CFU-GM	1
CS-85	BFU-E	5
AzdU (CS-87)	CFU-GM	10
AzdU (CS-87)	BFU-E	1-100[b]
D$_4$T	CFU-GM	20-100[c]
D$_4$T	BFU-E	10
FddT	CFU-GM	10
FddT	BFU-E	1
2'-deoxy-3'-thiacytidine	CFU-GM	10
(BCH-189)	BFU-3	5
ddC	CFU-GM	10
ddC	BFU-E	1
ddA	CFU-GM	100
ddA	BFU-E	10
ddI	CFU-GM	100
ddI	BFU-E	500

[a] Human bone marrow cells obtained from human health volunteers were cultured as described in FIG. 1. Assay conditions were similar to those previously described to study the effects of AZT on human myeloid and erythroid colony-forming cells.[4] The 50% inhibitory concentration (IC$_{50}$) was obtained by using least-squares linear regression analysis of the logarithm of drug concentrations versus CFU-GM or BFU-E survival fraction. These values were calculated from at least three experiments with different marrow donors.

[b] A steady state at the IC$_{50}$ was observed for concentrations between 1 and 100 μM.

[c] Important variations were detected following investigations in at least eight experiments with different marrow donors.

highly sensitive and specific techniques as DNA polymerase assays.[20] Inhibition of DNA elongation *in vitro* by chain termination has been also suggested as a potential mechanism of activity and/or toxicity,[21] but no study has yet demonstrated whether, and to which extent, AZT incorporates into cellular DNA using an intact cell system.

Our recent studies have demonstrated that AZT, at a pharmacologically meaningful concentration of 10 μM, is indeed incorporated into DNA of human bone marrow cells. Furthermore, for the first time, a direct correlation between AZT toxicity and a biochemical event can be demonstrated. FIGURE 3 illustrates the relationship between

TABLE 2. Inhibition of Hemoglobin Synthesis by AZT in Butyric Acid Induced-K-562 Cells after 96 Hour Exposure

	Control	10	25	100	250
Inhibition, B+[a] (%)	—	6.2 ± 12.8	3.5 ± 4.9	37.3 ± 5.6	54.6 ± 9.0
Inhibition, B+ cells/mL[b] (%)	—	−1.1 ± 17.9	1.4 ± 12.7	56.3 ± 4.2	72.6 ± 8.2

[a] Percent of benzidine-positive cells. Percentage values of benzidine-positive cells ranged from 0.6 to 4.2 in uninduced culture and from 29.0 to 51.6 in induced culture.

[b] Percent inhibition of benzidine-positive cells corrected for cell-growth inhibition.

AZT incorporation in DNA and the clonogenic survival fraction after exposure of bone marrow cells for 24 h to varying amounts of AZT. The decline in the survival fraction (by 50% inhibition of CFU-GM colony formation) was proportional to the amount of AZT incorporated into DNA, demonstrating that AZT incorporation into DNA is one mechanism responsible for cell toxicity. AZT was not detected in DNA, however, at concentrations ≤ IC_{50}, which further suggests that another mechanism(s) of toxicity may be involved, such as the effect on the expression of specific cellular genes as demonstrated above. Of importance, our group has demonstrated that imbalance of deoxyribonucleotide pools by AZT was not a critical factor in AZT inhibition of DNA synthesis in human bone marrow cells.[22]

Some authors[23] have recently suggested that intracellular levels of the active triphosphate derivative may be an important factor in determining the cytotoxicity of these nucleosides, whereas others[24] have suggested that high intracellular levels of these triphosphate metabolites did not necessarily result in an increased cellular toxicity.

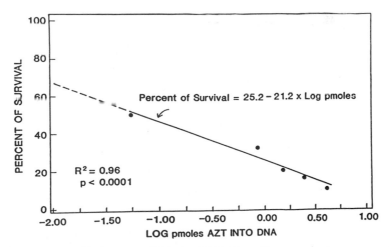

FIGURE 2. Relationship between AZT-induced inhibition of human granulocyte-macrophage clonal growth and incorporation of AZT in cellular DNA (pmoles/μg DNA). Human bone marrow cells were exposed for 24 h to AZT concentrations ranging from 1 to 25 μM. Effects of AZT on human bone marrow cells were assessed by a colony-forming assay (FIG. 1). Values shown are the mean of two experiments with values varying less 10% at each studied concentration.

TABLE 3 illustrates the relationship between intracellular concentration of 5'-triphosphate metabolites of dideoxynucleosides in human bone marrow cells and cellular toxicity as assessed by inhibition of cell proliferation. It can be seen that AZT triphosphates accumulated to the lowest extent as compared to other dideoxynucleosides, but the major cellular toxicity was observed with AZT, further demonstrating that toxicity is the result of several mechanisms, including inhibition of hemoglobin synthesis for AZT-induced myelosuppression.

PROTECTION FROM TOXICITY

Of particular interest is the need to develop pharmacologic approaches that can improve the chemotherapeutic selectivity of anti-HIV drugs. Such improvement can theoretically be obtained by three major modes. These include synergistic combination chemotherapy, as demonstrated with recombinant human granulocyte-macrophage colony-stimulating factor (rGM-CSF),[25,26] alpha A interferon,[27] and castanospermine;[28] combination chemotherapy of anti-HIV agents with different major sites of toxicity, as suggested for AZT and ddC or, more recently, for AZT and ddI; and probably the most appealing concept, which can be viewed as a selective "protection" or "rescue" combination chemotherapy. Here, the modulation is exerted by pharmacologically inactive compounds, *per se,* which are given at a time and a dosage that counteract (protection) or reverse (rescue) the toxic effects in the host cell without impairment of the chemotherapeutic activity of the anti-HIV drug. This concept has been successfully

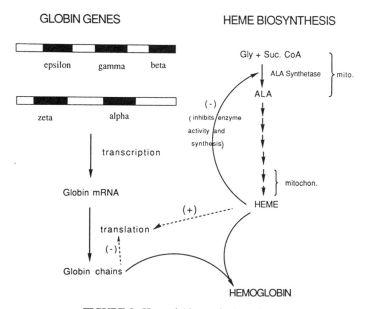

FIGURE 3. Hemoglobin synthesis pathway.

TABLE 3. Relationship between Intracellular Concentration of 5'-Triphosphate
Metabolites of Dideoxynucleosides in Human Bone Marrow Cells and Toxicities[a]

Compound	5'-Triphosphate concentration (pmol/10^6 cells)	IC$_{50}$ (μM)		Inhibition of hemoglobin synthesis
		CFU-GM	BFU-E	
AZT	0.08 ± 0.04	1	1-5	+ + +
D4T	0.30 ± 0.20	20-100	10	−
AzdU	Not detected	20	1-100	+
2'-deoxy-3'-thyacytidine	2.4 ± 1.1	10	5	−

[a] Human bone marrow cells (2 × 10^6 cells/mL) were suspended in McCoy's 5A medium that was supplemented with nutrients, and 10% dialyzed heat-inactivated fetal bovine serum, at 37° C in a 5% CO_2 incubator. The experiment was initiated with the addition of 10 μM ^{3}H dideoxynucleoside, and cells were exposed to drug for 24 h. Neutralized acid-soluble fractions were analyzed by HPLC, as previously described.[22]

used in cancer chemotherapy,[29] against protozoan infections,[30] in treatment of schistosomiasis,[31] and may also be of great interest for the treatment of AIDS.

Use of high doses of deoxycytidine have been reported to protect *in vitro* AZT toxicity for human bone marrow cells.[32] No data, however, were reported whether this combination was selective against HIV-infected cells. Until very recently, before completion of our recent studies,[22] inhibition of DNA synthesis induced by depletion of endogenous dTTP pools was considered a significant factor of AZT-induced toxicity. Therefore, Richman *et al.*[2] suggested that administration of thymidine sequentially with AZT might reverse the toxic effects of this drug. Based on that hypothesis, we investigated the capacities of several natural nucleosides to protect or reverse AZT toxicity in human bone marrow cells.[33] Thymidine could not reverse AZT toxicity, suggesting that AZT-induced toxicity of human bone marrow cells may not be associated with a decrease of dTTP pools. Final demonstration of this hypothesis was described in a recent study.[22] An unexpected finding was the discovery that complete reversal (and protection) was achieved with nontoxic concentrations of uridine (50-100 μM) and to a lesser extent with cytidine, probably acting as a uridine prodrug. Of particular importance was that the anti-HIV activity of AZT was unaffected by the presence of uridine in combination with AZT at a molar ratio (uridine/AZT) as high as 10,000. These studies provided the first evidence that uridine, an endogenous nucleoside, could directly and selectively rescue or protect human bone marrow cells *in vitro* against the toxic effects of AZT. Therefore clinical regimens of AZT in combination with uridine may have potential therapeutic benefit in the treatment of AIDS.

ACKNOWLEDGMENTS

We thank D. R. F. Schinazi for providing AZT, CS-85, and AzddU (CS-87). D4T, FddT, ddC, ddA, and ddI were supplied by Dr. I. Ghazzouli from Bristol-Myers Pharmaceutical Research and Development Division. 2'-Deoxy-3'-thiacytidine (BCH-189) was obtained from Dr. M. Stern from IAF Biochem, Montreal, Canada.

REFERENCES

1. YARCHOAN, R., K. J. WEINHOLD, H. K. LYERLY, E. GELMANN, R. M. BLUM, G. M. SHEARER, H. MITSUYA, J. M. COLLINS, C. E. MYERS, R. W. KLECKER, P. D. MARKHAM, D. T. DURACK, S. LEHRMAN, D. W. BARRY, M. A. FISCHL, R. C. GALLO, D. P. BOLOGNESI & S. BRODER. 1986. Administration of 3'-azido-3'-deoxythymidine, an inhibitor of HTLV III/LAV replication, to patients with AIDS or AIDS-related complex. Lancet i: 575-580.

2. RICHMAN, D. D., M. A. FISCHL, M. H. GRIECO, M. S. GOTTLIEB, P. A. VOLBERDING, O. L. LASKIN, J. M. LEEDOM, J. E. GROOPMAN, D. MILDVAN, M. HIRSCH, G. G. JACKSON, D. T. DURACK, S. NUSINOFF-LEHRMAN & THE AZT COLLABORATIVE WORKING GROUP. 1987. The toxicity of azidothymidine (AZT) in the treatment of patients with AIDS and AIDS-related complex. N. Engl. J. Med. 317: 192-197.

3. GIL, P. S., M. RARICK, R. K. BRYNES, D. CAUSEY, C. LOUREIRO & A. M. LEVINE. 1987. Azidothymidine associated with bone marrow failure in the acquired immunodeficiency syndrome (AIDS). Ann. Intern. Med. 107: 502-505.

4. SOMMADOSSI, J.-P. & R. CARLISLE. 1987. Toxicity of 3'-azido-3'-deoxythymidine and 9-(1,3-dihydroxy-2-propoxymethyl)guanine for normal human hematopoietic progenitor cells in vitro. Antimicrob. Agents Chemother. 31: 452-454.

5. SOMMADOSSI, J.-P., D. W. BARNES, L. R. MILLER, M. A. MARKIEWICZ & R. J. WHITLEY. 1987. Novel pharmacologic strategies in the treatment of life-threatening infections: clinical experience with 9-(1,3-dihydroxy-2-propoxy-methyl)-guanine (DHPG). Clin. Res. 35(3): 491A.

6. MITSUYA, H., K. J. WEINHOLD, P. A. FURMAN, M. H. ST. CLAIR, S. NUSINOFF-LEHRMAN, R. C. GALLO, D. BOLOGNESI, D. W. BARRY & S. BRODER. 1985. 3'-Azido-3'-deoxythymidine (BW A509U): an antiviral agent that inhibits the infectivity and cytopathic effect of human T-lymphotropic virus type III/lymphadenopathy-associated virus in vitro. Proc. Natl. Acad. Sci. USA 82: 7096-7100.

7. MITSUYA, H. & S. BRODER. 1986. Inhibition of the in vitro and cytopathic effect of human T-lymphotropic virus, type III/lymphadenopathy-associated virus (HTLV-III/LAV) by 2',3'-dideoxynucleosides. Proc. Natl. Acad. Sci. USA 83: 1911-1915.

8. MITSUYA, H. & S. BRODER. 1987. Strategies for antiviral therapy in AIDS. Nature 325: 773-778.

9. CHU, C. K., R. F. SCHINAZI, B. H. ARNOLD, D. L. CANNON, B. DOBOSZEWSKI, V. B. BHADTI & Z. GU. 1988. Comparative activity of 2',3'-saturated and unsaturated pyrimidine and purine nucleosides against human immunodeficiency virus type I in peripheral blood mononuclear cells. Biochem. Pharmacol. 36: 311-316.

10. LIN, T.-S., J.-Y. GUO, R. F. SCHINAZI, C. K. CHU, J.-N. XIANG & W. H. PRUSOFF. 1988. Synthesis and antiviral activity of various 3'-azido analogues of pyrimidine deoxyribonucleosides against human immunodeficiency virus (HIV-I, HTLV III/LAB). J. Med. Chem. 31: 336-340.

11. HERDEWIJN, P., J. BALZARINI, M. BABA, R. PAUWELS, A. V. AERSHOT, G. JANSSEN & E. DE CLERCQ. 1988. Synthesis and anti-HIV activity of different sugar-modified pyrimidine and purine nucleosides. J. Med. Chem. 31: 2040-2048.

12. MANSURI, M. M., J. E. STARRETT JR., I. GHAZZOULI, M. J. M. HITCHCOCK, R. Z. STERZYCKI, V. BRANKOVAN, T.-S. LIN, E. M. AUGUST, W. H. PRUSOFF, J.-P. SOMMADOSSI & J. C. MARTIN. 1989. 1-(2,3-Dideoxy-D-glycero-pent-2-enofuranosyl) thymine. A highly potent and selective anti-HIV agent. J. Med. Chem. 32: 461-466.

13. JOHNSON, M., T. CAIAZZO, J.-M. MOLINA, R. DONAHUE & J. GROOPMAN. 1988. Inhibition of bone marrow myelopoiesis and erythropoiesis in vitro by anti-retroviral nucleoside derivatives. Br. J. Haematol. 70: 137-141.

14. WEIDNER, D. A. & J.-P. SOMMADOSSI. 1989. Mechanism of toxicity of 3'-azido-3'-deoxythymidine (AZT): Evidence of inhibition of hemoglobin (Hb) synthesis in butyrate-induced K-562 cells. Proc. Am. Assoc. Cancer Res. 30: 2352.

15. FURMAN, P. A., S. NUSINOFF-LEHRMAN, J. A. FYFE, M. H. ST. CLAIR, K. L. WEINHOLD, J. L. RIDEOUT, G. A. FREEMAN, D. P. BOLOGNESI, S. BRODER, H. MITSUYA & D. W.

BARRY. 1986. Phosphorylation of 3'-azido-3'-deoxythymidine and selective interaction of the 5'-triphosphate with human immunodeficiency virus reverse transcriptase. Proc. Natl. Acad. Sci. USA **83:** 8333-8337.

16. BALZARINI, J., D. A. COONEY, S. BRODER & D. G. JOHNS. 1987. Biochemical basis for the cytostatic effects of the potent anti-HIV (human immunodeficiency virus) drug 3'-azido-2',3'-dideoxythymidine (AZT). Arch. Int. Physiol. Biochim. **95:** B-52.

17. FRICK, L. W., D. J. NELSON, M. H. ST. CLAIR, P. A. FURMAN & T. A. KRENITSKY. 1988. Effects of 3'-azido-3'-deoxythymidine on the deoxynucleotide triphosphate pools of cultured human cells. Biochem. Biophys. Res. Commun. **154:** 124-129.

18. HAO, Z., D. A. COONEY, N. R. HARTMAN, C. F. PERNO, A. FRIDLAND, A. L. DEVICO, M. G. SARNGADHARAN, S. BRODER & D. G. JOHNS. 1988. Factors determining the activity of 2',3'-dideoxynucleosides in suppressing human immunodeficiency virus *in vitro*. Mol. Pharmacol. **34:** 431-435.

19. BHALLA, K., M. BIRKHOFER, S. GRANT & G. GRAHAM. 1989. The effect of recombinant human granulocyte-macrophage colony-stimulating factor (rGM-CSF) on 3'-azido-3'-deoxythymidine (AZT)-mediated biochemical and cytotoxic effects on normal human myeloid progenitor cells. Exp. Hematol. (N.Y.) **17:** 17-20.

20. HUNTING, D. & J. F. HENDERSON. 1981. Determination of deoxyribonucleoside triphosphates using DNA polymerase: a critical evaluation. Can. J. Biochem. **59:** 723-727.

21. ST. CLAIR, M. H., C. A. RICHARDS, T. SPECTOR, K. J. WEINHOLD, W. H. MILLER, A. J. LANGLOIS & P. A. FURMAN. 1987. 3'-Azido-3'-deoxythymidine triphosphate as an inhibitor and substrate of purified human immunodeficiency virus reverse transcriptase. Antimicrob. Agents Chemother. **31:** 1972-1977.

22. SOMMADOSSI, J.-P., R. CARLISLE & Z. ZHOU. 1989. Cellular pharmacology of 3'-azido-3'-deoxythymidine with evidence of incorporation into DNA of human bone marrow cells. Mol. Pharmacol. **36:** 9-14.

23. BLAKLEY, R. L., F. C. HARWOOD & K. D. HUFF. 1990. Cytostatic effects of 2',3'-dideoxyribonucleosides on transformed human hemopoietic cell lines. Mol. Pharmacol. **37:** 328-332.

24. HAO, Z., D. A. COONEY, D. FARQUHAR, C. F. PERNO, K. ZHANG, R. MASOOD, Y. WILSON, N. R. HARTMAN, J. BALZARINI & D. G. JOHNS. 1990. Potent DNA chain termination activity and selective inhibition of human immunodeficiency virus reverse transcriptase by 2',3'-dideoxyuridine-5'-triphosphate. Mol. Pharmacol. **37:** 157-163.

25. HAMMER, S. C. & J. M. GILLIS. 1987. Synergistic activity of granulocyte-macrophage colony-stimulating factor and 3'-azido-3'-deoxythymidine against human immunodeficiency virus *in vitro*. Antimicrob. Agents Chemother. **31:** 1046-1050.

26. PERNO, C.-F., R. YARCHOAN, D. A. COONEY, N. R. HARTMAN, D. S. A. WEBB, Z. HAO, H. MITSUYA, D. G. JOHNS & S. BRODER. 1989. Replication of human immunodeficiency virus in monocytes-granulocyte/macrophage colony-stimulating factor (GM-CSF) potentiates viral production yet enhances the antiviral effect mediated by 3'-azido-2',3'-dideoxythymidine (AZT) and other dideoxynucleoside congeners of thymidine. J. Exp. Med. **169**(3): 933-951.

27. HARTSHORN, K. L., M. W. VOGT, T.-C. CHOU, R. S. BLUMBERG, R. BYINGTON, R. T. SCHOOLEY & M. S. HIRSCH. 1987. Synergistic inhibition of human immunodeficiency virus *in vitro* by azidothymidine and recombinant alpha A interferon. Antimicrob. Agents Chemother. **31:** 168-172.

28. JOHNSON, V. A., B. D. WALKER, M. A. BARLOW, T. J. PARADIS, T. C. CHOU & M. S. HIRSCH. 1989. Synergistic inhibition of human immunodeficiency virus type 1 and type 2 replication *in vitro* by castanospermine and 3'-azido-3'-deoxythymidine. Antimicrob. Agents Chemother. **33:** 53-57.

29. CAPIZZI, R. L., R. C. DE CONTI, J. C. MARSH & J. R. BERTINO, JR. 1970. Methotrexate therapy of head and neck cancer: improvement in therapeutic index by the use of leucovorin "rescue". Cancer Res. **30:** 1782-1788.

30. ALLEGRA, C. J., B. A. CHABNER, C. V. TUAZON, D. OGATA-ARAKAKI, B. BAIRO, J. C. DRAKE, J. T. SIMMONS, E. E. LACK, J. H. SHELHAMER, F. BALIS, R. WALKER, J. A. KOVACS, H. C. LANE & H. MANSUR. 1987. Trimetrexate for the treatment of *Pneumocystis carinii* pneumonia in patients with the acquired immunodeficiency syndrome. N. Engl. J. Med. **317:** 978-985.

31. EL KOUNI, M. H., D. DIOP, P. O'SHEA, R. CARLISLE & J.-P. SOMMADOSSI. 1989. Prevention of tubercidin host toxicity by nitrobenzylthioinosine 5'-monophosphate for the treatment of schistosomiasis. Antimicrob. Agents Chemother. **33:** 824–827.
32. BHALLA, K., J. COLE, M. BIRKHOFER, W. MACLAUGHLIN, S. GRANT & G. GRAHAM. 1987. Reversal of 3'-azido-3'-deoxythymidine (AZT) and 2',3'-dideoxycytidine (DDC) medicated cytotoxicity by deoxycytidine in cultured normal human myeloid progenitor cells. Blood **70:** 148a.
33. SOMMADOSSI, J.-P., R. CARLISLE, R. F. SCHINAZI & Z. ZHOU. 1988. Uridine reverses the toxicity of 3'-azido-3'-deoxythymidine in normal human granulocyte-macrophage progenitor cells *in vitro* without impairment of antiretroviral activity. Antimicrob. Agents Chemother. **32:** 997–1001.

Synergistic Drug Combinations in AIDS Therapy

Dipyridamole / 3'-Azido-3'-Deoxythymidine in Particular and Principles of Analysis in General[a]

JOHN N. WEINSTEIN,[b] BARRY BUNOW,[c]
OWEN S. WEISLOW,[d] RAYMOND F. SCHINAZI,[e]
SHARON M. WAHL,[f] LARRY M. WAHL,[f] AND
JANOS SZEBENI [b]

[b]National Cancer Institute
Bethesda, Maryland 20892

[c]Civilized Software, Inc.
Bethesda, Maryland 20814

[d]National Cancer Institute
Frederick Cancer Research Facility
and Program Resources, Inc.
Frederick, Maryland

[e]Veterans Affairs Medical Center
Department of Pediatrics
and Emory University School of Medicine
Atlanta, Georgia 30033

[f]Laboratory of Immunology
National Institute of Dental Research
Bethesda, Maryland 20892

INTRODUCTION

Combination chemotherapy has been prominent for more than a generation in the treatment of such diseases as cancer, hypertension, and bacterial infections. In the case of viral infections, combinations are coming rapidly into focus for the human immunodeficiency virus (HIV).[1-11] Reasons for combination chemotherapy of HIV

[a]R. Schinazi is supported in part by USPHS Grant AI 26055 and the Department of Veterans Affairs. The work of J. N. Weinstein and J. Szebeni was supported in part by the National Institutes of Health Intramural Targeted AIDS Antiviral Program.

367

include synergy of antiviral effects, antagonism of toxicities, distribution of toxicities among organ systems, prevention of emergence of resistant variants, enhancement of immune function, and treatment of concurrent opportunistic infections.

Despite its obvious importance, the conceptual basis for combination therapy has been fraught with confusion. Arguments about the proper meaning of such terms as additivity, potentiation, synergy, and antagonism often take on an almost metaphysical flavor. As with most apparently metaphysical problems, however, this one yields to careful definition of terms and their relationships. In the present paper two stories will be intertwined: a brief summary of our studies on combinations of the drug dipyridamole (DPM) with 3'-azido-3'-deoxythymidine (zidovudine, AZT) and other 2',3'-dideoxynucleosides; and presentation of a new approach to the analysis of drug combinations, as embodied in a computer program package called COMBO.

COMBINATION CHEMOTHERAPY WITH DIPYRIDAMOLE AND DIDEOXYNUCLEOSIDES

DPM (FIG. 1) is a potent inhibitor of "carrier-mediated" nucleoside transport.[12-16] In clinical practice DPM (Persantin™) is best known as an oral agent widely used for cardiovascular conditions because of its platelet antiaggregant and vasodilator activities (reviewed by FitzGerald[17]). Largely in that context, it accrued over 4,000 references in Index Medicus between 1966 and 1990. Specific indications have included secondary prevention of myocardial infarction, secondary prevention of transient cerebral ischemia and stroke, preservation of patency after coronary artery bypass, prevention of occlusion in obliterative arterial diseases of the lower limbs, prevention of venous thrombosis and thromboembolism, and prevention of thromboembolic complications of cardiac valve disease. It is not clear, however, that DPM, as generally administered in combination with aspirin, is preferable to aspirin alone.[17]

DPM inhibits nonenergy dependent, "facilitated diffusion" transport of nucleosides across cell membranes.[15,18,19] The inhibitory constant (K_i) is generally about 10-50 nM (free drug) for human cells. This transport is thought to be mediated by 45-65 kDa intrinsic membrane glycoproteins structurally similar to the sugar transporters. Through transport inhibition, DPM can affect the cellular uptake and efflux of physiological nucleosides and nucleoside drugs. Hence, in the last few years, it has been studied for cancer chemotherapy in combination with inhibitors of *de novo* nucleotide synthesis and other antitumor agents.[20-25] The essential idea is to block both *de novo* and "salvage" pathways, thereby increasing the potency of therapy. Weber[26] proposed that refractory tumors, by virtue of their reliance on nucleotide salvage pathways, might be more responsive than normal cells to therapy combining a cytotoxic antimetabolite with an agent that blocks salvage. DPM has been combined for antitumor effect *in vitro* with acivicin,[27] quinazoline (CB3717),[28] vincristine and vinblastine,[29] methotrexate,[25,30] N-phosphonacetyl-L-aspartate (PALA),[21,22] 2'-deoxyuridine,[31] adriamycin,[32] 3'-deazauridine,[33] and 5-fluorouracil.[34,35] Phase I clinical studies on DPM-acivicin,[36] DPM-PALA,[24] and DPM-methotrexate[37] combinations have been reported. DPM-methotrexate has been carried to phase II in colorectal carcinoma.[38]

DPM has also been reported to inhibit replication of various RNA and DNA viruses[39,40] and to have a therapeutic effect in patients with herpes simplex viruses.[41] No retroviruses were included in those studies, and the mechanism of antiviral action was not defined. DPM has been reported to induce interferon-α production in several cell types, and that could, in principle, contribute to the antiviral activity.[42–45]

Our own interest in DPM began with a serendipitous finding. We wanted to use DPM as a tool for inhibition of nucleoside transport in experiments with liposomes containing dideoxynucleotide drugs.[46] In control configurations with unencapsulated drug, however, DPM potentiated the activity of AZT and of dideoxycytidine (ddC) against HIV-1. That result led to the studies of antiviral activity, cell toxicity, and mechanism of action to be described next.

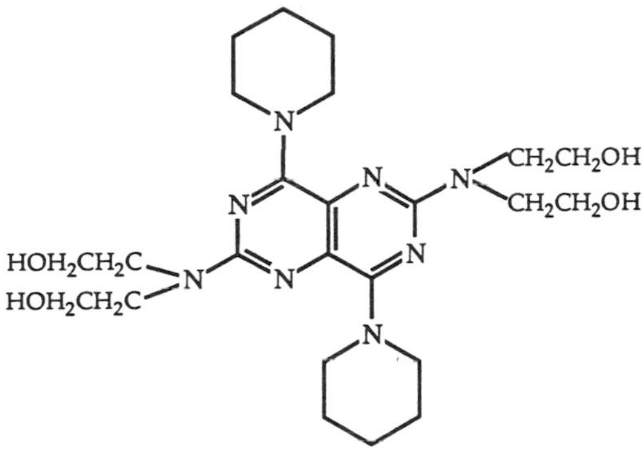

FIGURE 1. Chemical structure of dipyridamole.

Monocyte/Macrophages

Antiviral Activity

Our initial studies[47] were done with cultured monocyte/macrophages (M/M), purified either by elutriation[48,49] or by adherence to plastic.[50] DPM by itself appeared to have a small, variable inhibitory effect on HIV-1 replication in those cells, as assayed by p24 viral antigen production. More significantly, DPM potentiated the anti-HIV activity of AZT, ddC, and ddC triphosphate. EC_{50} and EC_{95} values for antiviral activity of the dideoxynucleosides were decreased at least 5-fold and 10-fold, respectively. TABLE 1 summarizes the results for AZT. DPM was not toxic to the M/M at concentrations < 10-$20~\mu$M as assessed by cell counts, Trypan blue exclusion, and the functional criterion of superoxide generation.[47]

Mechanism(s) of Action

Any of several different mechanisms of action reported for DPM[47] in various cell types could, in principle, explain the antiviral activity: increased cytoplasmic cyclic-

AMP, either by inhibition of cyclic-AMP phosphodiesterase or by effects on prostanoid metabolism; induction of interferon; nonspecific alteration of cell-surface properties; and "differential transport inhibition." Preliminary studies (Szebeni et al., unpublished data) have found no evidence in the M/M system for the first two mechanisms above. The third mechanism would probably require higher concentrations of DPM than those used in our antiviral studies.

The most intriguing possibility is the last one. Because AZT is more lipophilic than the physiological nucleosides, it might be expected to bypass the nucleoside transporter and enter cells by passive diffusion. This effect has been demonstrated for lymphocytes and red blood cells by Zimmerman and co-workers.[51,52] The normal deoxynucleosides (dNs) compete with AZT for phosphorylation and, as triphosphates, for reverse transcription.[6,53–57] Perno et al.[58] have emphasized the importance to antiviral potency of increased cytoplasmic ratios of dideoxy- to deoxy- nucleoside triphosphates. Therefore, DPM's potentiating effect on the antiviral action of AZT can be rationalized by differential inhibition of uptake and/or metabolic activation of the competing physiological nucleoside thymidine (dThd). The possible relationships are shown schematically in FIGURE 2.

TABLE 1. Levels of AZT Required to Inhibit HIV-1 p24 Antigen Expression in Adherence-Purified Human Monocyte-Macrophage Cultures in the Presence and Absence of DPM

	AZT (μM)		
Treatment	EC_{50}[a]	EC_{95}	r[b]
AZT alone	0.63 (100%)	5.99 (100%)	0.99
AZT + .08 μM DPM	0.30 (47%)	2.55 (43%)	0.99
AZT + 0.4 μM DPM	0.23 (37%)	0.74 (12%)	0.94
AZT + 2 μM DPM	0.11 (18%)	0.50 (8%)	0.96
AZT + 10 μM DPM	0.11 (18%)	0.72 (12%)	0.97

[a] EC_{50} and EC_{95} are the 50% and 95% effective antiviral concentration levels of AZT in the mixture.
[b] r is the linear regression coefficient for each calculation. Percentages in parentheses relate the EC_{50} and EC_{95} values to those of AZT alone.[47]

To examine these possibilities, we[59] incubated M/M with [³H]dThd or [³H]AZT under conditions similar to those of the antiviral studies. As shown in FIGURE 3, 2 μM DPM had no effect on [³H]AZT uptake in one-minute incubations. By contrast, DPM inhibited [³H]dThd uptake by approximately 60% if it was added simultaneously with the [³H]dThd and by approximately 90% if the cells had also been preincubated with DPM for 10 minutes prior to addition of the nucleoside. This effect of preincubation argues against simple competitive inhibition of nucleoside transport; it is consistent with the hypothesis that DPM partitions into the membrane and interacts with hydrophobic domains of the transporter protein.[15,31] In sum, these transport studies support the hypothesis that differential inhibition of the cellular uptake of dThd, as opposed to AZT, contributes to DPM's potentiating effect on the antiviral activity of AZT.

Next, we asked how DPM influences the accumulation of salvaged nucleotides in longer-term incubations with [³H]dThd and [³H]AZT.[59] The high-performance liquid

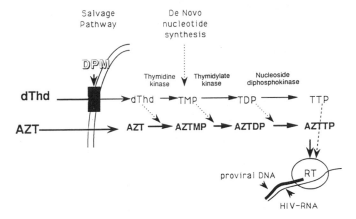

FIGURE 2. A working hypothesis for the mechanism of DPM's potentiating effect on the anti-HIV activity of AZT. dThd competes with AZT for phosphorylation and, as the triphosphate, for viral reverse transcriptase. Differential inhibition by DPM of dThd's entry in the cell and/or phosphorylation is expected to suppress any antagonistic influence of dThd on AZT's antiviral activity. As discussed in the text, however, it is hard to reconcile all of the experimental findings with a single metabolic mechanism such as this.

chromatogram in FIGURE 4a shows that the amounts of [3H]dThd mono-, di-, and triphosphate were reduced by DPM, whereas the dThd peak was at least as large as that in the control with no DPM. By contrast, FIGURE 4b shows that 2 μM DPM had no effect on the accumulation of [3H]AZT's phosphorylated forms. Hence, differential inhibition of phosphorylation of dThd is also apparent in the M/M system. FIGURE 4a shows an additional effect of DPM: enhanced incorporation of 3H into an unidentified peak (X), which eluted from the nucleotide column between [3H]dThd and

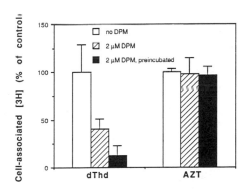

FIGURE 3. The effect of DPM on uptake of [3H]dThd and [3H]AZT by adherent monocyte-macrophages. The cells were exposed to isotope in the presence or absence of DPM. After 1 minute of incubation, they were washed and processed for liquid scintillation counting. Black bars indicate preincubation for 10 minutes prior to adding nucleoside, striped bars represent simultaneous addition of drugs, and open bars indicate untreated controls. Means ± SD are shown for 2-3 independent experiments, normalized to average of untreated controls.[59]

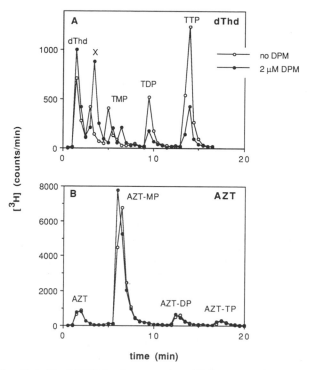

FIGURE 4. The effect of 2 μM DPM on incorporation of [³H]dThd (**A**) and [³H]AZT (**B**) counts into the nucleoside and nucleotide pools in adherent monocyte-macrophages. Typical HPLC chromatograms were recorded after 3 hours of incubation at 37°C. Filled and empty circles indicate DPM-treated and control cells, respectively. X in panel **A** is an unidentified metabolite. dThd, thymidine; MP, DP, and TP represent mono-, di-, and triphosphate, respectively.[59]

[³H]dThd monophosphate. This peak was present and increased in 3 out of 4 experiments, whereas nothing resembling peak X was seen in cells treated with [³H]AZT. The identity of this metabolite and its possible role in the antiviral effect of DPM are currently under study.

dThd appears to antagonize the antiviral activity of AZT,[6,53–57] and the observations presented here lend support to the hypothesis that differential inhibition of nucleoside transport and/or phosphorylation plays a role in DPM's potentiation of AZT activity. The relationship between transport and phosphorylation, however, is unclear. In particular, it is not obvious that inhibition of transport should decrease the steady-state production of phosphorylated nucleosides. Carrier-mediated transmembrane flux of nucleosides can equilibrate intracellular and extracellular concentrations within minutes, and, in the case of dThd, does not appear to be rate-limiting to the subsequent phosphorylation process.[15] We observed little or no decrease in salvaged dThd levels in DPM-treated cells at times when the [³H]dThd phosphates were substantially decreased. This last observation suggests a direct influence of DPM on dThd phosphorylation, although it does not necessarily reflect total pool sizes. Clearly, a great deal remains to be understood about the mechanism(s) of the antiviral activity. As will become evident in the following paragraphs, the picture becomes even harder to explain in terms of a single effect on nucleoside levels when we take into account the influences of DPM on AZT's cytotoxicity.

Stimulated T Lymphocytes

Mononuclear cells from healthy volunteers were grown in the presence of phytohemagglutinin (5 μg/mL) for 2 days and then stimulated with interleukin-2. After 3 days the cells were infected with HIV-1_{IIIb} for 90 minutes at 37°C. They were then washed, plated, treated with drug, and incubated for 10 days (with refeeding of medium and drug every 2-3 days); p24 production was measured by ELISA. TABLE 2 shows that DPM by itself inhibited p24 production only modestly. However, DPM greatly potentiated the activity of AZT, even at a concentration of 74 nM (Weinstein *et al.*, manuscript in preparation).

T-Lymphoblastoid Cells

Cells of the CD4$^+$ CEM-SS T-lymphoblastoid line were infected with HIV$_{IIIb}$ and incubated with drug in 96-well microtiter plates for 7 days at 37°C in RPMI-1640 with 10% fetal calf serum. The cells were then assessed for cytopathic effects of virus and drugs using the tetrazolium dye assay described by Weislow *et al.*[60] Uninfected cells, or those protected by drug and continuing to proliferate, convert the tetrazolium salt XTT into a soluble orange formazan dye that can be measured by an optical plate reader. As shown in FIGURE 5, low concentrations of AZT protect the cells from HIV-1, but high concentrations are toxic. There appears to be a modest potentiation (approx. 3-fold at 2.5 μM) of the antiviral effect by DPM. More strikingly, DPM protects the cells by more than an order of magnitude against the cytotoxicity of AZT (Weinstein *et al.*, manuscript in preparation). Thus, the therapeutic index is greatly increased. This is a reproducible finding. It emphasizes that different cell types are likely to show different apparent responses to a combination such as this and that the mechanisms involved may be complex. It is hard to explain this combination of results

TABLE 2. Potentiation by DPM of AZT's Anti-HIV Activity in Phytohemagglutinin Stimulated Human T Lymphocytes[a]

AZT (μM)	DPM (μM)					
	0	0.074	0.222	0.667	2.0	6.0
0.0	635	1423	1251	597	255	172
0.156	470	24	9	5	5	1
0.625	147	6	5	2	2	1
2.5	19	1	4	6	5	6
10.0	[b]	[b]	[b]	[b]	[b]	[b]

[a] Numbers in Table are p24 levels.
[b] Cell toxicity.

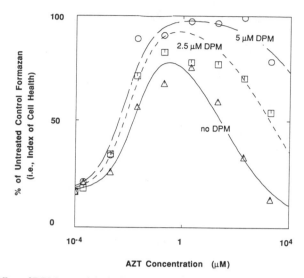

FIGURE 5. Effect of DPM on antiviral efficacy and toxicity of AZT in CEM-SS T-lymphoblastoid cells. DPM enhanced the antiviral potency of AZT severalfold and decreased the concentration required for toxicity by more than an order of magnitude, thereby greatly increasing the *in vitro* therapeutic index. Curves represent iso-effect contours of the best-fitting surface calculated according to an "Eff-Tox" model using COMBO. Modified from Weinstein *et al.* (manuscript in preparation.) Some conclusions from the "EFF-TOX" analysis:

Q: Does AZT have intrinsic antiviral activity? Cytotoxic effect?
A: Yes ($p < 0.01$); Yes ($p < 0.01$).
Q: What is the therapeutic index of AZT alone?
A: The best estimate is a 3,300-fold difference between EC_{50} and IC_{50}. There is a 95% chance that the "true" value lies between 800- and 8,300-fold.
Q: Does DPM potentiate the antiviral activity of AZT?
A: Yes ($p < 0.01$).
Q: Does DPM antagonize the cytotoxicity of AZT?
A: Yes ($p < 0.01$).
Q: Does DPM increase the therapeutic index?
A: Yes ($p < 0.01$), a 12.4-fold increase for 1 μM DPM.

on the basis simply of changes in nucleotide salvage or pool sizes. The nature of the assay virtually excludes the possibility that host cell heterogeneity could explain the opposite effects of DPM on antiviral and toxic activities. The results suggest a potentially exploitable dissociation of DPM's potentiating effect on the anti-HIV activity of a dideoxynucleoside drug and its antagonistic effect on the drug's cytotoxicity. These findings also illustrate the need for a framework of data analysis and interpretation that goes beyond simple potentiation, synergy, and antagonism.

Bone Marrow Progenitor Cells

Another important type of therapeutic index relates the antiviral efficacy to the limiting toxicity, that is, to bone marrow toxicity in the case of AZT.[61] To assess the bone marrow effect of AZT-DPM combinations, CFU_{GM} (granulocyte-monocyte colony forming unit) assays were performed on marrow samples from 7 healthy donors.[47] The mean inhibitory concentration (IC_{50}) of AZT, calculated from pooled values as described elsewhere,[47] was 0.6 ± 0.1 μM (SEM, n=21). DPM alone inhibited colony formation only at high, nonpharmacological doses ($IC_{50} = 10.0 \pm 4.5$ μM; n=19). With respect to both toxicity and antiviral activity, it should be noted that DPM is less highly protein-bound in cell culture medium than in human plasma[62] and that there will be less free drug in plasma for a given total concentration. Most important, DPM did not appear to potentiate the toxic effects of AZT. These results together with the antiviral data suggest that if AZT is combined with ≤ 2 μM DPM, it may be possible to obtain identical antiviral effects with less toxicity for bone marrow progenitor cells than with AZT alone. It is important to note that DPM is not reported to be marrow-toxic clinically. DPM is also not reported as neurotoxic, an important consideration with respect to its possible use with ddC.

THE DIDEOXYINOSINE - DIPYRIDAMOLE COMBINATION

The DPM-dideoxyinosine (ddI) combination was studied in CEM-SS cells using the same methods as with DPM-AZT. FIGURE 6 shows the results of an experiment that indicated another important type of drug combination that is possible whether or not one sees formal synergy in the antiviral activity. DPM had no effect on the cellular

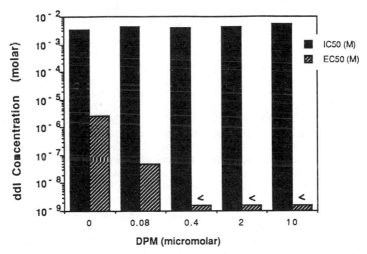

FIGURE 6. The antiviral activity and cytotoxicity of ddI and DPM in CEM-SS T-lymphoblastoid cells. IC_{50} (black bars) indicates the 50% cell toxic concentration of ddI. EC_{50} (hatched bars) indicates the concentration of ddI required for 50% protection of the cells against HIV. < indicates that the ddI concentration for 50% effect was below the lowest tested. The assay was performed essentially identically to that in FIG. 5.; 0.08 μM DPM reduced by 50-fold the concentration of ddI required for antiviral effect but did not affect the cell toxicity. Thus, the *in vitro* therapeutic index was larger for the combination.

cytotoxicity of dideoxyinosine, as indicated by the 50% cell inhibitory concentration (IC_{50}). However, 0.08 μM DPM increased the observed antiviral potency 50-fold. That is, the 50% virus inhibitory dose (EC_{50}) was greatly decreased. Thus, as in the case of DPM-AZT, the *in vitro* therapeutic index was considerably enhanced by addition of DPM.

A CONCEPTUAL FRAMEWORK AND COMPUTER "TOOLBOX" FOR ANALYSIS OF DRUG COMBINATIONS

In the introduction, we referred to the almost metaphysical arguments over concepts in drug interaction and to our view that those arguments are largely resolvable by proper attention to definitions and context. Here, let us consider three relevant points, leaving a more general analysis to be presented elsewhere:

(1) In certain simple circumstances, the concept of *additivity* is well-defined, and it forms a logical null hypothesis against which to judge interaction of drug efficacies (or toxicities). In more complex circumstances, the concept of additivity is elusive and must be divided up into more explicit quantitative concepts (*e.g., robust additivity, vide infra*).

(2) Confusion over the terms *potentiation* and *synergy* is easily resolved by paying attention to the syntax of their use: When we say that two drugs are synergistic, a mutuality of effect is stressed; when we say that one drug potentiates another, there is an asymmetry. Synergy can often be expressed mathematically as a "mutual potentiation." Some of the antiviral data sets summarized here are consistent with a pure potentiating ("modulatory") effect of DPM. Other data sets suggest that DPM has intrinsic activity and also that the interaction should be described as synergistic.

(3) It is sometimes very important to state whether a given drug combination displays formal potentiation, synergy, or antagonism, that is, whether a null hypothesis of additivity can be rejected. It is by no means, however, the only important question. Obviously, therapeutic indices must also be considered. In the experiments on DPM - AZT and DPM - ddI in CEM-SS cells, changes in the therapeutic index for the given experiment had implications for mechanism and suggested a dissociation of DPM's antiviral influence and effects on the cell toxicity of nucleoside drugs. Most important with relation to clinical therapy is the relationship between doses required for antiviral activity and the dose-limiting toxicity. We have also had occasion to analyze combinations in which the usual vocabulary for expressing drug interaction is inadequate and it is necessary to develop entirely new terminology.

Currently available methods of data analysis, principally the multiple-drug effect method of Chou and Talalay,[63] have been useful in the development of drug combinations for HIV infection. To supplement the available approaches, however, we decided to develop a computer toolbox for flexible analysis of combinations. The twin aims were to provide statistically satisfactory tools to handle the simpler instances of potentiation, synergy, and antagonism; and to provide tools for designing new quantitative models related to therapeutic indices and more complex types of interaction. The result is a prototype program package called COMBO. Because COMBO is described elsewhere in this volume by Bunow and Weinstein,[64] it will be discussed only briefly here.

Overview of COMBO

Although much of the statistical apparatus is more general, COMBO starts by projecting the classical logistic dose response curve into a third dimension to accommodate a second drug. The toolbox is used to explore a number of enzyme-kinetics based pseudomolecular models that we have found appropriate for analyzing data on drug combinations.

Briefly, the COMBO algorithm currently uses iteratively reweighted nonlinear least squares techniques for data fitting (robust regression and maximum likelihood approaches are also being included). If desired, the weights are computed by a gaussian windowing technique based on estimated responses. Statistical diagnostics available[64] include the weighted sum of squares, normal theory standard error estimates, variance-covariance matrix, parameter dependency values, root mean square weighted deviation errors, mean deviation/data fraction, residuals, and weighted residuals. Various graphical outputs are generated for summary of data fits, residuals, and statistics. COMBO offers the following features: (1) constant drug dose ratios are not necessary; (2) overlapping efficacy and toxicity can be analyzed simultaneously; (3) all data points can generally be used without editing or censoring; (4) global parameters are computed for potentiation, synergy, antagonism, and (if appropriate) therapeutic index; (5) a flexible choice of data models can be invoked; (6) a flexible choice of error structures is provided (including automatic error model estimation by gaussian windowing on the data set itself); (7) distribution-free confidence intervals on model parameters are obtained by a new Monte Carlo technique related (but not identical) to the Bootstrap method of Efron;[65,66] (8) statistical criteria for outliers can be calculated; and (9) experimental designs with fewer replicates are facilitated.[64] The most significant disadvantage of the COMBO toolbox is that the Monte Carlo methods and outlier selection algorithms are computer-intensive. COMBO operates in the MLAB computing environment (Civilized Software, Inc., Bethesda, MD) on mainframes and PCs.

The "Robust Potentiation" Model

Using a combination of ideas arising from the theory of multiple inhibitors in enzyme kinetics and the isobologram representation of Berenbaum,[67] we obtained the following effect equation[64] for a pair of drugs, one or both of which is intrinsically active:

$$1 = (1/z - 1)^{-1/B_1}(c_1/IC_1)(1 + (c_2/PC_2)^{BP_2})$$

$$+ (1/z - 1)^{-1/B_2}(c_2/IC_2)(1 + (c_1/PC_1)^{BP_1}) \tag{1}$$

where $z = (a - y)/(a - d)$ is the normalized effect; y, the measured p24 level in natural units, defines a surface over c_1 and c_2; c_1 and c_2 are the concentrations of the two drugs; IC_1 and IC_2 are the 50%-effect concentrations (generally called IC50s or

EC50s, but the "50" has been left out to simplify the notation); B_1 and B_2 are the 50%-effect slopes for the two drugs acting individually; PC_1 and BP_1 are the 50%-effect concentration and slope for the potentiation of drug 2 by drug 1; PC_2 and BP_2 are the 50%-effect concentration and slope for the potentiation of drug 1 by drug 2; a is p24 in the absence of drug; d is p24 at indefinitely high drug levels. PC_i is defined as the concentration of drug i required to increase the apparent potency of the other drug (i.e., decrease its apparent IC) by a factor of 2 (beyond what would be expected on the basis of the intrinsic activity of drug i). The lower the value of PC_i, the stronger the potentiation; additivity corresponds to PC_1 and PC_2 approaching infinity. Note that this equation reduces to an explicit expression for z if $B_1 = B_2$.

In the absence of interaction, equation 1 is equivalent to that of Syracuse and Greco.[68] The two differ when interaction is present, however. An additional difference is that the equation in reference 68 contains only one interaction parameter, α. Equation 1 above is a more general form containing 4 interaction parameters, although it can be simplified in the obvious way to include 0, 1, 2, or 3 interaction parameters as required (and/or justified) by the data. This flexibility allows for analysis of more complex interactions and better fitting of a wide range of experimental data. It also emphasizes the relationship between synergy and mutual potentiation. To date the most useful models have included interaction parameters PC_1 and BP_1 or PC_2 and BP_2, but not both sets simultaneously. It is often important to include the slope parameter.

FIGURE 7 shows application of the robust potentiation model to an experiment on reverse transcriptase production in stimulated T lymphocytes infected with HIV-1 and treated with DPM-AZT. The surface representing drug effect as a function of the two drug doses can be viewed conveniently as a set of isoeffect contours, as in the usual isobologram methods.[67] The analysis of this particular data set is shown because the experiment yielded less drug interaction than those done under the conditions of TABLE 2, and the proper conclusions to be drawn from the experiment were not obvious by inspection. In particular, it was not clear prior to analysis how statistically robust the potentiation would prove to be. FIGURE 7 includes a dialogue illustrating some of the bottom-line conclusions and statistical inferences available from COMBO for this experiment.

The Eff-Tox model

The fitted curves in FIGURE 5 were calculated using what we term an Eff-Tox model, which takes account of simultaneous, overlapping antiviral efficacy and cell toxicity.

The equations are

num =
$$av + (c_1/ICe_1)^{Be_1}(1 + (c_2/PCe_2)^{BPe_2})(1 + (c_1/ICt_1)^{Bt_1}(1 + (c_2/PCt_2)^{BPt_2})) \quad \textbf{(2a)}$$
den =
$$1 + (c_1/ICe_1)^{Be_1}(1 + (c_2/PCe_2)^{BPe_2})(1 + (c_1/ICt_1)^{Bt_1}(1 + (c_2/PCt_2)^{BPt_2})) \quad \textbf{(2b)}$$

where $z = num/den = (y - d)/(a - d)$ is the normalized formazan level. y is the measured formazan level in natural units; a is the formazan level in the absence of virus and drug; d is the formazan level at indefinitely high drug concentrations; ICe, Be, PCe, and BPe are parameters related to the antiviral efficacy and defined as were their equivalents in the robust potentiation model; ICt, Bt, PCt, and BPt are similar parameters related to the call toxicity; av is the normalized formazan level at zero drug. The above pair of equations may look complex, but it arises naturally from an enzymological model that has quite general application. In this data set, it was important to consider both limbs of the dose-response curve simultaneously inasmuch as the response variable, an index of cell health, reflects both damage by the virus and damage by the drugs. In other cases, the mixing of viral and toxic effects might be more subtle, when, for example, cell toxicity diminishes viral production of measured p24 or reverse transcriptase.

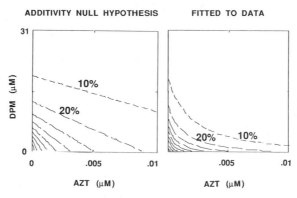

FIGURE 7. Iso-effect contours from the robust potentiation model for an experiment on AZT and DPM in phytohemagglutinin-stimulated primary human T lymphocytes. Percentages indicate the levels of HIV-1 reverse transcriptase observed, relative to untreated controls. The left-hand panel shows straight-line contours for the null hypothesis of additivity; the right-hand panel shows the best fit to the data set (with weights determined by gaussian windowing). Modified from Bunow *et al.*[64] Some conclusions from the robust potentiation analysis:

Q: Does AZT alone have intrinsic antiviral activity?
A: Yes (p < 0.01).
Q: Does DPM have intrinsic antiviral activity?
A: Yes (p < 0.01).
Q: Does DPM potentiate the antiviral activity of AZT?
A: Probably yes (p = 0.07).

CONCLUDING REMARKS

In summary, DPM potentiates the activity of AZT against HIV-1 in cultured monocytes and T lymphocytes, that is, the two-cell lineages considered as principal hosts for the virus. In some experiments, but not all, DPM also appears to have intrinsic antiviral activity, perhaps correlated with introduction of the drug early in infection. Investigation of the mechanism of activity in monocytes reveals potent inhibition of dThd transport and also an apparent inhibition at the level of phosphorylation. By contrast, the transport and metabolism of AZT are unaffected. We do not yet know, however, if either the differential transport inhibition or differential effects on metabolism explain the antiviral activity.

The studies with CEM-SS T-lymphoblastoid cells indicate a surprising dissociation of DPM's influence on AZT's antiviral and cytotoxic activities. The net effect is to increase the *in vitro* therapeutic index for that cell type. DPM modestly potentiates the antiviral activity of AZT and, at the same time, greatly antagonizes its cytotoxicity. With ddI in CEM-SS cells, DPM does not affect the cytotoxicity but increases the antiviral potency by several orders of magnitude, thereby increasing the *in vitro* therapeutic index. These studies suggest that more than one mechanism of activity is at work and that the balance of effects can depend on cell type and experimental conditions. Good tools of analysis will be required to put these phenomena into proper perspective, and the COMBO algorithms are being used for that purpose.

In the CFU_{GM} assay, DPM does not appear to potentiate the cytotoxic effects of AZT, and it is not reported to be marrow-toxic in its own right. Hence, there is reason for optimism that it would not exacerbate the dose-limiting toxicity of AZT and that improved therapeutic indices could be achieved *in vivo*. It is not possible to predict the clinical efficacy or safety of such combinations in the absence of careful trials. The extensive medical experience with both DPM and AZT provides important background for this effort, and clinical trials are planned.

ACKNOWLEDGMENTS

We are grateful to M. Corcoran for preparing elutriated cells, L. Muenz for advice on the statistics, S. Gartner and M. Popovic for their work on the early monocyte studies, R. Kiser and S. Thompson for assistance with antiviral experiments in CEM-SS cells, D. A. Cooney and D. G. Johns for advice on the biochemistry, S. Patel and G. Betageri for biochemical pharmacology experiments, J. E. Dahlberg and E. Hunter for studies in T lymphocytes, and R. L. Fine for work on the CFU_{GM} assays.

REFERENCES

1. BHALLA, K., M. BIRKHOFER, L. GONGRONG, S. GRANT, W. MacLAUGHLIN, J. COLE, G. GRAHAM & D. J. VOLSKY. 1989. 2'-Deoxycytidine protects normal human bone marrow progenitor cells *in vitro* against the cytotoxicity of 3'-azido-3'-deoxythymidine with preservation of antiretroviral activity. Blood **74:** 1923-1928.
2. HAMMER, S. M. & J. M. GILLIS. 1987. Synergistic activity of granulocyte-macrophage colony-stimulating factor and 3'-azido-3'-deoxythymidine against human immunodeficiency virus *in vitro*. Antimicrob. Agents Chemother. **31:** 1046-1050.
3. HARTSHORN, K. L., M. W. VOGT, T.-C. CHOU, R. S. BLUMBERG, R. BYINGTON, R. T. SCHOOLEY & M. S. HIRSCH. 1987. Synergistic inhibition of human immunodeficiency virus *in vitro* by azidothymidine and recombinant alpha A interferon. Antimicrob. Agents Chemother. **31:** 168-172.
4. JOHNSON, V. A., M. A. BARLOW, T.-C. CHOU, R. A. FISHER, B. D. WALKER, M. S. HIRSCH & R. T. SCHOOLEY. 1989. Synergistic inhibition of human immunodeficiency virus type 1 (HIV-1) replication *in vitro* by recombinant soluble CD4 and 3'-azido-3'-deoxythymidine. J. Infect. Dis. **159:** 837-844.
5. KOVACS, J. A., L. DEYTON, R. DAVEY, J. FALLOON, K. ZUNICH, D. LEE, J. A. METCALF,

J. W. BIGLEY, L. A. SAWYER, K. C. ZOON, H. MASUR & A. S. FAUCI. 1989. Combined zidovudine and interferon-alpha therapy in patients with Kaposi's sarcoma and the acquired immunodeficiency syndrome (AIDS). Ann. Intern. Med. **111:** 280-287.

6. SOMMADOSSI, J.-P., R. CARLISLE, R. F. SCHINAZI & Z. ZHOU. 1988. Uridine reverses the toxicity of 3'-azido-3'-deoxythymidine in normal human granulocyte-macrophage progenitor cells *in vitro* without impairment of antiretroviral activity. Antimicrob. Agents Chemother. **32:** 997-1001.

7. VOGT, M. W., K. L. HARTSHORN, P. A. FURMAN, T.-C. CHOU, J. A. FYFE, L. A. COLEMAN, C. CRUMPACKER, R. T. SCHOOLEY & M. S. HIRSCH. 1987. Ribavirin antagonizes the effect of azidothymidine on HIV replication. Science **235:** 1376-1379.

8. VOGT, M. W., A. G. DURNO, T.-C. CHOU, L. A. COLEMAN, T. J. PARADIS, R. T. SCHOOLEY, J. C. KAPLAN & M. S. HIRSCH. 1988. Synergistic interaction of 2',3'-dideoxycytidine and recombinant interferon-alpha on replication of human immunodeficiency virus type 1. J. Infect. Dis. **158:** 378-385.

9. ERIKSSON, B. F. H. & R. F. SCHINAZI. 1989. Combinations of 3'-azido-3'-deoxythymidine (Zidovudine) and phosphonoformate (Foscarnet) against human immunodeficiency virus type I and cytomegalovirus replication *in vitro*. Antimicrob. Agents Chemother. **33:** 663-669.

10. SCHINAZI, R. F., D. L. CANNON, B. H. ARNOLD & D. MARTINO-SALTZMAN. 1988. Combinations of isoprinosine and 3'-azido-3'-deoxythymidine in lymphocytes infected with human immunodeficiency virus type I. Antimicrob. Agents Chemother. **32:** 1784-1787.

11. SCHINAZI, R. F. Combined chemotherapeutic modalities for viral infections: Rationale and clinical potential. *In* Synergism and Antagonism in Chemotherapy. T.-C Chou & D. C. Rideout, Eds. Academic Press. Orlando, FL. In press.

12. PATERSON, A. R. P., E. Y. LAU, E. DAHLIG & C. E. CASS. 1980. A common basis for inhibition of nucleoside transport by dipyridamole and nitrobenzylthioinosine. Mol. Pharmacol. **18:** 40-44.

13. PATERSON, A. R. P., N. KOLASSA & C. E. CASS. 1981. Transport of nucleoside drugs in animal cells. Pharm. Ther. **12:** 515-536.

14. PATERSON, A. R. P. & C. E. CASS. 1986. Transport of nucleoside drugs in animal cells. *In* Membrane Transport of Antineoplastic Agents. I. D. Goldman, Ed.: 309-329. Pergamon Press. Oxford.

15. PLAGEMANN, P. G. W., R. M. WOHLHUETER & C. WOFFENDIN. 1980. Permeation of nucleosides, nucleic acid bases, and nucleotides in animal cells. Curr. Top. Membr. Transp. **14:** 225-330.

16. PLAGEMANN, P. G. W., R. M. WOHLHUETER & C. WOFFENDIN. 1988. Nucleoside and nucleobase transport in animal cells. Biochim. Biophys. Acta **947:** 405-443.

17. FITZGERALD, D. 1987. Dipyridamole. N. Engl. J. Med. **316:** 1247-1257.

18. WOFFENDIN, C. & P. G. W. PLAGEMANN. 1987. Interaction of ^{3}H-dipyridamole with the nucleoside transporters of human erythrocytes and cultured animal cells. J. Membr. Biol. **98:** 89-100.

19. GII, M. M & I. D. YOUNG. 1986. ^{3}H-Dipyridamole binding to nucleoside transporters from guinea-pig and rat lung. Biochem. J. **240:** 879-883.

20. NELSON, J. A. & S. DRAKE. 1984. Potentiation of methotrexate toxicity by dipyridamole. Cancer Res. **44:** 2493-2496.

21. CHAN, T. C. K., B. YOUNG, M. E. KING, R. TAETLE & S. B. HOWELL. 1985. Modulation of the activity of N-phosphonacetyl-L-aspartate by dipyridamole. Cancer Treat. Rep. **69:** 425-430.

22. CHAN, T. C. K. & S. B. HOWELL. 1985. Mechanism of synergy between N-phosphonacetyl-L-aspartate and dipyridamole in a human ovarian carcinoma cell line. Cancer Res. **45:** 3598-3604.

23. GREM, J. L. & P. H. FISCHER. 1986. Alteration of fluorouracil metabolism in human colon cancer cells by dipyridamole with a selective increase in fluorodeoxyuridine monophosphate levels. Cancer Res. **46:** 6191-6199.

24. MARKMAN, M., T. C. CHAN, S. CLEARY & S. B. HOWELL. 1987. Phase 1 trial of combination chemotherapy of cancer with N-phosphonacetyl-L-aspartic acid and dipyridamole. Cancer Chemother. Pharmacol. **19:** 80-83.

25. MUGGIA, F. M., P. SLOWIACZEK & M. H. N TATTERSALL. 1987. Characterization of conditions in which dipyridamole enhances methotrexate toxicity in L1210 cells. Anticancer Res. **7:** 161-166.

26. WEBER, G., H. N. JAYARAM, K. PILLWEIN, Y. NATSUMEDA, M. A. REARDON & Y.-S. ZHEN. 1983. Salvage pathways as targets of chemotherapy. Cancer Res. **43:** 3466-3492.

27. ZHEN, Y.-S., M. S. LUI & G. WEBER. 1983. Effects of acivicin and dipyridamole on hepatoma 3924A cells. Cancer Res. **43:** 1616-1619.

28. CURTIN, N. J. & A. L. HARRIS. 1988. Potentiation of quinazoline antifolate (CB3717) toxicity by dipyridamole in human lung carcinoma, A549, cells. Biochem. Pharmacol. **37:** 2113-2120.

29. HIROSE, M., E. TAKEDA, T. NINOMIYA, Y. KURODA & M. MIYAO. 1987. Synergistic inhibitory effect of dipyridamole and vincristine on the growth of human leukaemia and lymphoma cell lines. Br. J. Cancer **56:** 413-417.

30. VAN MOUWERIK, T. J., C. A. PANGALLO, J. K. V. WILLSON & P. H. FISCHER. 1987. Augmentation of methotrexate cytotoxicity in human colon cancer cells achieved through inhibition of thymidine salvage by dipyridamole. Biochem. Pharmacol. **36:** 809-814.

31. GREM, J. L. & P. H. FISCHER. 1989. Enhancement of 5-fluorouracil's anticancer activity by dipyridamole. Pharm. Ther. **40:** 349-371.

32. KUSUMOTO, H., Y. MACHARA, H. ANAI, T. KUSUMOTO & K. SUGIMACHI. 1988. Potentiation of adriamycin cytotoxicity by dipyridamole against HeLa cells *in vitro* and sarcoma 180 cells *in vivo.* Cancer Res. **48:** 1208-1212.

33. MOYER, J. D., N. MALINOWSKI & R. L. CYSYK. 1986. The effect of 3-deazuridine and dipyridamole on uridine utilization by mice. Eur. J. Cancer Clin. Oncol. **22:** 323-327.

34. GREM, J. L. & P. H. FISCHER. 1985. Augmentation of 5-fluorouracil cytotoxicity in human colon cancer cells by dipyridamole. Cancer Res. **45:** 2967-2972.

35. GREM, J. L. & P. H. FISCHER. 1986. Modulation of fluorouracil metabolism and cytotoxicity by nitrobenzylthioinosine. Biochem. Pharmacol. **35:** 2651-2654.

36. WILLSON, J. K. V., P. H. FISCHER, K. TUTSCH, D. ALBERTI, K. SIMON, R. D. HAMILTON, J. BRUGGINK, J. M. KOELLER, D. C. TORMEY, R. H. EARHART, A. RANHOSKY & D. L. TRUMP. 1988. Phase I clinical trial of a combination of dipyridamole and acivicin based upon inhibition of nucleoside salvage. Cancer Res. **48:** 5585-5590.

37. SUBAR, M. & F. M. MUGGIA. 1986. Phase I trial of low dose daily methotrexate with inhibition of rescue by dipyridamole. Proc. Am. Soc. Clin. Oncol. **5:** 165.

38. WADLER, S., M. SUBAR, M. D. GREEN, P. H. WIERNIK & F. M. MUGGIA. 1987. Phase II trial of oral methotrexate and dipyridamole in colorectal carcinoma. Cancer Treat. Rep. **71:** 821-824.

39. TONEW, M., E. TONEW & R. MENTEL. 1977. The antiviral activity of dipyridamole. Acta Virol. (Prague) (Engl. Ed.) **21:** 146-150.

40. TONEW, E., M. K. INDULEN & D. R. DZEGUZE. 1982. Antiviral action of dipyridamole and its derivatives against influenza virus A. Acta Virol. **26:** 125-129.

41. GUNTHER, W., S.-R. WASCHKE, H. MEFFERT, M. H. EL BASHIR, W. DIEZEL & N. SONNICHSEN. 1977. Untersuchungen zum therapeutischen Einsatz von Dipyridamol bei Herpesvirus-Infektionen. Dtsch. Gesundheitses. **32:** 1955-1959.

42. GALABOV, A. S. & M. MASTIKOVA. 1982. Dipyridamole is an interferon inducer. Acta Virol. (Prague) (Engl. Ed.) **26:** 137-147.

43. GALABOV, A. S. & M. MASTIKOVA. 1982. Interferon-inducing activity of dipyridamole in mice. Acta Virol. (Prague) (Engl. Ed.) **27:** 356-358.

44. GALABOV, A. S. & M. MASTIKOVA. 1984. Dipyridamole induces interferon in man. Biomed. Pharmacother. **38:** 412-413.

45. GALABOV, A. S., A. V. ITKES, M. MASTIKOVA, V. L. TUNITSKAYA & E. S. SEVERIN. 1985. Dipyridamole-induced interferon production in mouse peritoneal leukocytes. Biochem. Int. **11:** 591-598.

46. SZEBENI, J., S. M. WAHL, G. V. BETAGERI, L. M. WAHL., S. GARTNER, M. POPOVIC, R. PARKER, C. D. V. BLACK & J. N. WEINSTEIN. 1990. Inhibition of HIV-1 in monocyte/macrophage cultures by 2',3'-dideoxycytidine-5'-triphosphate, free and in liposomes. AIDS Res. Hum. Retroviruses **5:** 691-702.

47. SZEBENI, J., S. M. WAHL, M. POPOVIC, L. M. WAHL, S. GARTNER, R. L. FINE, U. SKALERIC, R. M. FRIEDMANN & J. N. WEINSTEIN. 1989. Dipyridamole potentiates

the inhibition by 3'-azido-3'-deoxythymidine and other dideoxynucleosides of human immunodeficiency virus replication in monocyte-macrophages. Proc. Natl. Acad. Sci. USA **86:** 3842-3846.

48. WAHL, S. M., I. M. KATONA, B. M. STADLER, R. L. WILDER, W. E. HELSEL & L. M. WAHL. 1984. Isolation of human mononuclear cell subsets by counterflow centrifugal elutriation (CCE) II. Functional properties of B-lymphocyte-, T-lymphocyte-, and mono-cyte-enriched fractions. Cell Immunol. **85:** 384-395.

49. WAHL, L. M., I. M. KATONA, R. L. WILDER, C. C. WINTER, B. HARAOUI, I. SCHER & S. M. WAHL. 1984. Isolation of human mononuclear cell subsets by counterflow centrifugal elutriation (CCE) I. Characterization of B-lymphocyte-, T-lymphocyte-, and monocyte-enriched fractions by flow cytometric analysis. Cell Immunol. **85:** 373-383.

50. GARTNER, S., P. MARKOVITS & D. M. MARKOVITZ. 1986. The role of mononuclear phago-cytes in HTLV-III/LAV infection. Science **233:** 215-219.

51. ZIMMERMAN, T. P., W. B. MAHONY & K. L. PRUS. 1987. An unusual nucleoside analogue that permeates the membrane of human erythrocytes and lymphocytes by nonfacilitated diffusion. J. Biol. Chem. **262:** 5748-5754.

52. DOMIN, B. A., W. B. MAHONY & T. P. ZIMMERMAN. 1988. 2',3'-Dideoxythymidine perme-ation of the human erythrocyte membrane by nonfacilitated diffusion. Biochem. Biophys. Res. Comm. **154:** 825-831.

53. BALZARINI, J., P. HERDEWIJN & E. DE CLERK. 1989. Differential patterns of intracellular metabolism of 2',3'-didehydro-2'3'-dideoxythymidine and 3'-azido-2',3'-dideoxythymi-dine, two potent anti-human immunodeficiency virus compounds. J. Biol. Chem. **264:** 6127-6133.

54. BHALLA, K., M. BIRKHOFER, S. GRANT & G. GRAHAM. 1989. The effect of recombinant human granulocyte-macrophage colony-stimulating factor (rGM-CSF) on 3'-azido-3'-deoxythymidine (AZT)-mediated biochemical and cytotoxic effects on normal human myeloid progenitor cells. Exp. Hematol. (NY) **17:** 17-20.

55. FURMAN, P. A., J. A. FYFE, M. H. CLAIR, K. WEINHOLD, J. L. RIDEOUT, G. A. FREEMAN, S. N. LEHRMAN, D. P. BOLOGNESI, S. BRODER, M. MITSUYA & D. W. BARRY. 1986. Phosphorylation of 3'-azido-3'-deoxythymidine and selective interaction of the 5'-triphos-phate with human immunodeficiency virus transcriptase. Proc. Natl. Acad. Sci. USA **83:** 8333-8337.

56. HAO, Z., D. A. COONEY, N. R. HARTMAN, C.-F. PERNO, A. FRIDLAND, A. L. DEVICO, M. G. SARNGADHARAN, S. BRODER & D. G. JOHNS. 1988. Factors determining the activity of 2',3'-dideoxynucleosides in suppressing human immunodeficiency virus *in vitro.* Mol. Pharmacol. **34:** 431-435.

57. YARCHOAN, R. & S. BRODER. 1987. Development of antiretroviral therapy for the acquired immunodeficiency syndrome and related disorders. N. Eng. J. Med. **316:** 557-564.

58. PERNO, C. F., R. YARCHOAN, D. A. COONEY, N. R. HARTMAN, S. GARTNER, M. POPOVIC, Z. HAO, T. L. GERRARD, Y. A. WILSON, D. G. JOHNS & S. BRODER. 1988. Inhibition of human immunodeficiency virus (HIV-1/HTLV-IIIBa-L) replication in fresh and cultured human peripheral blood monocyte/macrophages by AZT and related 2',3'-dideoxynucleo-sides. J. Exp. Med. **168:** 1111-1125.

59. BETAGERI, G. V., J. SZEBENI, K. HUNG, S. S. PATEL, M. CORCORAN & J. N. WEINSTEIN. 1990. Effect of dipyridamole on transport and phosphorylation of thymidine and 3'-azido-3'-deoxythymidine in human monocyte/macrophages. Biochem. Pharmacol. **40:** 867-870.

60. WEISLOW, O. S., R. KISER, D. L. FINE, J. BADER, R. H. SHOEMAKER & M. R. BOYD. 1989. New soluble formazan assay for HIV-1 cytopathic effects: Application to high-flux screening of synthetic and natural products for AIDS-antiviral activity. J. Natl. Cancer Inst. **81:** 577-586.

61. RICHMAN, D. D., M. A. FISCHL, M. H. GRIECO, M. S. GOTTLIEB, P. A. VOLBERDING, O. L. LASKIN, J. M. LEEDOM, J. E. GROOPMAN, D. MILDVAN, M. S. HIRSCH, G. G. JACKSON, D. T. DURACK & S. NUSINOFF-LEHRMAN. 1987. The toxicity of azidothymi-dine (AZT) in the treatment of patients with AIDS and AIDS-related complex. N. Engl. J. Med. **317:** 192-197.

62. SZEBENI, J. & J. N. WEINSTEIN. 1991. Dipyridamole binding to proteins in human plasma and in tissue culture media. J. Lab. Clin. Med. In press.

63. CHOU, T.-C. & P. TALALAY. 1984. Quantitation analysis of dose-effect relationships: the combined effects of multiple drugs or enzyme inhibitors. Adv. Enzyme Regul. **22:** 27-55.
64. BUNOW, B. & J. N. WEINSTEIN. COMBO: A new approach to the analysis of drug combinations *in vitro.* Ann. N. Y. Acad. Sci. This volume.
65. EFRON, B. D. 1979. Bootstrap methods: Another look at the jackknife. Ann. Statistics **7:** 1-26.
66. EFRON, B. & G. GONG. 1983. A leisurely look at the bootstrap, the jackknife, and cross-validation. Am. Statistician **37:** 36-48.
67. BERENBAUM, M. C. 1978. A method for testing for synergy with any number of agents. J. Infect. Dis. **137:** 122-130.
68. SYRACUSE, K. C. & W. R. GRECO. 1986. Proc. Biopharm. Sec. Am. Stat. Assoc. 127-132.

Antiretroviral Activity, Biochemistry, and Pharmacokinetics of 3'-Azido-2',3'-Dideoxy-5-Methylcytidine[a]

R. F. SCHINAZI,[b,e,f] C. K. CHU,[c] B. F. ERIKSSON,[b,e]
J.-P. SOMMADOSSI,[d] K. J. DOSHI,[c]
F. D. BOUDINOT,[c] B. OSWALD,[b] AND
H. M. McCLURE [e]

[b]Veterans Affairs Medical Center
Decatur, Georgia 30033
and Department of Pediatrics
Emory University School of Medicine
Atlanta, Georgia 30322

[c]College of Pharmacy
University of Georgia
Athens, Georgia 30602

[d]Department of Pharmacology
Division of Clinical Pharmacology
University of Alabama at Birmingham
Birmingham, Alabama 35294

[e]Yerkes Regional Primate Research Center
Emory University
Atlanta, Georgia 30322

INTRODUCTION

Several nucleoside analogues containing a 3'-azido function in the 2',3'-dideoxyribose ring have been shown to have specific antiretroviral activity.[1-3] Prominent members of this group of compounds are 3'-azido-3'-deoxythymidine (AZT), 3'-azido-2',3'-dideoxyuridine (AzddU, AZDU, CS-87), 3'-azido-2',3'-dideoxyguanosine (AzddG),

[a]This work was supported by Public Health Service Grants AI 26055 (R. Schinazi and C. Chu), AI 25899 (R. Schinazi, C. Chu, and F. D. Boudinot), HL 42125 (J. Sommadossi), AI 25784 (J. Sommadossi), and RR00165 (H. McClure) from the National Institutes of Health, and the Department of Veterans Affairs (R. Schinazi). J. P. Sommadossi is the recipient of a Junior Faculty Award from the American Cancer Society.
[f]Mailing address: Veterans Affairs Medical Center (Atlanta), Medical Research - 151, 1670 Clairmont Road, Decatur, GA 30033.

and 3'-azido-2',3'-dideoxy-5-chlorouridine.[4–10] AZT has been approved for the treatment of AIDS in adults, and clinical trials with AzddU have been initiated.

A compound related to AZT and AzddU is 3'-azido-2',3'-dideoxy-5-methylcytidine (AzddMeC, CS-92). An initial evaluation in human immunodeficiency virus type 1 (HIV-1)-infected primary lymphocytes of this compound demonstrated a median effective concentration (EC_{50}) of 5.1 μM, and no apparent toxicity was observed when tested up to 100 μM.[8] Additional studies in human peripheral blood mononuclear (PBM) cells infected with HIV-1 confirmed that CS-92 was active and found to be even more potent than originally reported, with an EC_{50} in the range of 0.081–0.22 μM.[5] The selective anti-HIV-1 effect of CS-92 has been confirmed in MT-4 cells.[11,12] The objective of the present study was to extend these early observations in order to determine the spectrum of antiviral activity and toxicity of CS-92, to study the interaction of the 5'-triphosphate of CS-92 and the HIV-1 reverse transcriptase and DNA polymerase α, to ascertain the chronic toxicity of CS-92 in mice, and to determine the pharmacokinetic parameters of this compound in rats and rhesus monkeys.

MATERIAL AND METHODS

Compounds

CS-92 and 3'-azido-2',3'-dideoxy-5-methyluridine (CS-85) were synthesized in our laboratory (UGA) by the method of Lin et al.[13] and Chu et al.[5] The nucleotide forms of AZT and CS-92 were synthesized as described previously.[9,14] 2',3'-Dideoxycytidine-5'-triphosphate was obtained from US Biochemical Corp., Cleveland, OH.

Antiviral and Cytotoxicity Assays

The nucleosides were evaluated for their ability to inhibit HIV-1 replication. The antiviral assays were conducted in mitogen-stimulated human PBM cells that were infected with HIV-1 (strain LAV), as described previously.[15] The drugs were added about 45 min after infection. Six days later, when virus production was at a maximum, the supernatant was clarified and the virus concentrated by high-speed centrifugation. The reverse transcriptase activity associated with the disrupted virus was determined. The effect of drug on the growth of uninfected human PBM cells was also established. Mitogen-stimulated PBM cells (3.8 $\times$ 10^5 per mL) were cultured in the presence and absence of drugs under similar conditions as those used for the antiviral assays described above. The cells were counted using a hemacytometer 6 days after initiation of treatment using the Trypan blue exclusion method.[16]

In Vitro Macrophage HIV-1 Infection Assay

Monocytes/macrophages were isolated from buffy coats of normal healthy blood donors. The cells were placed in Teflon culture vessels (Savillex, Minnetonka, MN) in

RPMI-1640 supplemented with 10% AB-positive (blood group) human serum at a density of 5×10^5 cells/mL. After 14 days in culture (a time when lymphocyte contamination was minimal), macrophages were exposed to HIV_{DV} at room temperature for one hour, as described previously.[17] Unbound virus was removed by washing with undiluted fetal calf serum. Cells were then resuspended and 10^5 cells/well added to a 96-well microdilution plate in the absence or presence of various drug dilutions in duplicate. Nine days after acute infection, supernatants were harvested, and HIV-1 p24 antigen was quantitated using the Abbott enzyme immunoassay (EIA).

Assay of Colony-Forming Unit Granulocyte-Macrophage (CFU-GM) for Drug Cytotoxicity Studies

Human bone marrow cells were collected by aspiration from the posterior iliac crest of normal healthy volunteers, treated with heparin, and the mononuclear population were separated by Ficoll-Hypaque gradient centrifugation, as described previously.[18] Cells were washed twice in Hanks' balanced salt solution and counted with a hemacytometer. Their viability was greater than 98% as assessed by Trypan blue exclusion. The culture assay for CFU-GM was performed using a bilayer soft agar or the methyl cellulose method. McCoy 5A nutrient medium supplemented with 15% dialyzed fetal bovine serum (heat inactivated at 56°C for 30 min) (Gibco Laboratories, Grand Island, NY) was used in all experiments. This medium was devoid of thymidine and uridine. Human recombinant GM-CSF (50 units/mL) (Genzyme, Boston, MA) or erythropoietin (1 unit/mL) (Connaught, Swiftwater, PA) was used as a colony-stimulating factor. After 14 days of incubation at 37°C in a humidified atmosphere of 5% CO_2 in air, colonies ($\geq$ 50 cells) were counted using an inverted microscope.

Experimental Design for Monkey and Rat Studies

Young adult male rhesus monkeys (Macaca mulatta) weighing 3-6 kg were used for the pharmacokinetic studies. The animals were maintained at the Yerkes Regional Primate Research Center of Emory University in accordance with guidelines established by the Animal Welfare Act and the NIH Guide for the Care and Use of Laboratory Animals.

The disposition of CS-92 was characterized after intravenous (iv) and oral (po) administration. Three monkeys were used to study CS-92 pharmacokinetics (RHD-1, RIJ-1, and RZO-1). Monkeys were administered 60 mg/kg CS-92 iv (6-7 mL) and, after a three week washout period, they received 60 mg/kg orally in 40-45 mL by gastric intubation. Blood samples were taken prior to and 0.25, 0.5, 1, 1.5, 2, 3, 4, 6, and 24 h after drug administration. A single cerebrospinal fluid (CSF) sample was taken from all monkeys 1 h after drug administration. Serum, CSF, and urine samples were frozen at $-20°C$ until analysis.

Six adult male Sprague-Dawley rats weighing 250-350 g were used for the study. External jugular vein cannulas were surgically implanted under light ether anesthesia the day before the experiment. Rats were administered 10 mg/kg CS-92 iv (1 mL). Blood samples were collected prior to and at 0.08, 0.25, 0.5, 0.75, 1, 1.5, 2, 3, 4, and 6 h after drug administration. Urine was collected for 24 h after drug administration. Serum and urine samples were frozen at $-20°C$ until analysis.

Analytical Methodology for Monkey and Rat Studies

CS-92 concentration in biological fluids was determined by high-performance liquid chromatography (HPLC). To measure nucleoside concentrations in serum, 100 μL serum sample, 10 μL CS-85 (50 μg/mL) as internal standard, and 100 μL 2 M perchloric acid as a protein precipitant were added to polypropylene microcentrifuge tubes (400 μL). Previous studies had indicated that perchloric acid did not affect the stability of CS-92. Tubes were thoroughly mixed for 30 s and centrifuged at 2,000 g for 5 minutes. Supernatant (15-150 μL) was injected onto the HPLC. For cerebrospinal fluid drug concentrations, 100 μL CSF was added to 20 μL internal standard and 80 μL water. One hundred μL was then injected onto the HPLC. For urine drug concentrations, 20 μL urine was added to 80 μL internal standard and 1.9 mL water. One hundred μL was then injected onto the HPLC. Chromatography was performed on an Alltech Hypersil ODS column (4.6 $\times$ 150 mm, 5 μm) using an isocratic mobile phase of 12% acetonitrile in 40 mM sodium acetate, pH 7.0, at a flow rate of 2 mL/minute. Compounds were detected at a UV wavelength of 283 nanometers. The retention times for CS-92, AZT, and CS-85 were 2.6, 4.1, and 8.3 min, respectively.

Pharmacokinetics

Area/moment analysis was used to calculate pharmacokinetic parameters for CS-92 and its metabolite as described previously.[19] Total clearance (Cl_T) was calculated from $Dose_{iv}$/area under the curve $(AUC)_{iv}$, steady-state volume of distribution (V_{SS}) from $Dose_{iv} \times AUMC_{iv}/AUC^2_{iv}$, and half-life ($t_{1/2}$) from $0.693/\lambda_Z$, where λ_Z is the terminal disposition slope. Renal clearance (Cl_R) was calculated from $Cl_T \times f_e$, where f_e is the fraction of the dose excreted unchanged in urine, and nonrenal clearance (Cl_{NR}) was calculated from Cl_T-Cl_R. Bioavailability (F) after oral and subcutaneous drug administration was calculated from $AUC_{PO,SQ} \times Dose_{iv}/AUC_{iv} \times Dose_{PO,SQ}$. For bioavailability calculations, Cl_T was assumed to be independent of dose.

Evaluation of ddCTP and CS-92 on Reverse Transcriptase and DNA Polymerase α

A recombinant 66 kDa HIV-1 reverse transcriptase, obtained from Dr. S. Hughes (National Cancer Institute, Frederick Cancer Research Facility, Frederick, MD), was used for these assays. This enzyme was recently reported to have an inhibition profile indistinguishable from the virion-derived enzyme when the effect of different antiviral agents were compared.[20] The standard reaction mixture (100 μL) for HIV-1 assays contained 100 mM Tris-Cl (pH 8.0), 50 mM KCl, 2 mM $MgCl_2$, 5 mM dithiothreitol, 400 μg/mL BSA, 0.05 U of $(rI)_n \cdot (dC)_{12-18}$ per mL (equivalent to 3.1 μg/mL), and 1 μM [^{3}H]dCTP (specific activity 25 Ci/mmol). DNA polymerase α was isolated from uninfected phytohemagglutinin (PHA)-stimulated PBM cells as reported previously.[9,21] PBM cell-DNA polymerase α activity was assayed in 100 μL reaction mixtures containing 100 mM Tris-Cl (pH 8.0), 6 mM $MgCl_2$, 5 mM dithiothreitol, 400 μg/mL BSA, 1 μM [^{3}H]dCTP (specific activity 25 Ci/mmol), 100 μM each of dATP, dTTP, and dGTP, and 200 μg of activated calf thymus DNA per milliliter. Reactions were started by the addition of 10 μL of enzyme. The reaction mixtures were incubated and processed as described previously.[20]

Data Analyses

The median effective (EC$_{50}$) and inhibitory (IC$_{50}$) concentrations were determined by the median effect method.[16]

RESULTS

Cell Culture

CS-92 is a potent and selective anti-HIV-1 compound with an EC$_{50}$ in HIV-1-infected human PBM cells of 0.09 μM. The compound was also effective against HIV-2 (TABLE 1). The compound appears to be selective for human retroviruses and was not active against herpes simplex virus type 1 and type 2 (HSV-1 and 2), coxsackievirus B4, and influenza A virus, but was weakly active against a Friend murine retrovirus (TABLE 1). CS-92 was also extremely active in human macrophages acutely infected with HIV-1, with an EC$_{50}$ of 0.006 μM. CS-92 was not toxic to exponentially growing PBM or Vero cells when tested up to 200 and 400 μM, respectively.

Because bone marrow toxicity has been demonstrated to be the limiting toxicity of certain nucleosides, the effect of CS-92 on these cells was determined (TABLE 1). CS-92 was significantly less toxic than AZT to human granulocyte-macrophage precursor cells (FIG. 1). Whereas AZT displayed a 50% suppression of colony formation at concentrations of 0.9 μM, CS-92 required a 40-fold or greater concentration to produce the same effect. CS-92 was at least 60-fold less toxic to erythroid precursor cells than was AZT (FIG. 2).

Biochemical Studies

The interaction of the 5'-triphosphate of CS-92 and the HIV-1 reverse transcriptase in synthesis directed by (rI)$_n$ · (dC)$_{12-18}$ as template indicated a competitive inhibition pattern with respect to deoxycytidine triphosphate (dCTP), and an affinity that was about 30-fold greater than that for ddCTP was observed (FIGURES 3 and 4). The values of the inhibition constant, K_{is}, as determined from the replot of slopes versus inhibitor concentration, were 0.0093 μM and 0.29 μM for CS-92-TP and ddCTP, respectively. The calculated mean K_m for dCTP was about 7.2 μM (range 5.3-9.1 μM). Kinetic studies of CS-92-TP and dideoxycytidine triphosphate (ddCTP) on cellular DNA polymerase α activity revealed that both compounds also were competitive inhibitors

TABLE 1. Antiviral Spectrum and Cytotoxicity of AzddMeC (CS-92) and AZT

	EC$_{50}$ or IC$_{50}$ (μM)	
	CS-92	AZT
Virus (Strain)		
HIV-1 (LAV) in PBM cells	0.09	0.002
HIV-1 (DV) in macrophages	0.006	0.0008
HIV-2 (ROD2) in PBM cells	0.016	0.005
HSV-1 (F) in Vero cells	> 100	> 100
HSV-2 (G) in Vero cells	> 100	> 100
Coxsackievirus (B4) in Vero cells	> 100	> 100
Friend retrovirus (EY-10) in SC cells	2.8	0.004
Influenza A[a] in MDCK cells	> 100	ND
Cells (Toxicity)		
Human PBM	> 200	> 100
Vero	> 400	29.0
MDCK	> 100	ND
Human bone marrow: CFU-GM	36	0.9
BFU-E	$\geq$ 100	1.6

[a] A Singapore 1157 (H2N2) and WI 3334-1 (H3N2).

with respect to the varied concentration of dCTP (data not shown). Significantly higher concentrations of the compounds were required, however, for a 50% reduction of DNA polymerase α activity. CS-92-TP inhibited HIV-1 RT by 50% at a concentration 6,000-fold lower than that required for a similar inhibition of DNA polymerase α (FIG. 5).

Mouse Studies

BALB/c mice were treated *ad libitum* orally with either AZT or CS-92 (0.1 mg/mL, equivalent to about 17.5 mg/kg per day). The continuous oral treatment with CS-

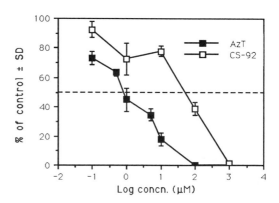

FIGURE 1. Effect of AZT and CS-92 on human granulocyte macrophage cells in a colony formation assay.

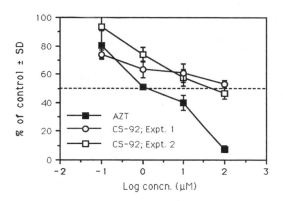

FIGURE 2. Effect of AZT and CS-92 on human erythroid precursor cells in a colony formation assay.

92 for 145 days produced no apparent toxicity. AZT produced an increase in mean corpuscular volume (MCV) of red cells as early as 34 days after treatment (MCV ± SD = 51.7 ± 0.3 fL versus 46.9 ± 0.4 fL for water-treated animals; n = 5). A similar effect was not seen with CS-92 (MCV = 46.9 ± 0.3 fL) even when the animals were evaluated 145 days after initiation of treatment (data not shown). None of the animals treated lost weight or failed to gain weight after treatment with either CS-92 or AZT when compared to untreated mice.

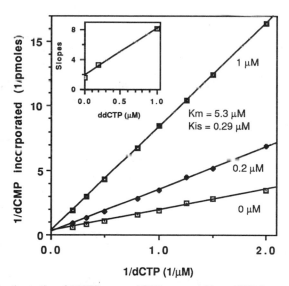

FIGURE 3. Kinetic studies of ddCTP versus dCTP on recombinant HIV-1 reverse transcriptase. Double-reciprocal plot of HIV-1 reverse transcriptase activity directed by $(rI)_n \cdot (dC)_{12-18}$ in the presence of ddCTP. The K_{is} value for ddCTP was calculated from the replot of the slopes versus inhibitor concentration (inset).

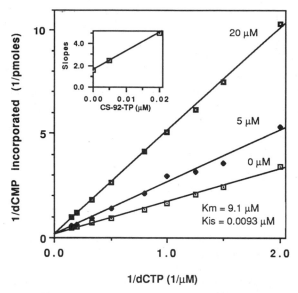

FIGURE 4. Kinetic studies of CS-92-TP versus dCTP on recombinant HIV-1 reverse transcriptase. Double-reciprocal plot of HIV-1 reverse transcriptase activity directed by $(rI)_n \cdot (dC)_{12-18}$ in the presence of CS-92-TP. The K_{is} value for CS-92-TP was calculated from the replot of the slopes versus inhibitor concentration (inset).

Pharmacokinetics in Rats and Monkeys

The pharmacokinetics of CS-92 after a single dose of 10 mg/kg iv to rats were determined. TABLE 2 shows the half-life, total clearance, and steady-state volume of distribution. The data indicated a mean half-life for the drug of 2.73 ± 2.47 hours. No new metabolite or AZT was detected after administration of a single bolus iv injection of the drug.

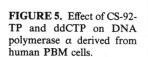

FIGURE 5. Effect of CS-92-TP and ddCTP on DNA polymerase α derived from human PBM cells.

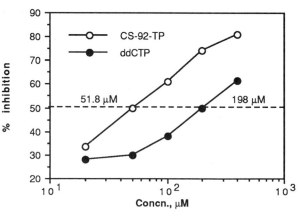

TABLE 2. Pharmacokinetic Parameters for 3'-Azido-2',3'-Dideoxy-5-Methylcytidine after Intravenous Administration of 10 mg/kg to Rats

Parameter	Mean (SD), n = 6
Weight, kg	0.272 (0.012)
$Cl_T,$[a] L/h/kg	2.33 (0.58)
$CL_R,$[b] L/h/kg	1.26 (0.44)
$CL_{NR},$[c] L/h/kg	1.07 (0.21)
$V_{SS},$[d] L/kg	0.92 (0.27)
$t_{1/2},$[e] h	2.73 (2.47)

[a] Cl_T, total clearance.
[b] Cl_R, renal clearance.
[c] Cl_{NR}, nonrenal clearance (*i.e.* metabolism and biliary excretion).
[d] V_{SS}, steady-state volume of distribution.
[e] $t_{1/2}$, half-life.

Pharmacokinetics studies after iv and oral administration of 60 mg/kg CS-92 in rhesus monkeys were also performed (TABLE 3). The mean half-life for CS-92 was 1.52 ± 0.73 and 1.74 ± 1.0 h after iv and oral administration, respectively. The oral bioavailability was about 21 ± 8 percent. A substantial amount of a new metabolite was detected in the monkey serum. The half-life of this uncharacterized component was 0.62 ± 0.11 h and 1.03 ± 0.49 h after iv and oral administration, respectively. Although CS-92 was not found in the CSF one hour after drug administration, the new metabolite could be detected. The CSF:serum concentration ratio after iv administration for this new metabolite was 0.06 ± 0.02 (TABLE 3). The retention time for this new peak was similar to that for AZT under a variety of HPLC separation methods. This peak (retention time = 4.1 min) was collected, and the ultraviolet spectrum indicated that the compound was a uracil or thymine analogue with a λ_{max} of 262 nm,

TABLE 3. Pharmacokinetic Parameters in Rhesus Monkeys after Intravenous (iv) or Oral (po) Administration of 60 mg/kg of CS-92

Parameter	Monkey					
	RHD-1		RIJ-1		RZO-1	
Route:	iv	po	iv	po	iv	po
Dose, mg/kg	60	60	60	60	60	60
AUC, mg·h/L	27.6	3.39	28.7	7.69	25.9	6.39
Cl_T, L/h/kg	2.17		2.09		2.32	
V_{SS}, L/kg	0.62		1.65		1.33	
$t_{1/2}$, h	0.68	0.68	1.98	2.66	1.89	1.87
F		0.12		0.27		0.25
AUC (X)[a] mg·h/l	13.4	1.39	13.5	2.09	9.99	1.61
$t_{1/2}$ (X) h	0.61	0.61	0.74	1.57	0.52	0.91
$\dfrac{AUC(X)}{AUC(CS\text{-}92)}$	0.49	0.41	0.47	0.27	0.39	0.25

[a] X, has not been fully characterized, (see text).

suggesting that deamination of CS-92 may have occurred in monkeys. The characterization of this metabolite awaits mass spectrum analysis.

DISCUSSION

Lin et al.[13] synthesized several 3'-azido and 3'-amino pyrimidine 2'-deoxyribonucleosides as potential anticancer agents. The amino analogues of these drugs proved to be more active than the corresponding 3'-azido analogues against L1210 and S-180 cells in vitro. In 1987, Lin et al.[22] reported on the activity of 3'-azido-2',3'-dideoxycytidine (AzddC, CS-91) and CS-92 against Moloney-murine leukemia virus, a mammalian T-lymphotropic retrovirus, and found them to be essentially inactive with EC_{50}s of 58 and 100 μM. Our group had already determined that AzddC and CS-92 had potent antiviral activity against HIV-1 in primary lymphocytes.[23] In initial evaluation in these cells, these two compounds had median effective concentrations of 1.2 and 5.1 μM with no apparent toxicity when evaluated up to 100 μM.[8] Additional studies confirmed that in PBM cells infected with HIV-1, CS-92 was more potent than originally thought, with an EC_{50} in the range of 0.081-0.22 μM.[5] However, because of the similarity in the bone marrow toxicity of AzddC and AZT using a GM-CSF clonogenic assay, AzddC was not considered further by us as a potential antiviral agent, and our attention focused on CS-92. Herdewijn et al.[24] initially reported that CS-92 was totally devoid of anti-HIV-1 activity in ATH8 cells. Later, the same group reported that CS-92 had an EC_{50} of 1.8 μM with no toxicity up to 1 mM in MT-4 cells.[12] These results emphasize the importance of testing compounds in cell culture systems that correlate well with primary lymphocytes that are highly susceptible to infection by HIV-1 in humans.[2,25]

In the present study, the EC_{50} for CS-92 in PBM cells infected with HIV-1 was 0.09 μM (TABLE 1), whereas the toxic dose for the host PBM and Vero cells was greater than 200 and 400 μM, respectively. The antiviral spectrum of this compound appeared to be limited to retroviruses, with greater potency towards human retroviruses. CS-92-TP is also a potent and selective inhibitor of HIV-1 reverse transcriptase, with a K_{is} of 0.0093 μM. The extent of phosphorylation of CS-92 in primary human PBM cells and in T cells is under investigation.

The data presented herein demonstrate that CS-92 is a selective antiviral agent with a therapeutic index greater than 1,000 in PBM cells. The therapeutic index measured in terms of the ratio of toxicity (IC_{50}) of granulocyte-macrophage precursor cells to the median effective antiviral concentration was 400, which is comparable to AZT with a therapeutic index of about 450. For erythroid precursor cells the therapeutic index was over 1,000 for CS-92 and 800 for AZT. CS-92 is probably not readily deaminated to AZT in bone marrow cells because its toxicity is significantly lower than is seen with AZT, regardless of how these cells are differentiated.

In summary, studies in cell culture indicate that CS-92 is a highly selective anti-HIV-1 agent that is significantly less myelosuppressive in bone marrow cells than AZT. Studies are in progress to evaluate the potential conversion of CS-92 to AZT or AZT-nucleotides in human PBM cells and bone marrow cells. Preliminary results with CS-92 indicate that the deamination of this drug in certain cells may modulate its activity and toxicity. The favorable antiviral selectivity, low bone-marrow toxicity in culture, lack of toxicity in mice, reasonable oral bioavailability, and long half-life in nonhuman primates compared to AZT[26] suggest that CS-92 may be a potentially useful antiviral agent for the treatment of HIV infections.

SUMMARY

3'-Azido-2',3'-dideoxy-5-methylcytidine (CS-92, AzddMeC) is an antiviral nucleoside analogue structurally related to 3'-azido-3'-deoxythymidine (AZT). CS-92 is a potent and selective inhibitor of HIV-1 reverse transcriptase and HIV-1 replication in human lymphocytes and macrophages. The EC_{50} for CS-92 in HIV-1-infected human PBM cells was 0.09 μM. In HIV-1-infected human macrophages, the EC_{50} was 0.006 μM. This compound was also effective against human immunodeficiency virus type 2 in lymphocytes. The replication of Friend murine virus was only weakly inhibited, and no effect was observed against herpes simplex virus type 1 and type 2 and coxsackievirus B4. CS-92 was not toxic to PBM or Vero cells when tested up to 200 μM and was, furthermore, at least 40 times less toxic to granulocyte-macrophage and erythroid precursor cells *in vitro* than was AZT. The interaction of the 5'-triphosphate of CS-92 with HIV-1 reverse transcriptase indicated competitive inhibition (the inhibition constant, K_{is}, was 0.0093 μM) with a 30-fold greater affinity for CS-92-TP than for ddCTP. CS-92-TP inhibited HIV-1 reverse transcriptase by 50% at a concentration 6,000-fold lower than that which was required for a similar inhibition of DNA polymerase α. Pharmacokinetic studies showed that CS-92 was not deaminated to AZT in rats, but this compound was found to have a half-life of 2.7 hours. In rhesus monkeys, however, a compound with a retention time and ultraviolet spectra characteristics similar to AZT was detected. The mean half-life in rhesus monkeys for CS-92 was 1.52 and 1.74 h after intravenous and oral administration, respectively, and the oral bioavailability was about 21 percent. Additional preclinical studies with CS-92 will determine the ultimate utility of this antiviral agent for the treatment of HIV-1 infections.

ACKNOWLEDGMENTS

We thank D. Cannon, V. Saalmann, and S. Sherry for their excellent technical assistance. We are also grateful to Dr. S. Wu (Centers for Disease Control, Atlanta) for performing the studies with influenza virus.

REFERENCES

1. HIRSCH, M. S. 1988. AIDS commentary. Azidothymidine. J. Infect. Dis. **157**: 427-431.
2. SCHINAZI, R. F. 1988. Strategies and targets for anti-human immunodeficiency virus type 1 chemotherapy. *In* AIDS in children, adolescents and heterosexual adults: an interdisciplinary approach to prevention. R. F. Schinazi & A.J. Nahmias, Ed.: 126-143. Elsevier-North Holland. New York.
3. YARCHOAN, R. & S. BRODER. 1989. Anti-retroviral therapy of AIDS and related disorders: General principles and specific development of dideoxynucleosides. Pharm. Ther. **40**: 329-348.
4. BALZARINI, J., A. VAN AERSCHOT, P. HERDEWIJN & E. DE CLERCQ. 1989. 5-Chloro-substituted derivatives of 2',3'-didehydro-2',3'-dideoxyuridine, 3'-fluoro-2',3'-dideoxyuridine and 3'-azido-2',3'-dideoxyuridine as anti-HIV agents. Biochem. Pharmacol. **38**: 869-874.

5. CHU, C. K., R. F. SCHINAZI, M. K. AHN, G. V. ULLAS & Z. P. GU. 1989. Structure-activity relationship of pyrimidine nucleosides as antiviral agents for human immunodeficiency type 1 in peripheral blood mononuclear cells. J. Med. Chem. 32: 612-617.

6. FISCHL, M. A., D. D. RICHMAN, M. H. GRIECO, M. S. GOTTLIEB, P. A. VOLBERDING, O. L. LASKIN, J. M. LEEDOM, J. E. GROOPMAN, D. MILDVAN, R. T. SCHOOLEY, G. G. JACKSON, D. T. DURACK, D. KING, & THE AZT COLLABORATIVE WORKING GROUP. 1987. The efficacy of azidothymidine (AZT) in the treatment of patients with AIDS and AIDS-related complex. A double-blind, placebo-controlled trial. N. Engl. J. Med. 317: 185-191.

7. HARTMANN, H., G. HUNSMANN & F. ECKSTEIN. 1987. Inhibition of HIV-induced cytopathogenicity in vitro by 3'-azido-2',3'-dideoxyguanosine. Lancet i: 40-41.

8. LIN, T.-S., J.-Y. GUO, R. F. SCHINAZI, C. K. CHU, J.-N. XIANG & W. H. PRUSOFF. 1988. Synthesis and antiviral activity of various 3'-azido analogues of pyrimidine deoxyribonucleosides against human immunodeficiency virus (HIV-1, HTLV-III/LAV). J. Med. Chem. 31: 336-340.

9. ERIKSSON, B. F. H., C. K. CHU & R. F. SCHINAZI. 1989. Phosphorylation of 3'-azido-2',3'-dideoxyuridine (CS-87, AzddU) and preferential inhibition of human and simian immunodeficiency virus reverse transcriptase by its 5'-triphosphate. Antimicrob. Agents Chemother. 33: 1729-1734.

10. SCHINAZI, R. F., C. K. CHU, M. K. AHN, J.-P. SOMMADOSSI & H. MCCLURE. 1987. Selective in vitro inhibition of human immunodeficiency virus (HIV) replication by 3'-azido-2',3'-dideoxyuridine (CS-87). J. Cell Biochem. 11D (Suppl.): 405.

11. DE CLERCQ, E. 1989. New acquisitions in the development of anti-HIV agents. Antiviral Res. 12: 1-20.

12. HERDEWIJN, P., J. BALZARINI, M. BABA, R. PAUWELS, A. VAN AERSCHOT, G. JANSSEN & E. DE CLERCQ. 1988. Synthesis and anti-HIV activity of different sugar-modified pyrimidine and purine nucleosides. J. Med. Chem. 31: 2040-2048.

13. LIN, T.-S., Y.-S. GAO & W. R. MANCINI. 1983. Synthesis and biological activity of various 3'-azido and 3'-amino analogues of 5-substituted pyrimidine deoxyribonucleosides. J. Med. Chem. 26: 1691-1696.

14. YOSHIKAWA, M., T. KATO & T. TAKENISHI. 1969. Studies of phosphorylation. III. Selective phosphorylation of unprotected nucleosides. Bull. Chem. Soc. Jap. 42: 3505-3508.

15. SCHINAZI, R. F., D. L. CANNON, B. H. ARNOLD & D. MARTINO-SALTZMAN. 1988b. Combinations of isoprinosine and 3'-azido-3'-deoxythymidine in lymphocytes infected with human immunodeficiency virus type 1. Antimicrob. Agents Chemother. 32: 1784-1787.

16. SCHINAZI, R. F., T.-C. CHOU, R. T. SCOTT, X. YAO & A. J. NAHMIAS. 1986. Delayed treatment with combinations of antiviral drugs in mice infected with herpes simplex virus and application of the median effect method of analysis. Antimicrob. Agents Chemother. 30: 491-498.

17. CROWE, S., J. MILLS & M. S. MCGRATH. 1987. Quantitative immunocytofluorographic analysis of CD4 surface antigen expression and HIV infection of human peripheral blood monocyte/macrophages. AIDS Res. Hum. Retroviruses. 3: 135-145.

18. SOMMADOSSI, J.-P., R. CARLISLE, R. F. SCHINAZI & Z. ZHOU. 1988. Enhancement of the antiretroviral activity of 3'-azido-3'-deoxythymidine by selective rescue of human bone marrow progenitor cells using metabolic modulation with uridine. Antimicrob. Agents Chemother. 32: 997-1001.

19. ROCCI, M. L. & W. J. JUSKO. 1983. LAGRAN program for area and moments in pharmacokinetic analysis. Comp. Prog. Biomed. 16: 203-216.

20. SCHINAZI, R. F., B. F. H. ERIKSSON & S. H. HUGHES. 1989. Comparison of inhibitory activity of various antiretroviral agents against particle derived and recombinant HIV-1 reverse transcriptase. Antimicrob. Agents Chemother. 33: 115-117.

21. ERIKSSON, B. F. H. & R. F. SCHINAZI. 1989. Combinations of 3'-azido-3'-deoxythymidine (zidovudine) and phosphonoformate (foscarnet) against human immunodeficiency virus type 1 and cytomegalovirus in vitro. Antimicrob. Agents Chemother. 33: 663-669.

22. LIN, T.-S., M. S. CHEN, C. MCLAREN, Y.-S. GAO, I. GHAZZOULI & W. H. PRUSOFF. 1987. Synthetics and antiviral activity of various 3'-azido, 3'-amino, 2',3'-unsaturated and 2',3'-

dideoxy analogues of pyrimidine deoxyribonucleosides against retroviruses. J. Med. Chem. **30:** 440-444.

23. CHU, C. K. & R. F. SCHINAZI. 3'-Azido-2',3'-dideoxy-5-methylcytidine. U.S. Patent. Application serial no. 016, 136 (filed February 18, 1987), and U.S. patent 4,681,933.
24. HERDEWIJN, P., J. BALZARINI, E. DE CLERCQ, R. PAUWELS, M. BABA, S. BRODER & H. VANDERHAEGHE. 1987. 3'-Substituted 2',3'-dideoxynucleoside analogues as potential anti-HIV (HTLV-III/LAV) agents. J. Med. Chem. **30:** 1270-1278.
25. CHU, C. K., R. F. SCHINAZI, B. H. ARNOLD, D. L. CANNON, M. K. AHN, B. DOBOSZEWSKI, V. B. BHADTI & Z. GU. 1988. Comparative activity of 2',3'-saturated and unsaturated pyrimidine and purine nucleosides against human immunodeficiency virus type 1 in peripheral blood mononuclear cells. Biochem. Pharmacol. **37:** 3543-3548.
26. BOUDINOT, F. D., R. F. SCHINAZI, J. M. GALLO, H. M. MCCLURE, D. C. ANDERSON, K. J. DOSHI, P. C. KAMBHAMPATHI & C. K. CHU. 1990. 3'-Azido-2',3'-dideoxyuridine (AzddU): comparative pharmacokinetics with 3'-azido-3'-deoxythymidine (AZT) in monkeys. AIDS Res. Hum. Retroviruses. **6:** 219-228.

Biochemical Pharmacology of Acyclic Nucleotide Analogues

JOANNE J. BRONSON, HSU-TSO HO,
HILDE DE BOECK, KATHLEEN WOODS,
ISMAIL GHAZZOULI, JOHN C. MARTIN, AND
MICHAEL J. M. HITCHCOCK

Bristol-Myers Squibb
Pharmaceutical Research and Development Division
Wallingford, Connecticut 06492-7660

In the search for selective antiviral agents, a common strategy has been to design inhibitors of enzymes that mediate viral DNA synthesis. Examples of such target enzymes include reverse transcriptase (RT) from human immunodeficiency virus (HIV) and DNA polymerase from herpesviruses. Efforts in this area have been directed primarily at the synthesis of nucleoside analogues and have led to the discovery of a number of highly effective antiviral agents.[1-3] The biological activity of a nucleoside analogue is typically associated with its intracellular conversion to a triphosphate derivative. The triphosphate analogue competes with natural deoxynucleoside triphosphates (dNTP) for binding to the viral polymerase, thus inhibiting the rate of viral DNA synthesis; the triphosphate analogue may also act as a substrate for the enzyme and lead to termination of viral DNA chain elongation. Phosphorylation of the nucleoside analogue to the key triphosphate derivative is a process mediated by viral and/or cellular enzymes, and the efficiency of this activation can be an important factor in the observed antiviral activity and specificity. Attention has turned to investigation of analogues of nucleoside phosphates, in part because these derivatives can bypass critical phosphorylation steps and thus offer the potential for increased potency and a broader spectrum of antiviral activity.[4]

De Clercq and Holy recently introduced a new series of acyclic nucleoside monophosphate analogues that are characterized by the presence of a phosphonylmethyl ether group $[O-CH_2-P(O)(OH)_2]$ in place of the phosphate moiety $[CH_2-O-P(O)(OH)_2]$.[5] The parent compound in this series, (S)-9-[3-hydroxy-2-(phosphonylmethoxy)propyl]adenine (HPMPA, FIG. 1), was reported to have antiviral activity against a wide range of DNA viruses, including thymidine kinase-deficient strains of herpes simplex virus. Initial biochemical studies have shown that HPMPA is converted by cellular enzymes to mono- and diphosphate esters (HPMPAp and HPMPApp) in infected and uninfected HEL and Vero cells.[6] These metabolites correspond to di- and triphosphate analogues respectively. HPMPA acts as a selective antiviral agent by inhibiting viral DNA synthesis at a much lower concentration than required to inhibit cellular DNA synthesis.[6] The broad-spectrum antiviral activity of a number of acyclic phosphonate derivatives related to HPMPA has been described.[7]

Two compounds from this series have been of particular interest for extended evaluation of their potential as antiviral agents. The adenine derivative 9-[(2-phosphonylmethoxy)ethyl]adenine (PMEA, FIG. 1) is structurally similar to HPMPA but lacks the hydroxymethyl appendage on the acyclic side chain.[8] PMEA shows *in vitro* antiviral activity against herpesviruses, although it is less potent than HPMPA, and also has good activity against retroviruses including HIV.[7,9,10] Several *in vivo* murine models of retrovirus infection have been used to evaluate PMEA in comparison to AZT. PMEA was more effective than AZT in inhibition of splenomegaly induced by infection of mice with Rauscher murine leukemia virus[10] and was also more potent than AZT in suppression of tumor formation in mice infected with Moloney sarcoma virus.[11] In a murine model of acquired immune deficiency syndrome (MAIDS) induced by infection of mice with LP-BM5 murine leukemia virus, PMEA showed antiretroviral activity comparable to AZT.[12] PMEA also appeared effective as a prophylactic treatment for preventing feline leukemia virus infection of cats.[13] In addition, the antiviral activity of PMEA has been demonstrated *in vivo* in a murine model of cytomegalovirus (CMV) infection.[10] Because CMV infection often occurs concurrently with HIV infection, the combination of activity against both retroviruses and CMV makes PMEA a particularly attractive candidate for AIDS chemotherapy.

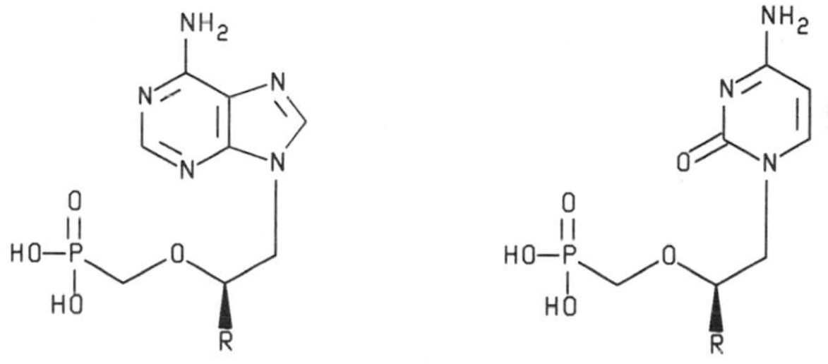

FIGURE 1. Structures of HPMPA, PMEA, HPMPC, and PMEC.

A second compound of interest, (*S*)-1-[3-hydroxy-2-(phosphonylmethoxy)propyl]-cytosine (HPMPC, FIG. 1) bears the same branched side chain as HPMPA, but has a cytosine ring in place of the adenine base. HPMPC displays potent antiherpesvirus activity *in vitro* with little cellular toxicity.[7,14-16] *In vivo*, HPMPC showed exceptional potency against systemic herpes simplex virus infections, giving a 50% survival rate (ED$_{50}$) at a dose of only 0.1 mg/kg per day in mice infected with HSV 1; by comparison, the ED$_{50}$ for acyclovir in this model was 50 mg/kg per day.[14,15] HPMPC was also more effective *in vivo* than ganciclovir against murine CMV.[15,17] Interestingly, the related cytosine derivative 1-[(2-phosphonylmethoxy)ethyl]cytosine (PMEC, FIG. 1) shows no *in vitro* activity against herpesviruses.[7,10,14]

The antiviral effectiveness of nucleotide analogues such as HPMPC and PMEA is most likely a complex function of their ability to interact with several host and virus-encoded enzymes. We have therefore initiated studies on the biochemical pharmacology of these phosphonate derivatives in order to better understand their mechanism(s) of action.

PMEA STUDIES

Metabolism in CEM Cells

Studies on intracellular metabolism of PMEA were carried out using compound labeled with ^{14}C at C-8 on the adenine ring. The human lymphocytic cell line CEM was used in initial experiments on PMEA metabolism because the anti-HIV activity of this nucleotide analogue has been demonstrated in these cells.[10] After incubation with 30 μM of labeled compound for 24 or 48 h, ion-exchange HPLC analysis of the cell extracts showed the presence of two peaks at 34 and 70 min, as well as a peak for PMEA at 9 min (TABLE 1). The total concentration of the intracellular species at both 24 and 48 h was 16% that of the extracellular drug concentration. These results show that PMEA is able to enter into cells despite its highly polar nature. The uptake of this nucleotide analogue, however, is clearly low in contrast with that of a typical nucleoside derivative that can equilibrate across the cell membrane within minutes.

The identification of the metabolites as PMEA-monophosphate (PMEAp) and PMEA-diphosphate (PMEApp) was based on a comparison with the HPLC retention times of authentic samples prepared by chemical synthesis (FIG. 2).[8] The structures of the synthesized metabolites were assigned on the basis of their ^{31}P NMR spectra: for PMEAp, two signals were seen at $+8$ ppm and -10 ppm for the phosphonate P and terminal phosphate P atoms respectively, whereas the ^{31}P NMR spectrum of PMEApp showed three peaks at $+9$ ppm, -10 ppm, and -23 ppm corresponding (in order) to the phosphorous atoms of the phosphonate, terminal phosphate, and internal phosphate groups.

Metabolism in MRC-5 Cells

The metabolism of PMEA in the human fibroblast cell line MRC-5 was more complex than in CEM cells. After a 24 h exposure to 34 μM of labeled compound, ion-exchange HPLC analysis of the cell extracts showed the presence of PMEA (9 min), PMEApp (70 min), and a new metabolite (53 min). The ratio of these peaks was

TABLE 1. Uptake and Phosphorylation of [^{14}C]PMEA in CEM Cells[a]

	Concentration of metabolites in cells (μM) Retention time		
Time of exposure (h)	PMEA 9 min	PMEAp 34 min	PMEApp 70 min
24	3.3	0.43	1.0
48	2.9	0.82	1.2

[a] [^{14}C]PMEA was present at 30 μM. HPLC analysis was carried out on a Whatman Partisil 10 SAX column, eluting with a 15 to 700 mM gradient of potassium phosphate buffer over 55 min and then at 700 mM for an additional 15 min.

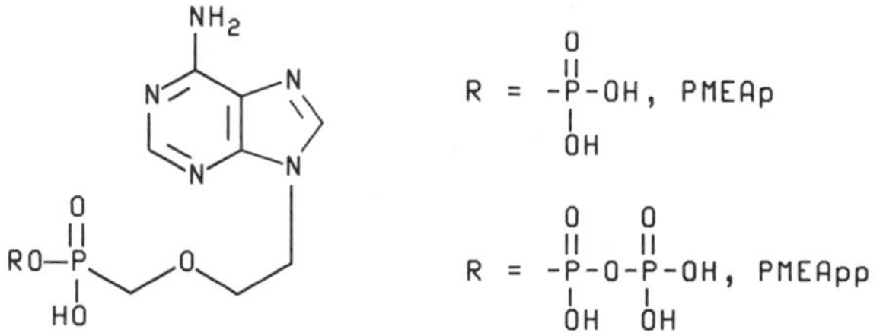

FIGURE 2. Structures of PMEAp and PMEApp.

2:1:2, and the total concentration of the intracellular species was only 3% that of the extracellular concentration of PMEA. When MRC-5 cells were incubated for 24 h with a higher concentration of PMEA (169 μM), a total of seven metabolites were seen by HPLC (elution times: 4, 7, 9, 30, 34, 53, and 70 min). The peaks at 9, 34, and 70 min correspond to PMEA, PMEAp, and PMEApp, respectively, and account for a total of 60% of the intracellular material (ratio = 7:1:4). The peak at 53 min constitutes an additional 30% of the labeled material in cells. The total concentration of the PMEA metabolites remained low (3%) relative to the external drug concentration.

Determination of the identity of the metabolites formed in MRC-5 cells in addition to PMEAp and PMEApp is underway. One possibility is that these products arise from deamination of PMEA or its phosphorylated forms to give the corresponding hypoxanthine derivatives. Similar deaminations are known to occur readily with 2',3'-dideoxyadenosine (ddA) and other adenine-based nucleoside analogues,[18,19] although Pauwels *et al.* have found that PMEA is resistant to deaminases derived from bovine intestine.[9] It should also be noted that PMEA differs from nucleoside analogues such as ddA in that the side chain is connected to the adenine base by an alkyl (N-C-C) linkage rather than a glycosidic (N-C-O) bond. As a result, PMEA should not be susceptible to cleavage of the adenine base by chemical hydrolysis or by degradation by enzymes such as purine nucleoside phosphorylase.

In further experiments, the effect of adenine or adenosine on the metabolism of PMEA was studied. MRC-5 cells were preincubated with 20 μM of adenine or adenosine for 3 h, and then coincubated with [^{14}C]PMEA for 24 h at 37 °C. HPLC showed no significant difference in the activation of PMEA under these conditions, thus ruling out the possibility that the unidentified metabolites in MRC-5 cells arise from liberated [^{14}C] adenine or from trace contamination of [^{14}C] adenine in the [^{14}C]PMEA, inasmuch as the proportions of these peaks would have been significantly lowered. These results also suggest that the enzymes responsible for phosphorylation of AMP to its di- and triphosphates are probably not involved in the metabolism of PMEA in MRC-5 cells. Identification of the enzyme(s) responsible for phosphorylation of PMEA to PMEAp and PMEApp is under investigation.

Reverse Transcriptase Inhibition Studies

The intracellular production of the di- and triphosphate analogues PMEAp and PMEApp from the nucleoside monophosphate analogue PMEA is similar to the activation process associated with nucleoside analogues, where the resulting triphosphate derivative exerts the antiviral effect by inhibition of viral DNA synthesis. In order to elucidate the possible mechanism of action of PMEA against retroviruses such as HIV, we examined the inhibitory effect of PMEApp on HIV reverse transcriptase. The RT inhibition assay was first carried out by using poly(rU):oligo(dA) as the RNA template/ primer pair and examining the effect of various concentrations of PMEApp on the incorporation of [³H]-dATP. The K_m for dATP in this system was 2 μM. Analysis of the inhibition data gave a K_i value for PMEApp of 15 μM (TABLE 2). Under the same conditions, the K_i value for ddATP was 8 μM. Because RT is known to have a DNA-dependent DNA polymerase function in addition to its RNA-dependent DNA polymerase activity, the assay was also performed using activated salmon sperm DNA as a template/primer system. In this case, the K_m for dATP was 0.31 μM, whereas the K_i values for PMEApp and ddATP were 0.23 μM and 0.08 μM, respectively. The results show that PMEApp acts as a competitive RT inhibitor with respect to dATP and that inhibition of the enzyme can be obtained at a concentration that is attainable in infected cells. These studies also show that PMEA is comparable to ddA in its ability to inhibit RT at the triphosphate level.

HPMPC STUDIES

Metabolism in MRC-5 Cells

HPMPC labeled with C-14 on the cytosine ring was prepared for cellular metabolism studies. MRC-5 cells were incubated with 200 μM of [¹⁴C]HPMPC, and cell extracts were then analyzed by ion-exchange HPLC for the presence of HPMPC and its metabolites at various time points (TABLE 3). In addition to the parent compound, three peaks were obtained with retention times of 14, 26, and 53 minutes. The concentrations of these metabolites did not change significantly after 24 h of incubation; however, the total concentration of intracellular species was only 7% that of the extracellular drug concentration. The metabolism of HPMPC was also examined in

TABLE 2. Inhibition of HIV-RT by PMEApp and ddATP[a]

Template/Primer	Concentration (μM)		
	K_m, dATP	K_i, PMEApp	K_i, ddATP
Poly(rU):oligo(dA)	2	15	8
Activated salmon sperm DNA	0.31	0.23	0.08

[a] The assay measures the incorporation of radiolabeled ATP into an acid-insoluble template-primer system. Reaction mixtures contained 50 mM Tris-HCl, pH 7.5, 0.1 mM KCl, 5 mM MgCl₂, 5 mM DTT, 10 μg BSA, 0.025 OD units of (rU)$_n$, 0.025 OD units of (dA)$_{12-18}$, and variable concentrations of [³H]dATP with variable concentrations of PMEApp or ddATP. The reaction was started by adding 10 μL of a diluted enzyme preparation, and 20 μL aliquots were removed after various periods of time. A Statistical Analysis Software (SAS) program was used to fit the data directly to the model for competitive inhibition; $v = (V_{max} \cdot S)/(S + K_m (1 + (I/K_i)))$. SAS Institute, Inc., P.O. Box 8000, Cary, NC 27511.

TABLE 3. Uptake and Phosphorylation of [14C]HPMPC in MRC-5 Cells[a]

	Concentration of metabolites in cells (μM) Retention time			
Time of exposure (h)	HPMPC 5 min	HPMPCp-choline 14 min	HPMPCp 26 min	HPMPCpp 53 min
6	3.8	0.21	0.38	0.32
12	4.8	1.2	0.45	0.75
24	8.4	2.7	0.67	1.6

[a] [14C]HPMPC was present at 200 μM. HPLC analysis was carried out on a Whatman Partisil 10 SAX column, eluting with a 15 to 700 mM gradient of potassium phosphate buffer over 55 min and then at 700 mM for an additional 15 min.

MRC-5 cells infected with HSV 1. There was no major difference in the concentration of HPMPC metabolites between infected and uninfected cells, indicating that neither viral enzymes nor viral-induced cellular enzymes are involved in the activation of HPMPC.

Based on a comparison with the intracellular activation of other cytosine-based nucleosides,[20–23] the metabolites obtained from HPMPC were tentatively assigned (in order of elution) as the monophosphate-choline adduct (HPMPCp-choline), HPMPC-monophosphate (HPMPCp), and HPMPC-diphosphate (HPMPCpp) (FIG. 3). Initial efforts to identify these peaks were based on their chemical and enzymatic stabilities. For example, the peaks at 26 and 53 min were collected and then treated with HCl to afford exclusively HPMPC, thus supporting the assignments of these metabolites as HPMPCp and HPMPCpp. To establish the identity of the peak at 14 min, labeled as HPMPCp-choline, the material was isolated and treated with alkaline phosphatase or snake venom phosphodiesterase. The sensitivity of the compound to only the latter enzyme is consistent with its assignment as the phosphate-choline adduct. Preparation of authentic samples of these metabolites directly from HPMPC initially proved problematic because the 3'-hydroxyl group readily participates in a cyclization reaction to provide the cyclic ester of HPMPC (FIG. 4). To circumvent this problem, a 3'-O-benzyl derivative of HPMPC was prepared and then converted under standard conditions to the corresponding mono- and diphosphate esters (FIG. 4). Removal of the benzyl protecting group by transfer hydrogenation provided authentic samples of HPMPCp and HPMPCpp; the structural assignments of the synthetic material were based on ^{31}P and ^{1}H NMR spectral data. Development of conditions for preparation of an authentic sample of HPMPCp-choline is underway.

In order to identify the enzymes responsible for HPMPC activation in cells, we have examined the metabolism of HPMPC after pretreatment of cells with various pyrimidine nucleosides. If the activation of HPMPC involves enzymes in the pyrimidine nucleoside activation pathway, there should be a suppression of HPMPC metabolism in the presence of the competing substrate. For example, deoxycytidine suppresses 2',3'-dideoxycytidine (ddC) activation because these two compounds are both dependent on deoxycytidine kinases for activation to the monophosphate.[22,24] MRC-5 cells were incubated with 20 μM of the nucleoside (cytidine, deoxycytidine, thymidine, or uridine) for 3 h and then treated with 200 μM labeled HPMPC for an additional 24 h; the concentration of the nucleoside was chosen because of the expected rapid equilibration across the cell membrane to give an intracellular concentration greater than that of HPMPC. Analysis of cell extracts by ion-exchange chromatography showed that

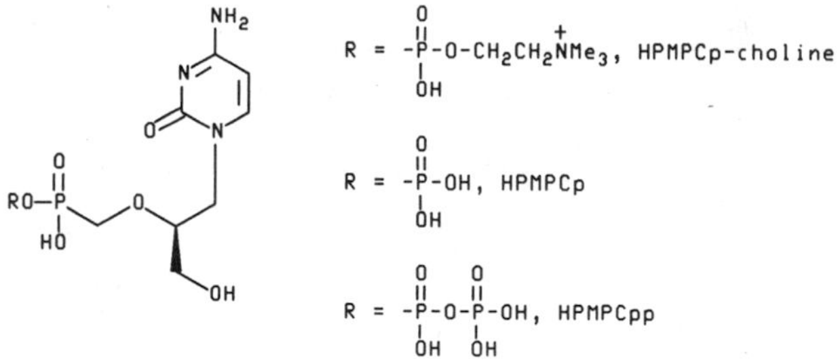

FIGURE 3. Structures of HPMPCp-choline, HPMPCp, and HPMPCpp.

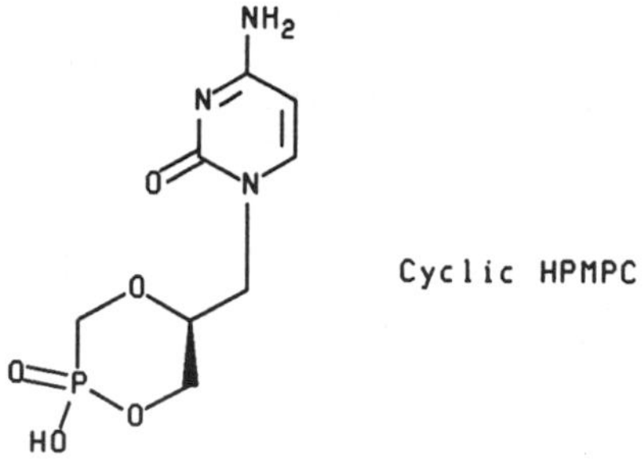

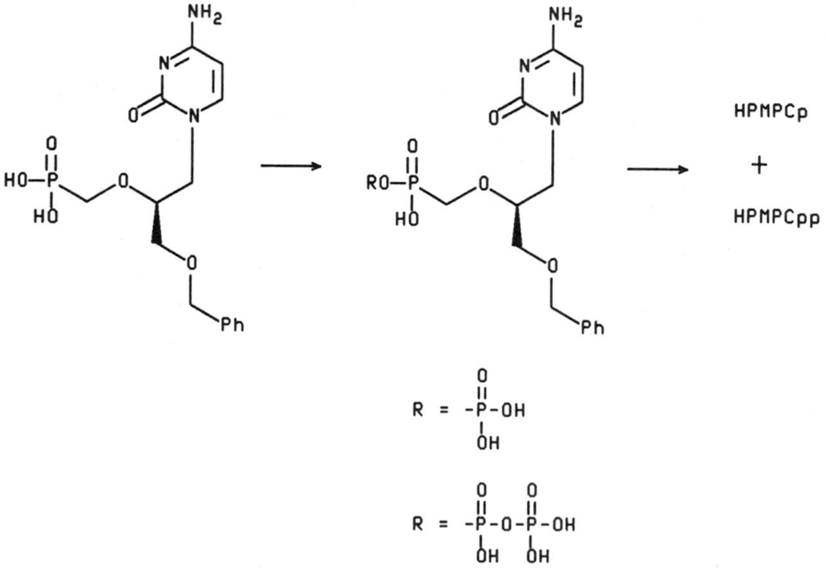

FIGURE 4. Synthesis of HPMPCp and HPMPCpp.

activation of HPMPC was not suppressed by the presence of any of the added nucleosides. These results were unexpected and suggest that phosphorylation of HPMPC is probably not catalyzed by CMP kinase (the enzyme responsible for phosphorylation of CMP, dCMP, and UMP) or TMP kinase (the monophosphate kinase responsible for phosphorylation of TMP and dUMP). The effect of competition with other nucleosides will be investigated.

In vivo, the extracellular concentration of drug falls due to clearance. Because the persistence of an antiviral effect is dependent on how rapidly activated forms of the drug are eliminated from cells, we have investigated the rate of decay of the intracellular species after removal of HPMPC from the cell medium. For these studies, MRC-5 cells were incubated with 200 μM labeled HPMPC for 24 h, and then the cells were washed and resuspended in fresh medium. Samples of cell extracts were analyzed after 6, 12, 24, and 48 h to determine the concentrations of the metabolites. These experiments showed the decay half-lives to be > 48 h for HPMPCp-choline, 6 h for HPMPCp, and 17 h for HPMPCpp. This suggests that dosing of HPMPC could be done on an infrequent basis because a prolonged antiviral effect would be possible due to the intracellular persistence of these activated species.

Effect of Dosing Schedule on in Vivo *Antiviral Efficacy*

Based on the biochemical results showing a slow rate of decay of HPMPC metabolites, *in vivo* studies were designed to explore the effectiveness of dosing with different frequencies of administration. An HSV 2 infection model in mice was used for these experiments,[14] and the antiviral effect of HPMPC was determined using five treatment schedules (TABLE 4). In each treatment regimen, HPMPC was administered intraperitoneally at a total dose over the course of the experiment of 50 mg/kg, 5 mg/kg, or 0.5 mg/kg. At the top dose of 50 mg/kg, HPMPC proved highly effective regardless of treatment schedule, providing complete protection even when administered once as a single 50 mg/kg dose. A single 5 mg/kg dose of HPMPC was as effective as a single dose at 50 mg/kg in reducing the mortality associated with HSV 2 infection. Furthermore, the single dose regimen at 5 mg/kg proved more efficacious than when this same total dose was administered in portions. The low dose of 0.5 mg/kg did not provide significant protection with any of the treatment schedules. These results indicate that infrequent dosing with HPMPC is still highly efficacious for the treatment of viral infections.

SUMMARY

Our studies have shown that the acyclic nucleotide analogues PMEA and HPMPC are able to penetrate into cells and are then activated to mono- and diphosphate derivatives. The latter correspond to triphosphate analogues and presumably serve an important role in the biological activity exerted by these antiviral agents. In support of this idea, the inhibitory effect of PMEApp on HIV reverse transcriptase has been demonstrated with both RNA and DNA template-primer systems. Further studies will be undertaken to determine the effect of HPMPCpp on viral DNA polymerases.

Whereas the metabolism of PMEA in CEM cells gives rise to only PMEAp and PMEApp, additional metabolites were obtained in MRC-5 cells; the identity of these metabolites remains to be determined. In the case of HPMPC, a third metabolite was obtained in addition to HPMPCp and HPMPCpp, which has been tentatively assigned as a phosphate-choline adduct by analogy with activation of cytosine-based nucleoside derivatives. The metabolism of HPMPC was unchanged between uninfected and infected cells, indicating that viral enzymes are not necessary for the activation of HPMPC. The long intracellular half-lives of the HPMPC metabolites may have implications for the antiviral efficacy of this compound. The persistence of activated metabolites suggests that infrequent dosing may be possible due to a prolonged antiviral effect. Our results on the effectiveness of infrequent dosing schedules with HPMPC in the treatment of HSV 2 infections in mice support this hypothesis. It is also possible that HPMPCp-choline may serve as a reservoir for HPMPC and therefore for the presumed active metabolite HPMPCpp.

TABLE 4. The Effect of Treatment Schedule on the Antiviral Efficacy of HPMPC against HSV 2 Systemic Infection in Mice[a]

| | Survivors (percent) Total dose: | | | |
Treatment schedule	50 mg/kg	5 mg/kg	0.5 mg/kg	Placebo
Day 1-5; b.i.d.	100[b]	70[b]	0	0
Day 1-5; once a day	90[b]	50[b]	10	
Days 1,3,5; once a day	100[b]	80[b]	—	
Days 1,3; once a day	90[b]	80[b]	20	
Day 1; once a day	100[b]	100[b]	0	

[a] Mice were inoculated intraperitoneally with 10^3 PFU/0.2 mL of HSV 2 (G strain) and divided into groups of 10 mice each. Intraperitoneal treatment with HPMPC was initiated 3 h postinfection using the treatment schedules described above. The experiment was terminated at day 21.

[b] Significance value as compared to placebo control, $p < 0.05$.

The enzymes responsible for activation of PMEA and HPMPC have not yet been identified. Further studies will address this question and will explore the possible mechanism(s) of action of these and related acyclic nucleotide analogues.

REFERENCES

1. MANSURI, M. M. & J. C. MARTIN. 1987. Annu. Rep. Med. Chem. **22:** 147-157.
2. MANSURI, M. M. & J. C. MARTIN. 1988. Annu. Rep. Med. Chem. **23:** 161-170.
3. DIANA, G. D., D. PEVEAR & D. C. YOUNG. 1989. Annu. Rep. Med. Chem. **24:** 129-137.
4. ROBINS, R. K. 1984. Pharm. Res. (NY) **1:** 11-18.
5. DE CLERCQ, E., A. HOLY, I. ROSENBERG, T. SAKUMA, J. BALZARINI & P. C. MAUDGAL. 1986. Nature **323:** 464-467.
6. VOTRUBA, I., R. BERNAERTS, T. SAKUMA, E. DE CLERCQ, A. MERTA, I. ROSENBERG & A. HOLY. 1987. Mol. Pharmacol. **32:** 524-527.

7. De Clercq, E., T. Sakuma, M. Baba, R. Pauwels, J. Balzarini, I. Rosenberg & A. Holy. 1987. Antiviral Res. **8:** 261-272.
8. Holy, A. & I. Rosenberg. 1987. Collect. Czech. Chem. Commun. **52:** 2801-2809.
9. Pauwels, R., J. Balzarini, D. Schols, M. Baba, J. Desmyter, I. Rosenberg, A. Holy & E. De Clercq. 1988. Antimicrob. Agents Chemother. **32** (7): 1025-1030.
10. Bronson, J. J., C. U. Kim, I. Ghazzouli, M. J. M. Hitchcock, E. R. Kern & J. C. Martin. 1989. *In* Nucleotide Analogues as Antiviral Agents. J. C. Martin, Ed. ACS Symposium Series **401:** 72-87. American Chemical Society. Washington, DC.
11. Balzarini, J., L. Naesens, P. Herdewijn, I. Rosenberg, A. Holy, R. Pauwels, M. Baba, D. G. Johns & E. De Clercq. 1989. Proc. Natl. Acad. Sci. USA **86:** 332-336.
12. Gangemi, J. D., R. M. Cozens, E. De Clercq, A. Matter & H-K. Hochkeppel. 1989. Collected abstracts of the 5th International Conference on AIDS (Montreal, Quebec): No. M.C.P.81. International Development Research Center. Ottawa, Ontario.
13. Mathes, L. E., C. L. Swenson, P. A. Polas, R. Sams, K. Hayes & G. Kociba. 1989. Collected abstracts of the 5th International Conference on AIDS (Montreal, Quebec): No. M.C.P.69. International Development Research Center. Ottawa, Ontario.
14. Bronson, J. J., I. Ghazzouli, M. J. M. Hitchcock, R. R. Webb II & J. C. Martin. 1989. J. Med. Chem. **32:** 1457-1463.
15. Bronson, J. J., I. Ghazzouli, M. J. M. Hitchcock, R. R. Webb II, E. R. Kern & J. C. Martin. 1989. *In* Nucleotide Analogues as Antiviral Agents. J. C. Martin, Ed. ACS Symposium Series **401:** 88-102. American Chemical Society. Washington, DC.
16. Snoeck, R., T. Sakuma, E. De Clercq, I. Rosenberg & A. Holy. 1988. Antimicrob. Agents Chemother. **32:** 1839-1844.
17. Kern, E. R. & P. E. Vogt. 1989. Collected abstracts of the 29th Interscience Conference on Antimicrobial Agents and Chemotherapy (Houston, TX): No. 751. American Society for Microbiology. Washington, DC.
18. Plunkett, W. & S. S. Cohen. 1975. Cancer Res. **35:** 1547-1554.
19. Cooney, D. A., G. Ahluwalia, H. Mitsuya, A. Fridland, M. Johnson, Z. Hao, M. Dalal, J. Balzarini, S. Broder & D. G. Johns. 1987. Biochem. Pharmacol. **36** (11): 1765-1768.
20. Lauzon, G. J., J. H. Paran & A. R. P. Paterson. 1978. Cancer Res. **38:** 1723-1729.
21. Lauzon, G. J., A. R. P. Paterson & A. W. Belch. 1978. Cancer Res. **38:** 1730-1733.
22. Cooney, D. A., M. Dalal, H. Mitsuya, J. B. McMahon, M. Nadkarni, J. Balzarini, S. Broder & D. G. Johns. 1986. Biochem. Pharmacol. **35:** (13): 2065-2068.
23. Heinemann, V., L. W. Hertel, G. B. Grindey & W. Plunkett. 1988. Cancer Res. **48:** 4024-4031.
24. Balzarini, J., D. A. Cooney, M. Dalal, G-J. Kang, J. E. Cupp, E. De Clercq, S. Broder & D. G. Johns. 1987. Mol. Pharmacol. **32:** 798-806.

Anabolism and Mechanism of Action of Ro24-5098, an Isomer of 2',3'-Dideoxyadenosine (ddA) with Anti-HIV Activity

KARL B. FRANK,[a] EDWARD V. CONNELL,[a]
MICHAEL J. HOLMAN,[a] DONNA M. HURYN,[a]
BARBARA C. SLUBOSKI,[a] STEVE Y. TAM,[a]
LOUIS J. TODARO,[a] MANFRED WEIGELE,[a]
DOUGLAS D. RICHMAN,[b] HIROAKI MITSUYA,[c]
SAMUEL BRODER,[c] AND IAIN S. SIM[a]

[a]Roche Research Center
Hoffmann-La Roche Inc.
Nutley, New Jersey 07110-1199
[b]University of California
San Diego, California
[c]National Cancer Institute
Bethesda, Maryland

INTRODUCTION

The potential of dideoxynucleosides as inhibitors of HIV replication has been demonstrated *in vitro* by Mitsuya and Broder.[1] This stimulated a great deal of interest in possible use of these compounds for therapy of HIV infections and led to clinical trials with 2',3'-dideoxycytidine (ddC)[2] and 2',3'-dideoxyinosine (ddI).[3]

One factor that may limit the clinical utility of dideoxypurine nucleosides is the instability of the glycosidic bond at low pH, resulting in destruction of a pharmacologically active compound. This creates difficulties when oral administration is desired. A second factor affecting the usefulness of ddA and ddI is biochemical catabolism. Studies in cell culture[4-7] revealed that ddA is readily converted to ddI by adenosine deaminase (ADA). A portion of ddI is then degraded by purine nucleoside phosphorylase (PNP),[8] whereas the remainder is anabolized, possibly by 5'-nucleotidase.[9] The end result of cellular anabolism of both ddA and ddI is ddATP, which interacts with HIV reverse transcriptase. Although ddA can be anabolized directly by deoxyadenosine kinase (dAK) and deoxycytidine kinase (dCK) to ddAMP, these reactions occur to a small extent compared to the indirect route of anabolism by way of ddI. Therefore, both ddI and ddA (following deamination) are subject to catabolism by PNP.

Among the goals of medicinal chemists working in this area are the development of dideoxypurine analogues that resist chemical degradation at gastric pH and are not subject to biochemical degradation by deaminases and phosphorylases. Furthermore, these compounds must retain substrate activity for the appropriate nucleoside kinases and be anabolized to a triphosphate that inhibits HIV reverse transcriptase selectively. With these objectives in mind, we have developed a series of purine dideoxynucleoside analogues that are currently being characterized in our laboratories.

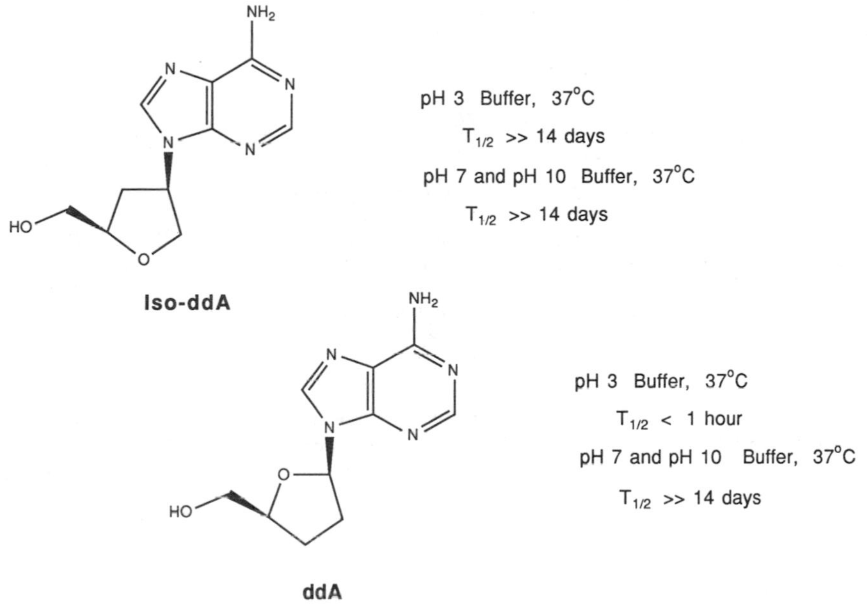

pH 3 Buffer, 37°C

$T_{1/2} \gg 14$ days

pH 7 and pH 10 Buffer, 37°C

$T_{1/2} \gg 14$ days

Iso-ddA

pH 3 Buffer, 37°C

$T_{1/2} < 1$ hour

pH 7 and pH 10 Buffer, 37°C

$T_{1/2} \gg 14$ days

ddA

FIGURE 1. The structure and acid-resistance of IsoddA is compared to ddA. Compounds were dissolved in buffer at pH 3, 7, and 10 and incubated at 37° C for 14 days. Aliquots were examined periodically by thin-layer chromatography.

CHEMICAL AND BIOCHEMICAL STABILITY

The structure of the isonucleoside IsoddA (Ro24-5098) is shown in FIGURE 1. The isonucleosides are synthesized using a novel isomer of 2',3'-dideoxyribose in which the positions of the 3' carbon and ring oxygen are transposed.[10] This new structural feature is designed to endow these compounds with improved stability at low pH. For example, IsoddA is stable at pH 3.0 (37° C) for more than two weeks, whereas the half-life of ddA under these conditions is less than one hour.

In addition to improved chemical stability, IsoddA is highly resistant to degradation by intracellular enzymes (FIG. 2). Incubation of adenosine, ddA, and IsoddA with ADA results in rapid deamination of the first two nucleosides to their inosine deriva-

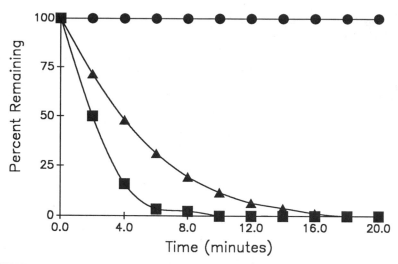

FIGURE 2. Resistance of IsoddA to catabolism by adenosine deaminase. Adenosine (■), ddA (▲), or IsoddA (●) at a concentration of 100 μM each were incubated for 20 min with 100 ng bovine ADA (Boehringer Mannheim), essentially as described.[11] Conversion to inosine derivatives was determined by measuring the change in optical density at 265 nm in a Beckman DU-7 spectrophotometer.

tives, whereas deamination of IsoddA is not detectable (< 1%). Furthermore, hydrolysis of IsoddA by PNP is undetectable (< 3%) under conditions in which hydrolysis of inosine is 90% complete (data not shown). Therefore, IsoddA may be highly resistant to catabolism *in vivo*.

ANTIVIRAL ACTIVITY

Antiviral potencies vary among different assay systems. Therefore, the antiviral activities of IsoddA, IsoddG (Ro24-5671), and IsoddI (Ro24-5669) were determined in several different anti-HIV assay systems to establish a concentration range over which each compound was active *in vitro* (TABLE 1). IsoddA was clearly the most potent of these compounds (ED_{50} range 4-20 μM). IsoddG was significantly less potent

TABLE 1. Inhibition of HIV Replication *in Vitro*[a]

	ED_{50} (μM)
IsoddA	4-20
IsoddG	10-50
IsoddI	> 100

[a] ED_{50} values indicate the ranges obtained in the following test systems: ATH8 (protection from cell killing)[1] and HT4-6C (plaque reduction assay).[12]

(ED$_{50}$ range 10-50 μM), whereas antiviral activity of IsoddI and a number of other isonucleoside analogues was not detectable in most assays. Antiviral selectivity cannot be calculated due to the extremely low cytotoxicities of these compounds (IC$_{50}$s > 200 μM).

Because of its antiviral potency, the anabolism of IsoddA was studied in CEM cell cultures and compared to that of ddA (FIG. 3). Cell cultures were incubated for up to 48 hours with various concentrations of compound; then cell extracts were analyzed

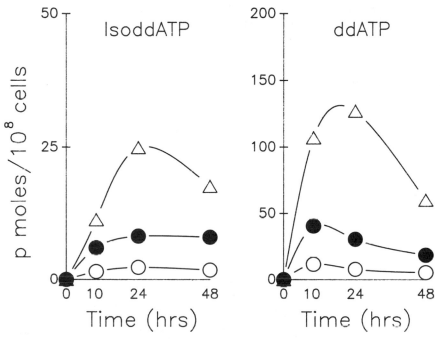

FIGURE 3. Phosphorylation of ddA and IsoddA by CEM cells. Radiolabeled ddA (Moravek) or IsoddA was added to produce concentrations of 3 (○), 10 (●), or 22 (▲) μM in CEM cell cultures that had been adjusted to a density of 10^6/mL in RPMI-1640 supplemented with 10% fetal calf serum, 2 mM L-glutamine, and 50 μg/mL gentamicin. Cells were incubated at 37° C for the times indicated. Then aliquots were removed, cells pelleted and washed, and nucleotides extracted with 60% methanol. Cell debris was removed by spinning in a microcentrifuge, and a sample of the supernatant was injected onto a SAX (Whatman) HPLC column. The column was eluted at 1.5 mL/minute over a period of 60 minutes with a linear gradient of 1% to 100% high salt buffer (500 mM KHPO$_4$, 1.0 M KCl) at pH 4.5 for analysis of IsoddATP and pH 5.0 for ddATP. One minute fractions were collected, and radioactivity was determined with a liquid scintillation counter.

by strong anion exchange (SAX) HPLC using conditions that clearly resolved all relevant purine nucleoside triphosphates. Radioactivity associated with these fractions was then quantitated. Formation of triphosphate from IsoddA was significant and increased almost linearly upon incubation for approximately 24 hours. By 48 hours the amount of intracellular triphosphate had declined, possibly due to crowding of cells or alteration of purine nucleoside pools. By contrast, phosphorylation of ddA did not increase much beyond the 10 hour point and had declined by 24 hours in cells exposed to 3 and 10 μM ddA. This may be due to extensive catabolism of ddA. In general, the amount of triphosphate produced from IsoddA was approximately one-third to one-fourth that produced from ddA at comparable times and concentrations.

Although it is not possible to predict relative anabolism of ddA and IsoddA *in vivo* from these data, the greater acid stability of IsoddA may have a significant impact. Furthermore, the resistance of IsoddA to deamination suggests that this compound is anabolized directly by a nucleoside kinase, rather than by way of the inosine derivative, as with ddA. Studies in animals and further biochemical investigations are planned.

By analogy to ddA, it is likely that IsoddA inhibits HIV replication by interaction with reverse transcriptase following anabolism to the triphosphate. Results obtained with purified HIV reverse transcriptase are consistent with this (FIG. 4). IsoddATP competitively inhibited incorporation of dATP into synthetic polynucleotide template/

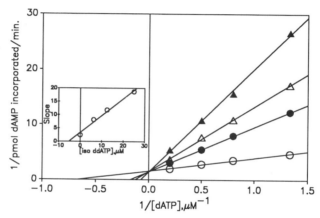

FIGURE 4. Inhibition of HIV reverse transcriptase by IsoddATP. Purified recombinant HIV reverse transcriptase[13] was assayed in 50 mM Tris-HCl (pH 8.0), 25 mM KCl, 8 mM MgCl$_2$, 0.05% Triton X-100, poly(rU)·oligo(dA)$_{12-18}$, and [^{3}H]dATP (New England Nuclear) at the concentrations indicated for 30 min at 37° C. IsoddATP was added to produce concentrations of 0 (○), 6.25 (●), 12.5 (△), and 25 μM (▲). Reactions were stopped by the addition of 10% trichloroacetic acid, and polynucleotide was collected on glass fiber filters (Whatman). Substrate incorporation was determined by liquid scintillation counting, and the results were analyzed by the method of Lineweaver and Burk.

primer, yielding K_m and K_i values of 1.6 μM and 5.2 μM for dATP and IsoddATP, respectively. In this assay, the K_i for ddATP was 0.22 μM.

Preferential interaction of a nucleoside analogue with viral reverse transcriptase may be desirable if toxicity is to be avoided. We found that DNA polymerase α from CEM cells was weakly inhibited by IsoddATP. Inhibition was competitive with dATP, producing a K_i of 300 μM for IsoddATP and a K_m of 3.2 μM for dATP. The K_i for ddATP was 210 μM. Therefore, DNA polymerase α is much more resistant to inhibition by IsoddATP than is HIV reverse transcriptase. Recently Cheng and co-workers[14,15] have suggested that the peripheral neuropathy observed in certain patients treated with ddC may be due, in part, to inhibition of mitochondrial DNA polymerase γ by ddCTP. We are currently examining the interaction of IsoddATP with mammalian DNA polymerases β and γ to determine the resistance of these enzymes.

CONCLUSION

IsoddA exhibits stability at low pH that is superior to ddA. Furthermore, IsoddA is highly resistant to enzymatic degradation and possesses moderate anti-HIV activity *in vitro*. In CEM cells, phosphorylation of IsoddA to the expected antiviral metabolite, the triphosphate, occurs approximately one-third to one-fourth as readily as phosphorylation of ddA. Greater chemical and biochemical stability of the isonucleoside, however, may provide greater antiviral potency *in vivo*. The triphosphate of IsoddA inhibits HIV reverse transcriptase selectively with respect to DNA polymerase α. Future development of this compound will depend upon the interaction of IsoddATP with mammalian DNA polymerases β and γ as well as toxicological studies in animals.

REFERENCES

1. MITSUYA, H. & S. BRODER. 1986. Inhibition of the *in vitro* infectivity and cytopathic effect of human T-lymphotrophic virus type III/lymphadenopathy-associated virus (HTLV-III/LAV) by 2′,3′-dideoxynucleosides. Proc. Natl. Acad. Sci. USA **83:** 1911-1915.

2. YARCHOAN, R., C. F. PERNO, R. V. THOMAS, R. W. KLECKER, J.-P. ALLAIN, R. J. WILLS, N. MCATEE, M. A. FISHCL, R. DUBINSKY, M. C. MCNEELY, H. MITSUYA, J. M. PLUDA, T. J. LAWLEY, M. LEUTHER, B. SAFAI, J. M. COLLINS, C. E. MYERS & S. BRODER. 1988. Phase I studies of 2′,3′-dideoxycytidine in severe human immunodeficiency virus infections as a single agent and alternating with zidovudine (AZT). Lancet i: 76-80.

3. YARCHOAN, R., H. MITSUYA, R. V. THOMAS, J. M. PLUDA, N. R. HARTMAN, C.-F. PERNO, K. S. MARCZYK, J.-P. ALLAIN, D. G. JOHNS & S. BRODER. 1989. *In vivo* activity against IIIV and favorable toxicity profile of 2′,3′-dideoxyinosine. Science **245:** 412-415.

4. AHLUWALIA, G., D. A. COONEY, H. MITSUYA, K. P. FLORA, Z. HAO, M. DALAL, S. BRODER & D. G. JOHNS. 1987. Initial studies on the cellular pharmacology of 2′,3′-dideoxyinosine, an inhibitor of HIV infectivity. Biochem. Pharmacol. **36:** 3797-3800.

5. COONEY, D. A., G. AHLUWALIA, H. MITSUYA, A. FRIDLAND, M. JOHNSON, Z. HAO, M. DALAL, J. BALZARINI, S. BRODER & D. G. JOHNS. 1987. Initial studies on the cellular pharmacology of 2′,3′-dideoxyadenosine, an inhibitor of HTLV-III infectivity. Biochem. Pharmacol. **36:** 1765-1768.

6. CARSON, D. A., T. HAERTLE, D. B. WASSON & D. D. RICHMAN. 1988. Biochemical genetic analysis of 2′,3′-dideoxyadenosine metabolism in human T lymphocytes. Biochem. Biophys. Res. Commun. **131.** 700 703.

7. JOHNSON, M. A., G. AHLUWALIA, M. C. CONNELLY, D. A. COONEY, S. BRODER, D. G. JOHNS & A. FRIDLAND. 1988. Metabolic pathways for the activation of the antiretroviral agent 2′,3′-dideoxyadenosine in human lymphoid cells. J. Biol. Chem. **263:** 15354-15357.

8. STOECKLER, J., C. CAMBOR & R. E. PARKS. 1980. Human erythrocyte purine nucleoside phosphorylase: Reaction with sugar-modified nucleoside substrates. Biochemistry **19:** 102-107.

9. JOHNSON, M. A. & A. FRIDLAND. 1989. Phosphorylation of 2′,3′-dideoxyinosine by cytosolic 5′-nucleotidase of human lymphoid cells. Mol. Pharmacol. **36:** 291-295.

10. HURYN, D. M., B. C. SLUBOSKI, S. Y. TAM, L. J. TODARO & M. WEIGELE. 1989. Synthesis of iso-ddA, member of a novel class of anti-HIV agents. Tetrahedron Lett. **30:** 6259-6262.

11. AGARWAL, R. P., T. SPECTOR & R. E. PARKS, JR. 1977. Tight-binding inhibitors—IV. Inhibitors of adenosine deaminases by various inhibitors. Biochem. Pharmacol. **26:** 359-367.

12. LARDER, B. A., G. DARBY & D. D. RICHMAN. 1989. HIV with reduced sensitivity to zidovudine (ACT) isolated during prolonged therapy. Science **243:** 1731-1734.

13. LE GRICE, S. F. J. & F. GRUNINGER-LEITCH. 1990. Rapid purification of homodimer and heterodimer HIV-1 reverse transcriptase by metal chelate affinity chromatography. Eur. J. Biochem. **187:** 307-314.

14. STARNES, M. C. & Y. C. CHENG. 1987. Cellular metabolism of 2′,3′-dideoxycytidine, a compound active against human immunodeficiency virus *in vitro.* J. Biol. Chem. **262:** 988-991.

15. CHEN, C. H. & Y. C. CHENG. 1989. Delayed cytotoxicity and selective loss of mitochondrial DNA in cells treated with the anti-human immunodeficiency virus compound 2′,3′-dideoxycytidine. J. Biol. Chem. **264:** 11934-11937.

Molecular Biology of
Pneumocystis carinii

MELANIE T. CUSHION, SUNG TAE HONG,
PAUL E. STEELE, SAUNDRA L. STRINGER,
PETER D. WALZER, AND JAMES R. STRINGER

University of Cincinnati College of Medicine
Cincinnati, Ohio 45267
and
Veterans Affairs Medical Center
Cincinnati, Ohio 45220

Pneumocystis carinii is an opportunistic pathogen that causes pneumonitis in immuno-compromised hosts[1] and is a leading cause of mortality in patients with AIDS.[2] The basic biology of the organism is poorly understood due in large part to a lack of adequate *in vitro* culture methods. The taxonomic status of *P. carinii* has been debated since its original identification, as a life-cycle stage of a trypanosome, by Chagas in 1909.[3] A protozoan or fungal identity has been suggested by different investigators, primarily based on morphological evaluations at the light microscopic and ultrastructural levels.[4-7] The ameboid appearance of the smaller form of *P. carinii*, the presence of tubular extensions interpreted as filopodia, and the fine structure of the mitochondria and cell pellicle/wall have been cited as supportive of a protozoan nature.[4-6] Studies emphasizing the morphologic similarities to fungi have found analogies with the sporogenous state of *P. carinii* and ascospore formation in yeast. The lack of any invasive organelles characteristic of parasitic protozoans (*e.g.* rhoptries) and the ultrastructural organization of the cyst wall are reminiscent of yeast envelopes.[7]

Other characteristics of the organism have also been used to support a fungal or protozoan identity, but these aspects cannot be considered as definitive taxonomic markers. The cyst stage of *P. carinii* stains with methenamine silver, a stain that typically stains fungi, but analyses of its membrane sterols indicate a lack of ergosterol, a major sterol found in fungi.[8,9] The lack of ergosterol may explain the insensitivity of *P. carinii* pneumonitis to amphotericin B, a standard antifungal agent. Response of *P. carinii* pneumonitis, however, to the antimicrobial agents pentamidine and trimethoprim-sulfamethoxazole is of little help in defining its taxonomic status. Certain fungi can acquire resistance to amphotericin B through mutations in sterol biosynthetic pathways, and some fungi are responsive to drugs traditionally used to treat protozoal infections.[10,11] Attempts to continually cultivate the organism in media and under conditions favoring protozoans or fungi have not met with success.[12]

Comparison of small ribosomal RNA (srRNA) sequences has become the molecular method of choice for determining the phylogenetic interrelatedness of organisms.[13,14] Use of 5s ribosomal RNA for such purposes is limited because of the relatively small number of nucleotides (~120) that can be used for comparison.[13] When *P. carinii* srRNA sequence was compared with corresponding sequences from fungi, slime molds, protozoans, plants, and mammals, it was found that this organism more closely resem-

415

bled representative microbes from the Fungi rather than from Protozoa.[15,16] In addition, isolation and sequencing of the thymidylate synthase and dihydrofolate reductase genes of *P. carinii* have shown that these enzymes are not bifunctional proteins on the same polypeptide chain as Protozoa possess, but exist as distinct monofunctional enzymes.[17,18] Recent morphological studies have also supported the fungal nature of this organism. The ultrastructure of *P. carinii* mitochondria was found to contain lamellar cristae, which is consistent with the cristae of most fungi.[19] The carbohydrate-rich surface of *P. carinii* reacted with the lectins Con A and wheat germ agglutinin (WGA), indicating an abundance of glucosyl/mannosyl and *N*-acetylglucosamine residues.[20] The outer cyst wall of the *P. carinii* cyst was cleaved by treatment with Zymolyase, a β-1, 3-glucanase.[21] All of these carbohydrates are important components of yeast cell walls, although not definitive in their presence. The structural organization of the *P. carinii* cyst wall resembles that of a yeast envelope; the electron-dense surface layer is separated from a typical plasma membrane by an electron-lucent layer, which may be analogous to the periplasmic space in yeast. As these data accumulate, the likelihood of *P. carinii* belonging to the Protozoa decreases.

The potential fungal nature of *P. carinii* has provided new strategies for approaching some of the unanswered questions concerning the basic biology of the organism. An important aspect of its life cycle has not been identified, the agent of transmission. An airborne route of transmission has been suggested, however, by a series of animal experiments involving close and distant contact of infected with noninfected animals.[22–24] Subclinical infection of many mammalian species and the positive antibody response of over 75% of the human population to *P. carinii* by age four indicate that this organism enjoys ubiquitous distribution within the environment.[25] Many investigators have postulated a reactivation of latent infection as the most likely mechanism leading to fulminant infection, but environmental reexposure is most certainly a factor.

Previous studies of the transmission of *P. carinii* were limited by techniques available at the time that were unable to differentiate among primary, latent, or recrudescent infections. With the development of pulsed field gradient electrophoresis (PFGE), electrophoretic karyotypes of microbes such as yeast and protozoans can now be defined and used as a method to help characterize clinical isolates. We applied this technique to *P. carinii* isolates obtained from rats and humans to evaluate the possibility of strain or species variations as a tool to initiate epidemiological and transmission studies.

Electrophoretic karyotyping by contour clamped homogeneous field electrophoresis (CHEF) and field inversion gel electrophoresis (FIGE) of *P. carinii* from rat and human sources has revealed genetic variation among the isolates.[26] *P. carinii* were derived from the lungs of individual immunosuppressed rats and also from pooled isolates housed in four physically separated animal facilities. Two colonies, A and B, housed Sprague-Dawley rats obtained from the same vendor source (Harlan, Madison, WI), and two colonies, C and D, housed Lewis rats obtained from two vendor sources (Charles River, Wilmington, MA and the National Cancer Institute). Each of the four colonies produced a distinct band pattern, but in all cases the bands ranged in size from 300 kb to 700 kb. Isolates from colonies A, B, and C produced FIGE patterns containing 15 bands, whereas individual animals from colony D consistently produced patterns of 22 bands (FIG. 1A). Two of the 15 bands from colony isolates A–C stained with twice the intensity expected for bands of their size, suggesting that the *P. carinii* haploid genome contains 17 chromosomes. Summation of the molecular sizes of the 15 FIGE bands suggests that the haploid genome of *P. carinii* contains approximately 1×10^7 base pairs. The complex band pattern of *P. carinii* isolates from colony D contained all the 15 bands present in isolates from colony C plus several additional bands, suggesting that colony D rats may have been simultaneously infected by two different strains of *P. carinii*.

Hybridization experiments using oligonucleotide probes specific for *P. carinii* srRNA gene supported the hypothesis that animals in colony D harbored a mixed infection. The srRNA oligonucleotides hybridized to a single 530 kb band in samples from colonies A and B, and a 505 kb band from colony C isolates (FIG. 2). By contrast, *P. carinii* from colony D contained two bands homologous to the probes at 505 kb and

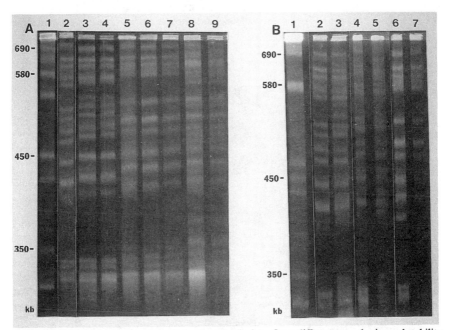

FIGURE 1. Variation among *Pneumocystis carinii* isolates from different rat colonies and stability of karyotype over time. FIGE parameters. 1% agarose gels, 105 v × 120 h, 50 s forward and 25 s back. Ethidium bromide visualization. **A:** Stability of karyotype. Different rat colonies were sampled over time. Lanes: (1) *Saccharomyces cerevisiae* size markers; (2) Sprague-Dawley rat from colony A, sampled Dec. 1988; (3) Sprague-Dawley rat from colony B, sampled May 1989; (4) Sprague-Dawley rat from colony B, sampled June 1989; (5) Lewis rat from colony C, sampled Jan. 1989; (6) Lewis rat from colony C sampled May 1989; (7) Lewis rat from colony C, sampled June 1989; (8) Lewis rat from colony D, sampled May 1989; (9) Lewis rat from colony D, sampled June 1989. **B.** Variation of karyotypes after mixing Lewis rats with Sprague-Dawley rats. Lewis rats from colony C were placed in colony A to evaluate effect on karyotype. Lanes: (1) *Saccharomyces cerevisiae* size markers; (2) Sprague-Dawley rat from colony A prior to introduction of Lewis rats; (3) Sprague-Dawley rat from colony A after introduction of Lewis rats; (4) Lewis rat mixed in with Sprague-Dawley rats of colony A; (5) same as 4; (6) and (7) Lewis rats from the same shipment as the mixed rats, but kept in colony C. (Hong *et al.* [26] With permission from the *Journal of Clinical Microbiology.*)

535 kb. Thus, it appears that these rats may have been infected by two strains of *Pneumocystis*, each harboring the srRNA locus on chromosomes of different sizes.

Whether single or mixed, the band pattern of *P. carinii* derived from a given colony remained the same over a five month period, during which time healthy animals were introduced into the colony, underwent immunosuppression, and subsequently developed *P. carinii* pneumonitis. When a group of Lewis rats were received in a single shipment from the same vendor (Charles River), and divided between colonies A and C, they ultimately produced an infection with a karyotype characteristic of the colony in which they were placed (FIG. 1B). Some Sprague-Dawley rats exposed to the Lewis rats, however, exhibited a karyotype unlike either *P. carinii* karyotype (from colony A or C) (FIG. 1B, lane 3). These data suggest that an important source of infection in immunosuppressed rats may be exogenous in addition to reactivation of latent or subclinical infection. It is also interesting to note that the same band pattern was consistently reproduced whether the isolates contained *P. carinii* obtained from a single

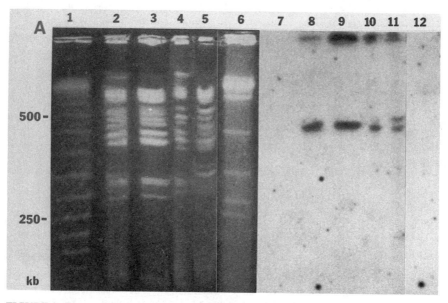

FIGURE 2. Electrophoretic karyotyping of rat *Pneumocystis carinii* by CHEF and hybridization with an oligonucleotide probe. CHEF conditions: 1% agarose gels, 90 V × 96 h, 50 to 100 s gradual switching. Ethidium bromide stained lanes (A): (1) lambda DNA 50 kb ladder; (2) Sprague-Dawley rat from colony A; (3) Sprague Dawley rat from colony B; (4) Lewis rat from colony C; (5) Lewis rat from colony D; (6) *Saccharomyces cerevisiae.* Hybridization lanes: lanes 7-12 correspond to lanes 1-6 above—hybridization of 26-mer oligonucleotides corresponding to unique srRNA sequence of *P. carinii.*[13,14] (Hong et al.[26] With permission from the *Journal of Clinical Microbiology.*)

rat or from two or more rats from the same colony. Even in the case of what appeared to be a mixed infection (colony D), the PFGE pattern was stable.

Electrophoretic karyotyping was applied to human-derived *P. carinii* obtained from five bronchoalveolar lavage fluids (BALFs) and two postmortem specimens. One BALF and one autopsy isolate produced clear band patterns by FIGE (data not shown). These two human isolates had karyotypes distinct from one another and from any of the rat karyotypes. The size range of the bands was similar to those produced by rat-derived *P. carinii*, although the number of chromosome bands was slightly lower (*i.e.* 10-12).

These data will provide a foundation for further studies of the transmission and epidemiology of infection caused by *P. carinii*. Identification of specific *P. carinii* strains will enable animal studies, with the ability to trace unique isolates through various methods of contact, including close and distant caging conditions, to be conducted. Likewise, it will be possible to analyze the source of recurrent *P. carinii* pneumonitis episodes in a single patient. Drug-resistant strains of *P. carinii* would be suggested by isolation of the same strain of *P. carinii* before and after treatment. Isolation of different strains of the organism would be suggestive of the environment as an important reservoir of infection.

REFERENCES

1. WALZER, P. D., D. P. PERL, D. J. KROGSTAD & P. G RAWSON. 1974. *Pneumocystis carinii* pneumonia in the United States: Epidemiologic, clinical, and diagnostic features. Ann. Intern. Med. **80**: 83-93.
2. MILLS, J. 1986. *Pneumocystis carinii* and *Toxoplasma gondii*: Infection in patients with AIDS. Rev. Infect. Dis. **8**: 1001-1011.
3. CHAGAS, C. 1909. Nova tripanomiazaea humana. Ueber eine neve trypanosomiasis de menschen. Mem. Inst. Oswaldo Cruz **1**: 159-218.
4. CAMPBELL JR., W. G. 1972. Ultrastructure of *Pneumocystis* in human lung. Arch. Pathol. **93**: 312-324.
5. VOSSEN, M. E. M. H., P. J. A. BECKERS, J. H. E. TH. MEUWISSEN & A. M. STADHOUDERS. 1978. Developmental biology of *Pneumocystis carinii*: an alternative life cycle of the parasite. Z. Parasitenkd. **55**: 101-118.
6. MATSUMOTO, Y. & Y. YOSHIDA. 1984. Sporogony in *Pneumocystis carinii*: Synaptonemal complexes and meiotic nuclear divisions observed in precysts. J. Protozool. **31**: 420-428.
7. VAVRA, J. & K. KUCERA. 1970. *Pneumocystis carinii* Delanoe, its ultrastructure and ultrastructural affinities. J. Protozool. **17**: 463-483.
8. YOSHIKAWA, H., H. MORIOKA & Y. YOSHIDA. 1987. Freeze fracture localization of filipinsterol complexes in plasma- and cyto-membranes of *Pneumocystis carinii*. J. Protozool. **34**: 131-137.
9. KANESHIRO, E. S., M. T. CUSHION, P. D WALZER & K. JAYASIMHULU. 1989. Analyses of *Pneumocystis* fatty acids. J. Protozool. (suppl.) **36**: 69s-72s.
10. WOODS, R. A. 1971. Nystatin-resistant mutants of yeast: alterations in sterol content. J. Bacteriol. **108**: 69.
11. ROLLO, I. M. 1980. Miscellaneous drugs used in the treatment of protozoal infections. *In* The Pharmacological Basis of Therapeutics, 6th ed., A. G. Gilman, L. S. Goodman & A. Gilman, Eds.: 1070-1079. Macmillan Publishing New York.
12. CUSHION, M. T. 1989. *In vitro* studies of *Pneumocystis carinii*. J. Protozool. **36**: 45-52.
13. STACKEBRANDT, E. & C. R. WOESE. 1981. Molecular and Cellular Aspects of Microbial Evolution. M. J. Carlile, J. F. Collins & B. E. B. Mosely, Eds.: 1-31. Cambridge University Press. Cambridge.
14. SOGIN, M. L., H. J. ELWOOD & J. H. GUNDERSON. 1986. Evolutionary diversity of eukaryotic small subunit rRNA genes. Proc. Nat. Acad. Sci. USA **83**: 1383-1387.
15. EDMAN, J. C., J. A. KOVACS, H. MASUR, D. V. SANTI, H. J. ELWOOD & M. L. SOGIN. 1988. Ribosomal RNA sequence shows *Pneumocystis carinii* to be a member of the fungi. Nature (London) **334**: 519-522.
16. STRINGER, S. L., J. R. STRINGER, M. A. BLASE, P. D. WALZER & M. T. CUSHION. 1989. *Pneumocystis carinii*: Sequence from ribosomal RNA implies a close relationship with Fungi. Exp. Parasitol. **68**: 450-461.
17. EDMAN, U., J. C. EDMAN, B. LUNDGREN & D. V. SANTI. 1989. Isolation and expression of the *Pneumocystis carinii* thymidylate synthase gene. Proc. Natl. Acad. Sci. USA **86**: 6503-6507.

18. EDMAN, J. C., U. EDMAN, M. CAO, B. LUNDGREN, J. A. KOVACS & D. V. SANTI. 1989. Isolation and expression of the *Pneumocystis carinii* dihydrofolate reductase gene. Proc. Natl. Acad. Sci. USA **86:** 8625-8629.
19. RUFFOLO, J. J., M. T. CUSHION & P. D. WALZER. 1989. Ultrastructural observations of life cycle stages of *Pneumocystis carinii*. J. Protozool. (suppl.) **36:** 53s-54s.
20. CUSHION, M. T., J. A. DeSTEFANO & P. D. WALZER. 1988. *Pneumocystis carinii*: Surface reactive carbohydrates detected by lectin probes. Exp. Parasitol. **67:** 137-147.
21. CUSHION, M. T., M. A. BLASE & P. D. WALZER. 1989. A method for isolation of RNA from *Pneumocystis carinii*. J. Protozool. (suppl.) **36:** 12s-14s.
22. HUGHES, W. T. 1989. Natural habitat and mode of transmission. *In Pneumocystis carinii* pneumonitis. **1:** 97-104. CRC Press, Inc. Boca Raton, FL.
23. HENDLEY, J.O. & T. H. WELLER. 1971. Activation and transmission in rats of infection with *Pneumocystis*. Proc. Soc. Exp. Biol. Med. **137:** 1401-1404.
24. WALZER, P. D., V. SCHNELLE, D. ARMSTRONG & P. P. ROSEN. 1977. Nude mouse: a new experimental model for *Pneumocystis carinii* infection. Science **197:** 177-179.
25. HUGHES, W. T. 1982. Natural mode of acquisition for *de novo* infection with *Pneumocystis carinii*. J. Infect. Dis. **145:** 842-847.
26. HONG, S. T., P. STEELE, M. T. CUSHION, P. D. WALZER, S. L. STRINGER & J. R. STRINGER. 1990. *Pneumocystis carinii* karyotypes. J. Clin. Microbiol. **28:** 1785-1795.

Development of Pentamidine Analogues as New Agents for the Treatment of *Pneumocystis carinii* Pneumonia[a]

RICHARD R. TIDWELL,[b] SUSAN K. JONES,[b,c]
J. DIETER GERATZ,[b] KWASI A. OHEMENG,[b]
CONSTANCE A. BELL,[d] BRADLEY J. BERGER,[d]
AND JAMES EDWIN HALL [d]

[b]*Department of Pathology*
[c]*Department of Pediatrics*
School of Medicine
University of North Carolina at Chapel Hill
Chapel Hill, North Carolina 27599-7525

[d]*Department of Parasitology*
School of Public Health
University of North Carolina at Chapel Hill
Chapel Hill, North Carolina 27599-7525

INTRODUCTION

The synthesis and antiprotozoal activity of 1,5-di(4-amidinophenoxy)pentane, pentamidine, was first reported in the late 1930s.[1] During the early 1940s hundreds of pentamidine analogues were synthesized and screened for their trypanocidal and bactericidal efficacy.[2] Pentamidine was the only diamidine compound to receive notable attention for clinical use and was first used in the 1940s for the treatment of African trypanosomiasis and leishmaniasis.[3] [f] The drug was reported to be an effective agent for the treatment of *Pneumocystis carinii* pneumonia (PCP) in 1958 by Ivady and Paldy.[6] Following this discovery, the drug continued to be used on a restricted basis for the treatment of PCP despite an extensive list of adverse effects that included nephrotoxicity, hepatotoxicity, hypotension, and sterile abscesses at the injection site.[7] Because of these adverse reactions the drug saw only limited use prior to the acquired immune deficiency syndrome (AIDS) epidemic.[8] Trimethoprim-sulfamethoxazole, the drug of choice in non-AIDS cases of PCP, was found to cause a high frequency of adverse reactions in AIDS-related PCP.[9,10] This observation, coupled with the finding

[a]These studies were funded by Public Health Service Contract NO1-A1-72648, NIH Grant HL-19171-13, and by Lyphomed, Inc., Rosemont, IL. Bradley J. Berger is a Howard Hughes Medical Institute pre-doctoral fellow.

421

that PCP is the leading cause of morbidity and mortality in AIDS patients,[11,12] has resulted in an increased use of pentamidine in the treatment of PCP. Recent clinical trials have shown that the toxicity of pentamidine can be greatly reduced if the drug is given by aerosol administration.[13] Despite this encouraging finding there remains an urgent need for an alternate drug for the treatment of PCP associated with AIDS.

Prior to our recent studies there were published records of only a handful of pentamidine-related compounds having been tested against PCP. An early study reported that a diamidine derivative, hydroxystilbamidine, was active against rat PCP,[14] whereas a more recent report showed that several dicationic molecules related to pentamidine were also active in the rat model of the disease.[15] This lack of information on the anti-PCP activity of pentamidine analogues is related to the difficulty of screening large numbers of compounds against the organism. This problem is due to the absence of a dependable *in vitro* assay system for *P. carinii,* and the resulting necessity to carry out structure-activity studies of anti-*P. carinii* drugs by using cumbersome and costly animal models. The standard animal model of disease involves the spontaneous generation of PCP in rats immunosuppressed by administration of corticosteroids.[14-16] Although not an ideal screening method, several studies have shown that the rat model of PCP is a good predictor of drug efficacy in humans.[14,15]

This paper describes our continuing investigation into the structure-activity relationship of pentamidine analogues against the rat model of PCP,[16-18] the mechanism of action of pentamidine and its analogues,[17] the distribution and metabolism of the parent drug,[19-21] and the efficacy of these compounds against other parasitic organisms.[22]

METHODS

Source of Compounds

All of the compounds for this study were synthesized in our laboratory and isolated as the mono- or dihydrochloride salts. The syntheses were carried out according to previously described methods.[16-18] The purity of the compounds was determined by high-performance liquid chromatography (HPLC), elemental analyses, and nuclear magnetic resonance (NMR) spectroscopy.

Animal Model of PCP

The induction and treatment of PCP was carried out, with only minor changes, according to reported methods.[14-16] Male Sprague-Dawley rats, barrier-raised, not certified virus-free, and weighing 150-200 g each, were obtained from Hilltop Laboratories (Scottsdale, PA). The individually caged animals were begun on a low protein (8%) diet (ICN Biomedicals, Cincinnati, OH) and drinking water containing tetracycline (0.5 mg/mL) and dexamethasone (1.0 µg/mL) immediately upon arrival. This regimen was continued for the next eight weeks with fluid intake monitored daily and animals weighed weekly. At the beginning of the sixth week, animals were divided into groups of eight or more, and the test compounds were administered by iv injection at a daily dose of 10 mg/kg in 0.4 mL of histidine-saline or the highest soluble or nontoxic dose for 14 days. The dose-response studies were accomplished in a similar manner, with animals receiving appropriate dosages of the compounds by either iv injection or gavage administration. Saline- and pentamidine-treated groups were included in each experiment as negative and positive controls, respectively. Animals were sacrificed at the end of eight weeks by chloroform inhalation. The right lung was inflated *in situ* with 10% formalin and fixed for histologic examination. The lung tissue was sectioned longitudinally and stained with Grocott's methenamine silver (GMS) stain, which selectively stains the walls of the *P. carinii* cysts. Stained sections were coded and each section scored by two examiners. The sections were scored according to the following system:

Score	Description
0.5	= Less than 10 cysts counted per two fully examined sections.
1	= Scattered cysts with less than 10% of lung involved.
2	= Scattered cysts with limited intense focal involvement and 10% to 25% of lung tissue involved.
3	= Scattered cysts with numerous intense areas of focal involvement and 26% to 50% of lung tissue involved.
4	= Cysts found throughout the tissue with numerous very intense focal areas of involvement and greater than 50% of lung involved.

The animals were observed closely for a ten- to fifteen-minute period following injection of the test drug for signs of hypotension. Their health and general well-being were observed and recorded on a daily basis for the remainder of the experiment. At necropsy, liver, spleen, kidneys, and pancreas were examined for histopathology. Toxicity of the test compounds was evaluated at 10 mg/kg or the highest soluble dose by the following criteria:

Score	Description
0	= No observed local, clinical, or histologic toxicity.
+	= All animals survived test dose without severe distress. Minimal or no signs of hypotension were observed. Some excess weight loss noted and/or mild signs of local toxicity at the injection site. No histopathology noted.
+ +	= All or most animals survived test dose with marked signs of hypotension. Animals were observed to have other clinical side effects and/or some histopathology. Many animals had severe lesions at injection site.
+ + +	= An acute toxic effect after single dose with symptoms compatible with severe hypotension and/or sharp decrease in animals' health after multiple doses. Death to 50% or less of the animals, resulting in a reduced screening dose.
+ + + +	= Death to greater than 50% of the animals with a resulting reduction in screening dose.

Method for Determining DNA Binding Affinity

The DNA binding of pentamidine and its analogues was measured, at low ionic strength, by determining the midpoint (ΔT_m) of the thermal denaturation curve of sonicated calf thymus DNA at a 1:10 drug to base ratio. The magnitude of the ΔT_m is approximately proportional to the binding constant of the compound under these conditions. The procedure has been described in detail.[23]

Statistical Studies

Student's t test was used to calculate the p values of each test group when compared to the saline-treated and drug-treated groups. The statistical analysis was carried out using the StatView 512+ software package (Brainpower, Inc., Calabasas, CA) on a Macintosh II computer.

Trypsin Inhibition Assay

The K_i values for the compounds against trypsin were determined graphically. All tests were carried out at 37° C and at a pH of 8.1. Details of the assay have been previously described.[24]

Thymidylate Synthetase Assay

Inhibitory activities of the compounds against both human (myeloid cells) and bacterial (*Lactobacillus casei*) enzymes were determined according to a published method.[25]

In Vitro *Assay of Analogues against* Giardia lamblia, Plasmodium falciparum, *and* Leishmania mexicana amazonensis

Plasmodium falciparum, clones W2 (Indochina III/CDC), chloroquine-resistant and mefloquine-sensitive, and D6 (Sierra Leone I/CDC), chloroquine-sensitive and mefloquine-resistant, were cloned and cultured in erythrocyte suspensions in modified RPMI-1640 culture medium as described.[26]*Leishmania mexicana amazonensis,* strain MHOM/BR/73/M2269 (WR669), promastigotes were cultured in Schneider's Drosophila medium supplemented with fetal bovine serum (FBS) as described.[27] *Giardia lamblia,* strain WB (ATCC #30957), was grown in TYI-S-33 medium supplemented with bile and FBS as described.[28] *In vitro* incorporation assays for antiplasmodial,[26,29] antileishmanial,[30] and antigiardial activity[31] have been previously described. Briefly, *in vitro* assays for antiparasitic activity were performed using an assay of incorporation of [³H]hypoxanthine (*P. falciparum*) and [³H]thymidine (*L. m. amazonensis* and *G. lamblia*) as a measure of parasite growth in the presence of the compounds to be tested. A microdilution technique was used in which serial dilutions of diamidines suspended in the appropriate culture media were prepared in duplicate rows of a 96-well microtiter plate to which was added the parasite suspension. The plates were then incubated for

24 hours under conditions appropriate for each organism after which time label was added. The plates were then incubated for 18 additional hours and harvested. Data on the uptake of [³H]hypoxanthine and [³H]thymidine were fitted to a logistic-logarithmic concentration response function by a nonlinear regression method, and drug concentrations required to inhibit 50% incorporation of [³H]hypoxanthine or [³H]thymidine were determined.[26,29]

Assay for Determining the Distribution of Pentamidine and Pentamidine Analogues

The tissue distribution of pentamidine in multiply dosed rats was determined by an HPLC method similar to previously described procedures.[19,32,33] Nonimmunosuppressed male Sprague-Dawley rats (Hilltop Laboratories) were injected iv with a daily dose of 10 mg/kg of pentamidine for 14 days. Rats were kept in metabolic chambers, and 24 hour urine and fecal samples were collected. After the final day of treatment, animals were sacrificed, heparinized blood was collected by cardiac puncture, and a variety of tissues were removed, weighed, and flash frozen. Concentrations of pentamidine were measured in body fluids and tissues by ion-modified reverse phase HPLC following solid phase extraction.[20] Two other groups of animals were given daily iv injections of either of two promising pentamidine analogues, compounds XI (5 mg/kg) or XXVI (2.5 mg/kg). Composite urine samples were used to obtain an approximation of the urinary excretion half-life for each compound.

Determination of **in Vitro** *Metabolism of Pentamidine*

Hepatic microsomal metabolism of pentamidine was examined using HPLC and liquid secondary ion mass spectrometry (MS). Nonimmunosuppressed male Sprague-Dawley rats were sacrificed, and then the livers were rapidly excised, weighed, and chilled to 4° C. Liver homogenate 9000 × g supernatants were prepared according to standard procedures.[34] Pentamidine was added to homogenates containing NADPH and MgCl₂ as cofactors and incubated at 37° C for varying times. Control incubations lacking cofactors, 9000 × g supernatants, or pentamidine were also examined. Reactions were terminated, and supernatants were extracted over C₁₈ solid phase extraction cartridges and analyzed by ion-modified reverse phase HPLC using a Zorbax RX column (Dupont, Wilmington, DE).[21]

MS was performed on a large-scale hepatic microsomal preparation. The hepatic preparation was extracted by C₁₈ solid-phase extraction and the volume reduced under a stream of air. Samples were analyzed by mass spectrometry/mass spectrometry (MS/MS) under liquid secondary ion MS conditions due to the relatively high level of background material in the samples. Samples were introduced via direct probe into a VG70-250 SEQ tandem hybrid MS/MS system (VG, Manchester, UK), using glycerol as the matrix and a Cs ion gun set at 35 kV and 8 kV source potential. Argon was used as the collision gas in an rf-only collision cell, with collision energy set at 4-7. eV The identities of two of the metabolites 1-(4'-(*N*-hydroxyamidino)phenoxy)-5-(4'-amidinophenoxyphenoxy)pentane and 1,5-bis(4'-(*N*-hydroxyamidino)phenoxy)pentane, FIG. 1) have been confirmed by chemical synthesis of the metabolites, co-elution of metabolic products with these synthesized standards in an HPLC system, and direct comparison of MS/MS of synthesized materials and metabolites.[21]

RESULTS AND DISCUSSION

Structure-Activity Studies of Pentamidine Analogues against PCP

Variation of the alkyl bridge connecting the 4-amidinophenoxy moieties from 3 through 6 carbons produced compounds that were all effective against rat PCP (TABLE

A.

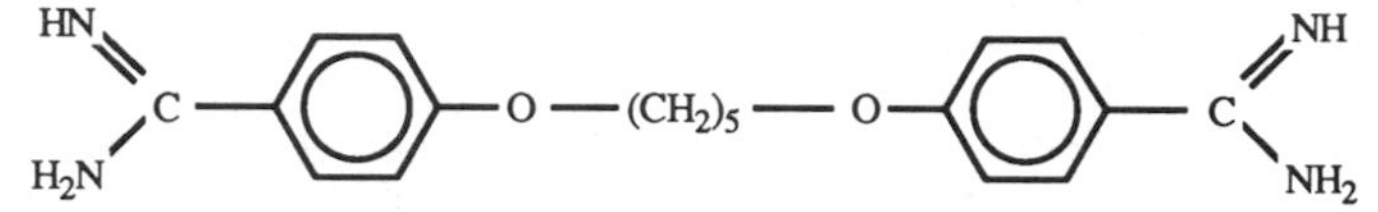

B.

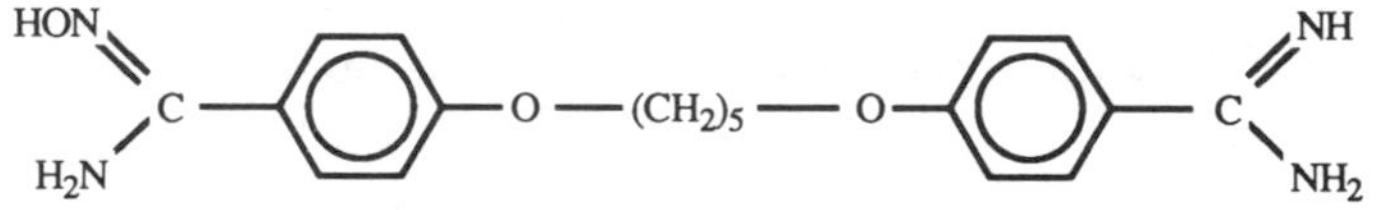

C.

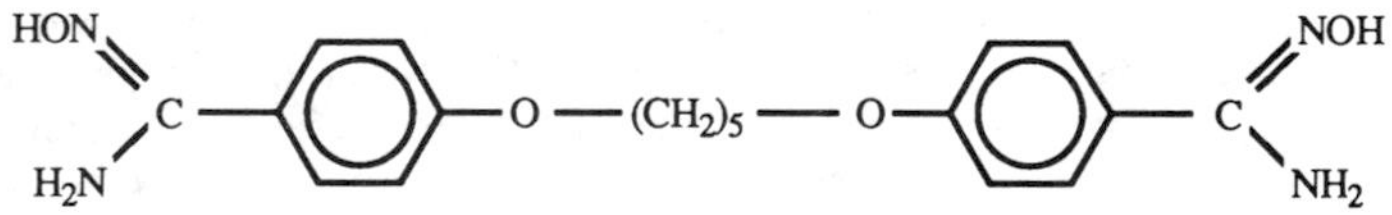

FIGURE 1. The structures of (A) pentamidine, (B) 1-(4′-(N-hydroxyamidino)phenoxy)-5-(4′-amidinophenoxy)pentane, and (C) 1,5-bis(4′-(N-hydroxyamidino)phenoxy)pentane.

1). The mean histologic scores of these derivatives were statistically lower than the scores from the saline-treated test group. Only the mean scores of the butamidine-treated group (compound II), however, proved to be significantly lower than the mean histologic scores seen with pentamidine. In addition, the 3 and 4 carbon chain derivatives exhibited less severe toxicity than pentamidine, whereas the 6 carbon analogue was apparently more toxic than the parent molecule.

The effects of various aromatic ring substituents on anti-PCP activity and toxicity in rats are shown in TABLE 2. Nitro substitution of one of the positions ortho to the ether bond on both aromatic rings (compounds IV and V) produced highly toxic compounds. Both nitro-substituted derivatives were found to be less potent than pentamidine at the highest nonlethal dose. Amino substitution in the same position (compounds VI and VII) resulted in highly active (potency equal to pentamidine) com-

TABLE 1. Effect of the Chain Length on Histologic Lung Scores of PCP and Toxicity in Rats

Compound no.	n	Histologic scores[a]						Mean score	Toxicity[b]
		Number of animals per scoring group							
		0.5	1	2	3	4			
I	3	3	4	1	0	0		0.9	+
II	4	28	4	0	0	0		0.6	0
Pentamidine	5	27	36	19	5	0		1.2	++
III	6	3	3	1	0	0		0.9	+++
Saline		1	2	14	41	58		3.3	0

[a] Efficacy determined at 10 mg/kg, unless noted.
[b] Toxicity determined at 10 mg/kg, unless noted. See text for symbol definitions.

TABLE 2. Effect of Aromatic Substitution on Histologic Lung Scores of PCP and Toxicity in Rats

| Compound no. | n | X | Histologic scores[a] | | | | | Mean score | Toxicity[b] |
| | | | Number of animals per scoring group | | | | | | |
			0.5	1	2	3	4		
IV[c]	5	$-NO_2$	0	2	4	2	0	2.0	++++
V[d]	4	$-NO_2$	0	0	3	1	4	3.1	++++
VI	5	$-NH_2$	8	5	1	1	0	0.9	+
VII	4	$-NH_2$	2	5	1	0	0	1.0	0
VIII	3	$-NH_2$	2	4	7	1	0	1.0	0
IX[c]	5	$-OCH_3$	2	4	1	1	0	1.6	++++
X[e]	4	$-OCH_3$	3	4	1	0	0	0.9	0[f]
XI[e]	3	$-OCH_3$	7	1	0	0	0	0.6	0[f]
XII[g]	5	$-Cl$	0	0	0	4	4	3.5	0[h]
XIII[g]	4	$-Cl$	0	1	2	3	2	2.8	0[h]
Pentamidine			27	36	19	41	0	1.2	++
Saline			1	2	14	41	58	3.3	0

[a] Efficacy determined at 10 mg/kg, unless noted.
[b] Toxicity determined at 10 mg/kg, unless noted.
[c] Tested at 5 mg/kg due to toxicity.
[d] Tested at 2.5 mg/kg due to toxicity.
[e] Tested at 5 mg/kg due to low solubility.
[f] Toxicity determined at 5 mg/kg.
[g] Tested at 2.5 mg/kg due to low solubility.
[h] Toxicity determined at 2.5 mg/kg.

pounds with somewhat reduced toxicity over the parent drug. Substitution of pentamidine with methoxy groups (compound IX) resulted in an increase in toxicity, but also gave a compound that showed good activity down to a dose of 5.0 mg/kg. More encouraging were the methoxy-substituted analogues with the 3 and 4 carbon chain links (compounds X and XI). Although these compounds were sparingly soluble and had to be tested at 5 mg/kg, they showed no toxicity and very good activity against PCP at this dose level. The 3 carbon chain analogue was significantly more potent than pentamidine at one-half the dose. Chloro-substitution (compounds XII and XIII) gave highly insoluble derivatives that showed no activity against PCP at the highest soluble dose (2.5 mg/kg).

The result of isosteric replacement of the ether oxygens with nitrogens is shown in TABLE 3. Replacement of oxygen with nitrogen in the 4 and 5 carbon chain analogues (compounds XV and XVI) gave compounds with highly increased toxicity. Animals in these two groups did not exhibit the anticipated acute hypotensive response, but their condition deteriorated over the course of the fourteen day dosing regimen. In the case of rats dosed with compound XV, half of the animals in this group died before completion of the experiment, and the remaining animals were in very poor condition. Although only one animal died in the group dosed with compound XVI, all of the remaining animals had severe weight loss and were generally found to be in very poor health. Surprisingly, the 3 carbon chain analogue (compound XIV) exhibited no detectable toxicity and did show significant anti-PCP activity. Whereas the 4 carbon analogue appears to be active against PCP, too few animals were evaluated to accurately analyze its effect. The mechanism of toxicity of the nitrogen isosteres is speculated to be the result of metabolic transformation of the 4 and 5 carbon chain derivatives to aniline products. The low toxicity observed in the corresponding 3 carbon chain analogue and in similar analogues with bulky substituents ortho to the anilino bridge (data not shown) would appear to be the result of steric hindrance of the metabolic conversion to the putative aniline products.

Moving the amidino group from the position para to the ether bridge to the meta position gave compounds (XVII-XXII, TABLE 4) with slightly reduced activity against PCP. The compounds, however, also appeared to be less toxic than the corresponding para-amidino derivatives. Methoxy substitution in the position para to the amidino group for the 3 carbon chain analogue (XXI) resulted in increased toxicity and no appreciable change in the potency. Placing a nitro para to the amidino (XXII) produced a nontoxic derivative but, in turn, gave a compound with no apparent effect on the rat PCP.

Replacement of the amidino groups with another cationic moiety (TABLE 5), the imidazoline group, resulted in a series of compounds that were observed to have enhanced potency relative to the corresponding diamidino compounds. As an example, when the 3 carbon chain imidazoline analogue (XXIII) was compared to the corresponding amidine (I) the imidazolino derivative was found to be significantly more potent against PCP and equally nontoxic. A very interesting series of compounds was obtained by placing a methoxy substituent meta to the imidazolino group (XXVI-XXVIII). The 3 carbon chain analogue (XXVI) of this series was found to be slightly more potent than pentamidine (TABLE 1) at one-quarter the dose of the parent compound. Unfortunately, toxicity for this compound could not be measured at higher doses due to the low solubility. XXVI, however, showed no toxicity at the dose level that produced a highly potent anti-PCP effect. Unaccountably, methylation of imidazoline nitrogens (XXIX and XXX) produced highly toxic compounds with the maximum nontoxic dose producing no anti-PCP activity. It should be noted that the promising activity of the imidazoline-substituted analogues against PCP has been previously observed.[15]

TABLE 3. Effect of Isosteric Replacement of the Ether Oxygens with Nitrogens on Histologic Lung Scores of PCP and Toxicity in Rats

Compound no.	n	Histologic scores[a]					Mean score	Toxicity[b]
		0.5	1	2	3	4		
XIV	3	5	1	2	0	0	0.9	0
XV	4	3	1	0	0	0	0.6	+++
XVI	5	1	2	3	1	0	1.6	+++
Pentamidine		27	36	19	5	0	1.2	++
Saline		1	2	14	41	58	3.3	0

Number of animals per scoring group

[a] Efficacy determined at 10 mg/kg, unless noted.
[b] Toxicity determined at 10 mg/kg, unless noted.

Dose-Response Studies and Oral Dosing of Promising Agents

Based on the results of the screening studies, three compounds were selected for oral dosing experiments and dose-response evaluation. The compounds selected were 1,4-di(4-amidinophenoxy)butane (II, butamidine), 1,3-di(4-imidazolinophenoxy)propane (XXIII), and 1,3-di(4-imidazolino-2-methoxyphenoxy)propane (XXVI).

A comparison of the dose-response curves of butamidine and pentamidine is shown in TABLE 6. At the highest daily dose level tested in the dose-response experiment (10

TABLE 4. Effect of Placing the Amidino-Group Meta to the Ether Bond on Histologic Lung Scores of PCP and Toxicity in Rats

Compound no.	n	X	Histologic scores[a]					Mean score	Toxicity[b]
			Number of animals per scoring group						
			0.5	1	2	3	4		
XVII	3	−H	2	1	4	1	0	1.6	0
XVIII	4	−H	2	1	1	3	0	1.9	0
XIX	5	−H	4	3	6	2	1	1.7	+
XX	6	−H	1	4	1	2	0	1.6	+
XXI[c]	3	−OCH$_3$	0	1	2	4	3	2.9	+++
XXII[d]	3	−NO$_2$	0	0	1	2	7	3.6	0[e]
Pentamidine			27	36	19	5	0	1.2	++
Saline			1	2	14	41	58	3.3	0

[a] Efficacy determined at 10 mg/kg, unless noted.
[b] Toxicity determined at 10 mg/kg, unless noted.
[c] Tested at 5 mg/kg due to toxicity.
[d] Tested at 5 mg/kg due to insufficient drug.
[e] Toxicity evaluated at 5 mg/kg.

mg/kg), butamidine (II) was found to be highly effective, significantly more potent and less toxic than the parent molecule. This finding closely correlated with the results from the initial drug screening study (TABLE 1). Dropping the daily dose of butamidine (II), however, to 1 mg/kg resulted in the loss of the drug's anti-PCP properties. A corresponding reduction of the pentamidine dose resulted in a similar loss of activity. An examination of the data in TABLE 6 reveals that the dose-response curves for pentamidine and butamidine (II) are almost identical. This finding was somewhat disappointing and seems to indicate that butamidine may enjoy only a modest advantage over pentamidine in the treatment of PCP.

TABLE 5. Effect of Replacing the Amidino-Group with an Imidazolino-Moiety on Histologic Lung Scores of PCP and Toxicity in Rats

| Compound no. | R | X | n | Histologic scores[a] | | | | | Mean score | Toxicity[b] |
| | | | | Number of animals per scoring group | | | | | | |
				0.5	1	2	3	4		
XXIII	—H	—H	3	7	0	0	0	0	0.5	0
XXIV[c]	—H	—H	4	1	2	3	1	0	1.6	+
XXV	—H	—H	5	5	3	0	0	0	0.7	0
XXVI[c]	—H	—OCH$_3$	3	8	5	2	0	0	0.9	0[d]
XXVII[c]	—H	—OCH$_3$	4	0	2	2	1	1	2.2	0[d]
XXVIII[e]	—H	—OCH$_3$	5	1	3	1	2	0	1.6	+++
XXIX[f]	—CH$_3$	—H	4	0	1	1	3	3	3.0	++++
XXX[f]	—CH$_3$	—H	5	0	0	2	4	2	3.0	++
Pentamidine				27	36	19	5	0	1.2	++
Saline				1	2	14	41	58	3.3	0

[a] Efficacy determined at 10 mg/kg, unless noted.
[b] Toxicity determined at 10 mg/kg, unless noted.
[c] Tested at 2.5 mg/kg due to low solubility.
[d] Toxicity evaluated at 2.5 mg/kg.
[e] Tested at 5 mg/kg due to toxicity.
[f] Tested at 2.5 mg/kg due to toxicity.

The dose-response data (iv) for XXIII compared to pentamidine are shown in TABLE 7. In addition, TABLE 7 details the effect of oral administration of XXIII. As with butamidine, the activity of XXIII against PCP in rats was greatly reduced and not statistically significant at a daily dose of 1.0 mg/kg. Both XXIII and pentamidine were observed to retain some anti-PCP activity when the daily dose was 5 mg/kg. Furthermore, XXIII was found to be inactive against PCP when given at 20 mg/kg per day by the oral route. Thus, this drug, as was the case with butamidine, appears to hold little hope of providing significant improvement over pentamidine.

Dose-response studies for XXVI are detailed in TABLE 8. Because of the low solubility of the drug, the highest dose administered by the iv route in this dose-response study was 2.5 mg/kg. This was the same dose that was evaluated in the

TABLE 6. Dose-Response Comparison of Compound II (Butamidine) with Pentamidine

		Histologic scores						
			Number of animals per scoring group					
Compound	Dose (mg/kg)	0.5	1	2	3	4	Mean score	Toxicity
(n = 5)	10.0	3	5	2	1	0	1.2	+ +
Pentamidine	1.0	1	0	3	5	3	2.8	0
	0.1	0	0	0	7	5	3.4	0
II	10.0	10	2	0	0	0	0.6	0
(n = 4)	1.0	0	1	3	5	3	2.8	0
Butamidine	0.1	0	0	4	5	2	2.8	0
Saline	—	0	0	2	5	5	3.3	0

original drug screen (TABLE 5). Comparison of the 2.5 mg/kg dose in the two experiments revealed a very close correlation. The mean histologic score achieved in the screening study by this dose was 0.9, whereas the 2.5 mg/kg dose in the dose-response experiment gave a mean score of 1.0. The dose-response study revealed that XXVI was only slightly less active when administered at 1.0 mg/kg and that the anti-PCP effect of the drug remained significant down to a daily iv dose of 0.5 mg/kg. Anti-PCP activity was lost when the daily iv dose was reduced to 0.25 mg/kg. In addition to the potent activity seen with iv injection of the drug, XXVI was found to be highly active when administered by a daily oral dosing regimen of 40 and 25 mg/kg. No drug toxicity was observed at the highest oral dose. Remarkably, XXVI was found to be equally active when administered orally every other day for two weeks.

Effect of Compounds on Other Organisms

The structure-activity relationship of pentamidine and the derivatives of pentamidine with respect to *in vitro* activity against *P. falciparum*, *L. m. amazonensis*, and *G. lamblia* has been examined.[22] Pentamidine had moderate activity against *G. lamblia*, whereas some of the less toxic derivatives had pronounced antigiardial activity in comparison to the parent compound. Pronounced antileishmanial activity was seen with virtually all of the compounds examined, but few were more potent than pentamidine. In general, *P. falciparum* was found to be very sensitive to pentamidine and many of the analogues. Differences were noted in the sensitivity to these compounds between *P. falciparum* clones that are chloroquine-resistant and mefloquine-sensitive (W2) and

TABLE 7. Oral Dosing of Compound XXIII and Dose-Response (iv) Comparison of Compound XXIII with Pentamidine

Compound XXIII

		Histologic scores						
		Number of animals per scoring group						
	Dose (mg/kg)	0.5	1	2	3	4	Mean score	Toxicity
Saline	—	0	0	4	14	24	3.5	0
Pentamidine	10.0	6	13	8	1	0	1.3	+ +
	5.0	1	3	7	1	0	1.7	0
	1.0	1	0	3	5	3	2.8	0
	0.1	0	0	0	7	5	3.4	0
Compound XXIII	10.0	7	0	0	0	0	0.5	0
	5.0	2	5	3	0	0	1.2	0
	1.0	0	0	4	4	2	2.8	0
	0.25	0	1	1	6	2	2.9	0
(oral)	20.0	0	1	1	6	2	2.9	0

those that are chloroquine-sensitive and mefloquine-resistant (D6). The 50% inhibitory concentration (IC_{50}) of selected compounds exhibiting highest activity against each parasite is reported in TABLE 9. These data point out our observations with a larger set of analogues that compounds with alkyl chain lengths of 3, 5, and 6 appear to be more potent against these organisms than do those with alkyl chains of 2 and 4. Compounds with a chain length greater than 3 and with the ether oxygens replaced by nitrogen have been observed to be toxic in the rat model. Thus, increased toxicity may correspond with the high antiprotozoan activity of compounds XVI and III. The placement of methoxy groups upon the aromatic rings of both 1,3-di(4-amidinophenoxy)propane (XI) and 1,3-di(4-imidazolinophenoxy)propane (XXVI) resulted in high activity against *P. falciparum* clone W2 and *G. lamblia* WB, respectively.

TABLE 8. Dose-Response Studies with Compound XXVI Administered by iv Injection or Gavage

	Dose (mg/kg)	Histologic scores					Mean score	Toxicity
		Number of animals per scoring group						
		0.5	1	2	3	4		
Compound XXVI (iv injection)	2.5	8	6	4	0	0	1.0	0
	1.0	3	6	3	0	0	1.1	0
	0.5	1	2	7	2	0	1.9	0
	0.25	0	1	3	4	4	3.0	0
Saline (iv injection)	—	0	0	2	8	10	3.4	0
Pentamidine (iv injection)	10.0	4	5	9	1	0	1.5	++
Compound XXVI (oral dosing, daily)	40.0	4	6	1	0	0	0.9	0
	25.0	4	8	3	1	0	1.2	0
	10.0	0	6	7	5	1	2.1	0
Saline (oral dosing, daily)	—	1	0	10	9	9	2.9	0
Compound XXVI (oral dosing, every other day)	25.0	5	6	2	3	0	1.3	0
	10.0	2	3	8	3	0	1.8	0
Pentamidine (oral dosing, every other day)	10.0	1	1	3	8	3	2.7	0
Saline (oral dosing, every other day)	—	1	0	10	9	9	2.9	0

TABLE 9. Antiprotozoan Activity of Pentamidine and Selected Derivatives of Pentamidine

Compound	Plasmodium falciparum W2 IC$_{50}$ (µM)	D6 IC$_{50}$ (µM)	Leishmania mexicana amazonensis IC$_{50}$ (µM)	Giardia lamblia IC$_{50}$ (µM)
Pentamidine	0.12	0.06	0.79	5.39
XXVI	**0.01**	0.27	2.46	1.89
XVI	0.07	**0.02**	0.55	5.15
III	0.11	0.09	**0.31**	5.53
XI	0.12	0.30	1.47	**0.60**

Enzyme Inhibition and DNA Binding Properties
of Selected Pentamidine Analogues

All of the molecules were found to bind to calf thymus DNA with ΔT_ms up to 16.3° C. Two of the most effective compounds (XI and XXVI) against rat PCP proved to be the strongest DNA binding agents based on the ΔT_m data (Table 10). The only real comparison, however, that could be made between the anti-PCP activity and DNA binding strength of the molecules was that all of the analogues tested bound DNA and exhibited at least minimal activity against PCP.

A large number of the compounds were examined for their inhibition of both human (myeloid cells) and bacterial (*Lactobacillus casei*) thymidylate synthetase. The results showed that the analogues inhibited the enzymes only at high concentrations ($\sim 10^{-3}$M). In addition, no structure-activity correlations or preference of the compounds for either the human or bacterial enzyme were observed.

From the K_i values of the pentamidine analogues against trypsin, it was observed that molecules with two amidine moieties were effective trypsin inhibitors (TABLE 10). The imidazoline derivatives, however, XV and XVI, were found to be devoid of antitrypsin activity and were effective agents in the treatment of rat PCP. This finding provides circumstantial evidence that the antiprotease activity of diamidines is not related to their activity against PCP.

Distribution of Pentamidine and Pentamidine Analogues

In agreement with reports from other investigators,[35,36] pentamidine was found to preferentially bind to certain organs (FIG. 2).[20] After multiple dosing for 14 days, the highest quantities of pentamidine per gram wet weight were found in kidneys (162.9 ± 53.2 μg/g) with relatively moderate levels in lungs, spleen/pancreas, heart, and stomach. Surprisingly low levels were detectable in the liver (4.8 ± 2.6 μg/g). Relatively low to negligible amounts were also detected in testes, brain, feces, and blood cells. Although not shown in FIGURE 2, terminal plasma concentrations were also low (1.1 ± 0.5 μg/mL). Urine levels of pentamidine were found to be low after the first dose and increased daily until an average of approximately 70 μg/24 hours was reached. Muscle and fat were not obtained from the initial groups of animals but were obtained from a later group of pentamidine-injected animals. Muscle contained moderately high quantities of pentamidine (37.9 ± 5.0 μg/g), whereas fat contained lower levels (14.0 ± 1.5 μg/g). The majority of the injected pentamidine could not be accounted for by the total amount of drug found in tissues or excretory samples. One possibility for such low recovery is that pentamidine undergoes metabolic transformation to products that were not detectable by the usual HPLC assays.

Urinary excretion of the two pentamidine analogues, 1,3-di(4-amidino-2-methoxyphenoxy)propane (XI) and 1,3-di(4-imidazolino-2-methoxyphenoxy)propane (XXVI), was measured in separate groups of animals. Compound XI was excreted at a concentration of 8.3 μg/mL after 24 hours, increasing to 14.7 μg/mL after 14 days of treatment. Compound XXVI was excreted fairly consistently throughout treatment, averaging approximately 11.2 μg/mL. This compared to the mean pentamidine urinary concentrations of 1.7 μg/mL after 24 hours of treatment, which increased to 10.3 μg/mL later. The excretion values after 24 hours were used to obtain an approximation of the urinary excretion half-life of each compound. Pentamidine was calculated to have a

TABLE 10. Trypsin Inhibitory Activity and DNA Binding Activity of Pentamidine and Selected Analogues

Compound	DNA binding ΔT_m, °C	Trypsin inhibition K_i (μM)	Mean histologic score against PCP
IX	12.0	1.3	1.6[a]
	10.7	2.3	1.1[b]
Pentamidine XI	16.3	1.3	0.6[c]
XVIII	8.1	1.8	1.9[b]
XXV	9.1	> 2000.0	0.7[b]
XXVI	14.5	> 2000.0	0.9[a]

[a] Tested at 2.5 mg/kg.
[b] Tested at 10 mg/kg.
[c] Tested at 5.0 mg/kg.

half-life of approximately 68 days, whereas XI had one of approximately 8 days and XXVI one of approximately 2 days.

In Vitro *Metabolism of Pentamidine*

Low recoveries of injected pentamidine in multiply dosed rats prompted initiation of studies examining hepatic microsomal metabolism of pentamidine. Short-term incubations of pentamidine with rat liver homogenate 9000 × g supernatants were found, upon HPLC assay, to contain 6 peaks not found in control incubations. Hydroxylation of the amidine groups of pentamidine was considered to be a likely metabolic transformation because benzamidine had been observed to be converted to N-hydroxybenzami-

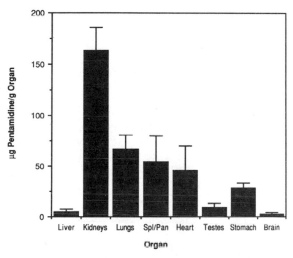

FIGURE 2. The distribution of pentamidine in the organs of multiply dosed rats.

dine by rat liver homogenates.[77] This speculation was confirmed when two of the peaks co-eluted with synthesized standards of 1-(4'-(N-hydroxyamidino)phenoxy)-5-(4'-amidinophenoxy)pentane and 1, 5-bis(4'-(N-hydroxyamidino)phenoxy)pentane.[21] The structures of these two metabolites were further confirmed by MS/MS. MS/MS used under liquid secondary ion mass spectrometry (LIMS) conditions performed on the standard compounds and a concentrated incubation extract gave spectra enriched for M + 1 ions, and the ions corresponding to the known molecular weight of the two pentane amidoximes were then selected for collisionally induced dissociation. Fragmentation of M + 1 = 357 1-(4'(N-hydroxyamidino)phenoxy)-5-(4'-amidinophenoxy)pentane and M + 1 = 373 1,5-bis(4'-N-hydroxyamidino)phenoxy)pentane ions in the liver supernatant preparations produced mass spectra that matched those for the standard compounds.[21] Further studies are in progress to identify the four other putative metabolites.

CONCLUSIONS

The data from the structure-activity studies clearly illustrate that strongly cationic molecules, such as the diamidines and di-imidazolines, are a potential source of new agents for the treatment of PCP. One of the compounds in this study, XXVI, was found to be as active as pentamidine at a 10-fold lower concentration for the iv treatment of rat PCP. Also XXVI was observed to be significantly active against PCP when administered by the oral route. There were few new data generated in this study that would pinpoint the mechanism of anti-PCP activity of pentamidine-like molecules. From this work, however, it appears highly unlikely that the antiprotease activity or thymidylate synthetase inhibition activity of these molecules is a contributing factor to their anti-PCP potency. A major finding of these studies is that pentamidine appears to be readily metabolized, and in the design of future analogues one must consider the metabolic fate of the molecule. The successful isolation and characterization of all of the metabolites of pentamidine will greatly enhance the success of future drug development for this class of molecules.

ACKNOWLEDGMENTS

We wish to thank M. Allen, V. Linga, and S. Morrison for technical assistance; Dr. M. Cory, Burroughs Wellcome Co., for the DNA-binding data; Dr. Y. Cheng for the thymidylate synthetase inhibition data; Dr. J. Charles and D. Marbury for mass spectra interpretation; and Dr. Dennis Kyle and Dr. Max Grogl, Walter Reed Army Institute of Research, for assistance with the antiplasmodial and antileishmanial assays.

REFERENCES

1. LOURIE, E. M. & W. YORKE. 1939. Ann. Trop. Med. Parasitol. **33:** 289-304.
2. ASHLEY, J. N., H. J. BARBER, A. J. EWINS, G. NEWBERY & A. D. H. SELF. 1942. J. Chem. Soc. Part I. **20:** 103-116.
3. LOURIE, E. M. 1942. Ann. Trop. Med. Parasitol. **36:** 113-131.
4. SAUNDERS, G. F. T., J. R. HOLDEN & M. H. HUGHES. 1944. Ann. Trop. Med. Parasitol. **38:** 159-168.
5. KIRK, R. & M. H. SATI. 1940. Ann. Trop. Med. Parasitol. **34:** 181-197.
6. IVADY, V. G. & L. PALDY. 1958. Monatsschr. Kinderheilkd. **106:** 10-14.
7. KAPUSNIK, J. E. & J. MILLS. 1988. *In* Antimicrobial Agents Annual 3. P. K. PETERSON & J. VERHOEF, Eds.: **3:** 299-311. Elsevier Science. Amsterdam.
8. WALZER, P. D., C. K. KIM & M. T. CUSHION. 1989. *In* Parasitic Infections in the Compromised Host. P. D. WALZER & R. M. GENTA, Eds.: 83-178. Marcel Dekker, Inc. New York.
9. JAFFE, H. S., D. I. ABRAMS, A. J. AMMANN, B. J. LEWIS & J. A. GOLDEN. 1983. Lancet **ii:** 1109-1111.
10. GORDIN, F. M., G. L. SIMON, C. B. WOFSY & J. MILLS. 1984. Ann. Intern. Med. **100:** 495-499.
11. NIEDT, G. W. & R. A. SCHINELLA. 1985. Arch. Pathol. Lab. Med. **109:** 727-734.
12. MOSKOWITZ, L., G. T. HENSLEY, J. C. CHAN & K. ADAMS. 1985. Arch. Pathol. Lab. Med. **109:** 735-738.

13. MONTGOMERY, A. B., J. M. LUCE, J. TURNER, E. T. LIN, R. J. DEBS, K. J. CORKERY, E. N. BRUNETTE & P. C. HOPEWELL. 1987. Lancet ii: 480-483.
14. FRENKEL, J. K., J. T. GOOD & J. A. SHULTZ. 1966. Lab. Invest. 15: 1559-1577.
15. WALZER, P. D., C. K. KIM, J. FOY, M. J. LINKE & M. T. CUSHION. 1988. Antimicrob. Agents Chemother. 32: 896-905.
16. TIDWELL, R. R., S. G. KILGORE, K. A. OHEMENG, J. D. GERATZ & J. E. HALL. 1989. J. Protozool. 36: S74-S76.
17. TIDWELL, R. R., S. K. JONES, J. D. GERATZ, K. A. OHEMENG, M. CORY & J. E. HALL. 1990. J. Med. Chem. 33: 1252-1257.
18. JONES, S. K., J. E. HALL, M. A. ALLEN, S. D. MORRISON, K. A. OHEMENG, V. V. REDDY & R. R. TIDWELL. 1990. Antimicrob. Agents Chemother. 34: 1026-1030.
19. BERGER, B. J., J. E. HALL & R. R. TIDWELL. 1989. J. Chromatogr. 494: 191-200.
20. BERGER, B. J., J. E. HALL & R. R. TIDWELL. 1990. Pharmacol. & Toxicol. 66: 234-236.
21. BERGER, B. J., R. J. LOMBARDY, G. D. MARBURY, C. A. BELL, C. DYKSTRA, J. E. HALL & R. R. TIDWELL. 1990. Antimicrob. Agents Chemother. 34: 1678-1684.
22. BELL, C. A., J. E. HALL, D. E. KYLE, M. GROGL, K. A. OHEMENG & R. R. TIDWELL. 1990. Anitmicrob. Agents Chemother. 34: 1381-1386.
23. CORY, M., D. D. MCKEE, J. KAGAN, D. W. HENRY & J. A. MILLER. 1985. J. Am. Chem. Soc. 107: 2528-2536.
24. GERATZ, J. D., A. C. WHITMORE, M. C.-F. CHENG & C. PIANTADOSI. 1973. J. Med. Chem. 16: 970-975.
25. DOLNICK, B. J. & Y.-C. CHENG. 1978. J. Biol. Chem. 253: 3563-3567.
26. ODUOLA, A. M. J., N. F. WEATHERLY, J. H. BOWDRE & R. E. DESJARDINS. 1988. Exp. Parasitol. 66: 86-95.
27. HENDRICKS, L. D., D. E. WOOD & M. E. HAJDUK. 1978. Parasitology 76: 309-316.
28. KEISTER, D. B. 1983. Trans. R. Soc. Trop. Med. Hyg. 77: 487-488.
29. DESJARDINS, R. E., C. J. CANFIELD, J. D. HAYNES & J. D. CHULAY. 1979. Antimicrob. Agents Chemother. 16: 710-718.
30. GROGL, M., A. M. J. ODUALA, L. D. C. CORDERO & D. E. KYLE. 1989. Exp. Parasitol. 69: 78-90.
31. BOREHAM, P. F. L., R. E. PHILLIPS & R. W. SHEPHERD. 1984. J. Antimicrob. Chemother. 14: 449-461.
32. LIN, J. M.-H., R. J. SHI & E. T. LIN. 1986. J. Liq. Chromatogr. 9: 2035-2046.
33. DUSCI, L. J., L. P. HACKETT, A. M. FORBES & K. F. ILETT. 1987. Ther. Drug Monit. 9: 422-425.
34. CLEMENT, B. & M. ZIMMERMANN. 1987. Xenobiotica 17: 659-667.
35. WAALKES, T. P., C. DENHAM & V. T. DEVITA. 1970. Clin. Pharmacol. Ther. 11: 505-512.
36. WALDMAN, R. H., D. E. PEARCE & R. A. MARTIN. 1973. Am. Rev. Respir. Dis. 108: 1004-1006.
37. CLEMENT, B. 1983. Xenobiotica 13: 467-473.

Treatment Strategies for Cryptosporidiosis

ROSEMARY SOAVE

Division of Infectious Diseases
The New York Hospital-Cornell Medical Center
New York, New York 10021

HISTORICAL BACKGROUND

Although *Cryptosporidium* has only been recognized as a significant pathogen for humans since the early 1980s, it is not a "new" organism. The coccidian protozoan parasite, first described by Tyzzer in 1907,[1] was regarded as a benign commensal for nearly half a century. In 1955 it was first linked to gastrointestinal disease in fowl.[2] Since the early 1970s, when *Cryptosporidium* was recognized as a significant pathogen for calves,[3] it has been found in many species of animals, and the economic consequences for agriculture have been more fully appreciated.[4-6] The first cases of human cryptosporidiosis were reported in 1976.[7,8] Because fewer than ten cases had been reported in humans prior to 1982, the disease was considered rare and the pathogen opportunistic. Detection of *Cryptosporidium* in patients with the acquired immunodeficiency syndrome (AIDS)[9] heightened physician awareness of its pathogenic potential for both the immunocompromised as well as the immunocompetent human host. Less than a decade later, there has been an explosion of publications and reviews on this aptly named [*Cryptosporidium* means "hidden spore" in Greek], enigmatic parasite.[10-15] *Cryptosporidium* is now regarded as a major public health problem worldwide.

THE ORGANISM

The *Cryptosporidium* oocyst contains four aflagellar but motile sporozoites with apical complexes that are believed to play a role in cell penetration. Thus, the organism has been assigned to the phylum Apicomplexa, class Sporozoasida, order Eucoccidiorida, suborder Eimeriorina (the true coccidia).[16]*Cryptosporidium* has been detected in all classes of vertebrates including mammals, birds, reptiles, and fish. Approximately twenty species of *Cryptosporidium* have been named for the host in which they were found. Recent cross-transmission studies however have invalidated many of the named species and suggest that there is little or no host specificity.[10,16,17] The precise number of *Cryptosporidium* species, and the nature of strain differences, have yet to be determined. Two species of *Cryptosporidium* affecting mammals, based on oocyst size, have recently been proposed by Upton and Current: (1) *C. parvum* (2.5 µm diameter) is thought to be the cause of disease in humans and cattle, and (2) *C. muris* (5-8 µm diameter) infects the stomach of mammals.[18] At present, most investigators use *C. parvum* or *Cryptosporidium sp.* to designate the species producing clinical illness in humans and other mammals. Future studies of host specificity and pathogenicity may lead to validation of other species.

Taxonomically, *Cryptosporidium* is related to other true coccidia (suborder Eimeriorina), including *Toxoplasma, Isospora, Eimeria,* and *Sarcocystis. Plasmodium sp.* are in the same order (Eucoccidiorida) but different suborder (Haemospororina) than *Cryptosporidium sp.* Morphologically, in its ability to parasitize the immunocompromised host, and in our inability to cultivate the parasite *in vitro, Cryptosporidium* resembles the unclassified pathogen, *Pneumocystis carinii.*

Studies by Tyzzer, Vetterling, Pohlenz, Iseki, and Angus have led to elucidation of the *Cryptosporidium* life cycle,[10] as have recent descriptions of the development of calf and human cryptosporidial isolates in suckling mice,[19] chicken embryos,[20] and cell culture[21] by Current. It appears that, as with other true coccidia, the *Cryptosporidium* life cycle can be divided into six major developmental phases: excystation (release of infective sporozoites from oocysts), merogony (asexual replication), gametogony (formation of gametes), fertilization, oocyst wall (zygote) formation, and sporogony (sporozoite formation). *Cryptosporidium* distinguishes itself from other coccidia in that the oocysts sporulate endogenously and are autoinfective. By contrast, *Eimeria, Isospora,* and *Toxoplasma* oocysts require a period outside the host for sporogony to occur, and *Sarcocystis* sporulates endogenously but does not autoinfect the host. In other studies, Current has reported that morphologic differences in the *Cryptosporidium* oocyst wall may correlate with the mode of transmission, that is, thick-walled oocysts are environmentally resistant, pass into the feces and, thus, to a new host, whereas thin-walled cysts are able to reinfect the same host.[20] The presence of autoinfective thin-walled cysts may contribute to the overwhelming nature of cryptosporidial infection that is seen in patients with immunodeficiency.

EPIDEMIOLOGY

Cryptosporidial infection has been reported in at least 35 countries spanning six continents.[10,14,22] Surveys of selected populations have revealed infection rates ranging from 0.6 to 20% in the developed world and 4 to 32% in the developing world.[10–15] The true prevalence of cryptosporidial infection is not known. Data obtained to date suggests that the parasite is a major cause of diarrhea worldwide. Prevalence studies have also revealed that higher infection rates are more common in young children and during the warm, humid months of the year.[10–15,22] Seroprevalence studies have shown higher than expected rates of seropositivity, suggesting that active or recent infection may be common in the general population.[23]

As of 1986, the Centers for Disease Control estimated that 3 to 4% of AIDS patients have cryptosporidiosis. In recent studies the parasite was detected in 15% of patients with AIDS and diarrhea at the National Institutes of Health,[24] and 16% of those at Johns Hopkins Hospital.[25] In Haiti and Africa, up to 50% of patients with AIDS have cryptosporidiosis. Whether cryptosporidiosis in AIDS patients is due to reactivation of past infection or *de novo* contamination is not known.

Zoonotic transmission of *Cryptosporidium* has been well-documented, but recent studies suggest that spread from person to person and through contaminated water may be more common.[10–15,22] Person-to-person transmission has been implicated in

Novel Pharmacological Strategies in the Treatment of Life-Threatening Cytomegalovirus Infections

Clinical Experience with Continuous Infusion 9-(1,3-Dihydroxy-2-Propoxymethyl) Guanine[a]

RICHARD J. WHITLEY,[b,e] JOAN CONNELL,[b]
MICHAEL A. MARKIEWICZ,[c] AND
JEAN-PIERRE SOMMADOSSI[d]

[b]Departments of Pediatrics, Microbiology, and Medicine
[c]Comprehensive Cancer Center
[d]Department of Pharmacology
Division of Clinical Pharmacology
University of Alabama at Birmingham
Birmingham, Alabama 35294

INTRODUCTION

Significant advances have been achieved in the development of antiviral agents for therapy of life- and sight-threatening herpesvirus infections. Among them, 9-(1,3-dihydroxy-2-propoxymethyl) guanine (DHPG, BW B759 U, 2′-NDG, BIOLF-62, ganciclovir), an acyclic nucleoside analogue of the guanine base, has demonstrated promising therapeutic effects in the treatment of cytomegalovirus (CMV) infections. Recently, this drug was licensed for severe CMV infections, major causes of morbidity and mortality in patients with the acquired immunodeficiency syndrome (AIDS), as well as other immunosuppressed patients.[1-5] Although both clinical and viral efficacy have been demonstrated with this drug, the side effects of neutropenia and thrombocytopenia have identified boundaries for the clinical utility of DHPG therapy. These effects have been observed after administration of 5-15 mg/kg/day of DHPG by iv bolus regi-

[a]Studies performed by the authors were initiated and supported under a Contract (NO1-AI-62554) with the Development and Applications Branch of the National Institute of Allergy and Infectious Diseases (NIAID), Grant CA-13148 (NCI), Grants from the General Clinical Research Center Program (RR-032), a Grant from Syntex, Inc. (USA), and a Junior Faculty Research Award from the American Cancer Society.
[e]Address correspondence to Richard J. Whitley, M.D., Professor of Pediatrics, Microbiology and Medicine, Suite 653, Children's Hospital Tower, 1600 7th Avenue South, Birmingham, Alabama 35294.

mens.[1–5] Likely, toxicity results from the dose and/or regimen used in these uncontrolled clinical investigations. Our studies were performed to develop a novel approach for the treatment of life- and sight-threatening CMV infections by the use of continuous drug infusion with a portable pump and the individualization of treatment regimens. Relationships between DHPG plasma levels, toxicity, and therapeutic effectiveness are presented in this report.

MATERIAL AND METHODS

Patients eligible for this study included those who were immunocompromised and had sight- or life-threatening cytomegalovirus infection as confirmed by virus isolation. Five patients were evaluated on therapeutic regimens for a range of therapy of 4 to 40 weeks of treatment. The demographic characteristics of the patients are summarized in TABLE 1.

TABLE 1. Characteristics of Patients Receiving Continuous Infusion Ganciclovir

Initials	Age	Diagnoses	CMV Disease	Virologic Profile at Onset of Therapy
PR	46	AIDS	Chorioretinitis Pneumonia	+ lung biopsy + urine + buffy coat
PK	32	AIDS	Chorioretinitis Pneumonia	+ lung biopsy + urine + buffy coat
RP	28	AIDS	Chorioretinitis Colitis	+ urine + buffy coat + colon biopsy
JR	34	AIDS	Chorioretinitis	+ urine + buffy coat
MD	6	Unknown T-cell deficiency	Chorioretinitis Colitis Pneumonia	+ lung biopsy + urine + buffy coat + colon biopsy

Informed consent was obtained prior to starting the study, according to institutional guidelines. A test dose of 2 mg/kg of DHPG (Syntex (USA), Inc., Palo Alto, CA) was infused intravenously over one hour on day one through a peripheral iv line. Venous blood samples (2 mL) were drawn into heparinized tubes before, at the end of drug administration (time 0), and at 5 min, 30 min, and 1, 2, 4, 6, 8, and 12 hours after the dose. After centrifugation at 5°C, plasma was separated and stored at −20°C until analysis. On day two, an indwelling central line was surgically placed in the subclavian vein. On day three continuous drug infusion was initiated using a portable pump (Provider 4000, Pancretec Inc., San Diego, CA). The daily dose of DHPG was diluted in 50 mL 5% dextrose and infused continually through the Broviac™ catheter. A sufficient amount of DHPG was provided in polyvinylchloride bags to allow bag exchange every two days, as recently suggested.[6] Plasma samples were obtained approximately every 48 to 72 hours during the continuous course of DHPG. Quantitation of DHPG was performed using a sensitive and specific high-performance liquid chromatography methodology.[7]

Pharmacokinetic parameters were calculated using noncompartmental analysis based on statistical moment theory.[8] Area under the curve (ACU) was calculated from time zero to the last time point using the trapezoidal rule with extrapolation to infinity. The total plasma clearance was calculated by dividing the dose by the AUC. The dose of DHPG to be administered during the long term iv infusion was calculated as follows: $D = C_P \times CL \times t$, where D = dose, C_P = desired plasma concentration, CL = total DHPG plasma clearance, and t = time. Antiviral activity of DHPG was evaluated in blood and urine by a plaque reduction assay.[9]

CASE REPORT

The following case illustrates the methodology and response to treatment. The patient was a six and one-half year old female born in March 1980. She was the six pound, six ounce product of an uncomplicated vaginal delivery. She became ill at two months of age with chronic diarrhea and failure to thrive. Small bowel biopsy at that time revealed villus atrophy with bacterial overgrowth. She was found to have lactose intolerance, and in July 1982 developed salmonella gastroenteritis. In December 1982 she developed CMV pneumonia and hepatitis, both proven by biopsy and confirmatory culture which prompted an immunologic workup. She was found to have a marked decrease in the absolute number of CD4$^+$ lymphocytes as well as decreased levels of IgA. An antibody test for human immunodeficiency virus, HIV, was subsequently shown to be negative on three occasions, as were HIV cultures. In April 1983, she developed hemiplegia and was found to have central nervous system lesions by computed tomography. Brain biopsy was nondiagnostic. She subsequently developed immune thrombocytopenic purpura in January 1984, which was eventually controlled with high-dose corticosteroids. An autoimmune hemolytic anemia followed, which again responded to steroids. In June 1986, the patient was admitted for evaluation of chronic diarrhea. A small bowel biopsy revealed CMV inclusions with cultures subsequently growing CMV, and she was also noted to have active CMV chorioretinitis.

Because of the progression of retinitis and deterioration of her general status, the patient was hospitalized on July 11, 1986. Before initiation of treatment of DHPG, CMV colitis was confirmed by biopsy. In addition elevated liver functions also were determined. The patient was febrile, with temperatures between 101° and 104°F. All cultures for CMV from urine and blood were positive. Funduscopic examination showed white, fluffy lesions with accompanying hemorrhages, showing chorioretinitis of the right eye (FIG. 1A), and an old, probably inactive area of chorioretinitis of the left eye. The visual acuity was $20/30^{-2}$ at the right eye and $20/30^{-2}$ at the left eye.

The patient (body weight = 13 kg) received a test dose of 2 mg/kg of DHPG as a one hour iv infusion on July 15, 1986. Using a calculated DHPG systemic clearance of 13.2 L/h, an infusion rate of 16 mg/24 h was selected to achieve a steady-state plasma concentration of 0.8 μM. Administration of DHPG as a continuous long-term intravenous infusion was initiated on July 17, 1986. After 11 days of continuous intravenous infusion, clinical improvement was observed with viremia, colitis, and hepatitis resolving as manifested by negative cultures for CMV from urine and blood, and defervescence. The retinitis was stable, and an area of healing was observed (FIG. 1B). The patient was discharged on July 31, 1986 (day 14), and therapy was continued on an outpatient basis. After 33 days all cultures remained negative, but widespread hemorrhage and retinitis of the right eye was detected (FIG. 1C), and the visual activity decreased to 20/40. On day 39, the dose of DHPG was increased to 32 mg/24 hours, and after three weeks of therapy the involved retinal area was stabilized, but no significant improvement was detected. DHPG therapy was further increased on August 25, 1986 (day 61) to 64 mg/24 hours. An eye exam performed two weeks later revealed that areas of white retinitis were largely resolved and improvement of the visual activity to 20/30 for both eyes was also observed. After 70 days with daily doses of 16 to 64 mg DHPG, no significant toxicity was observed, with absolute neutrophils remaining > 1000/mm^3. In order to establish the dose (and plasma levels) at which toxicity occurred, the dose of DHPG was increased to 80 mg/24 hours of DHPG. After one week, neutropenia (with neutrophil counts of 630/mm^3) was observed with DHPG plasma levels $\geq$ 4 μM. Therapy was discontinued for two days and lower doses reinitiated with neutrophil counts returning to previous levels of approximately 1300/mm^3 within three weeks. All clinical and laboratory tests did not change from baseline normal during the 85 day drug therapy.

The patient and her family elected to discontinue DHPG therapy. Reactivation of disease with progression of chorioretinitis was observed with positive bone marrow cultures (urine cultures were still negative). Her terminal admission was complicated by *Candida albicans* pneumonia and *Pseudomonas aeruginosa* sepsis. She died shortly thereafter.

RESULTS

FIGURE 2 summarizes the pharmacological, toxicological, and virological data over the course of the study in the case report detailed. Plasma levels of DHPG approximated the predicted values after administration of low doses (16 and 32 mg/24 h), whereas some differences were observed with high doses (64 and 80 mg/24 h). Neutrophil counts correlated with DHPG plasma levels (r = 0.77 with p < .01). A total dose of 64 mg/24 h (with steady-state plasma levels of approximately 2.5 μM) was the maximum nontoxic dose in this regimen. Neutropenia was observed with plasma levels $\geq$ 4 μM. Of note was the disappearance of viremia, colitis, and hepatitis with plasma levels of approximately 1 μM, whereas plasma levels approximately 2.5-fold higher were required to resolve the chorioretinitis.

TABLE 2 summarizes the results for all patients entered into the trial. Clinical improvement was noted in four of the five patients (PR, JR, RP, and MD). The fifth patient died from CMV pneumonia. Inasmuch as chorioretinitis was a primary disease manifestation for four patients, it was serially followed. Improvement in visual acuity was noted after two weeks of therapy in three patients at DHPG plasma levels of 2.5 μM to 4.2 μM. In the fourth patient, there was stabilization of visual acuity at a plasma level of 2.2 μM, but the patient died from complications of AIDS.

Neutropenia was the only laboratory abnormality encountered. Only one patient had neutropenia that was attributed directly to DHPG therapy. With the other patients, HIV infection with bone marrow involvement was thought to be the case, because dosage and plasma level stabilization had occurred for a minimum of three weeks.

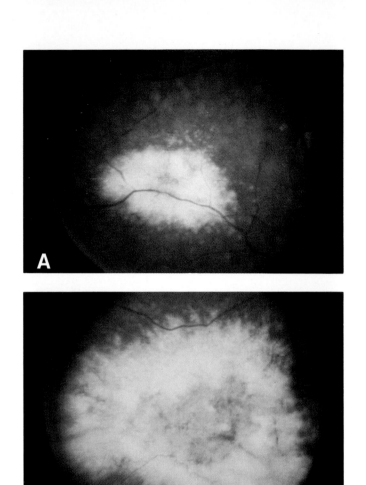

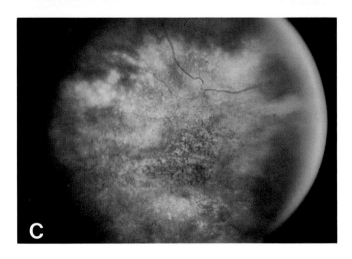

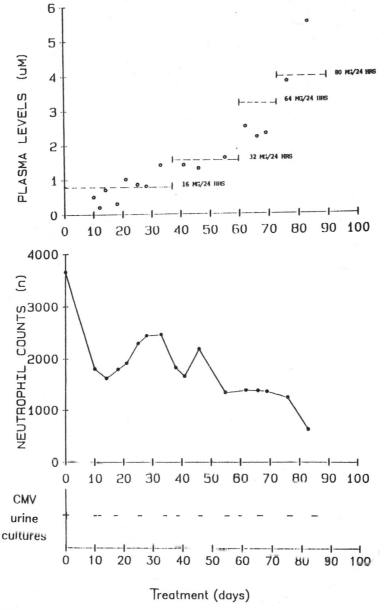

FIGURE 2. Pharmacological, toxicological, and virological data during DHPG therapy by continuous infusion.

FIGURE 1 A: Baseline photograph showing active cytomegalovirus retinitis with hemorrhage of the left eye. **B:** Day 33 of treatment, demonstrating extension of retinitis during a continuous therapy of DHPG at steady-state plasma levels of approximately 0.8 μM. **C:** Day 70 of treatment, demonstrating resolution of retinitis with DHPG plasma levels of approximately 2.5 μM.

No adverse effects were attributed to continuous administration through the central line. Specifically, no secondary infectious complications were encountered.

DISCUSSION

This report describes a novel pharmacological strategy in the treatment of life-threatening infections that combines a continuous drug therapy using a portable pump with an individualized regimen based on a test dose.[10] The feasibility of this approach was evaluated with a novel antiviral drug, DHPG, a compound that has shown promising therapeutic effects against disseminated CMV infections in patients with AIDS and in patients immunosuppressed for other reasons. Preliminary uncontrolled clinical trials with this drug have shown that administration of 2.5 to 15 mg/kg/day of DHPG by a one hour intravenous infusion over a two week induction course either eliminates or

TABLE 2. Treatment Outcome

Initials	Duration therapy	Toxicity	Outcome	Reason treatment terminated
PR	1 year	Neutropenia $ANC^a = 150$	Resolved Pneumonia acuity improved	Refractory Neutropenia
PK	3 weeks	None	Died from CMV pneumonia	Death
RP	1 year	$ANC = 700$	Improved acuity; resolved colitis	Death from AIDS
JR	2 months	$ANC = 700$	Improved visual acuity	Death for AIDS
MD	3 months	$ANC = 630$	Improved acuity; resolved pneumonia and colitis	Death from *Pneumocystis carinii* pneumonia

^{a}Absolute neutrophil count.

markedly reduces viral excretion, CMV colitis, retinitis, and gastrointestinal diseases.[1-5] These data have prompted the recent licensure of this drug by the Food and Drug Administration. Current DHPG regimens, however, have been limited because therapeutic CMV is not eradicated, and virtually all patients relapse within a few weeks after completion of induction therapy. Maintenance regimens of 5-7.5 mg/kg/day, 5 days/week, following the initial therapy, have been investigated recently; however, toxic side effects consisting of neutropenia and thrombocytopenia have limited the long-term use of this drug, reflecting the critical need to develop novel suppressive regimens. In addition, relapse occurs ultimately in virtually all patients.

Inasmuch as we reasoned that DHPG-induced toxicity resulted in part from the dose and/or regimen, we investigated the use of a continuous low-dose regimen using a portable pump associated with an individualized regimen to predict the dose with which desired steady-state plasma levels could be achieved. The individualization of DHPG therapy appears advisable because of the narrow therapeutic index of this drug and the significant variation in the total plasma clearance observed in patients with normal renal function after intravenous administration of DHPG.[11]

In this study, cessation of CMV colitis and viremia was observed following administration of a very low dose of DHPG (16 mg/24 hours), which resulted in steady-state plasma levels of approximately 1 μM in the studied patients. Complete resolution of the chorioretinitis, however, was accomplished only with steady-state plasma levels of approximately 2.5 μM of DHPG in three of the four patients. Whereas both plasma steady-state levels (*i.e.* 1 and 2.5 μM) approximated the mean 50% inhibitory dose (ID_{50}) of 2.57 ± 1.25 μM for DHPG recently reported in 33 CMV isolates,[12] this difference at various target organ sites may result from a noncomplete penetration of DHPG and/or a different quantitative activation of DHPG to its active triphosphate derivative at the sites of infection. Of particular importance was also that at these plasma levels no significant adverse toxicity occurred. Indeed, a major advantage of this approach was the elimination of fluctuating plasma levels of drug that peaked at toxic concentrations as shown in this study and had trough plasma levels at a subtherapeutic concentration. The necessity to avoid transient high plasma levels with DHPG is emphasized by our recent demonstration that direct and continuous exposure of DHPG consistently inhibited human granulocyte-macrophage colony-forming cells *in vitro* with an ID_{50} of 2.7 ± 0.5 μM.[13]

This report suggests that suppressive DHPG therapy with continuous administration of low doses of DHPG approaching the ID_{50} for CMV isolates might translate into a greater clinical efficacy and safety regimen. The possibility of providing an effective regimen not requiring continuous hospital care is an additional advantage of this novel approach.

The use of continuous infusion of DHPG by portable pump merits further investigation. This should provide a possible way to achieve desired DHPG plasma concentrations at the target site for long-term suppressive anticytomegalovirus maintenance therapy without potential toxic side effects.

SUMMARY

Two novel antiviral pharmacologic strategies were used for therapy of life- and sight-threatening cytomegalovirus (CMV) infection; these were continuous drug infusion by portable pump and individualized patient regimen. 9-(1,3-Dihydroxy-2-propoxymethyl)-guanine (DHPG), an active and recently licensed antiviral drug against cytomegalovirus infection, was administered to five immunocompromised patients with chorioretinitis (all patients), colitis (two), and pneumonitis (three). Through dosage escalation, correlations between plasma levels, toxicity (*i.e.*, myelosuppression), and clinical benefit were ascertained for therapy of acute disease (pneumonitis) as well as long-term therapy (chorioretinitis). Resolution of viremia, pneumonitis, colitis, and chorioretinitis was accomplished with steady-state plasma levels of DHPG approximating the mean ID_{50} of CMV isolates. The most notable clinical benefit was survival from CMV pneumonia and stabilization of vision. Although no adverse toxicity occurred during the DHPG continuous long-term therapy, survival was limited by the underlying disease.

ACKNOWLEDGMENT

The authors would like to thank Dr. William C. Buhles, Syntex (U.S.A.), Inc. for sharing helpful information.

REFERENCES

1. BACH, M. C., S. P. BAGWELL, N. P. KNAPP, K. M. DAVIS & P. S. HEDSTROM. 1985. 9-(1,3-Dihydroxy-2-propoxymethyl) guanine for cytomegalovirus infections in patients with the acquired immunodeficiency syndrome. Ann. Intern. Med. **103:** 381-382.
2. COLLABORATIVE DHPG TREATMENT STUDY GROUP. 1986. Treatment of serious cytomegalovirus infections with 9-(1,3-dihydroxy-2-propoxymethyl) guanine in patients with AIDS and other immunodeficiencies. N. Engl. J. Med. **314:** 801-805.
3. FELSENSTEIN, D., N. J. D'AMICO & M. S. HIRSH et al. 1985. Treatment of cytomegalovirus retinitis with 9-(2-hydroxy-1-(hydroxymethyl)ethoxymethyl) guanine. Ann. Intern. Med. **103:** 377-380.
4. MASUR, H., H. C. LANE, A. PALESTINE et al. 1986. Effect of 9-(1,3-dihydroxy-2-propoxymethyl) guanine on serious cytomegalovirus disease in eight immunosuppressed homosexual men. Ann. Intern. Med. **104:** 41-44.
5. PALESTINE, A. G., G. STEVENS, H. C. LANE et al. 1986. Treatment of cytomegalovirus retinitis with dihydroxy propoxymethylguanine. Am. J. Ophthalmol. **101:** 95-101.
6. VISOR, G. C., L.-H. LIN, S. E. JACKSON, J. S. WINTERLE, G. LEE & R. A. KENLEY. 1986. Stability of ganciclovir sodium (DHPG sodium) in 5% dextrose of 0.9% sodium chloride injections. Am. J. Hosp. Pharm. **43:** 2810-2812.
7. SOMMADOSSI, J. P. & R. BAVEN. 1987. High performance liquid chromatographic method for the determination of 9-(1,3-dihydroxy-2-propoxymethyl) guanine in human plasma. J. Chromatogr. **414:** 429-433.
8. GIBALDI, M. & D. PERRIER. 1982. Pharmacokinetics. 2nd edit. Marcel Dekker Inc. New York.
9. QUINNAN, G. V., JR., H. MASUR, A. H. ROOK et al. 1984. Herpesvirus infections in the acquired immune deficiency syndrome. J. Am. Med. Assoc. **252:** 72-77.
10. SOMMADOSSI, J. P., C. AUBERT, J. P. RIGAULT & S. MONJANEL. 1980. La rationalization des posologies: ses avantages et ses limites. Therapie (Paris) **35:** 391-393.
11. SOMMADOSSI, J. P., R. BEVAN & T. LING et al. 1988. Clinical pharmacokinetics of ganciclovir (DHPG) in patients with normal and impaired renal function. Rev. Infect. Dis. **10**(Suppl 3): S507-S514.
12. COLE, N. L. & H. BALFOUR. 1985. Does cytomegalovirus become more resistant during antiviral therapy? In Abstract 128 of the 25th Interscience Conference on Antimicrobial Agents and Chemotherapy. Minneapolis, MN. Sept. 29-Oct. 2, 1985.
13. SOMMADOSSI, J. P. & R. CARLISLE. 1987. Toxicity of 3'-azido-3'deoxythymidine and 9-(1,3-dihydroxy-2-propoxymethyl) guanine for normal human hematopoietic progenitor cells in vitro. Antimicrob. Agents Chemother. **31:** 452-454.

Fungal Infections in HIV Patients

CHARLES H. KIRKPATRICK

Conrad D. Stephenson Laboratory for Research in Immunology
Division of Allergy and Clinical Immunology
Department of Medicine
National Jewish Center for Immunology and Respiratory Medicine
Denver, Colorado 80206

INTRODUCTION

Fungal infections are very common events in HIV-infected patients. The development of oral candidiasis in association with other symptoms such as unexplained fever, night sweats, weight loss, and diarrhea in an HIV-seropositive subject usually leads to the diagnosis of AIDS-related complex (CDC group IV, subgroup C-2).[1] In the Walter Reed Classification for clinical staging of HIV infections, the development of oral candidiasis advances a patient to stage WR5 or WR6, depending on the coexistence of anergy or other opportunistic infections (TABLE 1).[2]

In the revised case definition of AIDS, fungal infections such as disseminated histoplasmosis or esophageal candidiasis in HIV-antibody positive patients are designated as adequate for the diagnosis of AIDS,[3,4] and other disseminated infections such as sporotrichosis and coccidioidomycosis have occurred in HIV-seropositive subjects.

With the recent reassignment of *Pneumocystis carinii* to the Fungi,[5] fungal infections become the most common opportunistic infections in HIV-infected persons. Prior to this report the taxonomic assignment of this organism had been uncertain, and its life cycle resembled both Protozoa and Fungi. From the sequences of 16S-like ribosomal RNAs, however, it was possible to identify *P. carinii* as a member of the Fungi (FIG. 1).

PROGNOSTIC SIGNIFICANCE OF FUNGAL INFECTIONS

Oral candidiasis has been shown to have prognostic significance for progression from less symptomatic stages of HIV infection to frank AIDS. Klein and associates[6] compared two groups of homosexual/bisexual men and/or male intravenous drug users that were similar for the presence of unexplained generalized lymphadenopathy and abnormal CD4/CD8 T-lymphocyte ratios, but that differed in the presence or absence of oral candidiasis. During the period of follow-up (5 to 21 months; median 12 months), none of the patients without oral candidiasis developed AIDS. By contrast, 13 of the 22 men with oral candidiasis (59 %) developed AIDS, as defined as a major opportunistic infection or Kaposi's sarcoma, during the period of follow-up (1 to 23 months) (p < 0.001). The median time from the onset of candidiasis to the development of AIDS

TABLE 1. The Walter Reed Staging Classification for HIV Infection

Stage	HIV Antibody or virus	Chronic lymphadenopathy	CD4 cells (per μL)	DTH[a]	Oral candidiasis	OI[b]
WR0	−	−	>400	intact	−	−
WR1	+	−	>400	intact	−	−
WR2	+	+	>400	intact	−	−
WR3	+	+ or −	<400	intact	−	−
WR4	+	+ or −	<400	partial defect	−	−
WR5	+	+ or −	<400	deficient	+	−
WR6	+	+ or −	<400	deficient	+ or −	+

[a] DTH = delayed-type hypersensitivity as defined by responses to tetanus toxoid, *Trichophyton*, mumps, and candida antigen.
[b] OI = opportunistic infections.

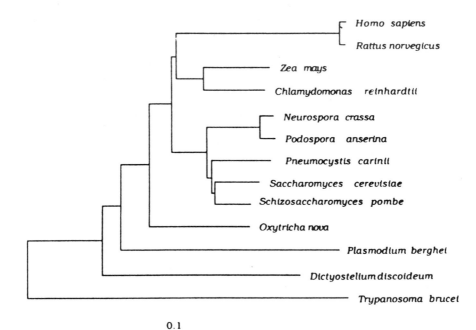

FIGURE 1. Phylogenetic tree that illustrates that *Pneumocystis carinii* is a member of the Fungi. The conclusions are based on sequence similarities of the 16S-like RNA. The sequence data were converted into an unrooted phylogenetic tree by distance matrix methods. The evolutionary distance between nodes of the tree is represented in the horizontal component of their separation in the figure. (Edman *et al.*[5] With permission from *Nature* © 1988. Macmillan Magazines Limited.)

was 3 months. CD4/CD8 values of 0.51 or less were additional risk factors for progression to AIDS; this observation is in concert with the recent report by Moss and coworkers[7] who noted that reduction of CD4 lymphocytes below $400/\mu L$ was accompanied by greater risk for progression to AIDS. Other reports[8,9] have independently confirmed the prognostic significance of oral candidiasis in HIV-infected patients.

FUNGAL INFECTIONS IN HIV-INFECTED PATIENTS (Table 2)

Pneumocystis carinii is a well-known cause of opportunistic pneumonias in patients with congenital and acquired immunodeficiency syndromes and in recipients of cytotoxic or immunosuppressive therapy. Pneumonia due to this organism is the most common fungal infection in HIV-infected patients. It establishes the definition of AIDS

TABLE 2. Fungal Infections in HIV-Infected Subjects

| | Sites of Infections | |
Etiology	Common	Uncommon
Candida sp.	buccal cavity esophagus	rectum vagina lungs
C. neoformans	meninges disseminated	lungs
Histoplasma capsulatum	disseminated	
C. immitis	disseminated	
Aspergillus sp.		lungs
Sporotrichium schenkii		lymphocutaneous
P. carinii	lungs	outside the lungs

in about 65% of cases and occurs at some time during the course of approximately 80% of AIDS patients.[10] Only rarely does *P. carinii* cause infections in extrapulmonary sites.

In contrast to the pneumonias of rapid onset and progression in patients with congenital immunodeficiency syndromes or recipients of organ transplants, in HIV-infected patients, pneumonia due to *P. carinii* may have a more insidious onset that is characterized by weeks of progressive exertional dyspnea and fatigue before the onset of cough and fever. Patients who are at risk for *Pneumocystis* pneumonia should be advised of the possible significance of these uncertain symptoms so they can be diagnosed and treated early. In the early stages, the chest X rays may be normal, and more invasive techniques may be required for making the correct diagnosis. The recent recommendations for prophylaxis of at-risk subjects with trimethoprim-sulfamethoxazole or inhaled pentamidine[11] may significantly reduce the frequencies of pneumonias due to this organism in HIV-infected subjects.

Mucosal and cutaneous candidiasis is the second most common fungal infection in HIV-infected patients. The infections of mucous surfaces tend to be persistent and recurrent. They are usually painful and may interfere with ingestion of salty, spicy, or acidic foods. Only rarely are infections due to *Candida* species the cause of systemic infections in patients with HIV infections; in this respect they differ from the *Candida* infections in patients who are neutropenic as a consequence of treatment with antineoplastic disease drugs.[12]

Oral candidiasis presents as plaques or ulcerations on mucous surfaces. They are usually painful. The diagnosis is readily made by microscopic examination of scrapings from lesions after digestion with 10% potassium hydroxide solution. The development of recurrent oral candidiasis in a patient who is not diabetic, is not using inhaled corticosteroids or broad-spectrum antibiotics, or who has not received immunosuppressive therapy should be a strong warning to the physician that the patient may have a defect in cell-mediated immunity. In certain individuals, such as gay or bisexual men, intravenous drug users, and hemophiliacs, HIV infection is the most common reason for this type of immunologic defect.

As mentioned above, Klein and associates[6] and others [8,9] have shown that oral candidiasis in HIV-infected subjects is often a prodrome to development of AIDS, and infections of the esophagus with *Candida* species are criteria for making the diagnosis of AIDS.

Cryptococcus neoformans is an important cause of meningitis, pneumonia, and disseminated infections in patients with AIDS. Cryptococcal infections occur in 7% of AIDS patients, and after HIV encephalopathy and toxoplasmosis, infections with *C. neoformans* rank third as a cause of neurological disease in patients with AIDS.[13] Extraneural infections with cryptococci are well-known and include pneumonia, arthritis, retinitis, dermatitis, and peritonitis. At autopsy, disseminated infections may be found. The recent evidence that the prostate may serve as a reservoir for *C. neoformans* even after apparently adequate treatment of meningitis or extraneural cryptococcosis may facilitate identification of patients who are at risk for posttreatment relapses.[14] It is probable that long-term maintenance treatment with antifungal drugs is necessary to maintain remission in AIDS patients with cryptococcal meningitis.[15]

Histoplasmosis and coccidioidomycosis are opportunistic infections that occur in AIDS patients from certain geographic areas.[16-18] Seven of the first 15 AIDS patients reported from Indiana had disseminated histoplasmosis.[16,17] Although rare in AIDS patients in general, 7 of 27 AIDS patients in Tucson developed coccidioidomycosis.[19]

A detailed review of the treatments used in disseminated fungal infections in HIV-infected patients is beyond the scope of this report. In general, superficial mucous membrane and cutaneous candidiasis respond well to topical therapy with clotrimazole troches. Treatment of deep-seated or disseminated infections is much more difficult and requires systemic medications and often combinations of antifungal agents.[20] Even then relapse rates are high, probably because the underlying defects in the host defense mechanisms that originally predisposed the patients to the infections are not affected by antifungal drug therapy.

HOST-DEFENSE MECHANISMS IN FUNGAL INFECTIONS

There is evidence that the mechanisms for clearing superficial fungal infections are different from those for deep mycoses. For example, Wilson and Sohnle[21] have examined mechanisms for clearance of cutaneous candida infections in mice that either do or do not develop delayed hypersensitivity to *C. albicans* as a consequence of the infection.

Both strains of mice developed neutrophilic microabscesses in the upper epidermis, and within three days these abscesses had been relocated to superficial sites. Epidermal proliferation appeared to be involved in the relocation process. Mice (C57BL/6) that developed delayed-type hypersensitivity to *C. albicans* showed more rapid clearance of the infections than the mice (C3H/He) that did not. Prior sensitization to Candida of low responder mice, however, resulted in more rapid clearance. These mechanisms are probably similar to the defects in patients with chronic mucocutaneous candidiasis who have impaired delayed hypersensitivity and lymphokine production to *C. albicans* and who have impaired clearance of cutaneous and mucous membrane infections with *C. albicans.*[22]

In deep fungal infections, neutrophil and monocyte-mediated oxidative reactions and cationic peptides appear to be more important for killing filamentous fungi such as Candida, Aspergillus, and Rhizopus.[23-25] Diamond and associates[26,27] have shown that neutrophils can attach to the pseudohyphae of *C. albicans* and release factors that injure the organisms. In some models, fungicidal activity of neutrophilic peptides is more effective if the organisms are metabolically active.[28]

A great number of abnormalities in host defense mechanisms have been identified in patients with HIV infections. especially if they have progressed to the diagnosis of AIDS (TABLE 3). Of these, certain abnormalities such as lymphopenia of CD4-bearing

TABLE 3. Immunologic and Host Defense Abnormalities in Patients with HIV Infections

Lymphopenia, especially of CD4$^+$ cells
T-cell fusion with syncytium formation
Impaired antigen presentation
Impaired IL-2 receptor expression
Autoantibody formation
Loss of delayed-type hypersensitivity
Impaired antibody responses to new antigens
Impaired chemotaxis of monocytes
Impaired bactericidal activity of monocytes and neutrophils

T cells are critical and have predictive significance.[7] Others such as formation of syncytia of CD4$^+$ cells, autoantibody production, and impaired neutrophil and monocyte functions are of uncertain clinical significance, although they could contribute to the immunodeficiency.

It seems clear that long-term management of patients with HIV infections will involve multiple therapies. The beneficial effects of antiretroviral therapy are impressive, especially in subjects who are asymptomatic. It is also noteworthy that recipients of azidothymidine (AZT) and dideoxyinosine (ddI) have shown improvement in immunologic functions, including increased numbers of circulating CD4$^+$ T cells and improved responses to skin tests for delayed-type hypersensitivity.[29,30] These findings indicate that recovery of immunologic functions is possible at least in some patients.

One group of agents that is capable of restoring immune functions in patients with certain immunodeficiency syndromes is transfer factors.[31] These molecules are families of polypeptides and have the property of inducing cell-mediated immune responses in recipients in an immunologically specific manner (FIG. 2). Only a few clinical studies have been done with transfer factors in HIV-infected patients. Carey *et al.*[32] administered a transfer factor-containing preparation from pooled dialysates of three normal persons with intact delayed hypersensitivity and three HIV-infected anergic donors to a group of patients with AIDS. In six of seven recipients of the transfer factor pool, one or more new delayed hypersensitivity responses were elicited by posttreatment skin testing.

We have observed clearance of chronic oropharyngeal candidiasis that was refractory to treatment with clotrimazole and ketoconazole in an AIDS patient after treat-

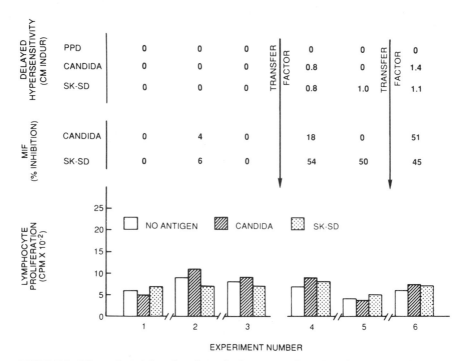

FIGURE 2. Effects of administration of transfer factors on cell-mediated immunologic functions in an anergic subject. Prior to treatment, the patient could not respond to skin tests with tuberculin (PPD), *Candida albicans,* or streptococcal proteins (SK-SD). Her T cells did not proliferate or secrete lymphokines (MIF) in response to Candida or SK-SD. The transfer factor donor had cell-mediated immunity to Candida and SK-SD but not to PPD. After receiving these transfer factors, the recipient developed delayed-type hypersensitivity (DTH) to Candida and SK-SD, but not to PPD, and her T cells produced MIF in response to these antigens. There were no changes in the lymphocyte proliferation responses. After a few months both DTH and MIF responses were lost (experiment 5), but they were restored after readministraton of more transfer factors (experiment 6).

ment with candida-specific transfer factor. The recipient also acquired delayed-type hypersensitivity to Candida. In another patient, treatment with bovine transfer factor that was specific for cytomegalovirus was effective in arresting progressive cytomegalovirus retinitis.

Louie *et al.*[33] have used a specific bovine transfer factor preparation for treatment of intestinal cryptosporidiosis in patients with AIDS. Five of eight subjects responded to this treatment.

These observations indicate that correction or improvement of cell-mediated immunity can be accomplished in some patients with HIV-mediated immunodeficiency, and that these treatments may produce clinical benefits. Controlled clinical trials with transfer factors are warranted.

REFERENCES

1. CENTERS FOR DISEASE CONTROL. 1986. Classification system for human T-lymphotrophic virus type III/lymphadenopathy associated virus infections. Morbid. Mortal. Weekly Rep. **35:** 334-339.
2. REDFIELD, R. R., D. C. WRIGHT & E. C. TRAMONT. 1986. The Walter Reed staging classification for HTLV III LAV infection. N. Engl. J. Med. **314:** 131-132.
3. CENTERS FOR DISEASE CONTROL. 1985. Revision of case definition of acquired immunodeficiency syndrome for national reporting—United States. Morbid. Mortal. Weekly Rep. **34:** 373-375.
4. CENTERS FOR DISEASE CONTROL. 1987. Human immunodeficiency virus infection in the United States: a review of current knowledge. Morbid. Mortal. Weekly Rep. **36**(Suppl. S-6): 1-48.
5. EDMAN, J. C., J. A. KOVACS, H. MASUR, D. V. SANTI, H. J. ELWOOD & M. L. SOGIN. 1988. Ribosomal RNA sequence shows *Pneumocystis carinii* to be a member of the Fungi. Nature **334:** 519-522.
6. KLEIN, R. S., C. A. HARRIS, C. B. SMALL, B. MOLL & M. LESSER. 1984. Oral candidiasis in high-risk patients as an initial manifestation of the acquired immunodeficiency syndrome. N. Engl. J. Med. **311:** 354-357.
7. MOSS, A. R., P. BACCHETTI, D. OSMOND, W. KRAMPF, R. E. CHAISSON, D. STITES, J. WILBER, J.-P. ALLAIN & J. CARLSON. 1988. Seropositivity for HIV and the development of AIDS or AIDS related condition: three year followup of the San Francisco General Hospital cohort. Br. Med. J. **296:** 745-750.
8. BARR, C. E. & J. P. TOROSIAN. 1986. Oral manifestations in patients with AIDS or AIDS-related complex. Lancet ii: 288.
9. TORSSANDER, J., L. MORFELDT-MANSON, G. BIBERFELD, A. KARLSSON, P.-O. PUTKONEN & J. WASSERMAN. 1987. Oral *Candida albicans* in HIV infection. Scand. J. Infect. Dis. **19:** 291-295.
10. KOVACS, J. A. & H. MASUR. 1988. Opportunistic infections. *In* AIDS. Etiology, Diagnosis, Treatment and Prevention. V. T. DeVita, Jr., S. Hellman & S. A. Rosenberg, Eds. Second Edition: 199-225. J. B. Lippincott. Philadelphia, PA.
11. CENTERS FOR DISEASE CONTROL. 1989. Guidelines for prophylaxis against *Pneumocystis carinii* pneumonia for persons infected with human immunodeficiency virus. Morbid. Mortal. Weekly Rep. **55:** 1-9.
12. BODEY, G. P. 1984. Candidiasis in cancer patients. Am. J. Med. **77:** 13-19.
13. DISMUKES, W. E. 1988. Cryptococcal meningitis in patients with AIDS. J. Infect. Dis. **157:** 624-628.
14. LARSEN, R. A., S. BOZZETTE, J. A. MCCUTCHAN, J. CHIV, M. A. LEAL, D. D. RICHMAN & THE CALIFORNIA COLLABORATIVE TREATMENT GROUP. 1989. Persistent *Cryptococcus neoformans* infection of the prostate after successful treatment of meningitis. Ann. Int. Med. **111:** 125-128.
15. CHUCK, S. L. & M. A. SANDE. 1989. Infections with *Cryptococcus neoformans* in the acquired immunodeficiency syndrome. N. Engl. J. Med. **321:** 794-799.
16. WHEAT, L. J., T. J. SLAMA & M. L. ZECKEL. 1985. Histoplasmosis in the acquired immune deficiency syndrome. Am. J. Med. **78:** 203-210.
17. BONNER, J. R., W. J. ALEXANDER, W. E. DISMUKES, W. APP, F. M. GRIFFIN, R. LITTLE & M. S. SHIN. 1984. Disseminated histoplasmosis in patients with the acquired immune deficiency syndrome. Arch. Intern. Med. **144:** 2178-2181.

18. JOHNSON, P. C., N. KHARDORI, A. F. NAJJAR, F. BUTT, P. W. A. MANSELL & G. A. SAROSI. 1988. Progressive disseminated histoplasmosis in patients with acquired immunodeficiency syndrome. Am. J. Med. **85:** 152-158.
19. BRONNIMANN, D. A., R. D. ADAM, J. N. GALGIANI, M. P. HABIB, E. A. PETERSEN, B. PORTER & J. W. BLOOM. 1987. Coccidioidomycosis in the acquired immunodeficiency syndrome. Ann. Intern. Med. **106:** 372-379.
20. SAAG, M. S. & W. E. DISMUKES. 1988. Azole antifungal agents: emphasis on new triazoles. Antimicrob. Agents Chemother. **32:** 1-8.
21. WILSON, B. D. & P. G. SOHNLE. 1986. Participation of neutrophils and delayed hypersensitivity in the clearance of experimental cutaneous candidiasis in mice. Am. J. Pathol. **123:** 241-249.
22. KIRKPATRICK, C. H. 1989. Chronic mucocutaneous candidiasis. Eur. J. Clin. Microbiol. Inf. Dis. **8:** 448-456.
23. LEHRER, R. I. & M. J. CLINE. 1969. Leukocyte myeloperoxidase deficiency and disseminated candidiasis: the role of myeloperoxidase in resistance to *Candida* infections. J. Clin. Invest. **48:** 1478-1488.
24. LEHRER, R. I. 1972. Functional aspects of a second mechanism of candidacidal activity by human neutrophils. J. Clin. Invest. **51:** 2566-2572.
25. LEHRER, R. I. 1975. The fungicidal mechanisms of human monocytes. I. Evidence for myeloperoxidase-independent candidacidal mechanisms. J. Clin. Invest. **55:** 338-346.
26. DIAMOND, R. D. & R. KRZESICKI. 1978. Mechanisms of attachment of neutrophils to *Candida albicans* pseudohyphae in the absence of serum, and of subsequent damage to pseudohyphae by microbicidal processes of neutrophils *in vitro*. J. Clin. Invest. **61:** 360-369.
27. DIAMOND, R. D., R. KRZESICKI & J. WELLINGTON. 1978. Damage of pseudohyphal forms of *Candida albicans* by neutrophils in the absence of serum *in vitro*. J. Clin. Invest. **61:** 349-359.
28. LEVITZ, S. M., M. E. SELSTED, T. GANZ, R. I. LEHRER & R. D. DIAMOND. 1986. *In vitro* killing of spores and hyphae of *Aspergillus fumigatus* and *Rhizopus oryzae* by rabbit neutrophil cationic peptides and bronchoalveolar macrophages. J. Infect. Dis. **154:** 483-489.
29. FISCHL, M. A., D. D. RICHMAN, M. H. GRIECO, M. S. GOTTLIEB, P. A. VOLBERDING, O. L. LASKIN, J. M. LEEDOM, J. E. GROOPMAN, D. MILDVAN, R. T. SCHOOLEY, G. G. JACKSON, D. T. DURACK, D. KING & THE AZT COLLABORATIVE WORKING GROUP. 1987. The efficacy of azidothymidine (AZT) in the treatment of patients with AIDS and AIDS-related complex. N. Engl. J. Med. **317:** 185-191.
30. YARCHOAN, R., H. MITSUYA, R. V. THOMAS, J. M. PLUDA, N. R. HARTMAN, C.-F. PERNO, K. S. MARCZYK, J.-P. ALLAIN, D. G. JOHNS & S. BRODER. 1989. *In vivo* activity against HIV and favorable toxicity profile of 2',3'-dideoxyinosine. Science **245:** 412-415.
31. KIRKPATRICK, C. H. 1988. Transfer factor. J. Allergy Clin. Immunol. **81:** 803-813.
32. CAREY, J. T., M. M. LEDERMAN, Z. TOOSSI, K. EDMONDS, S. HODDER, L. H. CALABRESE, M. R. PROFFITT, C. E. JOHNSON & J. J. ELLNER. 1987. Augmentation of skin test reactivity and lymphocyte blastogenesis in patients with AIDS treated with transfer factor. J. Am. Med. Assoc. **257:** 651-655.
33. LOUIE, E., W. BORKOWSKY, P. H. KLESIUS, T. B. HAYNES, S. GORDON, S. BONK & H. S. LAWRENCE. 1987. Treatment of cryptosporidiosis with oral bovine transfer factor. Clin. Immunol. Immunopathol. **44:** 329-334.

Summary of Part VIII

An Overview of Opportunistic Infections in AIDS Patients

DAVID LOEBENBERG, JEROME SCHWARTZ, AND
FRANCIS J. BULLOCK

Schering-Plough Research
Bloomfield, New Jersey 07003

Infectious diseases represent the most life-threatening problem associated with AIDS. Presently, innovative research is directed not only towards understanding the pathology of the HIV infection, but also towards new efforts to delineate improved ways to deal with the opportunistic infections that are its consequence. Such efforts include (1) better understanding of the pathophysiology of infectious agents such as *Pneumocystis carinii, Toxoplasma gondii* and fungi; (2) better exploitation of known prophylactic and chemotherapeutic agents, such as pentamidine and its analogues for *Pneumocystis* and ganciclovir for cytomegalovirus infection; (3) attempts to identify novel means of dealing with opportunistic infections, such as through immune enhancement; and (4) the search for new drugs with clear advantages over existing therapies.

Pneumocystis carinii pneumonia (PCP) is the most common opportunistic infection in AIDS patients. Management of PCP with agents such as aerosolized pentamidine and trimethoprim-sulphamethoxazole (TMP/SMZ) continues to be the procedure of choice, although both have serious side effects that limit their utility. In addition, there continues to be a population of nonresponding PCP-infected patients with existing AIDS.[1] The clinical utility of inhaled pentamidine as prophylaxis for PCP is currently being evaluated. The work of M. T. Cushion from the University of Cincinnati College of Medicine demonstrates that potential drug-resistant strains of *Pneumocystis* can be identified. This has implications for designing the best treatment modality for individual AIDS patients and also for identifying important reservoirs of these resistant strains in the population. The paper by R. R. Tidwell and associates from the University of North Carolina at Chapel Hill identifies derivatives of pentamidine with potentially better activity against PCP. The molecules were evaluated in a rat model of PCP. This model may be an accurate predictor of activity of new molecules in PCP infections in humans, but full toxicological evaluation of these entities remains to be completed.

Cryptococcosis, a deep-seated yeast infection, has been recognized as the cause of a frequently subclinical form of non-PCP respiratory disease that may occur sporadically. In AIDS patients, however, between 6 and 13% develop symptomatic cryptococcal infection of varying severity, including meningitis. Treatment of the disease with currently available drugs such as amphotericin B and ketoconazole is not sufficient due to possible appearance of resistant organisms in monotherapy and poor drug penetration into the central nervous system.[2] SCH 39304, a new orally active triazole antifungal crosses the blood brain barrier in mice,[3] rabbits,[4] and rhesus monkeys,[5] and has a very long cerebrospinal fluid (CSF) half-life. It significantly prolongs survival and reduces the level of infecting organisms in those infection models. These properties confer distinct potential clinical advantages to SCH 39304 over existing treatments for cryptococcal infection. The host immune response appears to play a key role in the suppression of disease during cryptococcal infection, and application of lymphokine therapy may be an important new development in this disease. R. Soave and colleagues from the New York Hospital-Cornell Medical Center have summarized clinical experiences with various treatment regimens in AIDS-related cryptococcal disease. The search continues, however, for antifungal agents with lower toxicity, a broader spectrum of activity, and a better pharmacokinetic profile.

Cryptococcal infection represents only one of an emerging group of serious fungal diseases being seen in AIDS patients.[6] *Candida* species cause a wide variety of pathogenic processes in AIDS patients, yet diagnosis remains problematic, and treatment is often accompanied by significant toxicities.[7,8] In experimental *Candida* infections in both normal and immunocompromised mice, SCH 39304 administered therapeutically or prophylactically was superior to fluconazole and ketoconazole in both survival and level of reduction of recoverable organisms.[9] In a rabbit model of endocarditis, pyelonephritis, and endophthalmitis, SCH 39304 sterilized many infected organs and significantly reduced the levels of organisms in other organs.[4] It is apparent from the paper by C. H. Kirkpatrick from the National Jewish Center for Immunology and Respiratory Medicine in Denver, Colorado, that therapeutic approaches to fungal infections in AIDS patients represent only a portion of a potential comprehensive therapeutic attack. Attempts at restoration of compromised immune function in AIDS patients is essential to derive maximum benefit from existing antifungal chemotherapy.

Toxoplasmosis is the most common cause of CNS mass lesions and consequent loss of neurologic function, occurring in 3 to 40% of AIDS patients, depending on the population group. Although sequential blockade of folic acid metabolism using the combination of pyrimethamine and sulfadiazine has been shown to be the most efficacious regimen for the disease, no therapy exists for patients who do not respond to these drugs or who undergo rapid relapse once therapy is terminated.[10] The initiation and spread of *Toxoplasma* infection relies on penetration of host cells by the intracellular parasite. The studies by J. D. Schwartzman and colleagues from the University of Virginia School of Medicine suggest that new agents that kill the bradyzoite stage, the most metabolically inactive stage, could potentially eradicate the latent parasites that are responsible for continued recrudescence of clinical infections in AIDS patients. Such basic studies of the pathology of opportunistic infections in AIDS are important to delineate new targets for potential pharmaceutical intervention.

Recent studies by D. J. Lang and colleagues from the University of Southern California and the Transfusion Safety Study Group confirm the high rate of active cytomegalovirus (CMV) infection among HIV seropositive individuals.[11] This infection becomes increasingly virulent as HIV infection progresses to AIDS, most frequently resulting in CMV retinitis and blindness, despite ganciclovir treatment.[12] R. J. Whitley and colleagues from the University of Alabama describe new pharmacological strategies using ganciclovir in the management of severe CMV infection in AIDS patients. Although these strategies result in stabilization of vision and increased survival from CMV pneumonia, survival of these patients continues to be limited by the underlying AIDS disease.

The question then remains, Where do we go for prevention and therapy of opportunistic infections in AIDS? At this session we saw advances being made in methods of administration of known therapeutic entities, such as ganciclovir in CMV infections, and in development of better analogues of known effective molecules such as pentamidine. Newer azole compounds such as fluconazole and SCH 39304, which penetrate the central nervous system, have excellent pharmacokinetics, and broad-spectrum anti-fungal activity are in clinical trials. In addition, we saw new research on mechanisms of drug resistance, new approaches to understanding the biology of *Toxoplasma,* and new studies that delineate the important role of an intact immune system in fighting opportunistic infectious diseases in AIDS. The potential application of lymphokines to restoration of immune function using molecules like granulocyte macrophage colony-stimulating factor (GM-CSF; ref. 13) seems most promising. In the feline model of AIDS (FeLV-AIDS) administration of interferon alpha 2b (Intron-A[R]) in combination with zidovudine is the only chemotherapeutic regimen that can completely block *de novo* infection.[14] Such studies demonstrate the potential importance of lymphokines in the management of AIDS. These new agents, used alone or in combination with prophylactic and therapeutic modalities, should favorably impact management of the life-threatening opportunistic infections in patients with AIDS.

REFERENCES

1. GAZZARD, B. G. 1989. *Pneumocystis carinii* pneumonia and its treatment in patients with AIDS. J. Antimicrob. Chemother. **23** Suppl. A: 67-75.
2. PERFECT, J. R. 1989. Cryptococcosis. Inf. Dis. Clin. N. Am. **3**: 77-102.
3. RESTREPO, B. I., J. AHRENS & J. R. GRAYBILL. 1989. Efficacy of SCH 39304 in murine cryptococcosis. Antimicrob. Agents Chemother. **33**: 1242-1246.
4. PERFECT, J. R., K. A. WRIGHT, M. M. HOBBS & D. T. DURACK. 1989. Treatment of experimental cryptococcal meningitis and disseminated candidiasis with SCH 39304. Antimicrob. Agents Chemother. **33**: 1735-1740.
5. WALSH, T. J., C. MCCULLEY, M. G. RINALDI, F. BALIS, J. LEE, P. A. PIZZO & D. POPLACK. 1989. Pharmacokinetics and penetration of SCH 39304 into cerebrospinal fluid of rhesus monkeys. 29th Interscience Conference on Antimicrobial Agents and Chemotherapy. Abstract 1361. American Society for Microbiology.
6. RINALDI, M. G. 1989. Emerging opportunists. Inf. Dis. Clin. N. Am. **3**: 65076.
7. MALE, O. 1989. Synopsis of mycotic infections in AIDS. Curr. Probl. Dermatol. **18**: 241-249.
8. CRISLIP, M. A. & J. E. EDWARDS, JR. 1989. Candidiasis. Inf. Dis. Clin. N. Am. **3**: 103-133.9.
9. LOEBENBERG, D., R. PARMEGIANI, A. CACCIAPOUTI, B. ANTONACCI, C. NORRIS, F. MENZEL, JR., E. L. MOSS, JR., T. YAROSH-TOMAINE, R. S. HARE & G. H. MILLER. 1988. SCH 39304, a new antifungal agent. I. Oral treatment of systemic infections in mice. 28th Interscience Conference on Antimicrobial Agents and Chemotherapy. Abstract 167. American Society for Microbiology.
10. TUAZON, C. U. 1989. Toxoplasmosis in AIDS patients. J. Antimicrob. Chemother. **23** Suppl. A: 77-82.
11. LANG, D. J., A. S. KOVACS, J. A. ZAIA & the TRANSFUSION SAFETY STUDY GROUP. 1989. Seroepidemiologic studies of cytomegalovirus and Epstein-Barr virus infections in relation to human immunodeficiency virus type 1 infection in selected recipient populations. J. AIDS **2**: 540-549.
12. CULBERTSON, W. W. 1989. Infections of the retina in AIDS. Int. Ophthalmol. Clin. **29**: 108-118.
13. RUEF, C. & D. L. COLEMAN. 1990. Granulocyte-macrophage colony-stimulating factor: Pleiotropic cytokine with potential clinical usefulness. Rev. Inf. Dis. **12**: 42-62.
14. ZEIDNER, N. S., M. H. MYLES, C. K. MATHIASON-DUBARD, M. J. DREITZ, J. I. MULLENS & E. A. HOOVER. 1990. Alpha interferon (26) in combination with zidovudine for the treatment of presymptomatic feline leukemia virus-induced immunodeficiency syndrome. Antimicrob. Agents Chemoth. **34**: 1749-1756.

Kinetics of ddI in Plasma, Brain, and CSF of Rats after Administration of ddI and an Ester Prodrug of ddI[a]

BRADLEY D. ANDERSON,[b]
BARBARA L. HOESTEREY,[b] DAVID C. BAKER,[c]
AND RAYMOND E. GALINSKY[b]

[b]Department of Pharmaceutics
University of Utah
Salt Lake City, Utah 84112

[c]Department of Chemistry
University of Alabama
Tuscaloosa, Alabama 35487

A progressive dementia, referred to as the AIDS dementia complex, occurs in as many as 60% of AIDS patients and is especially common in advanced stages of HIV infection.[1] The clinical course of AIDS dementia complex can be correlated with HIV replication in the CNS,[2] suggesting a need for antiviral drugs that readily cross the blood-brain barrier. Although dideoxynucleosides have been detected in cerebrospinal fluid (CSF) after intravenous doses,[3-4] the extent to which these relatively polar molecules cross the blood-brain barrier is unclear.[4] Lipophilic derivatives that undergo conversion to the active parent drug in brain tissue may enhance the CNS delivery of dideoxynucleosides. The present study was undertaken to characterize the pharmacokinetic parameters of dideoxyinosine (ddI) in plasma, brain, and CSF after administration of ddI and to compare these with the same parameters obtained after administration of ddI-5'-butyrate ester.

A recent study of the uptake kinetics of ddI into brain and CSF of rats after intravenous infusions indicates that the brain uptake of ddI is very inefficient.[5] During a two hour infusion of ddI in male Sprague-Dawley rats at a rate of 130 mg/kg/h, steady-state plasma concentrations of 50 μg/mL were obtained within 30 minutes. A systemic clearance of 2.4 L/kg/h was estimated from these data. After the infusions were terminated, ddI declined biphasically from plasma with α $t\frac{1}{2}$ = 3 minutes and β $t\frac{1}{2}$ = 5 minutes. As illustrated in FIGURE 1, steady-state concentrations of ddI in brain tissue and CSF were 4.7% and 1.5% of plasma concentrations, respectively. The higher percentage found in brain tissue was attributed primarily to the contribution of vascular blood in brain tissue (ca. 4%). Thus, the concentration of ddI in brain parenchyma attained during intravenous infusions is less than 1% of the plasma concentration at steady state. These low ratios are a result of the fact that elimination of ddI from the

[a]This work was supported by NIH/NIAID Contract NO1-AI-82680.

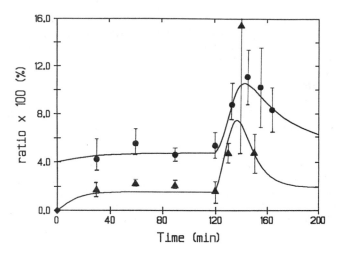

FIGURE 1. Ratio (in percent) of ddI in brain tissue or CSF to plasma versus time during and after intravenous infusions of ddI. The solid lines represent the best fit of the data according to the model described in ref 5. ●, brain tissue; ▲, CSF.

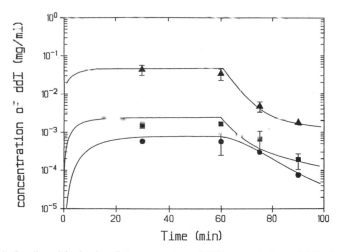

FIGURE 2. Semilogarithmic plot of plasma, brain, and CSF concentrations of ddI after infusions of ddI-5′-butyrate. The solid lines were generated using parameters obtained from infusions of ddI and therefore are the curves predicted if the butyrate ester hydrolyzes instantaneously after its administration. ▲, plasma; ■, brain tissue; ●, CSF.

CNS due to the combined contributions of CSF bulk flow, passive and active transport, and metabolism is more rapid than its entry. Dideoxyinosine, therefore, appears to be a suitable candidate for prodrug modification to enhance its rate of brain uptake.

To explore the feasibility of using lipophilic derivatives for targeting ddI to the brain, a series of 5'-aliphatic acid esters varying in chain length from 2 to 5 carbons was synthesized. These derivatives exhibited increased lipophilicities (octanol/water partition coefficients) ranging from 2- to 80-fold compared to ddI. A preliminary evaluation of their bioconversion in rat plasma indicated rapid hydrolysis to the parent compound in plasma ($t\frac{1}{2} \leq 1$ min), which may limit their utility in targeting ddI to the brain. To test this possibility *in vivo*, the 5'-butyrate of ddI was infused into rats at a rate of 165 mg/kg/h, which was equivalent to the molar rate employed in a previous study of ddI.[5] Shown in FIGURE 2 are the concentrations of ddI found in plasma, brain tissue, and CSF at various times during and after 60 minute infusions of ddI 5'-butyrate. The solid lines were generated from data obtained after infusions of ddI.[5] Agreement between these experimental points and the theoretical curve indicates that ddI 5'-butyrate behaves similarly to an injection of ddI. Synthesis of prodrug derivatives with reduced plasma bioconversion rates will be necessary to evaluate the true potential of lipophilic esters for enhancing the delivery of dideoxynucleosides to the brain.

REFERENCES

1. PRICE, R. W. & B. J. BREW. 1988. J. Infect. Dis. **158:** 1079-1083.
2. PRICE, R. W., B. BREW, J. SIDTIS, M. ROSENBLUM, A. C. SCHECK & P. CLEARY. 1988. Science **239:** 586-592.
3. KLECKER, R. W., J. M. COLLINS, R. YARCHOAN, R. THOMAS, J. F. JENKINS, S. BRODER & C. E. MYERS. 1987. Clin. Pharmacol. Ther. **41:** 407-412.
4. TERASAKI, T. & W. M. PARDRIDGE. 1988. J. Infect. Dis. **158:** 630-632.
5. ANDERSON, B. D., B. L. HOESTEREY, D. C. BAKER & R. E. GALINSKY. 1990. J. Pharmacol. Exp. Ther. **253:** 113-118.

Mechanism of Uptake of 3'-Deoxythymidin-2'-ene (d4T) in Human Lymphocyte H9 Cells[a]

E. MICHAEL AUGUST AND WILLIAM H. PRUSOFF

Department of Pharmacology
Yale University School of Medicine
New Haven, Connecticut 06510

Physiological nucleosides, as well as most nucleoside analogues, permeate mammalian cells by using one or more of several carrier proteins that possess broad specificities.[1] Recent evidence, however, has shown that some nucleoside analogues, most notably several of those shown to be potent inhibitors of the replication of human immunodeficiency virus (HIV-1), permeate the cell membrane independent of this carrier by nonfacilitated diffusion. These include 3'-azido-3'-deoxythymidine,[2] 2',3'-dideoxycytidine and 2',3'-dideoxyadenosine,[3] and 2',3'-dideoxythymidine.[4] This unique property has been attributed to an increase in lipophilicity relative to the parent nucleoside, although it has also been observed that the murine erythrocyte nucleoside transporter is sensitive to substrate alterations at the 3'-position,[5] a characteristic that these compounds share.

In light of the potent and selective antiviral activity of 3'-deoxythymidin-2'-ene against HIV-1,[6-8] and as a part of our ongoing studies of the cellular pharmacology of d4T, we have investigated the mechanism of uptake of d4T in the human lymphocyte cell line H9. The uptake of [^{3}H]d4T by H9 cells was linear for at least the first 8-10 seconds and was nonconcentrative, approaching equilibrium with the extracellular drug concentration. The initial rates of d4T uptake were a linear function of concentration over the range from 1 μM to 5 mM, with no evidence of uptake by a saturable mechanism. The uptake of [^{3}H]d4T was insensitive to the nucleoside transport inhibitors nitrobenzylthioinosine and dipyridamole under conditions where the uptake of thymidine was inhibited by 90 percent. The uptake of [^{3}H]d4T was likewise not inhibited by a 1000-fold excess of thymidine, AZT, adenine (which permeates the cell by way of a specific nucleobase carrier), and d4T itself. These data suggest that d4T permeates the cell membrane of human lymphocytes by the noncarrier-mediated process of passive diffusion. Moreover, d4T is not a substrate for the nucleoside transport protein(s) responsible for the entry of physiological nucleosides and numerous nucleoside analogues.[1]

[a]This work was supported by NCI Grants CA-05262 and CA-45410, NIAID Grant AI-26055, and an Unrestricted Research Grant from the Bristol-Myers Squibb Co.

ACKNOWLEDGMENTS

The authors are grateful to E. M. Birks for her technical assistance and R. Kirck for assistance in the preparation of this manuscript.

REFERENCES

1. PATERSON, A. R. P., N. KOLASSA & C. E. CASS. 1981. Transport of nucleoside drugs in animal cells. Pharm. Ther. **12:** 515-536.
2. ZIMMERMAN, T. P., W. B. MAHONEY & K. L. PRUS. 1987. 3'-Azido-3'-deoxythymidine: An unusual nucleoside analogue that permeates the membrane of human erythrocytes and lymphocytes by nonfacilitated diffusion. J. Biol. Chem. **262:** 5748-5754.
3. PLAGEMANN, P. G. W. & C. WOFFENDIN. 1989. Permeation and salvage of dideoxyadenosine in mammalian cells. Mol. Pharmacol. **36:** 185-192.
4. DOMIN, B. A., W. B. MAHONEY & T. P. ZIMMERMANN. 1988. 2',3'-Dideoxythymidine permeation of human erythrocyte membrane by nonfacilitated diffusion. Biochem. Biophys. Res. Commun. **154:** 825-831.
5. GATI, W. P., H. K. MISRA, E. E. KNAUS & L. I. WIEBE. 1984. Structural modifications at the 2'- and 3'-positions of some pyrimidine nucleosides as determinants of their interaction with the mouse erythrocyte nucleoside transporter. Biochem. Pharmacol. **33:** 3325-3331.
6. LIN, T.-S., R. F. SCHINAZI & W. H. PRUSOFF. 1987. Potent and selective *in vitro* activity of 3'-deoxythymidin-2'-ene (3'-deoxy-2',3'-didehydrothymidine) against human immunodeficiency virus. Biochem. Pharmacol. **36:** 2713-2718.
7. HAMAMOTO, Y., H. NAKASHIMA, T. MATSUI, A. MATSUDA, T. UEDA & N. YAMAMOTO. 1987. Inhibitory effect of 2',3'-didehydro-2',3'-dideoxynucleosides on infectivity, cytopathic effects, and replication of human immunodeficiency virus. Antimicrob. Agents Chemother. **31:** 907-910.
8. BABA, M., R. PAUWELS, P. HERDEWIJN, E. DECLERCQ, J. DESMYTER & M. VANDEPUTTE. 1987. Both 2',3'-dideoxythymidine and its 2',3'-unsaturated derivative (2',3'-dideoxythymidinene) are potent inhibitors of human immunodeficiency virus *in vitro*. Biochem. Biophys. Res. Commun. **142:** 128-134.

Continuous Optical Assays for DNA Polymerases and Reverse Transcriptases

JEAN G. BAILLON, NASHAAT T. NASHED,
JANE M. SAYER, AND DONALD M. JERINA

Laboratory of Bioorganic Chemistry
National Institute of Diabetes and Digestive and Kidney Diseases
The National Institutes of Health
Bethesda, Maryland 20892

Standard assay methods for DNA-polymerizing enzymes are based on the incorporation of radiolabeled deoxynucleotides into polynucleotides. Such assays, although highly sensitive, are time-consuming and require extensive manipulations, and thus are inconvenient for rapid screening of potential enzyme inhibitors. Furthermore, the discontinuous nature of these methods presents a drawback to their use in kinetics studies, because many such single-point assays are required to define adequately the time course of a single reaction. A recently described continuous assay for DNA polymerases based on light scattering[1] overcomes the above disadvantages, but the intensity of the scattered light exhibits a square dependence on the molecular weight of the polymeric product; and thus the experimentally measured quantity is not directly proportional to the extent of reaction. Both the ultraviolet absorption (UV) and circular dichroism (CD) spectra of nucleic acids are sensitive to the extent of complementary double helix formation, and thus assays based on these optical properties should be capable of measuring the extent of enzymatic transcription of a primed DNA or RNA template into a duplex. In the present study we describe two such optical assays for the measurement of DNA polymerization catalyzed by the reverse transcriptase of human immunodeficiency virus type 1 (HIV-1 RT) and the Klenow fragment of *E. coli* DNA polymerase I.

It is well-recognized that enzymatic polymerization of nucleic acids is associated with a decrease in UV absorption.[2] The use of microspectrophotometric cells (50 or 100 μL, path length 1 cm), as described by us for a microassay of retroviral proteases,[3] has made it practical to base assay methods for DNA-polymerizing enzymes on this absorbance change. The synthetic oligomer $p(dA)_{40-60}$ primed with $p(dT)_{20}$ is a substrate for both the Klenow fragment of *E. coli* DNA polymerase I and HIV-1 RT. FIGURE 1A shows the time dependence of the UV spectra observed upon reaction of this substrate with deoxythymidine triphosphate (dTTP) in the presence of the Klenow fragment. Similarly, the formation of secondary structure during the course of primer elongation by this enzyme results in a time-dependent change in the observed CD spectrum, as shown in FIGURE 1B. For routine assays, typical conditions were as follows: 37°C, 50 mM MOPS buffer (pH 7.4), 50 mM KCl, 10 mM $MgCl_2$, 1 mM DTT, 0.5 mM EGTA, 50 μg/mL bovine serum albumin (nuclease- and protease-inhibited),

1.6 μM p(dA)$_{40-60}$/p(dT)$_{20}$, and 100 μM dTTP. The CD change at 248 nm or the UV absorbance change at 275 nm was monitored as a function of time.

The shapes of the progress curves for transcription of p(dA)$_{40-60}$ primed with p(dT)$_{20}$, as measured by both CD and UV assays, are identical to each other and to that of the curve corresponding to the time dependence of incorporation of ^{3}H-labeled

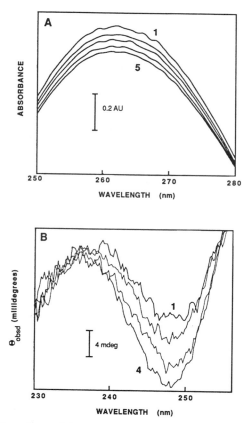

FIGURE 1. Time dependence of the UV and CD spectra observed upon duplex formation from p(dA)$_{40-60}$ primed with p(dT)$_{20}$, catalyzed by the Klenow fragment of *E. coli* DNA polymerase I. Concentrations of enzyme, template/primer, and dTTP were 1.76 nM, 1.6 μM, and 104 μM, respectively. Other assay conditions were as described in the text. Absorbances at time zero were 1.7 and 1.3 AU at 262 and 275 nm, respectively. UV scans (panel A) were obtained at time zero, 5, 10, 20, and 60 min (decrease in absorbance). CD scans (panel B) were obtained at time zero, 6, 20, and 60 min (decrease in absolute magnitude of the ellipticity.)

dTTP into polymeric material as measured by the standard filtration assay. Complete reaction of 1.6 μM p(dA)$_{40-60}$/p(dT)$_{20}$ with excess dTTP catalyzed by the Klenow fragment gave an average CD change, $\Delta\Theta_{248}$, of 13 millidegrees, or an absorbance change, ΔA_{275}, of 130 mAU. If the assumption is made that the p(dA)$_{40-60}$ is fully transcribed, an average of 48 μmoles dTTP should be incorporated in the presence of

1.6 μmoles template/primer upon completion of reaction; thus incorporation of 1 μmoles dTTP would correspond to a $\Delta\Theta_{248}$ of 0.27 millidegrees or a ΔA_{275} of 2.7 mAU. Quantitative radiochemical experiments are in progress to test the validity of this assumption. Transcription of poly(rA) primed with p(dT)$_{12-18}$, catalyzed by HIV-1 RT, can also be measured in the same way by following the time-dependent changes in the CD signal at 248 nm or the UV absorption at 275 nm.

REFERENCES

1. JOHNSON, K. A., F. R. BRYANT & S. J. BENKOVIC. 1984. Anal. Biochem. **136:** 192-194.
2. SCHACHMAN, H. K., J. ADLER, C. M. RADDING, I. R. LEHMAN & A. KORNBERG. 1960. J. Biol. Chem. **235:** 3242-3249.
3. NASHED, N. T., J. M. LOUIS, J. M. SAYER, E. M. WONDRAK, P. T. MORA, S. OROSZLAN & D. M. JERINA. 1989. Biochem. Biophys. Res. Commun. **163:** 1079-1085.

Potent and Selective Anti-HIV Activity of 5-Chloro-Substituted Derivatives of 3'-Azido-2',3'-Dideoxycytidine, 3'-Fluoro-2',3'-Dideoxycytidine, and 2',3'-Didehydro-2',3'-Dideoxycytidine

JAN BALZARINI, ARTHUR VAN AERSCHOT,
PIET HERDEWIJN, AND ERIK DE CLERCQ

Rega Institute for Medical Research
Katholieke Universiteit Leuven
Minderbroedersstraat 10
B-3000 Leuven, Belgium

Several 2',3'-dideoxynucleoside analogues exhibit potent and selective activity against human immunodeficiency virus (HIV) *in vitro* (for an overview, see ref. 1).

We synthesized a series of novel 5-chloro-derivatives of 3'-azido-2',3'-dideoxycytidine (AzddCyd), 3'-fluoro-2',3'-dideoxycytidine (FddCyd), and 2',3'-didehydro-2',3'-dideoxycytidine (d4Cyd) and evaluated these compounds for their antiviral activity against HIV-1 (FIG. 1, TABLE 1). The 5-chloro-substituted AzddCyd, FddCyd, and d4Cyd analogues proved inhibitory against HIV-1 replication in MT-4 cells at a 50% effective dose (ED_{50}) ranging between 9 and 26 μM, whereas their 50% cytotoxic (cytostatic) dose (CD_{50}) was considerably higher. Based on their selectivity index (ratio of CD_{50} to ED_{50}), AzddClCyd and FddClCyd could be considered as selective inhibitors of HIV-1 replication, as d4Cyd and ddCyd are more selective than d4ClCyd. The 5-chloro-substituted ddCyd derivatives were also inhibitory to HIV-2 replication in MT-4 cells.

If intracellular phosphorylation by dCyd kinase of the 5-chloro-substituted ddCyd congeners is a prerequisite for their antiretrovirus (and cytotoxic) activity, the addition of high concentrations of dCyd should prevent the biological activity of the ddCyd derivatives. Indeed, addition of 1000 μM dCyd resulted in a marked decrease of the anti-HIV activity of the 5-chloro-substituted ddCyd analogues. The K_i/K_m values of FddClCyd and AzddClCyd for MT-4 dCyd kinase were 334 and 270, respectively. This suggests a relatively poor substrate affinity for dCyd kinase. Yet, FddClCyd and AzddClCyd showed a 2- to 3-fold higher affinity for their activating enzyme than did the parent compound ddCyd.

Combination of the test compounds with tetrahydrouridine (THU) and tetrahydrodeoxyuridine (dTHU), two potent inhibitors of dCyd deaminase and dCMP deaminase,

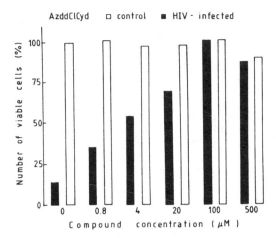

FIGURE 1. Inhibition by AzddClCyd of the cytopathic effect of HIV-1 on MT-4 cells. □, cell cultures treated with compound only. ■, cell cultures treated with compound after infection with the virus.

also resulted in a marked decrease of the antiviral activity. These findings could be explained in two ways. First, the 5-chloro-substituted ddCyd derivatives act as prodrugs and must be converted to the corresponding ddUrd analogues to exert their antiretroviral activity. Second, the antiretrovirus action of the 5-chloro-substituted ddCyd derivatives is counteracted when the intracellular pool size of dCMP, dCDP, and dCTP expands as a consequence of dCyd (dCMP) deaminase inhibition. The fact that addition of 200 μM dThd had no effect on the antiviral (or cytotoxic) effects of FddClCyd, AzddClCyd, and d4ClCyd argues against the prodrug hypothesis. Our observations thus suggest that, under our experimental conditions, the 5-chloro-ddCyd analogues do not act as prodrugs of the corresponding (deaminated) ddUrd metabolites, but may be antivirally active in their own right. The 5-chloro-substituted ddCyd derivatives

TABLE 1. Inhibitory Potency and Selectivity of 2',3'-Dideoxycytidine Analogues against HIV-1 Replication in MT-4 Cells

Compound	ED_{50} (μM)	CD_{50} (μM)	Selectivity index[a]
d4Cyd	0.13	7.9	61
d4ClCyd	22	185	8.4
AzddCyd	7.6	160	21
AzddClCyd	9	877	97
FddCyd	16	26	1.6
FddClCyd	26	> 1000	> 38

[a] Ratio of CD_{50} to ED_{50}.

should be considered as an interesting group of antivirals that should be further pursued in the treatment of AIDS.

REFERENCE

1. DE CLERCQ, E., A. VAN AERSCHOT, P. HERDEWIJN, M. BABA, R. PAUWELS & J. BALZAR-INI. 1989. Anti-HIV-1 activity of 2',3'-dideoxynucleoside analogues: structure-activity relationship. Nucleosides & Nucleotides 8: 659-671.

An Improved Sulfurization Reagent for the Synthesis of Sulfur-Containing Oligonucleotides

SERGE L. BEAUCAGE, RADHAKRISHNAN P. IYER,
WILLIAM EGAN, AND JUDITH B. REGAN

Division of Biochemistry and Biophysics
Center for Biologics Evaluation and Research
Food and Drug Administration
Bethesda, Maryland 20892

Oligodeoxynucleoside phosphorothioates are isosteric analogues of natural phospho-diesters in which one of the oxygen atoms that does not participate in the internucleo-tidic linkage is replaced by a sulfur atom.[1] This modification has enhanced the resistance of these oligonucleotides against degradation by nucleases[1] and has promoted their usefulness as "antisense" molecules in the regulation of gene expression.[2] It has been shown that phosphorothioates complementary to the messenger RNA of the HIV-1 *rev* gene inhibited the cytopathic effect of the virus in chronically infected H9 cells.[3] These results suggested that these oligonucleotides may represent a new class of thera-peutic agents. Our efforts at improving their preparation are reported herein.

The automated synthesis of phosphorothioates[4,5] according to the "deoxynucleoside phosphoramidite" approach[6] involves a stepwise sulfurization reaction effected by elemental sulfur (S_8). This reaction is slow (7.5 min)[5] and has often led to instrument failure as a result of the insolubility of S_8 in most organic solvents. To circumvent these problems, various polysulfides were tested as potential sulfur-transfer reagents. Specifically, the thiosulfonate **3**,[7] (FIG. 1) prepared in ca. 50% yield by the oxidation of the benzodithiol **1**[8] using trifluoroperoxyacetic acid,[9] was used as a 0.2 M solution in acetonitrile (MeCN) to sulfurize **4** (FIG. 2) during a period of 30 seconds. After standard deprotection, HPLC analysis indicated that **7** was generated in greater than 99% yield as a mixture of diastereoisomers.[1] Under similar conditions, a phosphoro-thioate complementary to the mRNA of the HIV-1 *rev* gene[3,a] was synthesized with a

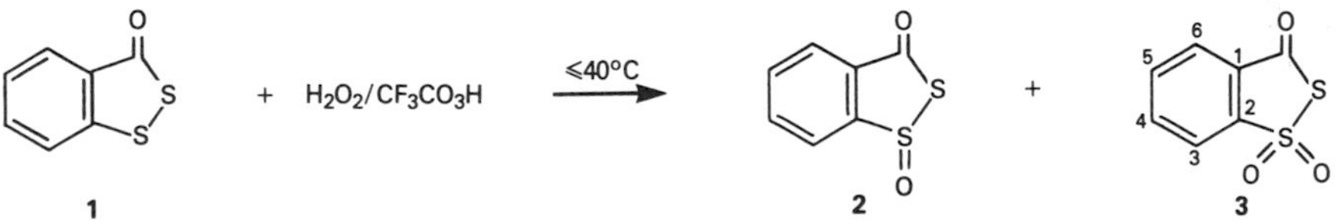

FIGURE 1.

[a] S-d(TCGTCGCTGTCTCCGCTTCTTCCTGCCA).

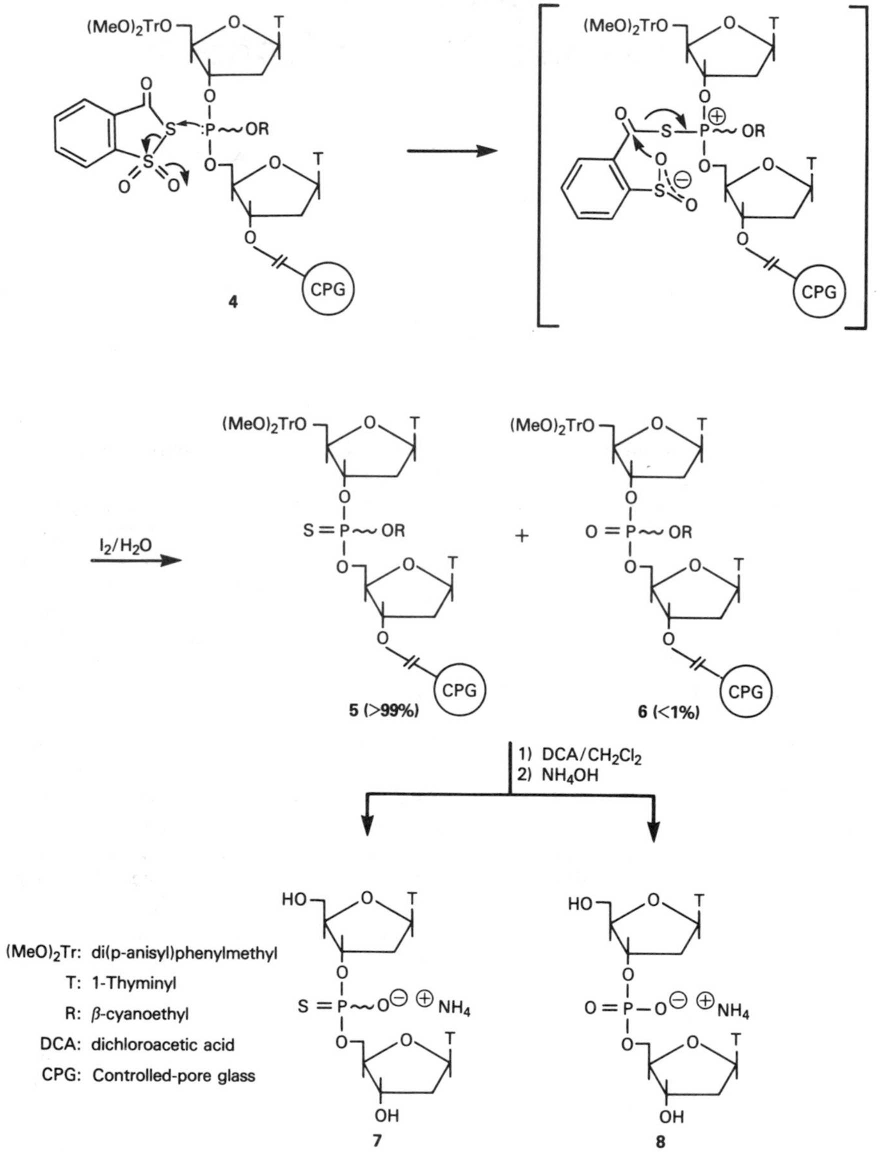

FIGURE 2. Sulfurization of a dinucleoside phosphite triester by 3*H*-1,2-benzodithiol-3-one-1,1-dioxide (3) as a model experiment to the preparation of oligodeoxynucleoside phosphorothioates.

99% stepwise yield according to "trityl color" determination. ^{31}P-NMR analysis of the fully deprotected and HPLC-purified oligonucleotide indicated that more than 96% of the resonances observed accounted for P(S) (δ 52 ppm) linkages, whereas less than 4% of the resonances corresponded to P(O) (δ -4 ppm) linkages. A similar oligomer bearing only two P(S) linkages at predetermined positions was also prepared.[b] ^{31}P-NMR analysis of the purified oligomer displayed the proper P(S) resonances in correct integrated ratio relative to the P(O) resonances.

Finally, a random DNA sequence[c] bearing exclusively P(O) linkages and equal numbers of the four nucleosidic bases was synthesized to assess potential nucleosidic modification during the sulfurization step. The fully protected oligomer covalently attached to the solid support was incubated with a 0.2 M solution of 3 in MeCN for 24 h at ambient temperature. After deprotection and purification, the oligomer was subjected to enzymatic degradation with snake venom phosphodiesterase and alkaline phosphatase. No evidence of nucleosidic base modification was detected from HPLC analysis of the hydrolysates, as only peaks corresponding to the four nucleosides were observed.

We have demonstrated that because of its rapid sulfurization kinetics, high efficiency, and facile automation, the thiosulfonate 3 is a superior reagent relative to S_8 for the preparation of oligodeoxynucleoside phosphorothioates by way of the phosphoramidite approach. One can then speculate that this technology may become the method of choice for the large-scale preparation of oligodeoxynucleoside phosphorothioates required for therapeutic applications.

REFERENCES

1. ECKSTEIN, F. 1985. Ann. Rev. Biochem. **54:** 367-402.
2. STEIN, C. A. & J. S. COHEN. 1988. Cancer Res. **48:** 2659-2668.
3. MATSUKURA, M., G. ZON, K SHINOZUKA, M. ROBERT-GUROFF, T. SHIMADA, C. A. STEIN, H. MITSUYA, F. WONG-STAAL, J. S. COHEN & S. BRODER. 1989. Proc. Natl. Acad. Sci. USA **86:** 4244-4248.
4. STEC, W. J., G. ZON, W. EGAN & B. STEC. 1984. J. Am. Chem. Soc. **106:** 6077-6079.
5. STEIN, C. A., C. SUBASINGHE, K. SHINOZUKA & J. S. COHEN. 1988. Nucleic Acids Res. **16:** 3209-3221.
6. BEAUCAGE, S. L. & M. H. CARUTHERS. 1981. Tetrahedron Lett. **22:** 1859-1862.
7. HORTMANN, A. G., A. J. ARON & A. K. BHATTACHARYA. 1978. J. Org. Chem. **43:** 3374-3378.
8. McKIBBEN, M. & E. W. McCLELLAND. 1923. J. Chem. Soc. 170-173.
9. VENIER, C. G., T. G. SQUIRES, Y-Y. CHEN, G. P. HUSSMANN, J. C. SHFI & B. F. SMITH. 1982. J. Org. Chem. **47:** 3773-3774.

[b] d(T_{PS}CGTCGCTGTCTCCGCTTCTTCCTGCC_{PS}A).
[c] d(TACCGTAGCTAAGGTCATGCAAGTTCCG).

Therapeutic Activity of Reverse Transcriptase Inhibitors in Murine Retrovirus Models[a]

PAUL L. BLACK,[b,e] MICHAEL A. USSERY,[c]
JAMES T. RANKIN JR.,[d] AND
MICHAEL A. CHIRIGOS [d]

[b]Southern Research Institute-Frederick Research Center
Frederick, Maryland 21701

[c]Food and Drug Administration
Rockville, Maryland 20857

[d]USAMRIID, Fort Detrick
Frederick, Maryland 21702

The Rauscher murine leukemia virus (RLV) has served as a primary *in vivo* model for screening of potential antiretroviral agents and biological response modifiers against human immunodeficiency virus (HIV). Infection of BALB/c female mice (4–6 weeks of age) with RLV rapidly produced splenomegaly, viremia, and hypergammaglobulinemia, all of which have been used as measures of disease progression. This murine retrovirus model has predictive value only for agents that act on viral or cellular functions common to both RLV and HIV, for example, reverse transcriptase (RT) inhibitors. 3'-Azido-3'-deoxythymidine (AZT) and 2',3'-dideoxycytidine (ddC), two RT inhibitors with established activity against HIV, provided a test of the validity of the RLV model. Both of these agents typically have shown therapeutic indexes (TI) of > 333 *in vitro* in repeated tests against HIV with MT-2 cells and against RLV by plaque inhibition in a UV-XC assay (TABLE 1). AZT had slightly better anti-HIV activity *in vitro* than did ddC, but AZT was much more active (TI > 10^6) than ddC against RLV *in vitro*. Similarly, AZT had antiviral activity in the RLV murine model *in vivo* at lower doses than ddC (FIG. 1), with AZT active at ≥ 30 mg/kg (qd, ip) and ddC active at ≥ 300 mg/kg (qd, ip). At the maximum tested doses of each, however, ddC had much greater antiviral activity than did AZT. At a dose of 100 mg/kg daily, AZT reduced viremia by approximately 10- to 30-fold (FIGURES 1 and 2), whereas ddC at 1000 mg/kg daily reduced viremia by > 10,000-fold (FIG. 2). Dose responses for ddI both *in vivo* and *in vitro* were almost identical to those for ddC.

The antiviral activity of AZT in the RLV model *in vivo* depended critically on schedule of administration. AZT was most effective when treatment was initiated prophylactically (20 h before virus inoculation) and became progressively less effective as the onset of treatment was delayed (FIG. 2). By contrast, both ddC and ribavirin retained much of their antiviral activity even when treatment did not begin until seven

[a]This research was supported in part by NCDDG 1U01AI25617-01 from NIAID.
[e]Address for correspondence: SRI-FRC, 431 Aviation Way, Frederick, MD 21701.

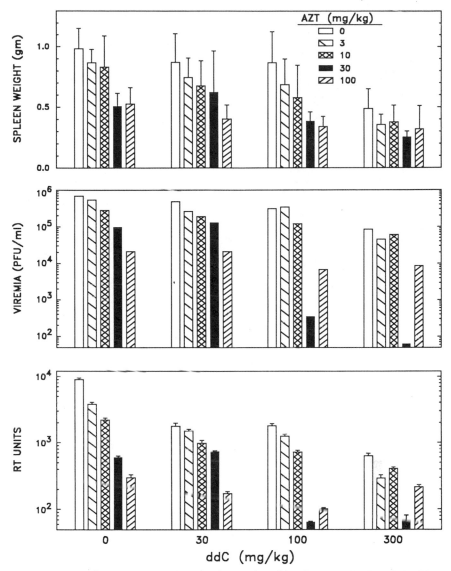

FIGURE 1. Combined treatment of RLV-infected mice with AZT and ddC. Female BALB/c mice, four to six weeks of age, were inoculated ip with RLV (approximately 10^5 plaque-forming units (PFU) as a cell-free splenic homogenate from infected mice) on day 0. Mice were treated ip daily from day −1 through day 13, and they were euthanized on day 14. Spleens were removed and weighed (top panel). Viremia was measured in serum by a UV-XC assay and is expressed as PFU/mL of serum (middle panel). RT activity in serum (bottom panel) was determined by incorporation of [^{3}H]dTTP into DNA using an oligo rAdT primer. RT units are expressed as picomoles of dTTP incorporated in 1 h by 1 mL of serum, and sera from uninfected mice had RT levels of <100 units.

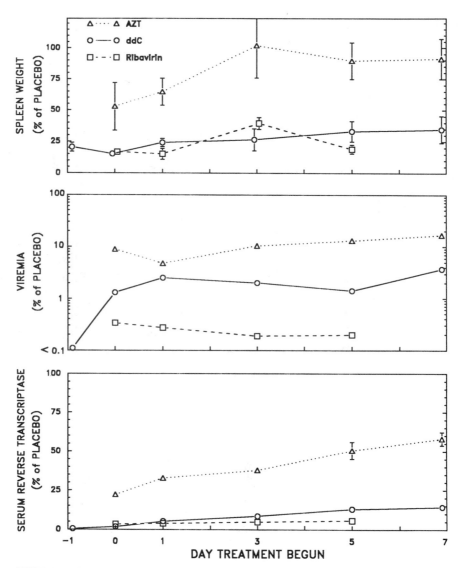

FIGURE 2. Effect of delaying the initiation of treatment with AZT, ddC, or ribavirin. Mice were infected with RLV as described in FIG. 1. Daily treatment by the ip route with AZT (100 mg/kg), ddC (1000 mg/kg), or ribavirin (100 mg/kg) was begun on the indicated days and continued through day 13. Mice were euthanized on day 14, and assays were performed as described in FIG. 1. Results are expressed as percent of placebo values so that different experiments can be compared. Placebo values for the experiments in FIG. 2 were as follows: spleen weight, 1.27 ($\pm$0.186) g for AZT and ribavirin and 0.98 ($\pm$0.171) g for ddC; viremia, 4.8 $\times$ 10^6 PFU/mL for AZT and ribavirin and 6.9 $\times$ 10^5 PFU/mL for ddC; RT, 6690 ($\pm$622) units for AZT and ribavirin and 8960 ($\pm$555) units for ddC.

days after virus inoculation (FIG. 2), by which time productive virus infection was well established. Therefore, in the RLV model ddC and ribavirin demonstrated therapeutic antiviral activity in addition to prophylactic activity. For both AZT and ribavirin, however, the frequency of drug administration determined efficacy. Treatment at least once a day was required for AZT, whereas ribavirin still had some activity if given every other day (data not shown).

Additionally, combined treatment with suboptimal doses of AZT and ddC improved antiviral activity (FIG. 1). This combination effect was most evident at the two higher doses of AZT (30 and 100 mg/kg). For example, the combination of ddC at 100 mg/kg, a dose that by itself had virtually no antiviral activity, with either of the

TABLE 1. *In Vitro* Tests of Antiviral Activity

Drug	Virus	ID_{50}[a] (μg/mL)	MTC_{50}[b] (μg/mL)	TI[c]
AZT	HIV	< 0.01	> 100	> 10^4
ddC	HIV	< 0.1	> 100	> 10^3
AZT	RLV	< 0.001	> 1000	> 10^6
ddC	RLV	1–3	> 1000	> 333
ddI	RLV	3	> 1000	> 333

[a] ID_{50} = dose producing 50% inhibition of virus production.
[b] MTC_{50} = dose producing 50% toxicity in uninfected cells.
[c] TI = MTC_{50}/ID_{50}.

two higher doses of AZT markedly reduced splenomegaly, viremia, and serum reverse transcriptase levels (FIG. 1). When splenomegaly was analyzed by the general linear models procedure using SAS statistical software (SAS Institute, Carg, NC), these combination effects were additive, not synergistic.

These results permit a comparison of *in vivo* murine screening models with clinical data. AZT, ddC, ddI, and ribavirin have all shown antiretroviral activity in the RLV model *in vivo*. AZT has been approved for the treatment of AIDS, and ddC and ddI have shown anti-HIV activity in clinical trials. Ribavirin, on the other hand, has not shown clinical activity consistent with its anti-RLV activity *in vivo*.

COMBO: A New Approach to the Analysis of Drug Combinations *in Vitro*[a]

BARRY BUNOW[b] AND JOHN N. WEINSTEIN[c]

[b]*Civilized Software, Inc.*
Bethesda, Maryland 20814

[c]*National Cancer Institute*
Bethesda, Maryland 20892

Combination chemotherapy has been a staple of cancer treatment for many years. Inasmuch as currently available agents for HIV infection are toxic, the idea of combination chemotherapy has become prominent in this field as well. The first step is generally to analyze candidate pairs of drugs for interaction *in vitro;* the median effect analysis of Chou and Talalay[1] has been useful for this purpose.

Our own investigation of several drug pairs for use against HIV infection[2] led us to develop a new approach to the analysis of data from experiments on combinations. We began by exploring enzyme kinetics-based models for drug interaction and found a number of them that appear particularly useful for analyzing this class of data. These models are all elaborations of the logistic dose-response curve that frequently characterizes the behavior of single drug assay systems. As indicated in FIGURE 1 (left panel), the single-drug logistic curve is characterized by four parameters: the zero-dose response (A), the high-dose response (D), the midpoint dose (*e.g.* the EC_{50}), and the midpoint slope (B).

With two drugs, the essential idea is to extend the logistic curve into an extra dimension (FIG. 1, right panel) to accommodate the second drug. Assuming no interaction, there are two new parameters, the midpoint dose and slope for drug 2. This is a variant of the isobologram (*e.g.* Berenbaum,[3] and Syracuse and Greco[4]). Assuming interaction, there are one or more additional parameters, and we refer to this as the "robust potentiation" model.

In precise analogy to the usual isobologram, the surface of effect as a function of dose of the two drugs can be viewed conveniently by plotting isoeffect contours. The right panel of FIGURE 2 shows such contours for additivity. The left panel of FIGURE 2 shows contours obtained from an experiment by R.F. Schinazi on reverse transcriptase production in stimulated T lymphocytes using the drug combination AZT-dipyridamole. The data were fitted to a modification of the robust potentiation model that contains two interaction parameters. The inward bowing of the isoeffect contours indicates potentiation of AZT by dipyridamole.

It is important to be able to quantitate drug interactions such as the potentiation shown in FIGURE 2 (left panel) and to determine confidence intervals for the parame-

[a]Partial support for this work came from the NIH Intramural Targeted AIDS Antiviral Program.

490

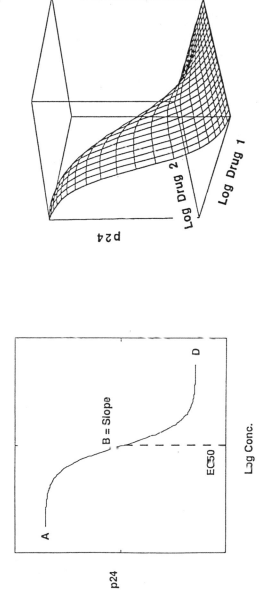

FIGURE 1. (Left panel) Logistic dependence of response to a single drug, showing zero dose response (A), high dose response (D), mideffect dose (EC_{50}), and mideffect slope (B). (Right panel) Surface of additivity; generalization of the logistic to two-drug combination.

ter(s) of interaction. To do this, we have developed an iteratively reweighted nonlinear least squares algorithm for fitting experimental data on drug combinations. Weights are computed by gaussian windowing techniques based on estimated response. Monte Carlo resampling methods related to those of Efron[5] are used to estimate confidence intervals for the best-fitting parameters. The results of the analysis may be displayed in several graphical formats, including those of FIGURE 2. Statistical summaries of the curve fits can be displayed in graphical and/or tabular form. Statistical diagnostics available include the weighted sum of squares, normal theory standard error estimates, variance-covariance matrix, parameter dependency values, root mean square weighted deviation errors, mean deviation/data fraction, residuals, and weighted residuals. The prototype program package COMBO developed to perform this analysis operates in the MLAB computing environment (Civilized Software, Inc.) and can be used on IBM-compatible personal computers.

COMBO offers the following features: (1) constant drug dose ratios are not necessary; (2) efficacy and toxicity can be analyzed simultaneously; (3) all data can be used without exclusion of points near 0 and 100% effect; (4) global parameters for potentiation, synergy, and antagonism are obtained; (5) a flexible choice of data models (which may be further generalized by the user if desired) is provided; (6) a flexible choice of error structures is provided, including automatic detection from the data itself; (7) confidence intervals on model parameters are obtained by Monte Carlo methods; and (8) statistical criteria for selection of outliers are generated.

Potential weaknesses of the approach: (1) it is computer-intensive, especially for confidence interval estimation, and (2) the assumption of global interaction parameters may not always be appropriate. This latter problem, however, can be circumvented by options available in COMBO.

We have used COMBO to evaluate data from several different laboratories and on several different drug combinations. In particular, analysis using COMBO has quantified the potentiation by dipyridamole of a number of nucleoside analogues (see also Szebeni *et al.* and Weinstein *et al.*, this volume). In simultaneous analysis of efficacy and toxicity by what we term the "eff-tox" model, dipyridamole was found both to

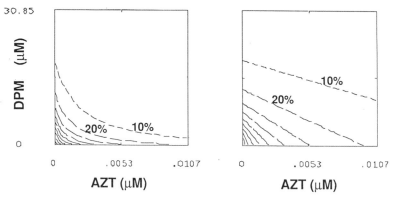

FIGURE 2. (Right panel) Isoeffect contours for additivity (null hypothesis). (Left panel) Isoeffect contours obtained by curve fitting to experimental data. Inward bowing of the contours indicates potentiation, in this case of AZT by dipyridamole. Fits to experimental studies of R.F. Schinazi (see Weinstein *et al.*, this volume, for details and fitting equations).

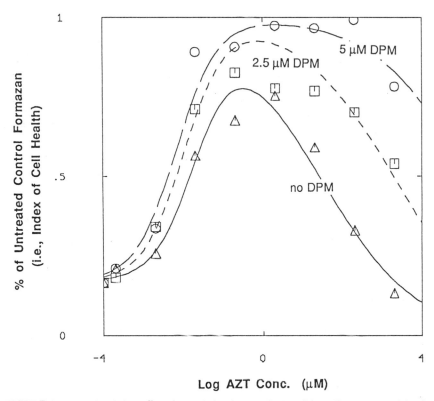

FIGURE 3. Curve fit of the "eff-tox" model simultaneously describing efficacy and toxicity for the drug combination AZT-dipyridamole. The FIGURE shows that in cultured cells dipyridamole both potentiates the anti-HIV effect of AZT and decreases the cellular toxicity of AZT. The assay[6] was based on colorimetric analysis of formazan dye produced by healthy cells. Information from experimental studies in collaboration with J. Szebeni and O.S. Weislow (manuscript in preparation). See Weinstein et al., this volume, for details and fitting equations.

potentiate the antiviral effect of AZT and to decrease the cellular toxicity of AZT for CEM T-lymphoblastoid cells, as shown in FIGURE 3 (manuscript in preparation). See Weinstein et al. (this volume) for fitting equations and definitions.

ACKNOWLEDGMENTS

We gratefully acknowledge Larry R. Muenz, for advice on the statistics, and J. Szebeni, R. F. Schinazi, and O. S. Weislow for experimental data.

REFERENCES

1. CHOU, T-C. & P. TALALAY. 1984. Adv. Enzyme Regul. **22:** 27-55.
2. SZEBENI, J., S. M. WAHL, M. POPOVIC, L. M. WAHL, S. GARTNER, R. L. FINE, U. SKALERIC, R. M. FRIEDMAN & J. N. WEINSTEIN. 1989. Proc. Natl. Acad. Sci. USA **86:** 3842-3846.
3. BERENBAUM, M.C. 1978. J. Infect. Dis. **137:** 122-130.
4. SYRACUSE, K. C. & W. R. GRECO. 1986. Proc. Biopharm. Sec. Am. Stat. Assoc. 127-132.
5. EFRON, B. D. 1979. Ann. Stat. **7:** 1-26.
6. WEISLOW, O. S., R. KISER, D. L. FINE, J. BADER, R. H. SHOEMAKER & M. R. BOYD. 1989. J. Natl. Cancer Inst. **81:** 577-586.

Brain Targeting of Anti-HIV Nucleosides

Synthesis and *in Vivo* Studies of Dihydronicotinyl Derivatives of AzddU (AZDU or CS-87) and AZT[a]

C. K. CHU, V. S. BHADTI, K. J. DOSHI, J. T. ETSE,
J. M. GALLO, F. D. BOUDINOT, AND
R. F. SCHINAZI [b]

*Department of Medicinal Chemistry and Pharmacognosy
and Department of Pharmaceutics
College of Pharmacy
The University of Georgia
Athens, Georgia 30602*

[b]*Department of Pediatrics
Emory University School of Medicine and
The VA Medical Center
Atlanta, Georgia 30033*

Patients with acquired immunodeficiency syndrome (AIDS) and AIDS-related complex frequently develop neurological complications due to the human immunodeficiency virus (HIV) infection in the brain.[1,2] Although the mechanism of HIV-induced CNS dysfunction is unknown, it is believed that HIV is carried into the brain by infected macrophages/monocytes.[3] Thus, it is essential that anti-HIV agents cross the blood-brain barrier (BBB) to suppress the viral replication in the brain. 3'-Azido-3'-deoxythymidine (AZT) has been demonstrated to penetrate into cerebrospinal fluid and partially reverse the neurological complications.[4,5] It has not been demonstrated, however, that AZT actually crosses the BBB or maintains the sufficient concentration in CNS by which it would be able to effectively suppress the viral replication in the brain.[6] Thus, it was of interest to develop antiviral prodrugs which could more readily penetrate the BBB than do the parent nucleosides. We have chosen two anti-HIV nucleosides, AZT and AzddU (AZDU, or CS-87). The latter is a compound of which anti-HIV activity was discovered in our laboratories,[7,8] and it is currently undergoing phase I clinical trials.

Among various methods of brain targeting of drugs, Bodor and co-workers' strategy[9] seems to be attractive. The approach uses a dihydropyridine-pyridinium salt redox

[a]This work was supported by U.S. Public Service Grants AI 25899 and AI 26055, and the Veterans Administration.

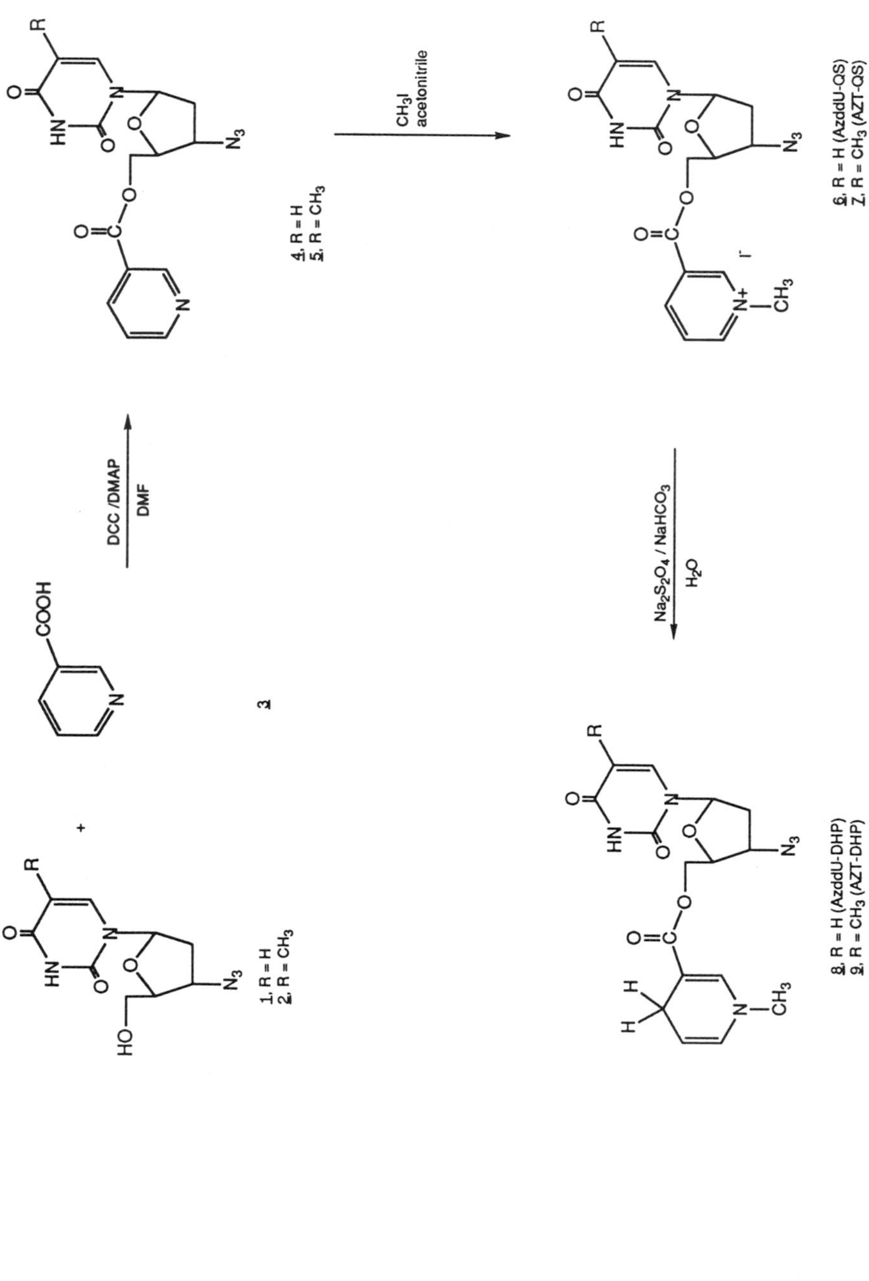
1, R = H
2, R = CH3
3
DCC /DMAP
DMF
4, R = H
5, R = CH3
CH3I
acetonitrile
6, R = H (AzddU-QS)
7, R = CH3 (AZT-QS)
Na2S2O4 / NaHCO3
H2O
8, R = H (AzddU-DHP)
9, R = CH3 (AZT-DHP)

SCHEME 1.

TABLE 1. Areas under the Serum and Brain Concentration-Time Curves (AUC) for Prodrugs, Quaternary Salts, and Parent Compounds after Administration of AZT-DHP and AzddU-DHP in Comparison to AzddU and AZT

Compound	AUC μg h/mL	
	Serum	Brain
AzddU-DHP	4.4	—
AzddU-QS (from AzddU-DHP)	1.2	3.9
AzddU (from AzddU-DHP)	25.8	11.4
AzddU (administered itself)	25.8	2.1
AZT-DHP	1.3	—
AZT-QS (from AZT-DHP)	0.6	1.2
AZT (from AZT-DHP)	25.4	11.2
AZT (administered itself)	26.6	1.2

system. Thus, dihydropyridine (DHP) derivatives of AzddU and AZT were synthesized as shown in SCHEME 1. The AzddU and AZT DHP derivatives *8* and *9* show the greatest stability in human serum, followed by mouse serum and brain homogenate. The extended half-lives of DHP derivatives in human serum (>4 h) would allow sufficient time to cross the BBB in humans. The *in vitro* degradation rates for the AzddU derivative *8* are higher than the corresponding reactions for the AZT derivative *9*. The studies of *8* and *9* in mice are shown in TABLE 1. The data suggest that DHP derivatives disappear rapidly from the mouse serum and brain as suggested by the *in vitro* data. Brain concentrations of the quaternary salt (QS) species could be measured for up to 2 h for AzddU-QS and up to 6 h for AZT-QS. The area under the curve (AUC) in serum for AzddU following prodrug administration is 25.8 μg·h/mL and 25.8 μg·h/mL for AzddU when it is administered. Analogously, the serum AUCs for AZT, when prodrug and parent compounds are administered, are 25.4 μg·h/mL and 26.6 μg·h/mL, respectively. The brain AUCs, however, for both AzddU and AZT derived from prodrug, being 11.4 μg·h/mL and 11.3 μg·h/mL, respectively, are greater than the brain AUCs for AzddU (2.1 μg·h/mL) and AZT (1.2 μg·h/mL) when the parent drugs are administered.

TABLE 2 shows the relative brain exposure (r_e) and apparent brain half-lives for AzddU and AZT. The r_e value of 5.5 for AzddU and 9.3 for AZT indicate a significant increase in exposure to these compounds following prodrug administrations. The

TABLE 2. Relative Brain Exposure (r_e) Values and Apparent Brain Elimination Half-lives ($t_{1/2}$) for AzddU and AZT

Compound	r_e[a]	$t_{1/2}$ (h)
AzddU (prodrug administered)	5.47	4.34
AzddU (administered itself)	—	0.84
AZT (prodrug administered)	9.32	15.8
AZT (administered itself)	—	0.54

[a] $r_e = (AUC)_{pd \to p}/(AUC)_p$; r_e values greater than one indicate favorable brain delivery of the parent nucleosides following prodrug administration. pd = prodrug; p = parent drug.

greater octanol/water partition coefficients of DHP derivatives (21.6 and 53.1 for AzddU-DHP and AZT-DHP, respectively) relative to the parent compounds (0.45 and 1.10 for AzddU and AZT, respectively) are consistent with the notion that the lipophilic DHP derivatives penetrate the BBB more readily than do the parent compounds. Comparison of the parent brain half-lives for AzddU (4.3 h vs 0.8 h) following prodrug administration indicates an increased retention of each compound in the brain following prodrug administration compared to the values obtained for parent drug.

Optimizing brain delivery of anti-HIV agents is an important criteria for successful treatment of AIDS. It appears that the chemical delivery system designed by Bodor *et al.* does work to a reasonable extent in mice. Certainly, similar CSF uptake studies are warranted in larger animals.

REFERENCES

1. KENNEDY, P. G. E. 1988. Postgrad. Med. J. **64:** 180 (a review).
2. BUDKA, H. 1989. Acta Neuropathol. **77:** 225. (a review).
3. HO, D. D., J. R. ROTA & M. S. HIRSCH. 1986. J. Clin. Invest. **77:** 1712.
4. FIALA, M., L. A. CONE, N. COHEN, D. PATEL, K. WILLIAMS, D. CASAREALE, P. SHAPSHOK & W. TOURTELOTTE. 1988. Rev. Infect. Dis. **10:** 250.
5. BRUNETTI, A., G. BERG, G. DI CHIRO, R. M. COHEN, R. YARCHOAN, P. A. PIZZO, S. BRODER, J. EDDY, M. J. FULHAM, R. D. FINN & S. M. LARSON. 1989. Clin. Sci. **30:** 581.
6. WEISBERG, L. A. & W. ROSS. 1989. Postgrad. Med. **86:** 213.
7. CHU, C. K., R. F. SCHINAZI, M. K. AHN, G. V. ULLAS & Z. P. GU. 1989. J. Med. Chem. **32:** 612.
8. ERIKSSON, B. F. H., C. K. CHU & R. F. SCHINAZI. 1989. Antimicrob. Agents Chemother. **33:** 1729.
9. BODOR, N., H. H. FARAG & M. E. BREWSTER. 1981. Science **214:** 1370.

Synthesis and Evaluation of a Triphenylcarbinol Related to the Incorrectly Assumed Structure of Aurintricarboxylic Acid[a]

MARK CUSHMAN AND
SUSEELA KANAMATHAREDDY

Department of Medicinal Chemistry and Pharmacognosy
Purdue University
West Lafayette, Indiana 47907

Treatment of a mixture of salicylic acid and formaldehyde with sulfuric acid and sodium nitrite results in the formation of a solid substance known as aurintricarboxylic acid (ATA).[1] This material was originally believed to have the triphenylmethane dye structure 1, and this structure has persisted in the current literature even though previous studies reported by González, Blackburn, and Schleich seem to indicate quite clearly that ATA is actually a heterogeneous mixture of polymers, which they represented schematically as structure 2.[2]

It was recently demonstrated that ATA prevents the cytopathic effect of HIV-1 in an ATH8 cell culture, as well as the expression of p24 in H9 cells infected with HIV-1; and it has been suggested that this effect may be due to the inhibition of HIV-1 reverse transcriptase[3] and/or to the blockade of the HIV/CD4 cell receptor.[4] In addition, it has been reported that the authentic triphenylmethane dye fuchsin acid, as well as ATA, inhibits the cytopathic affect of HIV-1 in MT-4 cells.[5] A variety of triphenylmethane-related dyes sharing the same skeletal structure as 1 have also been reported to inhibit Raucher leukemia virus reverse transcriptase.[6] These results pose the question of whether or not a compound having the commonly accepted, incorrect structure 1 of ATA would have any potential as an anti-AIDS agent. In order to answer the latter question, as well as to gain further insight into the true chemical nature of ATA, a synthesis of the compound having structure 1 was attempted.

A three-step synthesis that gave the triphenylcarbinol 6 was devised, as depicted in SCHEME 1. This is the covalent hydrate of the hypothetical structure 1, which we could not obtain under various conditions. In preliminary screening at the National Cancer Institute, compounds 6 and 8 were found to reproducibly afford high levels of protection (89% and 112% at 164 and 144 μg/mL, respectively) against the cytopathic effect of HIV-1 in CEM cells in culture, with little or no evidence of cytotoxicity to the cells. In comparison, ATA polymer 2 afforded complete protection at around 10 μg/mL, with little or no accompanying cytotoxicity. Both the trimethyl ester 7 and methylenedisalicylic acid 5 were inactive. Synthesis and comparison of biologically active structural analogues of 6 are in progress and will be reported.

[a]This research was supported by NCI, DHHS NO1-CM-87268 and NO1-CM-67699.

Two methods for the synthesis of ATA have been reported in the literature. One involves the previously mentioned treatment of salicylic acid with formaldehyde, sulfuric acid, and sodium nitrite.[1] The other involves the oxidative condensation of supposedly pure methylenedisalicylic acid with salicylic acid, which was claimed by Smith *et al.* to give pure ATA (structure 1).[7] The methylenedisalicylic acid used by Smith, however, was later shown to be a mixture of 6-8 components,[8] and a resynthesis of ATA by the method of Smith was shown to give at least eight products.[9] The present work demonstrates that the oxidative condensation of methylenedisalicylic acid with salicylic acid in fact gives the covalent hydrate of the incorrect structure of ATA. It also points out the fact that the incorrect structure 1 of ATA is not only incorrect in the sense that it does not represent the true structure of ATA, but it is also incorrect in the sense that the substance does not exist in the quinone methide form 1: it exists as the covalent hydrate 6.

The present work is also in agreement with the polymeric structure of ATA as indicated by the previous work of González, Blackburn, and Schleich.[2] Comparison of the properties of 6 with those of ATA verifies that they are not the same substance.

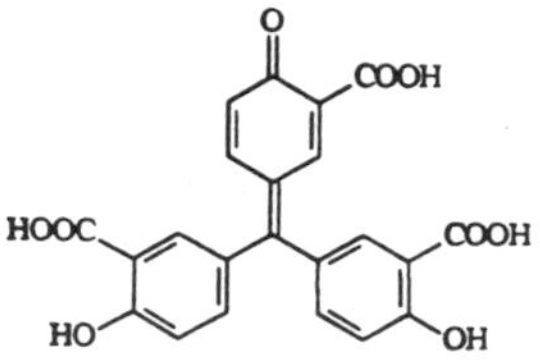

1

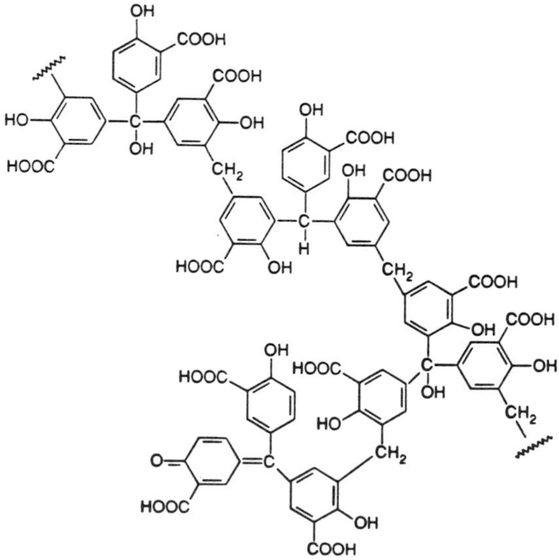

2

STRUCTURES 1 and 2.

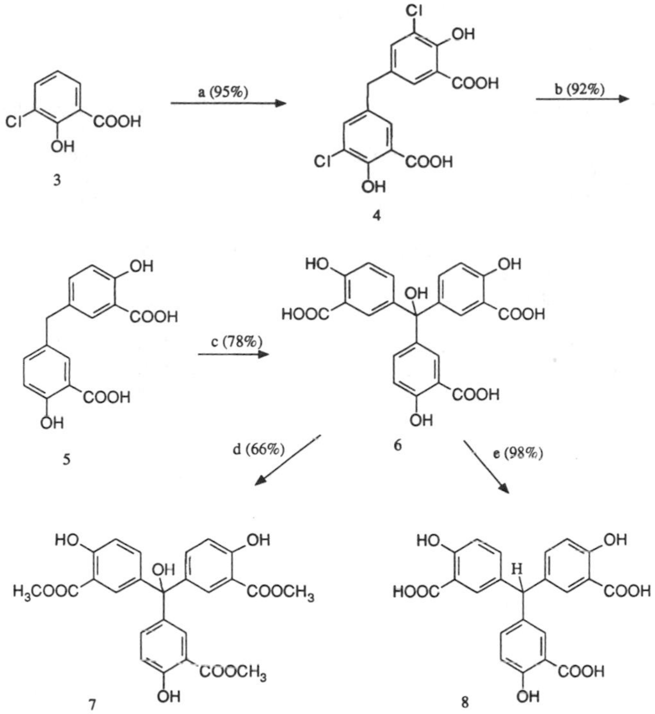

SCHEME 1. a, H_2SO_4, CH_2O, $-5°$ C to $0°$ C (2 h), room temperature (24 h); b, H_2, palladium on charcoal Pd/C (10%), EtOH, Et_3N, room temperature (48 h); c, salicylic acid, H_2SO_4, NaONO, room temperature (24 h); d, diazomethane, Et_2O, $5°$ C (48 h); e, H_2 (80 psi), Pd/C (10%), EtOH, room temperature (72 h).

Our preliminary work on the gel permeation chromatography (gpc) of ATA definitely shows that it is a very complex, heterogeneous mixture of polymers, and that there is very little, if any, triphenylcarbinol **6** present in ATA, which is also in agreement with the previously reported study.[2] Further work on the fractionation of ATA is in progress.

Whereas ATA prevents the binding of the OKT4A monoclonal antibody to the CD4 receptor and inhibits HIV-1 reverse transcriptase, both **6** and **8** do not. It therefore appears that the substances prepared in this study that prevent the cytopathic affect of HIV in cell cultures are not acting by the same mechanism(s) of action as ATA but are instead acting by an as yet unidentified mechanism. In this sense, the low molecular weight ATA monomer analogues prepared in this study provided a new lead, distinct from polymeric ATA, for further anti-HIV drug development.

ACKNOWLEDGMENTS

We are grateful to Dr. Edward M. Acton, Dr. Rudiger D. Haugwitz, and Dr. Ven L. Narayanan, NCI, for helpful discussions.

REFERENCES

1. CARO, N. 1892. Ber. **25:** 939.
2. GONZÁLEZ, R. G., B. J. BLACKBURN & T. SCHLEICH. 1979. Biochim. Biophys. Acta **562:** 534.
3. BALZARINI, J., H. MITSUYA, E. DE CLERQ & S. BRODER. 1988. Biochem. Biophys. Res. Commun. **136:** 64.
4. SCHOLS, D., M. BABA, R. PAUWELS, J. DESMYTER & E. DE CLERQ. 1989. Proc. Natl. Acad. Sci. USA **86:** 3322.
5. BABA, M., D. SCHOLS, R. PAUWELS, J. BALZARINI & E. DE CLERQ. 1988. Biochem. Biophys. Res. Commun. **155:** 1404.
6. LIAO, L.-L., S. B. HORWITZ, M.-T. HUANG, A. P. GROLLMAN, D. STEWARD & J. MARTIN. 1975. J. Med. Chem. **18:** 117.
7. SMITH, M. H., E. E. SAGER & I. J. SIEWERS. 1949. Anal. Chem. **21:** 1334.
8. DAVISON, C. & R. T. WILLIAMS 1968. J. Pharm. Pharmacol. **20:** 12.
9. TSUTSUI, K., S. SEKI, K. TSUTSUI & T. ODA. 1978. Biochem. Biophys. Acta **177:** 91.

An Approach to the Synthesis of HIV Protease Inhibitors

Stereochemically Pure Peptide Substrate Analogues Containing [Phe-ΨCH₂N-Pro] Linkages[a]

MARK CUSHMAN,[b] YOUNG-IM OH,[b]
TERRY D. COPELAND,[c] STUART W. SNYDER,[c] AND
STEPHEN OROSZLAN[c]

[b]Department of Medicinal Chemistry and Pharmacognosy
Purdue University
West Lafayette, Indiana 47907

[c]Laboratory of Molecular Virology and Carcinogenesis
BRI-Basic Research Program
NCI-Frederick Cancer Research Facility
Frederick, Maryland 21701

HIV-1 and HIV-2 proteases cleave the gag and pol precursor polyproteins into the functional proteins of the mature viruses. *In vitro* mutagenesis that produces protease-defective virus results in the formation of uninfective, immature forms of the virus.[1,2] Therefore, inhibition of the protease constitutes a rational strategy for the development of potential anti-AIDS agents.

A highly conserved cleavage site of retroviral polyproteins is between Tyr or Phe and Pro. It is also known that relatively small peptide fragments containing the cleavage sites of the gag and pol polyproteins are substrates for HIV protease.

Because HIV protease is an aspartic protease, initial studies on the design and synthesis of potential HIV protease inhibitors have taken advantage of the fact that there is a large body of information available on the design and synthesis of inhibitors of proteases of this class, including renin. The basic strategy is to replace the cleaved amide bond in a minimum peptide substrate with a noncleavable moiety that is isosteric with the transition state of the enzymatic hydrolysis reaction. One possibility that is presently being investigated is the aminomethylene (-CH₂NH-) isostere.[3,4]

A general method for the introduction of aminomethylene (-CH₂NH-) linkages into peptides involves the reductive alkylation of an amine with an aldehyde in the presence of sodium cyanoborohydride.[5] BOC-L-phenylalaninal (1) was added to the resin-bound proline in *N,N*-dimethylformamide (DMF) containing 1% acetic acid followed by

[a]This research was supported, in part, by NCI, DHHS NO1-CM-87268, and also by NCI, DHHS, NO1-CO-74101 with BRI.

BOC-Phe-CHO   +   ProIleSer(OBzl)-OResin $\xrightarrow[\text{1\% AcOH}]{\text{NaBH}_3\text{CN, DMF}}$

   1   **2**

BOC-Phe-ψCH$_2$N-ProIleSer(OBzl)-OResin $\xrightarrow[\text{3. HF}]{\substack{\text{1. TFA}\\\text{2. ABI Synthesizer}}}$

                3

ThrLeuAsnPhe-ψCH$_2$N-ProIleSer

   4

SCHEME 1.

sodium cyanoborohydride to give the resin **3**. The peptide resin **3** was deprotected, and the ThrLeuAsn segment was added automatically on the peptide synthesizer. The peptide ThrLeuAsnPhe-ψCH$_2$N-ProIleSer (**4**) was cleaved from the resin using anhydrous hydrofluoric acid (HF) (SCHEME 1). Using this methodology, the peptide Leu-AsnPhe-ψCH$_2$N-ProIle (**18**) (TABLE 1) was also prepared. In both cases, the crude peptides were contaminated by diastereomers, which prevented a certain configurational assignment and complicated the purification process (FIGURE 1). An investigation of this problem led to the conclusion that racemization during aldehyde synthesis[6] was not the sole cause of diastereomer formation inasmuch as the diastereomeric ratio of the peptides (D-Phe/L-Phe) was always higher than the corresponding enantiomeric ratio of the aldehyde. A possible explanation might be that proline, being a secondary amine, forms an enamine intermediate (upon its reaction with the aldehyde), which results in loss of chirality in the phenylalanine residue (SCHEME 2).

Alternatively, a stereochemically pure reduced dipeptide derivative BOC-PheψCH$_2$N-Pro-OH (**9**) was synthesized (SCHEME 3) and incorporated into the peptide chain (SCHEME 4). Proline methyl ester hydrochloride **6a** was reacted with BOC-L-phenylalanine and benzotriazolyloxytris(dimethylamino)-phosphonium hexafluorophosphate (BOP) to give the dipeptide **7a**, which was reduced with diborane in tetrahydrofuran to the dipeptide **8a**.[7] In a parallel sequence, the dipeptide BOC-D-Phe-ψCH$_2$N-Pro-OMe was prepared from BOC-D-phenylalanine and proline methyl ester hydrochloride. HPLC analysis of both BOC-L-Phe-ψCH$_2$N-Pro-OMe **8a**

TABLE 1. Inhibition of HIV-1 Protease by Reduced Peptide Analogues

Inhibitor		Concentration μg/mL	Percent Inhibition[a]
Phe-ψCH$_2$N-Pro-OBz	**14**	250	inactive
Phe-ψCH$_2$N-Pro	**15**	250	inactive
Phe-ψCH$_2$N-ProIleSer	**12**	250	20
AsnPhe-ψCH$_2$N-ProIle	**16**	250	inactive
LeuPhe-ψCH$_2$N-ProIle	**17**	250	inactive
LeuAsnPhe-ψCH$_2$N-ProIle	**18**	250	21
AsnPhe-ψCH$_2$N-ProIleSer	**13**	250	54
ThrLeuAsnPhe-ψCH$_2$N-ProIleSer	**4**	6	100
ThrLeuAsnDPhe-ψCH$_2$N-ProIleSer	**19**	250	inactive

[a] ValSerGlnAsnTyrProIleValGln was used as a substrate.

and BOC-D-Phe-ΨCH₂N-Pro-OMe confirmed that the diborane reduction did not result in epimerization of the Phe asymmetric center. The methyl ester of **8a** was saponified with 1N NaOH to give the dipeptide BOC-L-Phe-ΨCH₂N-Pro-OH (**9**) without any detectable epimerization, as evidenced by HPLC analysis. Although this procedure did not result in epimerization, the chemical yield was unacceptably low (37%)

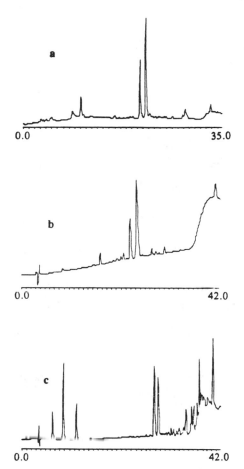

FIGURE 1. Analytical HPLC traces of the crude peptides obtained by reductive alkylation method. (a) ThrLeuAsnPheΨ[CH₂N]ProIleSer; (b) LeuAsnPheΨ[CH₂N]ProIle; (c) CysThrLeuAsnPheΨ[CH₂N]ProIleSerProIle.

due to the complicated workup. The use of a benzyl ester protecting group and hydrogenolysis for deprotection gave the dipeptide **9** in high yield (94%). When the dipeptide **9** was manually coupled to the peptide resin **10** in the presence of DCC and HOBt, the peptide resin **11** was obtained. The resin **11** was deprotected, the ThrLeuAsn segment added automatically on the peptide synthesizer, and the resulting pure diastereomer **4** was cleaved from the resin using HF (SCHEME 4).

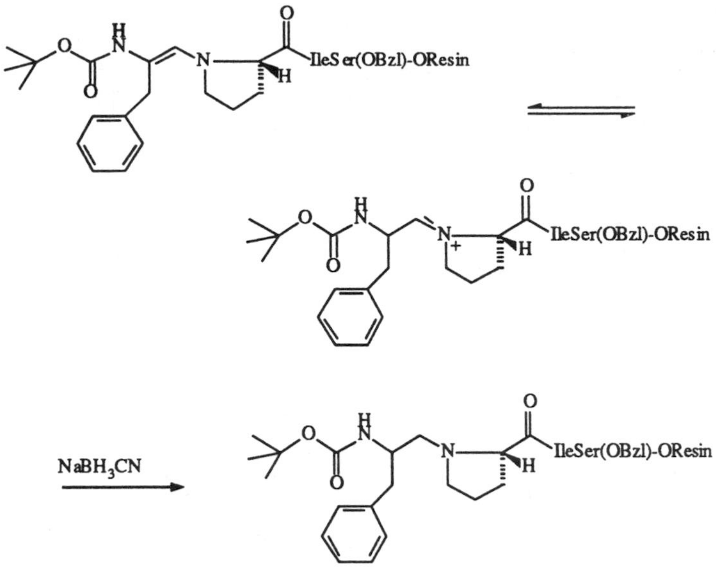

SCHEME 2.

$$\text{BOC-Phe-OH} + \text{Pro-OR.HCl} \xrightarrow[\text{CH}_3\text{CN}]{\text{BOP, Et}_3\text{N}} \text{BOC-PhePro-OR} \xrightarrow[\text{THF}]{\text{B}_2\text{H}_6}$$

5   **6 a,b**   **7 a,b**

$$\text{BOC-Phe-}\psi\text{CH}_2\text{N-Pro-OR} \xrightarrow{\text{i or ii}} \text{BOC-Phe-}\psi\text{CH}_2\text{N-Pro-OH}$$

8 a,b   **9**

(a) R = Me; (b) R = Bzl. (i) 1N NaOH, MeOH; (ii) H$_2$, Pd/C, MeOH

SCHEME 3.

$$\text{BOC-Phe-}\psi\text{CH}_2\text{N-Pro} + \text{IleSer(OBzl)-OResin} \xrightarrow{\text{DCC, HOBt, DMF}}$$

9   **10**

$$\text{BOC-Phe-}\psi\text{CH}_2\text{N-ProIleSer(OBzl)-OResin}$$

11

1. TFA
2. ABI Synthesizer
3. HF

Phe-ψCH$_2$N-ProIleSer   **12**

and   AsnPhe-ψCH$_2$N-ProIleSer   **13**

and   ThrLeuAsnPhe-ψCH$_2$N-ProIleSer   **4**

SCHEME 4.

All the peptides that were shorter than 7 amino acids in length were either inactive or very poor inhibitors when assayed by the published method.[8] On the other hand, the heptapeptide **4** showed good inhibitory activity, completely inhibiting the enzyme at a concentration of 6 μg/mL. Its D-Phe diastereomer, however, was inactive (TABLE 1). This heptapeptide **4** was also tested against HIV-2 protease and showed good inhibitory activity against HIV-2 protease, reaching up to 84% at an inhibitor concentration of 9 mg/assay.[8]

REFERENCES

1. KRAUSSLICH, H. C., S. OROSZLAN & F. WIMMER. 1989. Current Communications in Molecular Biology: Viral Proteinases as Targets for Chemotherapy. Cold Spring Harbor Laboratory.
2. OROSZLAN, S. & R. B. LUFTIG. 1990. Curr. Top. Microbiol. Immunol. **157:** 153.
3. BILLICH, S., M.-T. KNOOP, J. HANSEN, P. STROP, J. SEDLACEK, R. MERTZ & K. MOELLING. 1988. J. Biol. Chem. **263:** 17905.
4. MOORE, M. L. *et al.* 1989. Biochem. Biophys. Res. Commun. **159:** 420.
5. COY, D. H. & Y. SASAKI. 1987. Peptides **8:** 119.
6. COY, D. H., S. J. HACART & Y. SASAKI. 1988. Tetrahedron **44:** 835.
7. BROWN, H. C. & P. HEIM. 1973. J. Org. Chem. **38:** 912.
8. COPELAND, T. D. & S. OROSZLAN. 1988. Gene Anal. Tech. **5:** 109.

Effect of Derivatized Nucleotide Antiviral Drugs on HIV-1 Replication in Cells of T-Lymphoblastoid and Monocyte/Macrophage Lineage in Vitro[a]

M. I. DAWSON,[b] H. ABRAMS,[c] A. SATYAM,[b]
S. TORKELSON,[b] B. ROSS,[c] A. SHIBA,[c] M. REEVE,[c]
D. GEORGE,[d] I. GASTON,[d] M. McGRATH,[d,e] AND
J. LIFSON[c]

[b]Stanford Research Institute International
Bioorganic Chemistry Laboratory
Menlo Park, California 94025

[c]Genelabs, Inc.
Redwood City, California

[d]San Francisco General Hospital
San Francisco, California
and
[e]University of California-San Francisco
San Francisco, California

2',3'-Dideoxycytidine (ddC) produces concentration-dependent inhibition of HIV-1 replication in acutely infected cultures of CD4-positive T-lymphoblastoid cells.[1] Clinical studies have been conducted with ddC as a potential treatment for AIDS. Significant and often dose-limiting toxicity, however, has been observed, with neuropathies being the most serious complication of ddC therapy.[2]

Selective delivery using targeted carriers could minimize systemic exposure and possible toxic side effects. Suitable derivatization could increase local drug concentrations and enhance availability of active forms of the drug to the cells, thereby improving drug efficacy in cells not yet infected by HIV. A carrier of sufficient molecular size was expected to be taken up preferentially by macrophages. Dextran (MW 9,000) was suitably derivatized with 6-aminohexylamino groups to permit multiple loading of the ddC derivative ddC-5'-(5-carboxypentyl)phosphate. ddC-5'-(5-carboxypentyl)-phosphate was designed for linkage to the polymer through an amide bond. With a 5'-phosphate diester group of sufficient stability to ensure delivery to the infected cells,

[a]This research was supported by USPHS Grant 1R01 AI25860 (M. I. Dawson).

the derivatized ddC, once internalized, could be enzymatically cleaved to release the free drug or its related 5'-phosphate.

The activities of these compounds were compared in acute HIV-1 infectivity assays using the HIV-1 isolate HIV-1$_{DV}$[3] and as target cells either the CD4-positive T-lymphoblastoid line VB[4] or primary peripheral blood-derived monocytes/macrophages prepared and cultured from HIV-seronegative healthy donors.[3] Antiviral effects were monitored by use of a capture immunoassay to measure HIV p24 protein in culture supernatants from infected VB cells or in cellular lysates of infected monocytes/macrophages. Cytotoxicity to uninfected VB cells was monitored by trypan blue dye exclusion.

In VB cells, ddC exhibited antiviral activity in the low nanomolar range, with marked cytotoxicity to uninfected cells at high drug concentrations (FIGURES 1A, B, and C). The observed inactivity of either ddC-5'-(5-carboxypentyl)phosphate or its (6-aminohexylamino)$_{11}$dextran conjugate (FIG. 1A) may be explained by lack of entry of these compounds into VB cells. In monocytes/macrophages, ddC or the dextran conju-

TABLE 1. Antiviral Activity of ddC and Its Derivatives in Acutely Infected Cells as Assessed by Inhibition of HIV-1 p24^{gag} Titers

| Compound | Antiviral Activity | | | |
| | In T-Lymphoblastoid VB Cells | | In Monocytes/ Macrophages | |
	IC$_{50}$ (μM)	IC$_{85}$ (μM)	IC$_{50}$ (μM)	IC$_{85}$ (μM)
ddC	0.009	0.04	<0.001	0.15
ddC-5'-(5-carboxypentyl)phosphate	IC$_{25}$ = 100		0.3	10
Conjugate of ddC-5'- (5-carboxypentyl)- phosphate with (6-amino- hexylamino)$_{11}$dextran[a]	30[b]	70[b]	0.01[b]	1.0[b]

[a] [ddC-5'-OP(O)(O$^-$)(CH$_2$)$_5$CONH(CH$_2$)$_6$NH]$_{6.7}$[H$_2$N(CH$_2$)$_6$NH]$_{4.3}$dextran.
[b] Expressed as equivalent ddC concentration.

gate of ddC-5'-(5-carboxypentyl)phosphate exhibited antiviral activity in the low nanomolar range, whereas, ddC-5'-(5-carboxypentyl)phosphate exhibited activity in the low micromolar range (FIG. 1D). Comparison of the antiviral efficacy (IC$_{50}$ and IC$_{85}$) of ddC and its derivatives in acutely infected T-lymphoblastoid and monocyte/macrophage lineage cells is presented in TABLE 1. Both ddC derivatives were more active in monocytes/macrophages than in VB cells by at least two orders of magnitude. The increased activity of the derivatives in monocytes/macrophages compared with that in the CD4-positive T-lymphoblastoid VB cell line may be attributed to their entry into phagocytic cells and/or their intracellular conversion to bioactive species of drug.

These results suggest that modifications to nucleoside antiviral drugs for improving activity and cellular bioavailability or for covalent linkage to targeting macromolecules may significantly affect antiviral efficacy. Such effects either may be operative at the level of cellular uptake, metabolism, compartmentalization, or intracellular conversion to a bioactive species, or, less likely, may reflect actual changes in the antiviral activity caused by derivatization.

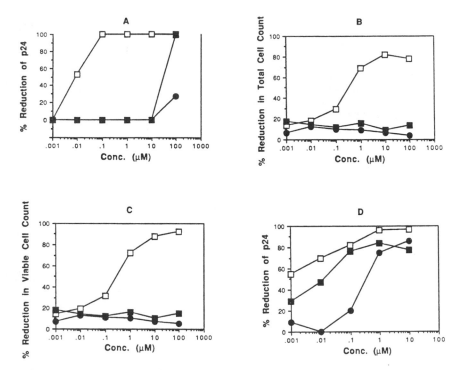

FIGURE 1. Comparison of antiviral activity (**A** and **D**) and cytotoxicity (**B** and **C**) of ddC (□), ddC-5'-(5-carboxypentyl)phosphate (●), and the modified dextran conjugate (■) of ddC-5'-(5-carboxypentyl)phosphate in T-lymphoblastoid VB cells acutely infected with HIV-1$_{DV}$ (**A**); uninfected VB cells (**B** and **C**); or monocytes/macrophages acutely infected with HIV-1$_{DV}$ (**D**). An input multiplicity of infection of approximately 0.005 or 5 HIV-1$_{DV}$ was used for VB cells or monocytes/macrophages, respectively. After adsorption of virus to cells and removal of unbound virions, cells were cultured in the presence or absence of test compound for 4 days (VB cells) or 9 days (monocytes/macrophages). Quantitation of HIV p24 antigen content in culture supernatants (from VB cells) or cell lysates (of monocytes/macrophages) was accomplished by use of commercially available capture immunoassays (Coulter microtiter plate assays for VB cell system; Abbott coated-bead assay for monocyte/macrophage system). Control value for untreated infected VB cells (**A**) was 2 μg of p24 per mL of supernatant. In repeated p24 ELISAs, control values for cell lysates of untreated infected monocytes/macrophages (**D**) ranged from 39.5 to 72.1 ng of p24 per mL. Molarity is expressed as ddC concentration.

REFERENCES

1. MITSUYA, H. & S. BRODER. 1986. Proc. Natl. Acad. Sci. USA **83:** 1911–1915.
2. YARCHOAN, R., R. THOMAS, J.-P. ALLAIN *et al.* 1988. Lancet **i:** 76–81.
3. CROWE, S., J. MILLS & M. MCGRATH. 1987. AIDS Res. Hum. Retroviruses **3:** 135–145.
4. LIFSON, J., G. REYES, M. MCGRATH, B. STEIN & E. ENGLEMAN. 1986. Science **232:** 1123–1127.

Porphyrins as Agents against the Human Immunodeficiency Virus[a]

DABNEY W. DIXON,[b] RAYMOND SCHINAZI,[c] AND
LUIGI G. MARZILLI [d]

[b]Department of Chemistry
Georgia State University
Atlanta, Georgia 30303

[c]VA Medical Center
Emory University School of Medicine
Decatur, Georgia 30033

[d]Department of Chemistry
Emory University
Atlanta, Georgia 30322

We have preliminary evidence that diverse types of porphyrins and metalloporphyrins are active against the human immunodeficiency virus in peripheral blood mononuclear (PBM) cells. Both natural porphyrins (*i.e.* those derived ultimately from protoporphyrin IX, the porphyrin found in hemoglobin) and the synthetic porphyrins (*i.e.* symmetrical porphyrins made in the laboratory from pyrrole and aldehydes, see FIG. 1) are active, many in the 0.1 to 10 μM range. TABLE 1 gives 10 of the compounds studied to date. Assays have been described previously.[1–3]

Many negatively charged porphyrins are active. Molecular models indicate that the porphyrin ring is comparable in size to a base pair in DNA or the DNA/RNA heteroduplex. The negative charges on the periphery of the porphyrin have a distance between them similar to the phosphate phosphate distance in the DNA base pair. Thus, these compounds might inhibit enzymes that bind to the growing DNA or DNA/RNA chain. TABLE 1 shows that these compounds have good reverse transcriptase inhibitory activity.

Some natural porphyrins also have good activity. These compounds may be reverse transcriptase inhibitors or control some aspect of cellular pharmacology that impinges on virus survival.

Readily oxidizable porphyrins (*i.e.* ones that can form free radicals) also have good activity. In the case of the phenolic compounds studied to date, however, the anti-HIV activity appears to reside in the reverse transcriptase inhibition rather than in any free radical chemistry.

Positively charged porphyrins also have good activity. This is presumably because they interact strongly with DNA as we[4,5] and others[5,6] have shown.

Porphyrins and metalloporphyrins have been used clinically in the treatment of porphyrias,[7] cancer by way of "photodynamic" therapy,[8] and neonatal hyperbilirubi-

[a]We thank the National Institutes of Health (1001A127196) for support of this work.

511

TABLE 1.

Drug name	HIV-1[a]	Toxicity in Vero[b]	Cell-free RT (rec)[b,c]	DNA pol α[b,c]
Tetra(4-sulfonatophenyl)porphyrin Na salt	<1.0	>100		
Tetra(2,6-dichloro-3-sulfonatophenyl)porphyrin, Na	≪1	0.31		
Mono(4-pyridyl)-tri(4-sulfonatophenyl)porphyrin, Na	≪1	0.40		
Tetra(4-hydroxyphenyl)porphyrin	0.6	3.7	3.0	100
Tetra(2-hydroxyphenyl)porphyrin	3.1	5.3	3.0	100
Tetra(3-hydroxyphenyl)porphyrin	5.37	3.79	5.0	100
5,15-Diphenyl-10,20-di-N-methyl-pyridylporphyrin Cl-	<1	0.84		
Tetra(N-ethyl-4-pyridyl)porphyrin chloride	2.0	5.9		
Mesoporphyrin IX dihydrochloride	0.95	0.44	2.1	
Hematoporphyrin IX	1.94	100		

[a] EC_{50}, μM.
[b] IC_{50}, μM.
[c] RT (rec), recombinant reverse transcriptase; pol, polymerase.

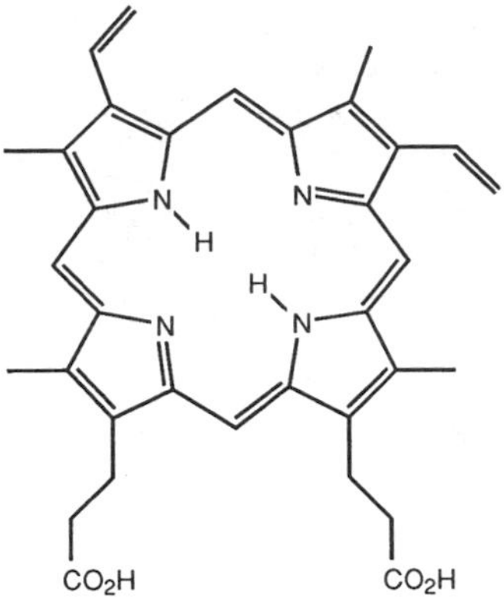

protoporphyrin IX 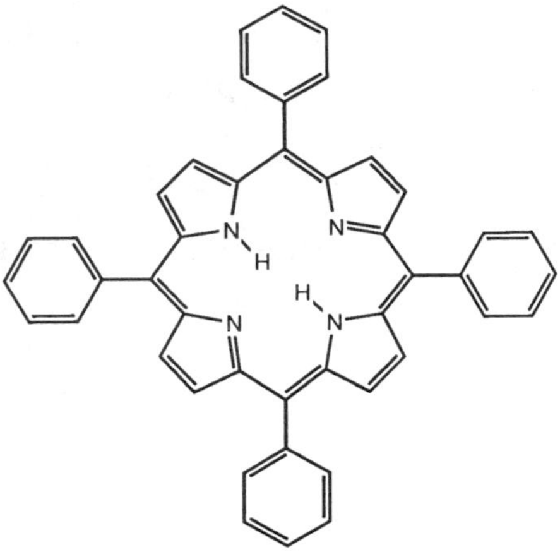   tetraphenylporphyrin

FIGURE 1.

nemia.[9] Our preliminary testing also indicates that these compounds often have low toxicity. Therefore, it is expected that these compounds could readily be introduced clinically.

REFERENCES

1. SCHINAZI, R. F., D. L. CANNON, B. H. ARNOLD & D. MARTINO-SALTZMAN. 1988. Antimicrob Agents Chemother. **32:** 1784-1787.
2. SCHINAZI, R. F., J. PETERS, C. C. WILLIAMS, D. CHANCE & A J. NAHMIAS. 1982. Antimicrob. Agents Chemother. **22:** 499-507.
3. SCHINAZI, R. F., B. F. H. ERIKSSON & S. H. HUGHES. 1989. Antimicrob. Agents Chemother. **33:** 115-117.
4. STRICKLAND, J. A., D. L. BANVILLE, L. G. MARZILLI & W. D. WILSON. 1987. Inorg. Chem. **26:** 3398-3406
5. MARZILLI, L. G. 1990. New J. Chem. **14:** 409-420.
6. GIBBS, E. J. & R. F. PASTERNACK. 1989. Semin. Hematol. **26:** 77-85.
7. MUSTAJOKI, P., R. TENHUNEN, C. PIERACH & L. VOLIN. 1989. Semin. Hematol. **26:** 1-9.
8. GOMER, C. J. 1989. Semin. Hematol. **26:** 27-34.
9. DRUMMOND, G. S. 1989. Semin. Hematol. **26:** 24-26.

Expression in *E. coli* and Purification of Human Immunodeficiency Virus Type 1 Major Core Protein, p24

LORNA S. EHRLICH, HANS-GEORG KRAÜSSLICH,[a]
ECKARD WIMMER, AND CAROL A. CARTER

Department of Microbiology
State University of New York
Stony Brook, New York 11794

Capsid protein (p24,CA) of human immunodeficiency virus type 1 (HIV-1) was expressed in *E. coli* and purified in a form able to self-associate. Expression was done in BL21(DE3) cells transformed with plasmid FS II, which allows translation of the *pol* gene in the *gag* reading frame, resulting in efficient processing of matrix (MA), capsid (CA), nucleocapsid (NC), and proteinase (PR) from one polyprotein.[1] Analysis of lysate from cells induced for expression with addition of isopropyl-β-D-thiogalactopyranoside (IPTG) showed mature CA to be the major induced protein (FIG. 1). Expressed CA is found in the soluble fraction of the cell lysate, is recognized by monoclonal antibodies directed against the HIV capsid protein, and has an N-terminus amino acid sequence identical to that of CA purified from HIV.[2] Purification was done under mild conditions where coexpressed HIV PR retains enzymatic activity. Milligram quantities of 90% pure capsid protein were obtained after chromatography of clarified cell lysate on DEAE cellulose followed by facilitated aggregation of capsid proteins in the unbound fraction. FIGURE 2 shows that when the concentration of the DEAE cellulose unbound fraction was increased to about 20 mg/ mL (lane 1), CA precipitated out in nearly homogenous form (see lane 3), whereas most of the other proteins remained in the supernate (lane 2). Aggregated CA readily dissolves in aqueous buffers and in solution exists in oligomeric form. This observation and the fact that CA precipitates at high concentration suggest an ability to self-associate, a property expected of a protein that forms the shell of the virus core[3] and shown to be true for the capsid protein (p30) isolated from Moloney murine leukemia virus.[4] This material should be useful in obtaining structure-function information that can guide the design of antiviral drugs targeted to events occurring during virus assembly.

[a] Present address: Institut für Virusforschung, Deutsches Krebsforschungzenbum, Im Nenenheimer Feld 280, D-69 Heidelberg, Federal Republic of Germany

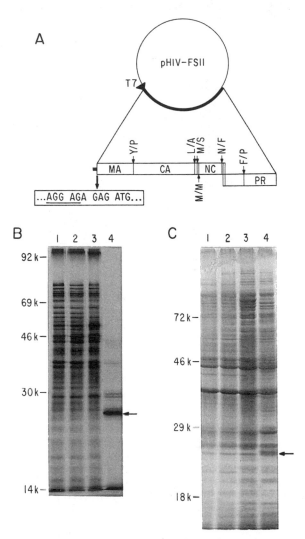

FIGURE 1. Expression of FS II in *E. coli.* A: Schematic drawing of the FS II plasmid[1] and the polyprotein translated from the HIV sequence. Processing of the polyprotein by HIV proteinase at the cleavage sites indicated by arrows generates mature proteins: MA, matrix; CA, capsid; NC, nucleocapsid; PR, proteinase. Shown in a boxed area on the bottom left is the ATG translation start site and the Shine Delgarno-like sequence (AGGAG). B: [35S]methionine labeled proteins from *E. coli* strain BL21(DE3) cells carrying FS II or PBR322. Cells were induced for expression in the presence of [35S]methionine as described in ref. 1. Total cell lysates were analyzed by SDS-PAGE and proteins visualized by autoradiography. Lane 1, lysate from uninduced PBR322-carrying cells; lane 2, lysate from induced PBR322-carrying cells; lane 3, lysate from uninduced FS II-carrying cells; and lane 4, lysate from induced FS II-carrying cells. Arrow indicates the 24 kDa major expressed protein. C: Coomasie stained proteins from total cell lysates prepared as described in **B.**

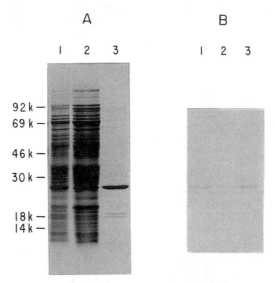

FIGURE 2. Facilitated aggregation of HIV capsid protein. Samples from the final stages of capsid purification were analyzed by SDS-PAGE (panel A) and Western blotting with monoclonal antibody directed against HIV capsid protein (panel B). Lane 1, DEAE cellulose unbound fraction at about 20 mg/mL total protein concentration; lane 2, supernate after removal of precipitated capsid protein; and lane 3, precipitated capsid protein.

REFERENCES

1. KRAÜSSLICH, H-G., H. SCHNEIDER, G. ZYBARTH, C. A. CARTER & E. WIMMER. 1988. Processing of *in vitro*-synthesized gag precursor proteins of human immunodeficiency virus (HIV) type 1 by HIV proteinase generated in *E. coli.* J. Virol. **62:** 4393-4397.
2. HENDERSON, L. E., T. D. COPELAND, R. C. SOWDER, A. M. SCHULTS & S. OROSZLAN. 1988. Analysis of proteins and peptides purified from sucrose gradient banded HTLV-III. *In* Human Retrovirus, Cancer and AIDS: Approaches to Prevention and Therapy. 135-147. Alan R. Liss, Inc. New York.
3. GELDERBLOM, H. R., E. H. S. HAUSMANN, M. OZEL, G. PAULI & M. A. KOCH. 1987. Fine structure of HIV and immunolocalization of structural proteins. Virology **156:** 171-176.
4. BURNETTE, W. N., L. A. HOLLADAY & W. MITCHELL. 1976. Physical and chemical properties of Moloney murine leukemia virus p30 protein: a major core structural component exhibiting high helicity and self-association. J. Mol. Biol. **107:** 131-143.

Metabolism, Toxicity, and Anti-HIV Activity of 2′-Deoxy-3′-Thia-Cytidine (BCH-189) in T and B Cell Lines

MICHAEL L. GREENBERG,[a] H. S. ALLAUDEEN,[b]
AND MICHAEL S. HERSHFIELD [a]

[a]Department of Medicine
Duke University Medical Center
Durham, North Carolina 27710
[b]Division of AIDS
National Institutes of Health
Rockville, Maryland

We examined the metabolism, cytotoxicity, and antiviral activity of BCH-189 (dTHC, 2′-deoxy-3′-thia-cytidine), a novel 3′-thia-ddC analogue. BCH-189 was efficiently converted to phosphorylated metabolites (BCH-189-XP) in cells possessing deoxycytidine kinase (dCK) activity (TABLE 1). CEM T cells converted BCH-189 to at least 6 nucleotides detected by radiochemical HPLC; essentially none was formed in a double-mutant lacking adenosine kinase (AK) and dCK. In wild-type cells, formation of a labeled product eluting in the dideoxynucleoside triphosphate region was linear with 1-5 μM BCH-189; the amount formed did not change between 4 and 24 hours. BCH-189 triphosphate had an extended half-life in CEM cells compared to ddCTP. We examined the effects of BCH-189 and ddC on the growth of wild type AK$^-$ or dCK$^-$ single and AK$^-$/dCK$^-$ double mutants of CEM T cell and WIL-2 B-cell lines over 3-4 days. The growth of dCK$^+$ T cells was inhibited by 50% with 1-5 μM ddC; slightly higher concentrations inhibited B cells similarly. By contrast, BCH-189 concentrations ranging from 25 to >250 μM were required to inhibit the growth of dCK$^+$ T and B

TABLE 1. Deoxycytidine Kinase Mediates Phosphorylation of BCH-189[a]

Cell Line	Kinase Status	pmol BCH-189-XP per 10⁶ cells
AG1a	Wild type	2.01
M1-1a	AK$^-$/dCK$^+$	2.87
ACO611a	AK$^+$/dCK$^-$	$\leq$0.03

[a] Cells were incubated with 2 μm [³H]BCH-189 for 4 hours.

517

cells. dCK⁻ T and B cells were resistant to growth inhibition by either nucleoside. Both BCH-189 and ddC inhibited replication of HIV-IIIB in CEM T cells and WIL-2-derived B cells at <0.5 μM, as indicated by assay of culture supernatant reverse transcriptase activity. Anti-HIV activity of both compounds required host-cell dCK. Our results suggest that BCH-189 may have an improved therapeutic index compared to ddC; further studies of the basis for improved selectivity and therapeutic potential of BCH-189 are warranted.

Ultrastructural and Cytochemical Analysis of the Loss of Envelope Glycoproteins (gp120) on Budding and Mature HIV-1 following Treatment with Soluble T4 (sT4)

TIMOTHY K. HART,[a] RICHARD KIRSH,[b]
ANNE M. KLINKNER,[a] DENNIS M. LAMBERT,[c]
S. R. PETTEWAY JR.,[c] HARMA ELLENS,[b] AND
PETER J. BUGELSKI[a]

[a]Department of Experimental Pathology
[b]Department of Drug Delivery
[c]Department of Anti-infectives
Smith Kline & French Laboratories
King of Prussia, Pennsylvania 19406-0939

The human immunodeficiency virus (HIV) infects cells that express the surface antigen CD4 (T4), a 55 kDa transmembrane glycoprotein expressed on the surface of CD4+ T lymphocytes and cells of the mononuclear phagocyte lineage.[1,2] HIV is believed to infect CD4+ cells following binding of the viral envelope glycoprotein gp120 to cellular CD4.[3,4]

Viral gp120 is noncovalently bound to gp41 on the surface of HIV-1 but can be visualized on the surface of HIV as 9 nm $\times$ 15 nm spikes by the tannic acid–lead citrate method of Gelderblom[5] or by immunocytochemical staining. These spikes, however, appear to be "spontaneously" shed from the virion after it has budded from the infected cell.[5]

Soluble T4 (sT4) is a recombinant soluble form of CD4 that inhibits both viral infectivity[6] and syncytia formation.[7] The mechanism of sT4 inhibition is not completely understood. Soluble CD4 constructs bind to gp120 and thus are believed to interfere with viral binding to CD4+ cells.[8]

We attempted to demonstrate the binding of sT4 to gp120 on HIV using electron microscopic cytochemistry. At concentrations of sT4 that inhibit infectivity and syncytia formation, however, we were unable to detect binding of horseradish peroxidase- and colloidal gold-labeled sT4 to HIV-1, strain IIIB virions. To examine this apparent lack of binding and to evaluate the loss of gp120 spikes from virions, we examined the spike distribution on CEM cells infected with HIV-1, strain IIIB before and after treatment with sT4.

On budding virions, distribution of spikes was highly periodic (FIG. 1A). After treatment with sT4 (10 μg/mL, FIG. 1B), there was an apparent decrease in the number of spikes. Morphometric analysis (FIG. 2A) of the distribution of spikes revealed a

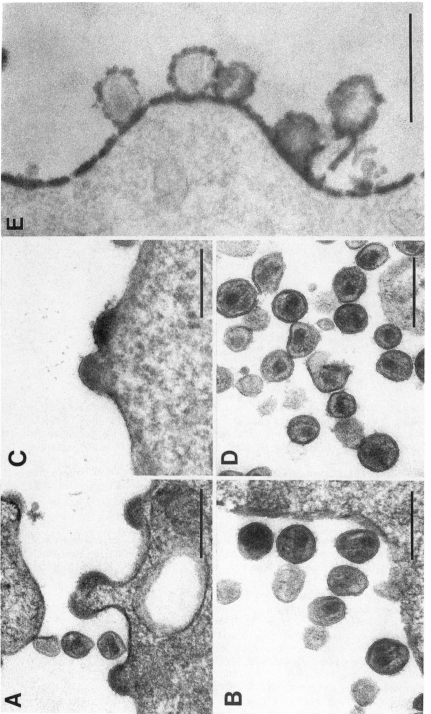

FIGURE 1. Electron micrographs of budding (**A** and **C**) and mature (**B** and **D**) HIV-1, strain IIIB virions. Envelope projections, spikes or gp120, are clearly visible over most of the surface of the 4 budding virions prior to sT4 treatment (**A**). Following sT4 treatment (10 μg/mL; **C**), the spikes are diminished in frequency on the surface of budding virions. Similarly, on mature untreated virions, spikes are visible, although decreased in number (**B**). Spikes are further reduced following treatment with sT4 (**D**). **E:** Immunocytochemical staining for HIV gp120. Spikes are revealed on the surface of virions as small balls of reaction product in a similar distribution as the tannic acid-revealed spikes. In addition, HRP reaction product is present in a uniform distribution over the cell plasma membrane. Bars = 250 nm.

significant decrease (p < 0.01) in the mean linear surface density (89 ± 2.75 to 61 ± 2.56 spikes/μm). On mature virions (FIG. 1C) the linear surface density of spikes was considerably less than that on budding virions, which is consistent with the reported spontaneous loss of surface spikes. Following treatment of mature virions with sT4 (FIG. 1D) there was a further and significant decrease (p < 0.01) in the linear surface density of spikes (39 ± 0.56 to 30 ± 0.65 spikes/μm; FIG. 2B).

To verify that the electron dense spikes correlated with gp120, HIV-infected cells were immunostained with an antibody to the hypervariable loop of gp120 (FIG. 1E), and the gp120 antibody was revealed with a horseradish peroxidase-labeled probe.

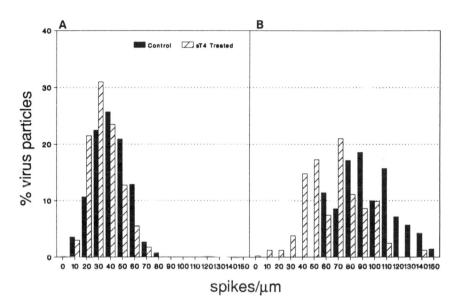

FIGURE 2. Morphometric analysis of the distribution of gp120 spikes on the surface of mature (A) and budding (B) HIV-1, strain IIIB virions. The percentage of mature or budding virions having a given range of spikes is plotted against the number of spikes per μm of viral membrane. Incubation with sT4 has shifted both the mature and budding viral population mean linear surface density of spikes to the right. Mature virions have a significant decrease (p < 0.01) from 39 ± U.56 to 30 ± 0.65 spikes per μm, and budding virions also significantly decrease (p < 0.01) from 89 ± 2.75 to 61 ± 2.56 spikes per μm (mean ⊥ 3ΣM).

Electron-dense patches corresponding to the distribution of spikes were visible on the surface of virions.

These data suggest that sT4 potentiates the loss of gp120 from the surface of HIV-1 and HIV-infected cells. This stripping of gp120 indicates that the previously believed mechanism of action of sT4, that is, coating of gp120 on the virus, may not in fact be the case. Furthermore, stripping of gp120 suggests that sT4 can act as a competitive irreversible inhibitor of HIV. The identification of this mechanism also provides insight into the interactions of gp120-gp41 and CD4 (sT4), as well as the importance of these molecules in the initial stages of HIV infection.

REFERENCES

1. MADDON, P. J., A. G. DALGLEISH, J. S. McDOUGAL, P. R. CLAPHAM, R. A. WEISS & R. AXEL. 1986. Cell **47:** 333-348.
2. KLATZMANN, D., D. E. CHAPAGNE, S. CHAMARET, J. GRUEST, D. GUETARD, T. HERCEND, J. C. GLUCKMAN & L. MANTAGNIER. 1985. Nature **312:** 767-768.
3. McDOUGAL, J. S., M. S. KENNEDY, J. M. SLIGH, S. P. CORT, A. MAWIE, & J. K. A. NICHOLSON. 1986. Science **231:** 382-385.
4. SCHMITTMAN, S. M., H. C. LANE, J. ROTH, A. BURROWS, T. M. FOLKS, J. H. KEHRI, S. KOENIG, P. BERMAN & A. S. FAUCI. 1988. J. Immunol. **141:** 4181-4186.
5. GELDERBLOM, H. R., H. S. HAUSMANN, M. OZEL, G. PAULI & M. A. KOCH. 1987. Virology **156:** 171-176.
6. SMITH, D. H., R. A. BYRN, S. A. MARSTERS, T. GREGORY, J. E. GROOPMAN & D. J. CAPON. 1987. Science **238:** 1704-1707.
7. HUSSEY, R. E., N. E. RICHARDSON, M. KOWELSKI, N. R. BROWN, H.-C. CHANG, R. F. SILICIANO, T. DORFMAN, B. WALKER, J. SODROSKI & E. L. REINHERZ. 1988. Nature **331:** 78-81.
8. TILL, M. A., V. GHETIE, T. GREGORY, E. J. PATZAR, J. P. PORTER, J. W. UHR, D. J. CAPON & E. S. VITETTA. 1988. Science **242:** 1166-1168.

Pharmacokinetic Study of Dextran Sulfate in Rats

NEIL R. HARTMAN, DAVID G. JOHNS, AND
HIROAKI MITSUYA

National Cancer Institute
National Institutes of Health
Bethesda, Maryland 20892

Dextran sulfate (DS) with a molecular weight of approximately 8000 has recently been shown to be active against HIV-1 *in vitro*.[1,2] In the phase I clinical trial, oral dextran sulfate appears to be well-tolerated;[3] however, no measurable evidence of systemic absorption of the compound in patients is yet available. To address this, we administered radiolabeled dextran sulfate ([3H]-labeled on the reducing end, molecular weight ≈ 8000, [3H]DS) to rats. Analysis of plasma from animals that were given [3H]DS intravenously revealed that the initial plasma half-life was about 30 minutes. When the molecular weight of the radiolabeled material was determined by size-exclusion HPLC, it was found that the majority of the [3H]DS left the circulation intact (FIG. 1), with breakdown products of MW ≈ 4000 seen in later time points. Eleven percent of [3H]DS administered was recovered in the urine in 24 hours; this material had a molecular weight of 4000, indicating minor breakdown. When orally administered, the apparent bioavailability of [3H]DS was about 7% based on the recovered radioactivity; however, the molecular weight of the radioactive material obtained from the plasma was all < 200, indicating that no detectable intact dextran sulfate was absorbed upon oral administration. Only 2% of orally administered [3H]DS was found in the 24 hour urine; this material also had a molecular weight < 200.

Further *in vitro* testing of antiviral activity revealed that DS fractions with molecular weight less than 4000 had decreased activity relative to the MW 8000 starting material, and that no anti-HIV effect was seen with fractions of MW < 2300 (FIG. 2). In the presence of high concentrations of human serum, more DS was required for antiviral effect. Under normal culture conditions, 5-10 $\mu g/mL$ DS was required for complete inhibition of HIV, whereas 20 $\mu g/mL$ was required in the presence of 50% normal human serum and more than 50 $\mu g/mL$ was required in the presence of 85% human serum.

These data suggest that oral administration of DS is unlikely to produce significant antiretroviral effect against HIV *in vivo*, and higher plasma levels of DS might be necessary than those inferred from earlier *in vitro* data.

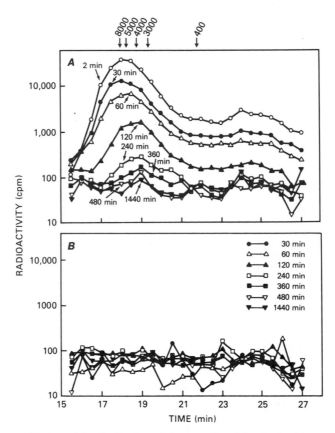

FIGURE 1. Molecular weight distribution of plasma radioactivity obtained from rats receiving [³H]DS. Ultrafiltered plasma samples were analyzed by size-exclusion HPLC. Radioactivity in half-minute fractions was determined by beta liquid scintillation counting. Void volume of the column was 12 mL, corresponding to an elution time of 15 min. **A:** intravenous [³H]DS; **B:** oral [³H]DS. Elution times of molecular weight standards are shown at the top of the graph. Note logarithmic ordinate axis.

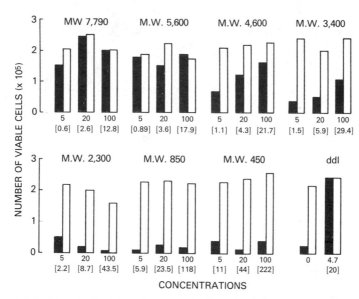

FIGURE 2. Inhibition of infectivity and cytopathic effect of HIV-1 by dextran sulfate of varying molecular weight. ATH8 cells (2×10^5) were exposed to HIV-1/III$_B$ (2.8×10^4 TCID$_{50}$) and cultured in the presence of various concentrations of dextran sulfate (solid column). Control cells (open column) were similarly treated but were not exposed to the virus. On day 7, total viable cells were counted. Concentrations are expressed in μg/mL (micromolarity shown in brackets). Under the same conditions, 20 μM ddI exerted a complete inhibition.

REFERENCES

1. UENO, R. & S. KUNO. 1987. Dextran sulfate, a potent anti-HIV agent *in vitro* having synergism with zidovudine. Lancet **1**: 1379.
2. MITSUYA, H., D. J. LOONEY, S. KUNO, R. UENO, F. WONG-STAAL & S. BRODER. 1988. Dextran sulfate suppression of viruses in the HIV family: Inhibition of virion binding to CD4$^+$ cells. Science **240**: 646-649.
3. ABRAMS, D. I., S. KUNO & R. WONG *et al.* 1989. Oral dextran sulfate (UA001) in the treatment of the acquired immunodeficiency syndrome (AIDS) and AIDS-related complex. Ann. Intern. Med. **110**: 183-8.

Recombinant Human Erythropoietin (rHuEPO) versus Placebo in Anemic AIDS Patients Taking AZT

Report on a Double-Blind Prospective Randomized Trial

DAVID H. HENRY[a]

Erythropoietin Study Group
Graduate Hospital
Philadelphia, Pennsylvania
and
R. W. Johnson Pharmaceutical Research Institute
Raritan, New Jersey

Anemia is common in AIDS patients and is frequently exacerbated by treatment with AZT. The anemia observed follows most closely the anemia of chronic disease (ACD). ACD occurs in the presence of any chronic inflammatory disease and is characterized by an underproductive bone marrow. Furthermore, there is a defect in iron re-utilization in the marrow, and there is generally an inadequate endogenous level of erythropoietin (EPO) for any given degree of anemia. To test the efficacy of EPO replacement therapy in AIDS-related anemia, a multicenter, prospective, double-blind trial was performed using either rHuEPO or placebo.

Sixty-three anemic patients with AIDS taking AZT were randomized to receive either 100 units/kilogram of rHuEPO or placebo IV, 3 times/week for 12 weeks or until reaching a target hematocrit of 38-40 percent. Safety, transfusion requirement, degree of anemia, and quality of life were measured in the study. The two patient groups were comparable and equally balanced with regard to age, sex, performance status, and AZT dosage.

Baseline endogenous EPO levels were measured on all patients at study entry. As expected, most patients (79%) had an endogenous EPO level inadequate for their degree of anemia; but some (21%) had a much higher than expected EPO level for their degree of anemia. Some of these patients had EPO levels > 1,000 mU/mL. Yet, they were still anemic. This phenomenon is only observed in those AIDS patients taking AZT and not in patients not on AZT.

A retrospective analysis of the baseline endogenous EPO levels proved to be predictive with regard to response to rHuEPO therapy. Those patients whose baseline EPO levels were < 500 mU/mL had a significant decrease in their transfusion requirement with rHuEPO therapy versus placebo (see TABLE 1). There was no difference in transfusion requirement in those patients whose baseline EPO levels were > 500 mU/

---

[a] Address for correspondence: Graduate Hospital, 1840 South St., Philadelphia, PA 19146.

TABLE 1. Units of Blood Transfused per Patient per Month

	Units/Patient/Month	
	Study Start	Study End
EPO $\leq$ 500 mU/mL[a] (n = 48)		
rHuEPO	1.31	0.84
Placebo	1.68	2.74
(p Value)	0.264	0.005[b]
EPO > 500 mU/mL[a] (n = 13)		
rHuEPO	3.10	3.50
Placebo	3.32	2.78
(p Value)	0.718	0.866

[a] Patient endogenous EPO level at start of study.
[b] Statistically significant.

mL. Throughout the course of the study, there was a trend toward a decrease in AZT dose in all patient groups, but there was no between-group difference in AZT dosage at any time.

There was a trend toward improvement in the quality of life in those patients receiving rHuEPO whose baseline endogenous EPO levels were < 500 mU/mL. There was no significant increase in side effects or in the tendency toward progression of disease in the rHuEPO versus placebo-treated groups.

These data suggest that rHuEPO at the doses employed in this study can significantly decrease transfusion requirement and demonstrate a trend toward improvement in the quality of life in AIDS patients on AZT whose endogenous baseline EPO levels are less than 500 mU/mL.

Anti-HIV-1, Cytotoxic, and Biological Properties of Selected Polyoxometalate Compounds[a]

C. L. HILL,[b] M. WEEKS,[b] M. HARTNUP,[b]
J-P. SOMMADOSSI,[c] AND R. F. SCHINAZI[d]

[b]Department of Chemistry
Emory University
Atlanta, Georgia 30322

[c]Department of Pharmacology
Division of Clinical Pharmacology
University of Alabama at Birmingham
Birmingham, Alabama 35294

[d]Veterans Affairs Medical Center and
Laboratory of Biochemical Pharmacology
Department of Pediatrics
Emory University School of Medicine
Atlanta, Georgia 30033

Polyoxometalate compounds, a large class of inorganic cluster-like compounds, are formed principally of oxide anions and early transition metal cations, usually in their d^0 electronic configurations.[1] Recent studies indicated that one compound of the polyoxometalate class, the French anti-HIV-1 agent, HPA-23 (molecular formula $(NH_4^+)_{17}(H^+)[NaSb_9W_{21}O_{86}^{18-}])$, exhibited activity against several viruses *in vitro* and *in vivo*.[2] Clinical studies in Europe and the USA, however, indicated that this particular compound was too toxic to be of serious interest as an anti-HIV-1 agent.[3] We report here the results from evaluation of 38 polyoxometalates of several structural categories: (1) the Keggin class (*e.g.* $\alpha\text{-}SiW_{12}O_{40}^{4-}$ = ST and $\alpha\text{-}BW_{12}O_{40}^{5-}$ = BT); (2) the Wells-Dawson class ($P_2W_{18}O_{62}^{6-}$); and (3) various fragments derived from these structures (*e.g.* $PW_{11}O_{39}^{7-}$ and $PW_9O_{34}^9$), the Keggin-derived sandwich compounds (*e.g.* $K_{10}Cu_4$-$(H_2O)_2(PW_9O_{34})_2)$, the hexametalates ($W_6O_{19}^{2-}$ and $Mo_6O_{19}^{2-}$), decatungstate ($W_{10}O_{32}^{4-}$), the Preyssler ion, $[NaP_5W_{30}O_{110}]^{14-}$, and different salt forms of these complexes.

The anti-HIV-1 activity of the compounds in infected peripheral blood mononuclear (PBM) cells was uniformly high; nearly 80% of the compounds tested had activity. Some of the most active compounds were ST, BT, and $W_{10}O_{32}^{4-}$ (EC_{50} values ~ 1 μM). The smaller polyoxometalates, generally those with 6 atoms or less, did not have appreciable anti-HIV-1 activity. The toxicity in PBM cells varied from high

[a]This work was supported by Public Health Service Grants AI 26055 (C. L. Hill and R. F. Schinazi) and AI 25784, AI 27767, and No 1 RR 0032 (J. P. Sommadossi) from the National Institutes of Health and by the Department of Veterans Affairs (R. F. Schinazi).

$(P_2W_{12}O_{40}{}^{6-}$; $IC_{50} \sim 2)$ to virtually nontoxic (80% of the compounds tested). There was no apparent correlation of toxicity in these cells with molecular electronic and structural parameters (shape, charge densities, and redox potential).

Five exemplary polyoxometalates, HPA-23, ST, BT, and the ammonium salt forms of the latter two were evaluated for toxicity in human bone marrow cells. The data (FIG. 1) reveal a number of heretofore unappreciated points: (1) HPA-23 is quite toxic in these key cell cultures and by far the most toxic compound examined; (2) both BT and ammonium BT were less toxic than the corresponding ST analogues; (3) replacement of the proton with ammonium cation reduced the toxicity by an order of magnitude for both ST and BT; and (4) the least toxic compound of the five tested, ammonium BT [NH$_4$BT in FIGURE 1 = $(NH_4)_5(\alpha\text{-}BW_{12}O_{40})$], has virtually no toxicity in these cell lines and substantially less than AZT $(IC_{50} = 1\ \mu M)$.

Three representative polyoxometalates (HPA-23, ST, BT) and three nucleosides (AzddU, AzddEtU, and AZT) were evaluated for their ability to prevent fusion of

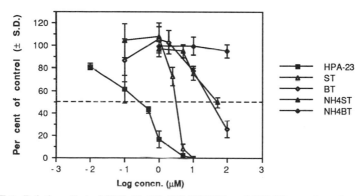

FIGURE 1. Relative effect of HPA-23, ST, BT, NH$_4$BT, and NH$_4$ST on colony formation of human granulocyte-macrophage precursor cells. Values represent the mean ± SD of at least three determinations.

infected lymphocytes to uninfected CD4$^+$cells. All three polyoxometalates were effective in completely preventing cell fusion at both 50 μM after 24 h or 150 μM after 72 h of incubation, whereas all three nucleosides were incffective. At 10 μM or lower concentration, no inhibition was observed by the three polyoxometalates.

REFERENCES

1. POPE, M. T. 1983. Heteropoly and Isopoly Oxometalates. Springer-Verlag. Berlin.
2. ROZENBAUM, W., D. DORMONT, B. SPIRE, E. VILMER, M. GENTILINI, C. GRISCELLI, L. MONTAGNIER, F. BARRE-SINOUSSI & J. C. CHERMAN. 1985. Lancet 1: 450-451.
3. MOSKOVITZ, B. L. & the HPA-23 COOPERATIVE STUDY GROUP. 1988. Antimicrob. Agents Chemother. 32: 1300-1303.

Synthesis and Anti-HIV Activity of a Novel Series of Isomeric Dideoxynucleosides

D. M. HURYN, B. C. SLUBOSKI, S. Y. TAM,

L. J. TODARO, M. WEIGELE, I. S. SIM,

K. B. FRANK, D. D. RICHMAN,[a] H. MITSUYA,[b]

AND S. BRODER[b]

Roche Research Center
Hoffmann-LaRoche Inc.
Nutley, New Jersey 07110-1199

[a]VA Medical Center
University of California San Diego
San Diego, California

[b]Clinical Oncology Program
National Cancer Institute
Bethesda, Maryland

Recently a class of potent inhibitors of the HIV reverse transcriptase, the 2',3'-dideoxy-nucleosides (e.g., ddA/ddI, ddC), has been described.[1] The therapeutic use of these compounds, particularly ddA and other dideoxypurine nucleosides, however, is limited by their rapid degradation through hydrolysis of the sugar-base linkage.[2] To overcome this deficiency we designed a modified dideoxynucleoside in which a more stable nucleoside linkage exists, e.g., iso-ddA, 1 (FIG. 1). The exchange of oxygen and carbon atoms, while maintaining an isomeric relationship with the model compounds, imparts stability at the sugar-base union.

Starting material for the synthesis of 1 was the erythro-pentofuranose derivative, 2 (FIG. 2). This compound, when treated with a 1% HOAc/methanol solution, initially yielded a mixture of the methyl glycoside, the ring-opened dimethyl acetal, and the desired cyclized product. With continued stirring, complete conversion to 3 was achieved in greater than 95% overall yield from 2.[c] Tosylation of 3 under standard conditions, followed by hydrolysis and reduction, provided the iso-sugar, 4.

The preparation of iso-ddA (1) was carried out by direct nucleophilic displacement of adenine on the iso-sugar unit, 4.[4] Other members of this class of compounds (e.g., iso-ddC (5) and iso-ddT (6)) could be similarly synthesized. Additional isomeric purine dideoxynucleosides were prepared by the use of standard purine transformations. TABLE 1 details their synthesis.

---

[c]This reaction represents an improvement over a solvolysis reaction of a related system reported by authors in ref. 3.

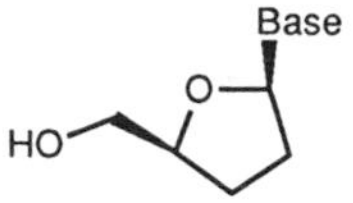

2',3'-Dideoxyadenosine (ddA): Base = Adenine
2',3'-Dideoxyinosine (ddI) :Base = Hypoxanthine
2',3'-Dideoxycytidine (ddC):   Base = Cytosine

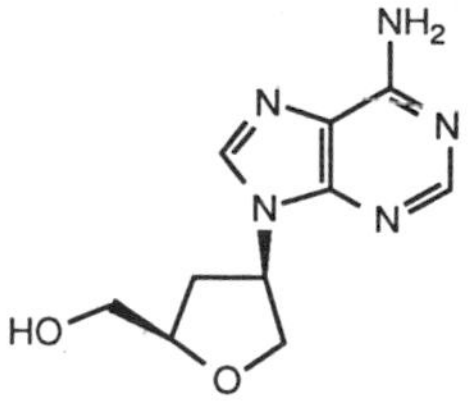

1: Isomeric Dideoxyadenosine
(Iso-ddA)

FIGURE 1.

All of these compounds were tested for anti-HIV activity in at least two cell lines. IC_{50}'s for iso-ddA in ATH-8[1] and HT4-6C[5] cells were 5-10 μM and 22 μM, respectively. Interestingly, iso-ddI (9) exhibited no antiviral activity. Iso-ddG (10) also showed anti-HIV activity; IC_{50}'s in the range of 10-50 μM were measured in ATH-8 cells; > 50 μM in HT4-6C cells. Neither of these compounds showed significant toxicities (TD_{50} > 200 μM in ATH-8 cells).

Due to the antiviral activity exhibited by iso-ddA, further studies were carried out. A single crystal x-ray structure was determined and is illustrated in FIGURE 3. Interestingly, the 2'-exo-3'-endo sugar conformation differs from that of other known nucleoside anti-HIV agents.[6] Stability studies show that, as designed, iso-ddA is considerably more stable than ddA. At 37°C in neutral and basic buffer solutions, both compounds showed similar stabilities (no appreciable decomposition after 14 days). In acid (pH 3 buffer), however, the half-life of ddA was measured at less than one hour; under identical conditions, iso-ddA was stable for over two weeks.

Their antiviral activity, along with enhanced acid stability, distinguish the isomeric dideoxynucleosides as an important new class of potential anti-HIV agents.

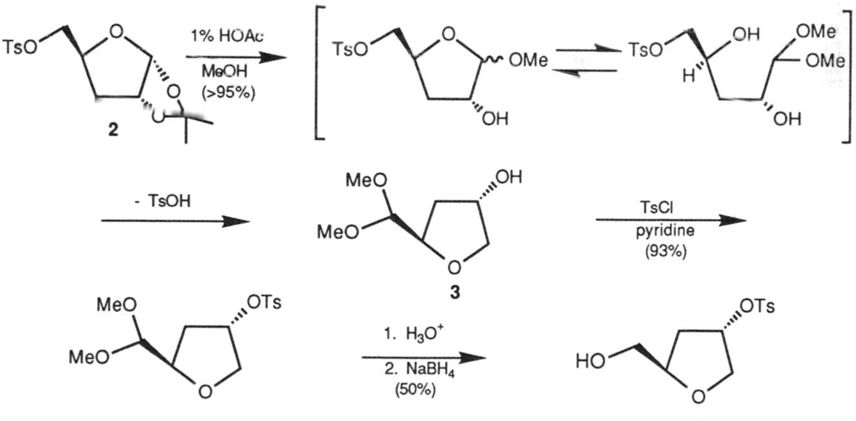

FIGURE 2.

TABLE 1.

Base	Compound Number	Starting Material	Reaction Conditions
	1	4	Adenine, K$_2$CO$_3$, 18-crown-6
	5	4	Cytosine, K$_2$CO$_3$, 18-crown-6
	6	4	Thymine, K$_2$CO$_3$, 18-crown-6
	7	4	6-chloro-purine, K$_2$CO$_3$, 18-crown-6
	8	4	2-amino-6-chloro-purine, K$_2$CO$_3$, 18-crown-6
	9	1	NaNO$_2$, HOAc
	10	8	HCl, H$_2$O
	11	7	H$_2$, Pd on C

TABLE 1. continued.

	12	8	H$_2$, Pd on C
	13	7	thiourea, propanol
	14	8	thiourea, propanol
	15	14	CH$_3$I, NH$_4$OH
	16	7	MeNII$_2$
	17	7	KF, Me$_3$N
	18	8	KF, Me$_3$N

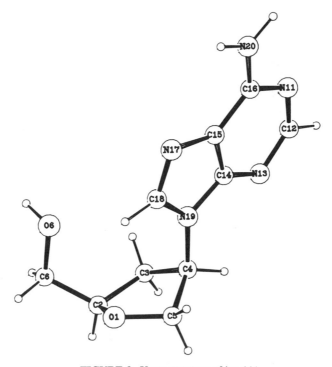

FIGURE 3. X-ray structure of iso-ddA.

REFERENCES

1. MITSUYA, H. & S. BRODER. 1986. Proc. Natl. Acad. Sci. USA **83:** 1911.
2. MARQUEZ, V. E., C. K.-H. TSENG, J. A. KELLEY, H. MITSUYA, S. BRODER, J. S. ROTH & J. S. DRISCOLL. 1987. Biochem. Pharmacol. **36:** 2719.
3. DEFAYE, J., D. HORTON & M. MUESSER. 1971. Carbohydr. Res. **20:** 305.
4. MEDICH, J. R., K. B. KUNNEN & C. R. JOHNSON. 1987. Tetrahedron Lett. **28:** 4131.
5. LARDER, B. A., G. DARBY & D. D. RICHMAN. 1989. Science **243:** 1731.
6. VAN ROEY, P., J. M. SALERNO, C. K. CHU & R. F. SCHINAZI. 1989. Proc. Natl. Acad. Sci. USA **86:** 3929.

Improved Synthesis of (−)-Carbovir, GR90352X, a Potent and Selective Inhibitor of HIV-1 *in Vitro*

M. F. JONES, C. L. MO, P. L. MYERS,
I. L. PATERNOSTER, R. STORER,
G. G. WEINGARTEN, AND C. WILLIAMSON

Microbiological Chemistry Department
Glaxo Group Research
Greenford, Middlesex, United Kingdom UB6 OHE

INTRODUCTION

(+/−)-Carbovir, a carbocyclic nucleoside, is a potent and selective inhibitor of HIV-1 *in vitro*,[1-3] of comparable activity with zidovudine (AZT). Activity may be mediated through competitive inhibition of HIV-encoded reverse transcriptase,[4] a prime target enzyme for the development of a drug candidate for AIDS.

It would be anticipated that the observed activity of racemic carbovir resides in only one enantiomer. This poster describes our synthesis of (−)-carbovir (9) (FIG. 1) from aristeromycin (1), a chiral carbocyclic nucleoside that is available as a secondary metabolite of *Streptomyces citricolor*.[5]

CHEMISTRY

In outline, the synthetic strategy we envisaged involved initial manipulation of the aristeromycin carbocycle by selective protection of the primary hydroxyl group, followed by the introduction of the olefin function from the 2,3-diol. Subsequent conversion of the adenine moiety into a guanine[6,7] would give the desired (−)-carbovir (9).

Reaction of aristeromycin (1) with thexyldimethylsilyl chloride allowed selective protection[8] of the primary 5'-hydroxyl group. The resulting silyl ether was converted into the cyclic orthoester (2) with trimethyl orthoformate in tetrahydrofuran at ambient temperature in the presence of catalytic amounts of pyridinium tosylate.[9] Treatment of the orthoester (2) with acetic anhydride followed by N-deacetylation with ammonia in methanol furnished the required 2',3'-cyclopentene (3).

The adenine (3) gave the N-oxide (4) on treatment with m-chloroperoxybenzoic acid. Addition of cyanogen bromide furnished the oxadiazole (5), which was isolated as its hydrobromide salt. Subsequent treatment with triethylamine gave an intermediate N6-cyanoadenine-N-oxide, which was methylated *in situ* to give the cyano-imine (6).

535

Rearrangement to the 2-amino-6-methoxyamino-purine (7) was effected with 1,8-diaz-abicyclo[5.4.0]undec-7-ene (DBU) in aqueous ethanol at reflux.

Reduction of the methoxyamino group was effected with aluminium amalgam,[10] and subsequent treatment with a 1:1 mixture of 3 N hydrochloric acid and ethanol at ambient temperature was employed for removal of the silyl group. Finally, enzymatic hydrolysis of the resulting diamine (8) with adenosine deaminase (EC 3.5.4.4) at pH

FIGURE 1. R = thexyldimethylsilyl. (*a.*) i. thexyldimethylsilylchloride, imidazole, dimethyl-formamide, 82%; ii. trimethyl orthoformate, cat. pyridinium tosylate, tetrahydrofuran, 90%. (*b.*) i. acetic anhydride, Δ; ii. ammonia, methanol, 85%. (*c.*) *m*-chloroperoxybenzoic acid, chloroform, 77%. (*d.*) cyanogen bromide, methanol, 99%. (*e.*) i. triethylamine, dimethylformamide; ii. iodo-methane, 65%. (*f.*) DBU, aqueoous ethanol, Δ, 92%. (*g*) i. aluminium amalgam, aqueous tetrahy-drofuran, 92%; ii. 3 N hydrochloric acid, ethanol, 94%. (*h.*) i. adenosine deaminase, pH 7.5; ii. water crystallization, 91%.

7.5 resulted in quantitative formation of (−)-carbovir (9), $[\alpha]_D$ −64° (*c* 0.4, methanol), isolated in 91% yield after crystallization from water.

Reaction of (−)-carbovir (9) with phosphorus oxychloride in trimethylphosphate[11] furnished the monophosphate, which was isolated as its ammonium salt, $[\alpha]_D$ −68° (water). This gave the morpholidate after coupling with morpholine in the presence of 1,3-dicyclohexyl-carbodiimide (DCC) in aqueous *tert*-butanol at reflux.[12] Condensation with bis(tributylammonium) pyrophosphate[13] provided the required triphosphate as its tris-ammonium salt, after chromatography on Sephadex A-25 (HCO3⁻ form, eluant aqueous ammonium bicarbonate).

BIOLOGICAL EVALUATION

In whole cell assays using MT-4 cells, (−)-carbovir had similar activity against HIV (RF strain) to AZT (IC_{50} = 0.0015 μg/mL and 0.001 μg/mL respectively).

The (−)-carbovir triphosphate was a potent inhibitor of the HIV reverse transcriptase, K_i's being approximately 50 nM for (−)-carbovir triphosphate (rCdG template/primer assay), and 25 nM for AZT triphosphate (rAdT template/primer assay).

ACKNOWLEDGMENTS

We wish to acknowledge J. M. Cameron, J. A. V. Coates, H. Inggall, D. C. Orr, and H. T. Figueiredo of the Virology Department of Glaxo Group Research, Greenford for the presentation of this data.

REFERENCES

1. VINCE, R. *et al.* 1988. Antiviral Res. **9**(1-2): 120.
2. VINCE, R. *et al.* 1988. Biochem. Biophys. Res. Commun. **156**(2): 1046.
3. YEOM, Y. H. *et al.* 1989. Antimicrob. Agents Chemother. **33**(2): 171.
4. WHITE, E. L. *et al.* 1989. Biochem. Biophys. Res. Commun. **161**(2): 393.
5. KUSAKA, T. *et al.* 1968. J. Antibiot. (Tokyo) (Ser. A) **21**(4): 255.
6. UEDA, T. *et al.* 1975. Chem. Pharm. Bull. (Tokyo) **23**(2): 464.
7. UEDA, T. *et al.* 1978. Chem. Pharm. Bull. (Tokyo) **26**(7): 2122.
8. WETTER, H. & K. OERTLE. 1985. Tetrahedron Let. **26**(45): 5515.
9. ANDO, M. *et al.* 1986. Chem. Let. 879.
10. KECK, G. E. *et al.* 1979. Synth. Commun. **9**(4): 281.
11. YOSHIKAWA, M., T. KATO & T. TAKENISHI. 1967. Tetrahedron Let. **50**: 5065.
12. MOFFATT, J. G. & H. G. KHORANA. 1961. J. Amer. Chem. Soc. **83**: 649.
13. MOFFATT, J. G. 1964. Can. J. Chem. **42**: 599.

Design of an Anti-HIV Prodrug

N^4-Dimethylaminomethylene-2',3'-Dideoxy-3'-Fluorocytidine (DDFC)

THOMAS I. KALMAN

Department of Medicinal Chemistry
State University of New York at Buffalo
Buffalo, New York 14260

The initial aim of this work was to design, synthesize, and study lipophilic, membrane permeable, prodrug derivatives of nucleoside analogue inhibitors of HIV replication. As a prototype of such prodrugs, DDFC (NSC-614989) was designed based on chemical principles, and biochemical and pharmacological considerations.

The choice of DDFC as a prototype is justified on the following bases: (a) 2',3'-dideoxycytidine is one of the most potent anti-HIV nucleoside analogues,[1] showing much lower toxicity to the bone marrow than AZT (zidovudine); it is more resistant to chemical and metabolic degradation than most of the dideoxynucleosides of purine bases; (b) the 3'-fluoro substitution disfavors the *3'-endo* sugar conformation prevalent in ribonucleosides and stabilizes the *2'-endo* sugar pucker most frequently assumed by 2'-deoxyribonucleosides; in addition, due to its electronegativity and its ability to accept H-bonds, it may better mimic the missing 3'-OH group in its interaction with the kinases required for phosphorylation and with the target enzyme reverse transcriptase; (c) the dimethylaminomethylene side chain increases the lipophilicity of the molecule, promoting diffusion across the blood brain barrier and decreasing the rate of elimination; (d) it can undergo slow, spontaneous hydrolysis, resulting in the sustained release of the parent drug, 2',3'-dideoxy-3'-fluorocytidine (3'-F-ddC).

DDFC was synthesized in a one-step reaction starting from 3'-F-ddC[2] using the dimethylacetal of DMF, essentially as described.[3] The molecular structure of DDFC was determined by single crystal X-ray diffraction techniques.[4] The analogue exists in the *anti*-conformation usually observed in pyrimidine nucleosides, and the van der Waals surface of the molecule reveals the additional bulk introduced by the side chain (see FIG. 1). Other notable structural features of DDFC include the coplanarity of the side chain with the pyrimidine ring, extending to the 1'-carbon. The coplanarity allows resonance stabilized delocalization of electrons from the side chain N to 2-O of the cytosine moiety, consistent with the strong H bond between the 2-O and the 5'-OH of a neighboring molecule observed in the crystal[4] and with the spectroscopic properties of DDFC. The side chain orientation with respect to the cytosine moiety corresponds to the *syn*-rotamer.

The dideoxyribofuranose ring conformation is of particular significance as it may be an important determinant of enzyme binding and substrate or inhibitory activity. Therefore, it is of interest that there is a remarkable overlap between the sugar conformation of DDFC and that of one of the two structures of AZT (AZTA) recently determined,[5] if the AZT molecule is superimposed upon the DDFC molecule by matching the positions of 1-*N*, 1'-C, 2'-C, and the furanose *O*. The electronegative fluorine atom of DDFC occupies the same position as the first electronegative N atom of the azido group of AZT at the 3'-position. By contrast, no match could be obtained when the structure of DDFC was superimposed upon the structure of ddC recently reported.[6] The significance of these findings remains to be determined.

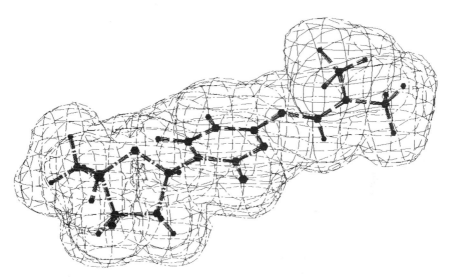

FIGURE 1. The molecular structure of DDFC.[4]

REFERENCES

1. YARCHOAN, R., H. MITSUYA, C. E. MYERS & S. BRODER. 1989. N. Engl. J. Med. **321:** 726.
2. HERDEWIJN, P., J. BALZARINI, E. DE CLERCQ, M. BABA, S. BRODER & H. VANDERHAEGHE. 1987. J. Med. Chem. **30:** 1270.
3. ŽEMLIČKA, J. & A. HOLÝ. 1967. Collect. Czech. Chem. Commun. **32:** 3159.
4. CODY, V. & T. I. KALMAN. In preparation.
5. VAN ROEY, P., J. M. SALERNO, W. L. DUAX, C. K. CHU, M. K. AHN & R. F. SCHINAZI. 1988. J. Amer. Chem. Soc. **110:** 2277.
6. BIRNBAUM, G. I., T.-S. LIN & W. H. PRUSOFF. 1988. Biochem. Biophys. Res. Commun. **151:** 608.

Chemistry and Biological Activity of the Anti-HIV Prodrug N^4-Dimethylaminomethylene-2′,3′-Dideoxy-3′-Fluorocytidine (DDFC)[a]

THOMAS I. KALMAN AND A. R. V. REDDY

Department of Medicinal Chemistry
State University of New York at Buffalo
Buffalo, New York 14260

This work was undertaken to demonstrate the feasibility of a prodrug approach to the improvement of the therapeutic effectiveness of existing anti-HIV dideoxynucleosides, aiming at more effective penetration into the central nervous system, prolonged duration of action, and decreased cellular and systemic toxicities. DDFC (NSC-614898) was designed and chosen as a representative of this class of agents.[1]

The kinetics of the hydrolysis of the dimethylaminomethylene side chain was investigated using reverse-phase HPLC. At 37°C and pH 7.4 in phosphate buffer, DDFC had a half-life of 4.8 hours. An intermediate containing a conjugated side chain with a retention time of 4.4 min, was observed to rapidly accumulate, reaching a maximum of 10% within 1.5 hours. On the basis of the similarity of its ultraviolet spectrum (determined by a diode-array detector during HPLC analysis) to that of N^4-acetylcytidine, the intermediate was identified as N^4-formyl-3′-F-ddC.

A plausible mechanism previously considered[2] for the hydrolysis of the dimethylaminomethylene side chain, consistent with our results, is outlined below:

$$R-N=CH-NMe_2 \rightleftharpoons R-NH-CH(OH)-NMe_2 \xrightarrow{-Me_2NH} R-NHCHO$$

$$\xrightarrow{H_2O} R-NH_2 \quad + \quad HCOOH$$

Reversible addition of H_2O to the double bond of the amidine side chain leads to the corresponding carbinolamine, which loses Me_2NH to form the formamide intermediate, which undergoes further hydrolysis to the unsubstituted 3′-F-ddC and formate. This mechanism provides for the spontaneous sustained release of the parent anti-HIV nucleoside analogue.

In the reverse-phase HPLC system used for the kinetic studies, DDFC and the parent 2′,3′-dideoxy-3′-fluorocytidine (3′-F-ddC) had retention times of 13.5 and 1.9

[a] This work was supported in part by Grant R01 AI27251 from the National Institute of Allergy and Infectious Diseases and by the Developmental Therapeutics Program, Division of Cancer Treatment, National Cancer Institute.

min, respectively, indicating the large increase in lipophilicity due to the introduction of the dimethylaminomethylene side chain.

In five different human cell lines (ATH8, CEM, C3-44, LDV-7, and MT-2), no cytotoxicity of DDFC was observed up to the highest concentration employed (200 μM). In the CEM cell line, complete protection against the cytopathic effect of HIV was achieved in the presence of 6 μM DDFC. The dose-dependent disappearance of p24 antigen detected by ELISA correlated well with the protection of the cells by DDFC against HIV.

It is concluded that DDFC is representative of a novel class of anti-HIV nucleoside prodrugs with no significant cytotoxicity. Due to its structural features and physicochemical properties, DDFC is expected to show a favorable pharmacokinetic profile, including efficient penetration into the central nervous system, warranting its further study and *in vivo* evaluation.

ACKNOWLEDGMENTS

The authors are indebted to Dr. R. F. Schinazi and Dr. J.-P. Sommadossi for their evaluation of the biological activity of 3'-F-ddC.

REFERENCES

1. KALMAN, T. I. 1990. Ann. N.Y. Acad. Sci. This volume.
2. HOLÝ, A. & J. ŽEMLIČKA. 1968. Collect. Czech. Chem. Commun. **34:** 2449.

Characterization of Tannins Containing Anti-HIV Activity

R. E. KILKUSKIE,[a] Y.-C. CHENG,[b] K.-H. LEE,[c]

G. NONAKA,[d] I. NISHIOKA,[d] M. NISHIZAWA,[c]

T. YAMAGISHI,[c] G. E. DUTSCHMAN,[b] AND

A. J. BODNER [a]

[a]Biotech Research Laboratories, Inc.
Rockville, Maryland 20850

[b]Yale University
New Haven, Connecticut

[c] University of North Carolina
Chapel Hill, North Carolina

[d]Kyushu University
Fukuoka, Japan

Because it plays a vital role in HIV-1 replication, reverse transcriptase has been an attractive target for developers of anti-HIV drugs. Nucleoside derivatives, including 3′-azido-2′,3′-dideoxythymidine and 2′,3′-dideoxycytidine, and pyrophosphate analogues, such as phosphonoformate, are well-known inhibitors of reverse transcriptase (RT).[1,2] Previously, tannins have been demonstrated to inhibit AMV-RT.[3] We have recently shown that a class of tannins, galloylquinic acids, are inhibitors of HIV-RT as well as HIV replication in culture.[4] Because the structures of galloylquinic acids are quite different from those of known HIV inhibitors, we have investigated other classes of tannins for their ability to inhibit HIV-RT and HIV replication in culture.

The tannin classes we screened for anti-HIV-RT activity have included gallotannins, ellagitannins, condensed tannins, complex tannins, and other related compounds. Fifty-one tannins were isolated from the plant materials by published methods. Reverse transcriptase inhibition assays were performed using affinity-purified HIV-1 RT according to the method described by Cheng et al.,[2] using poly $rA \cdot (oligo\ dT)_{10}$ as the substrate. Among the fifty-one tannins tested, twelve compounds inhibited HIV-RT by $> 40\%$ at 20 μg/mL (data not shown). We evaluated six of these compounds for inhibition of HIV replication in H9 lymphocytes using the procedures previously described.[4] Briefly, H9 lymphocytes were incubated with HIV-1 (0.01-0.1 $TCID_{50}$/cell) for one hour at 37°C. Cells were washed to remove unadsorbed virions, then incubated in the presence of drug for three days at 37°C. The amount of HIV released into the supernatant of infected cells over the three days was measured by a p24 antigen capture assay. Cell counts of uninfected, drug-treated cultures were used to measure cytotoxicity. All six tannins inhibited HIV replication by 50% in this assay at 5-10 μg/mL. Three of the six compounds were toxic to uninfected H9 cells ($> 30\%$ growth inhibition) at 20 μg/mL.

We characterized the anti-HIV effect of one ellagitannin, punicalin (structure shown in FIG. 1), further. This compound was not toxic to H9 cells at concentrations

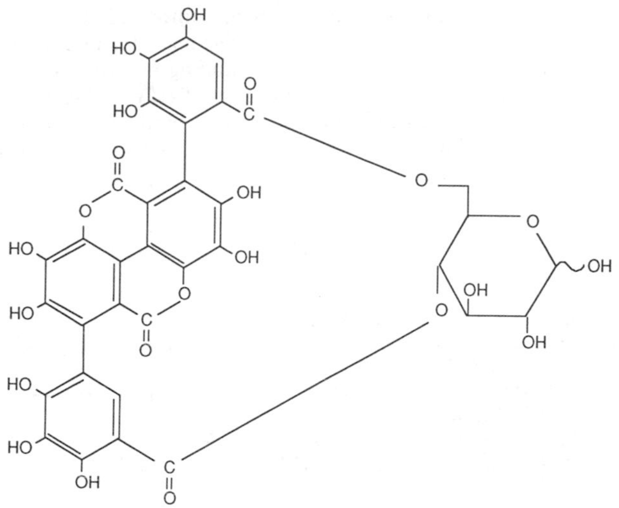

FIGURE 1. Structure of punicalin.

that had substantial anti-HIV activity. Virions were preincubated with 10 μg/mL (12 μM) punicalin for one hour at 37°C and then diluted tenfold into a suspension of H9 cells for infection. The infection step, using these virions or untreated virions, was conducted with or without additional punicalin included (at 12 μM). Following infection and washing, the various infected cultures were incubated in the presence or absence of punicalin (12 μM) for three days at 37°C. TABLE 1 shows that a maximum anti-HIV effect occurs when punicalin is present during the infection step. Preincubation of virus with punicalin did not inhibit HIV replication. Punicalin present only during the three day culture inhibited HIV replication to a lesser extent than did its addition during infection. These results suggest that punicalin possibly inhibits binding of virus to H9 cells.

TABLE 1. Characterization of HIV-1 Inhibition by Punicalin[a]

Punicalin Present			
Virus preinfection	Infection step	Culture	Percent inhibition
███████████			0
███████████		███████	58
████████████████████████			77
███████████	██████		86
	████████		99
		███████	60

[a] Punicalin was added to HIV inhibition experiments at different times. Percent inhibition was calculated compared to an untreated, infected culture using p24 antigen capture. See text for details.

In summary, we have identified a new class of compound that can inhibit HIV reverse transcriptase and HIV replication *in vitro*. The mechanism of HIV-1 inhibition by one active tannin (punicalin) was studied. Our finding was that punicalin does not inactivate HIV virions but shows maximum inhibition of HIV replication when present during the infection of H9 cells. Punicalin may inhibit binding of HIV-1 to H9 cells. The mechanism of HIV inhibition by other active tannins is presently being studied.

REFERENCES

1. DeClerq, E. J. 1986. J. Med. Chem. **29:** 1561.
2. Cheng, Y.-C., G. E Dutschman, K. F. Bastow, M. G. Sarngadharan & R. C. Y. Ting. 1987. J. Biol. Chem. **262:** 2187.
3. Kakiuchi, N., M. Hattori, T. Namba, N. Nishizawa, T. Yamagishi & T. Okuda. 1985. J. Nat. Prod. (Lloydia) **48:** 614.
4. Nishizawa, N., T. Yamagishi, G. E. Dutschman, W. B. Parker, A. J. Bodner, R. E. Kilkuskie, Y.-C. Cheng & K. H. Lee. 1989. J. Nat. Prod. (Lloydia) **52:** 762.

Effect of Membrane-Active Ether Lipid (EL) Analogues on Human Immunodeficiency Virus Production Measured by Plaque Assay[a]

LOUIS S. KUCERA, NATHAN IYER, EVA S. LEAKE,
ADAM RABEN, LARRY W. DANIEL,
EDWARD J. MODEST,[b] AND CLAUDE PIANTADOSI[c]

The Bowman Gray School of Medicine of Wake Forest University
Winston-Salem, North Carolina 27103

[b]*Boston University*
Boston, Massachusetts

[c]*University of North Carolina*
Chapel Hill, North Carolina 27599

Recent findings in our laboratory indicate that a novel class of membrane interactive[1] ether lipid (EL) analogues of platelet-activating factor has potent activity against replication of infectious HIV-1 and associated pathogenesis. Data are provided indicating that anti-HIV-1 EL compounds cause production of defective virus that is unable to initiate new rounds of infection and produce cytopathology.

Human CEM-SS T lymphocytes in monolayer or suspension culture were used to determine effects of type A phosphorus and type B inverse choline EL analogues on HIV-1 syncytial plaque formation, cell cytotoxicity ([3H]TdR incorporation into DNA), and reverse transcriptase activity.

Results indicated that both type A and type B EL inhibit HIV plaque formation in a dose-dependent manner when treatment was started as late as 2 days after infection. Type A EL (IC_{50} range = 0.14 to 1.4 μM) with a thioalkyl or amidoalkyl group at position 1 and type B (IC_{50} range = 0.13 to 0.63 μM) with an inverse choline at position 3 have anti-HIV activity that is 5- to 53-fold below IC_{50} values for cell cytotoxicity. Because the plaque assay has recently been introduced as a method for evaluating antiviral agents, we evaluated the effect of AZT and dideoxyinosine (ddI) on HIV-1 plaque formation and CEM-SS cell growth. The results indicated that the IC_{50} for AZT and ddI against HIV-1 plaque formation is 0.004 μM and 1.0 μM, respectively. The IC_{50} for cell growth was 6.2 μM for AZT and > 100 μM for ddI.

Both type A (compound 1) and type B (compound 5) EL inhibited infectious HIV-1 production and RT activity in a concentration-dependent manner at 8 and 10 days after infection and treatment, compared with untreated controls (TABLE 1). At 13 days infectious HIV-1 production was still markedly inhibited, but RT activity in

[a]This work was supported in part by the Cancer Center of Wake Forest University, Grant CA 12197, and BRS Grant RR 05404 from the United States Public Health Service.

TABLE 1. Effect of Representative Type A and Type B EL Compounds on Infectious HIV-1 Multiplication and Reverse Transcriptase Activity[a]

Compounds[b]	Concn. (μM)	Percent of control at days after infection						Ratio: RT/plaque count at 13 days	Fold increase in ratio
		Plaque-forming units/mL × 10²			RT dpm/mL × 10⁻⁶				
		8	10	13	8	10	13		
Control	0	100(2)[c]	100(45)	100(85)	100(18.4)	100(78.4)	100(84.4)	9.9×10^3	0
Type A									
1 (ET-18-OMe)	0.2	395	287	89	54	192	94	1.0×10^4	1.0
	0.4	25	30	35	15	90	161	4.6×10^4	4.6
	2.0	0	33	30	6	6	174	5.8×10^4	5.9
Type B									
5 (CP-7)	0.2	100	143	100	33	85	133	1.3×10^4	1.3
	0.4	75	23	47	10	43	155	3.3×10^4	3.3
	2.0	0	49	18	18	30	102	5.7×10^4	5.8

[a] CEM-SS cells were infected with HIV-1 (multiplicity of infection = 0.003 plaque-forming units per cell). After 1 h virus attachment the cells were pelleted (450 × g, 5 min) and resuspended in fresh growth medium (5×10^5 cells/mL) with or without added compound. Culture fluids were harvested at every 2 or 3 days and assayed for infectious virus production by plaque count and reverse transcriptase activity.

[b] Structures:

1 (ET-18-OMe)

5 (CP-7)

[c] Numbers outside the parentheses are percent of control. Numbers inside the parentheses are plaque-forming units/mL $\times 10^{-2}$ or RT dpm/mL $\times 10^{-6}$.

treated cultures was equal to or greater than RT activity in nontreated controls. The ratio of RT to plaque count was increased 1.3- to 5.9-fold compared to untreated controls (TABLE 1). In HIV-1-infected T cells the virus is often seen budding at the plasma membrane[2] (FIG. 1). In EL-treated HIV-1-infected cells there was marked

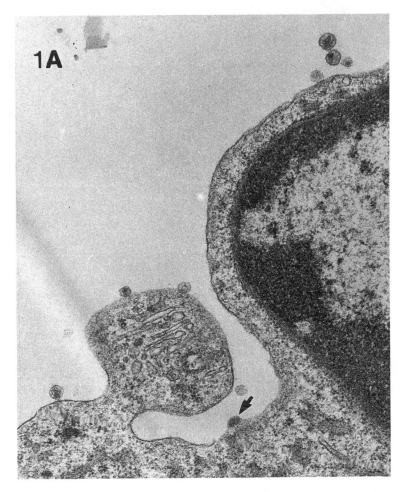

FIGURE 1. Effect of compound 5 on budding of virus particles at the plasma membrane. **A:** Representative HIV-1-infected and untreated CEM-SS cell 10 days after infection; ×30,460. **B:** Representative HIV-1-infected CEM-SS cell treated with 2.0 μM compound 5 for 10 days after infection; ×23,970.

inhibition of HIV-1 assembly by budding at the plasma membrane but presence of intracytoplasmic vacuolar virus particles (FIG. 1). Together, these data suggest that EL treatment induces defective virus production and causes a shift in virus assembly from the plasma membrane to intracytoplasmic vacuoles. Being membrane interactive,

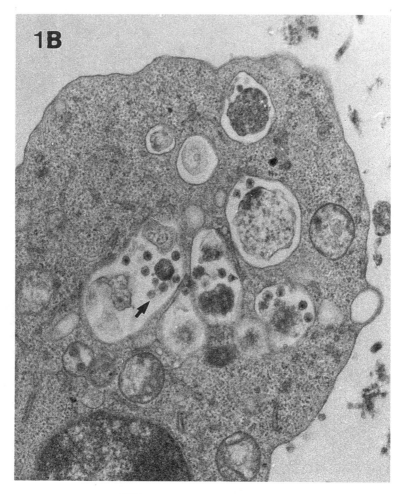

FIGURE 1B. See legend on p.547.

EL are ideally suited for combination chemotherapy with DNA interactive anti-HIV nucleoside analogues.

REFERENCES

1. NOSEDA, A., P. L. GODWIN & E. J. MODEST. 1988. Effects of antineoplastic ether lipids on model and biological membranes. Biochim. Biophys. Acta **945:** 92-100.
2. GALLO, R. 1985. Human T-cell leukemia (lymphotropic) retroviruses and their causative role in T-cell malignancies and acquired immune deficiency syndrome. Cancer **55:** 2317-2323.

Improved Clinical Evaluation of Prospective Vaccines and New Therapies against AIDS

VADIM I. KVITASH[a] AND ROBERT M. SCHMIDT

Center for Preventive Medicine and Health Research
Pacific Presbyterian Medical Center
San Francisco State University
San Francisco, California 94115

Our objective is to improve the design and evaluation of AIDS-related clinical trials by elimination of avoidable biases in patient selection. We propose a better stratification of prognostically identical individuals with HIV infection for controlled clinical trials.

MATERIAL

Initial laboratory data for six immunological (WBC, TC#, BC#, T4#, T8#, T4/T8) and seven metabolic variables (uric acid, BUN, glucose, cholesterol, triglycerides, SGOT, alk. phos.) were obtained from the San Francisco Men's Health Study data base for 130 homosexual/bisexual men. Within the following 24 months, 29 HIV Ab(−) asymptomatics and 29 HIV Ab(+) asymptomatics did not develop symptoms. Thirty HIV Ab(+) ARC patients did not develop AIDS, and 42 HIV Ab(+) ARC patients progressed to AIDS.

METHODS

In a blind retrospective study, two immunobalascopy patterns were used to predict a clinical outcome for each of the 130 above subjects[1] after 24 months (FIGS. 1 and 2). Immunobalascopy is a first-generation cognitive expert system for detection, quantification, and mapping of multidimensional relational abnormalities among given immunological and metabolic variables in their total interrelatedness.[2-4]

---

[a] Address for correspondence: Balascopy Institute, 369 Upper Terrace, San Francisco, CA 94117.

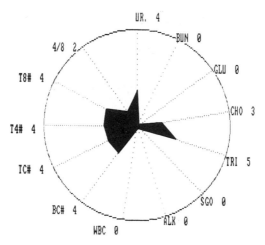

FIGURE 1. Pattern of AIDS-resistant ARC.

RESULTS

Immunobalascopy confirmed the existence of identifiable subpopulations of patients with ARC: AIDS-resistant ARC and ARC progressing to AIDS. Each subpopulation exhibits characteristic patterns of abnormal immunometabolic relationships. Statistical evaluation of predictive performance of immunometabolic patterns in early individual identification of AIDS-resistant ARC versus ARC actually progressing to AIDS demonstrated the following: sensitivity, 95%; specificity, 92%; predictive value of positive

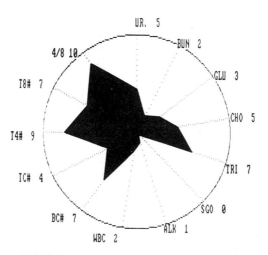

FIGURE 2. Pattern of ARC progressing to AIDS.

results, 84.4%; predictive value of negative results, 95.3%; and efficiency of identification, 91.5%.

CONCLUSIONS

Two identifiable subpopulations of ARC patients exist: AIDS-resistant ARC, and ARC actually progressing to AIDS within 24 months. Early definitive identification of individuals with ARC who are actually progressing to AIDS can be done by immunobalascopy based on routine laboratory tests. Immunobalascopy avoids the pitfalls of heterogeneity in AIDS clinical trials by identifying more prognostically homogenous patient cohorts.

REFERENCES

1. KVITASH, V. I. & R. M. SCHMIDT. 1989. Forecasting individual rates of progression from ARC to AIDS using routine clinical laboratory tests. Collected abstracts of the V International Conference on AIDS, Montreal, Quebec, Canada, 4-9 June 1989. 364.
2. SCHMIDT, R. M. & V. I. KVITASH. 1987. Behavioral, immunological and biochemical patterns in ARC and AIDS. Collected abstracts of the III International Conference on Acquired Immunodeficiency Syndrome (AIDS), Washington, D.C., June 1-5, 1987. 95.
3. KVITASH, V. I., R. M. SCHMIDT & H. S. KAUFMAN. 1986. Immunodeficiency: Novel immuno-metabolic mechanisms. Collected abstracts of the Sixth International Congress of Immunology, Toronto, Canada, 6-11 July, 1986. 455.
4. KVITASH, V. I. 1983. Balascopy as a tool for heuristic diagnosis. AAMSI Congress 83. Collected abstracts of the Proceedings of the Congress on Medical Informatics, San Francisco, California. 1983. 121-125.

Synthetic Inhibitors of HIV-1 Protease Block Processing of Pr55^{gag} and Pr160$^{gag-pol}$ Polyproteins in Infected T Lymphocytes

D. M. LAMBERT,[a] T. D. MEEK,[b] G. B. DREYER,[b]
T. K. HART,[c] T. J. MATTHEWS,[d] J. J. LEARY,[a]
P. J. BUGELSKI,[c] B. W. METCALF,[b] AND
S. R. PETTEWAY JR.[a]

*Departments of [a]Anti-Infectives, [b]Medicinal Chemistry, and
[c]Experimental Pathology
Smith Kline & French Laboratories
King of Prussia, Pennsylvania 19406-2799
and
[d]Department of Surgery
Duke University Medical School
Durham, North Carolina 27710*

Retroviruses, including HIV-1, the causative agent of AIDS, contain a protease responsible for processing the initial translation products of their *gag* and *pol* genes into functional proteins. In HIV-1, these genes are translated as two polyproteins, Pr55^{gag} and Pr160$^{gag-pol}$, the latter protein resulting from a ribosomal frameshift between the *gag* and *pol* reading frames. Pr55^{gag} is subsequently cleaved into the four structural proteins of the virion core (p17, p24, p7, and p6), whereas these gag proteins as well as the enzymes essential for retrovirus replication (protease, reverse transcriptase (RT), ribonuclease H, and endonuclease) result from processing of Pr160$^{gag-pol}$. The virus-encoded protease responsible for this processing is apparently capable of catalyzing its own cleavage from Pr160$^{gag-pol}$. In principle, inhibition of the protease within HIV-1 and other retroviruses should inhibit maturation of both the virion core and the retroviral enzymes. Thus, inhibition of the protease of HIV-1 presents an attractive yet unproven strategy for the development of antiviral agents useful for the treatment of AIDS.

Toward the goal of developing specific inhibitors of HIV-1 protease, SmithKline Beecham scientists have (1) subcloned and expressed the protease in *E. coli,* (2) purified and characterized the recombinant enzyme in terms of its primary and quaternary structure, (3) characterized oligopeptides (6-9 amino acids) of the type R-Ser-Gln-Asn-Tyr-Pro-Val-R' as substrates of the protease, (4) characterized the enzyme kinetically with respect to irreversible inactivation by 1,2-epoxy-3-(4-nitrophenoxy)propane (EPNP) and pH rate profiles of the substrates.[1–3] From these results, HIV-1 protease appears to be an aspartyl protease that is formed by dimerization of identical 11 kDa monomers.[2,4] Accordingly, we have designed and synthesized peptide analogues based on the structure of the substrates to act as competitive inhibitors of the protease.[3,5] We have analyzed the effects of these inhibitors on the processing of virion polyproteins within a T-lymphocyte culture chronically infected with HIV-1. Studies described in this report used three hydroxyethylene isostere inhibitors, compounds 1 (Cbz-AFΨGVV-OMe), 2 (AAFΨGVV-OMe), and 3 (Cbz-AAFΨGVV-OMe).

RESULTS

HIV-1 gag Processing

Using Western blot and pulse chase/radioimmunoprecipitation techniques, inhibition of the proteolytic processing of both Pr55^{gag} and Pr160$^{gag-pol}$ was observed in the infected T lymphocytes upon treatment with protease inhibitors. Treatment with HIV-specific protease inhibitor resulted in an accumulation of Pr55^{gag} and Pr160$^{gag-pol}$ as well as processing intermediates (data not shown). In addition, there was a corresponding decrease in amounts of mature protein products (p24 and p17).

Virion Morphology

Electron microscopy revealed that most of the virion particles produced from inhibitor-treated cells were of an aberrant morphology that temporally correlated with the inhibition of polyprotein processing (FIG. 1).

Virus Infectivity

Two of the three HIV protease inhibitors used here prevented the spread of virus in acutely infected Molt-4 cells treated immediately after infection. At seven days postinfection, dramatically lower levels of reverse transcriptase activity, p24 antigen, and syncytial formation were observed in cultures treated with compounds 1 and 3 (TABLE 1).

CONCLUSIONS

Rationally designed peptide analogue inhibitors of HIV protease block Pr55^{gag} and Pr160$^{gag-pol}$ processing in chronically infected T lymphocytes without evidence of

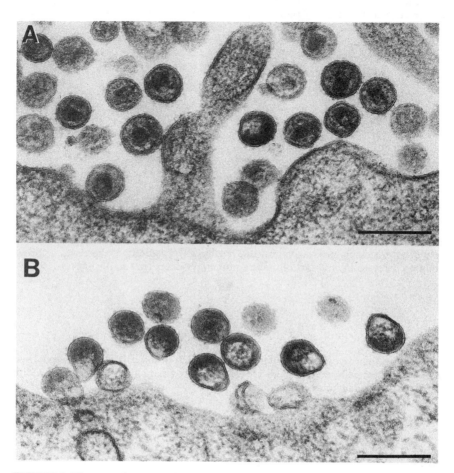

FIGURE 1. Electron microscopy. CEM cells infected with HIV_{IIIB} treated with HIV protease inhibitor. **A:** Infected cell following 24 hours in vehicle (media + 1% DMSO). Almost all virions are mature and contain a nuclear core. Nuclear cores appear as dark circles or cone shaped bodies in virions. Immature virions are distinguished by the absence of cores and a retention of a dense plaque in a "C" pattern on the viral membrane. **B:** Cell treated with compound 3 (25 μM in media + 1% DMSO) for 24 hours. All virions associated with the cell are immature in appearance, that is, they do not contain nuclear cores. Unprocessed nuclear material remains associated with the viral membrane to give the various images seen here. Many particles appear somewhat "cone"-shaped with the membrane opposite the nuclear plaque bulging out. Magnification = $\times$ 144,000; reduced by 6% (bar = 250 nm). Methods: Cells were treated for 24 hours with or without HIV protease inhibitor in 1% DMSO; fixed in 2.5% glutaraldehyde in 0.1 M phosphate buffer; postfixed in 1% OsO_4; 1% tannic acid; 1% aqueous uranyl acetate; dehydrated in ethanol and embedded in EMBed 812. Thin sections were stained with lead citrate and examined in a JEOL 100CX.

TABLE 1. Effects of Compounds 1, 2, and 3 on Spread of HIV_{111B} Infection in Molt-4 Cells

Culture Components[a]	Inhibitor (μM) at		Syncytial formation[b]		Percent inhibition	
	Day 1	Day 7	With Inhibitor	Without Inhibitor	RT	p24
Molt-4 cells			− − −	−		
Molt-4/Virus			− − −	+ + + + +		
Molt-4/Virus/1	10	1.7	+ + + + +	+ + + + +	47	0
	25	4.2	+ +	+ + + + +	88	70
	100	17	−	+ + + + +	96	99
Molt-4/Virus/2	10	1.7	+ + + + +	+ + + + +	28	0
	25	4.2	+ + + + +	+ + + + +	8	0
	100	17	+ + + + +	+ + + + +	0	0
Molt-4/Virus/3	10	1.7	+ + + + +	+ + + + +	76	2
	25	4.2	−	+ + + + +	98	99
	100	17	−	+ + + + +	97	98

[a] 1, 2, 3 = compounds 1, 2, and 3, respectively.
[b] − − − = no cytotoxicity or CPE; − = no syncytia; + + + + + = > 50 syncytia in a single microscopic field, 40× magnification.

cytotoxicity. Aberrant particle formation was observed in treated chronically infected T-lymphocyte cultures. Two inhibitors blocked virus spread in uninfected cultures of T lymphocytes. These results provide an encouraging foundation for the development of protease inhibitors as antiretroviral agents.

REFERENCES

1. DEBOUCK, C. *et al.* 1987. Proc Natl. Acad. Sci. USA **84:** 8903-8906.
2. MEEK, T. *et al.* 1989. Proc. Natl. Acad. Sci. USA **86:** 1841-1845.
3. MOORE, M. *et al.* 1989. Biochem. Biophys. Res. Commun. **159:** 420-425.
4. STRICKLER, J. E. *et al.* 1989. Proteins. **6:** 139-154.
5. DREYER, G. *et al.* 1989. Proc. Natl. Acad. Sci. USA **86:** 9752-9756.

Hypericin as an Antiretroviral Agent

Mode of Action and Related Analogues

GAD LAVIE,[a] YEHUDA MAZUR,[b] DAVID LAVIE,[b]
BRANDI LEVIN,[a] YITZHAK ITTAH,[b] AND
DANIEL MERUELO[a]

[a]Department of Pathology and Kaplan Cancer Center
New York University Medical Center
New York, New York 10016

[b]Department of Organic Chemistry
The Weizmann Institute of Science
Rehovot 76 100, Israel

We have recently reported on the antiretroviral activity and mechanism of action of two polycyclic aromatic naphthodianthrones, hypericin and pseudohypericin.[1,2] Hypericin and pseudohypericin interfere with the assembly of mature viral particles from infected cell lines and also inactivate retroviruses directly.[1,2] These compounds occur naturally in plants of the genus *Hypericum* (St. Johns wort). Hypericin, the more potent one, has been chosen for development as a potential therapeutic agent. It is currently being synthesized from emodin.

The present manuscript reports studies that begin to evaluate the structural features of hypericin essential for antiretroviral activity. Numerous molecular analogues and precursors of hypericin have been examined for activity in two *in vitro* and one *in vivo* biological assays. The results of these studies support the notion that the quinone group and certain side chain groups are important for the antiretroviral activity of hypericin.

METHODS AND MATERIAL

Direct Inactivation of Retroviruses in Vitro

Five to ten milliliters of tissue culture supernatants from murine cell lines producing radiation leukemia virus (RadLV) were incubated on ice for 30 minutes with the indicated concentration(s) of compound(s) (*e.g.* hypericin). At the end of 30 minutes viruses were pelleted at $100,000 \times g$ for 1 hour and assayed for reverse transcriptase activity as previously described.[1]

In Vitro *Inhibition of Virus Budding*

Tissue-culture adapted, virus-producing cells were incubated with the indicated amount(s) of compounds(s) for 30 minutes at 37°C. After 30 minutes the cells were washed three times with Dulbecco's modified Eagle medium (DMEM) supplemented with fetal calf serum, growth factors, and antibiotics and grown for 24 to 48 hours. The cells are then harvested and the culture supernatants assayed for reverse transcriptase activity as described elsewhere.[1,2]

In Vivo *Inhibition of Friend Virus Splenomegaly*

BALB/c mice were first inoculated intravenously with 10^6 focus-forming units (FFU) of NB tropic[a] Friend virus (FV) capable of inducing significant erythroleukemia and enlargement of the spleen within 10-14 days. Virus inoculation was followed within 1-2 hours with an intravenous injection of the tested agent at various concentrations. Animals were sacrificed 10-14 days after FV inoculation and their spleen weight determined.

RESULTS

FIGURES 1A-1C display results obtained with hypericin and the various hypericin analogues tested in each of our standard assays. TABLE 1 provides the molecular structures and a summary of results obtained for all analogues studied in the three antiretroviral assays: (1) direct inactivation of virions, (2) inhibition of proper virus assembly from infected cells *in vitro,* and (3) interference with Friend virus-induced splenomegaly. It is apparent that different analogues vary in their levels of effectiveness, and that compounds that are highly active in some assays are less so in other assays. Only hypericin, pseudohypericin, and desmethyl-hypericin show a high degree of activity in more than one assay.

Removal of the carbonyl groups from hypericin (*e.g.,* desoxohypericin) results in a significant loss of the reverse transcriptase inhibitory activity. This loss of activity is also evident when the activities of the hexaacetate derivative of hypericin are compared with those of the desoxo-hexaacetate derivative. These observations suggest that the quinone structure is of vital importance for the antiviral activity of polycyclic aromatic diones, preferably when structured on a naphthodianthrone backbone.

Triplet carbonyl groups have been found to play a role in transferring energy that excites efficient acceptors (such as oxygen) to their singlet state.[3] Indeed singlet oxygen quenchers such as sodium azide and β-carotene obviate the inhibitory activity of hypericin in direct retrovirus inactivation studies of the type described herein (data not shown).

Bianthrone and hypericin dicarboxylate were unable to affect the release of intact RadLV from AQR cells. Intravenous injection of hypericin and its various analogues to Friend virus-infected BALB/c mice has shown pseudohypericin and hypericin to be very effective in inhibiting splenomegaly development. Whereas several of the other

[a] NB tropic = viruses which can replicate in NIH or BALB/c derived cells.

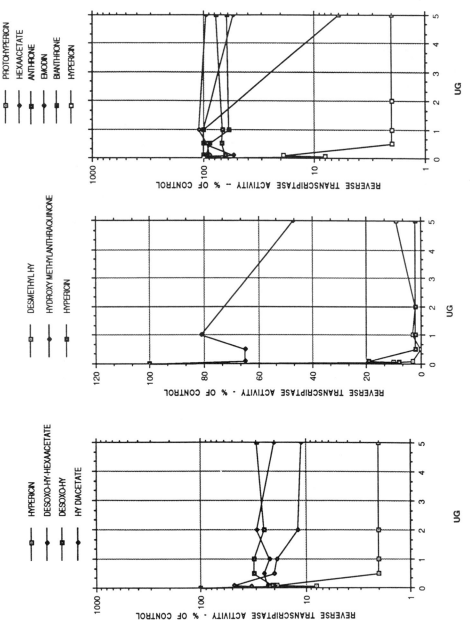

FIGURE 1A. *In vitro* direct inactivation of virions.

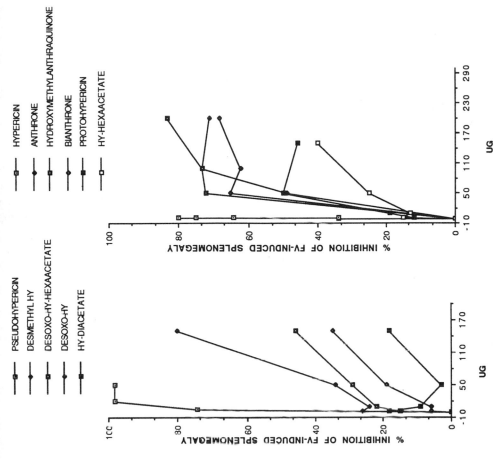

FIGURE 1C. *In vivo* experiments with Friend virus.

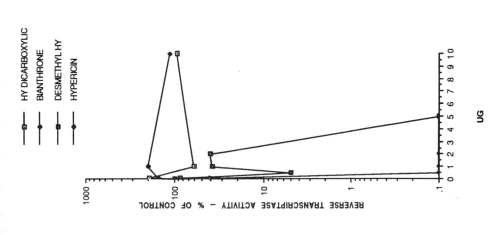

FIGURE 1B. *In vitro* budding experiments.

TABLE 1. Antiretroviral Activity of Several Hypercin Analogues

Compound	Formula	EC_{80} (μM) for direct inactivation of virions	EC_{50} (μM) for production of defective budded virions	EC_{50} (μM) for FV-induced splenomegaly
Hypericin		0.06	0.2	0.12
Protohypericin		7.90		98
Pseudohypericin				3.8
Hypericin-dicarboxylic acid			>100	
Hypericin-diacetate		0.85		>255
Hypericin-hexaacetate		12.90		>199

Compound			
Desmethyl-hypericin	174	2	0.07
Hydroxy-desmethylhypericin			>19.60
Desoxohypericin	>316		>21
Desoxohypericin-hexaacetate	>242		6.90
Emodin			>37
Hydroxymethylanthraquinone	145		>41
Anthrone	267		>51
Bianthrone	98	>100	>26

analogues can decrease FV-induced splenomegaly, they do so only at much higher doses.

DISCUSSION

Differences in the activities of hypericin-related analogues can be used to focus on the structural elements of the hypericin backbone required for the antiretroviral activity. Most significantly carbonyl groups (as quinones) on a naphthodianthrone backbone seem essential for the antiretroviral activity of these molecules. This suggests that the same elements of the molecule involved in the photodynamic action may play a role in its antiviral mechanism. This association between the two activities is also supported by the finding that quenchers of singlet oxygen reactions also interfere with the antiretroviral activity of hypericin-like molecules.

In addition, replacement of the methyl side chains by more polar groups such as carboxylic, acetoxy, or hydroxy side groups diminishes the antiviral activity as seen in hypericin dicarboxylic acid, the di- and hexaacetate, and hydroxy-desmethyl derivatives of hypericin.

Failure of various analogues to demonstrate equal activities in the different assays implies that the actions of hypericin-like agents at the various stages of the retrovirus replication cycle are distinct (albeit, related mechanisms may underlie all of these effects). These studies combined with ongoing biochemical and physicochemical analyses of hypericin's interaction with a variety of viral and cellular components should help determine the exact mode of hypericin's antiretroviral/antiviral activities. The identification of new antiretroviral agents within this group of direct inactivators of retroviruses, such as desmethyl-hypericin, is another desirable outcome of this type of work.

REFERENCES

1. MERUELO, D., G. LAVIE & D. LAVIE. 1988. Proc. Natl. Acad. Sci. USA **85:** 5230-5234.
2. LAVIE, G., F. VALENTINE, B. LEVIN, Y. MAZUR, G. GALLO, D. LAVIE, D. WEINER & D. MERUELO. 1989. Proc. Natl. Acad. Sci. USA **86:** 5963-5967.
3. CILENTO, G. 1980. Photochem. Photobiol. **5:** 199-228.

Stable Transformed Human Cell Lines Exhibiting tat-Directed Expression of Tissue Plasminogen Activator

S. K. MALCOLM, T. W. THAIS, P. A. HEFFERNAN,
S. R. JASKUNAS, J. TANG, J. M. COLACINO, AND
B. R. WARREN

Departments of Molecular Biology and Virology Research
Lilly Research Laboratories
Indianapolis, Indiana 46285

The *trans*-activation protein tat encoded by HIV-1 is required for the production of genomic RNA, viral proteins, and virus.[1,2] Because it appears to act by a unique mechanism and is virally encoded, inhibitors of tat may be useful as antiviral drugs for individuals infected by HIV. Therefore, stable cell lines were constructed to identify inhibitors of tat-dependent *trans*-activation. Such cell lines may be more analogous to HIV-infected cells than transiently transfected cells. Derivatives of HeLa cells were constructed that expressed tat and a reporter gene whose expression was dependent on tat. Tissue plasminogen activator (tPA) was used as the reporter enzyme because it is secreted into the medium, is stable, and can be easily assayed.[3,4]

To generate cell lines in which the expression of tPA was dependent on tat, a plasmid (pL606) was constructed in which a cDNA gene for tPA was placed under control of the HIV-1 long terminal repeats (LTR) promoter that contained the *trans*-activation response (TAR) sequence required for tat-dependent *trans*-activation.[5] Another plasmid (pL570) was constructed in which the tat gene was expressed from a derivative of the adenovirus major late promoter designated BL,[6] which was known to be a relatively weak promoter in HeLa cells.[7]

The desired cell lines were constructed in two steps, by first introducing the tat plasmid and then the LTR-tPA plasmid, or in the reverse order. Several cell lines were tested at each step to confirm their phenotype with respect to tat *trans*-activation. The cell line designated 1B2, which only contained the tat plasmid, was found to be capable of TAR-dependent *trans*-activation of a chloramphenicol acetyltransferase (CAT) reporter gene. The cell line designated LT35, which only contained the LTR-tPA plasmid, could be *trans*-activated by plasmids that encode tat or by tat protein produced in *E. coli.*

The expression of tPA in cell lines containing both pL570 and pL606 (LT35-tat12 and 1B2L12) was dependent on tat. *Trans*-activation resulted in a dramatic increase (> 100X) in the level of steady-state tPA mRNA, and in the secretion of functional tPA, without amplification of the LTR-tPA hybrid gene (see FIG. 1). Results of transient transfection experiments with an LTR-CAT plasmid indicated that the level

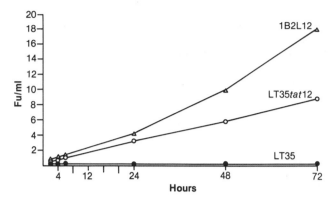

FIGURE 1. tPA production. Cells were plated at 5×10^4/mL into a 24-well dish. Growth medium was Dulbecco's modified Eagle medium containing 10% FBS and 50 μg/mL gentamicin. Media (10 μL) containing the secreted tPA was removed at the indicated time points and assayed for tPA levels using a spectrophotometric assay.[4]

of expression of CAT in LT35-tat12 and 1B2L12 was limited by the level of tat, suggesting that the level of expression of tPA also may be limited by the level of tat (see TABLE 1).

A control cell line (1B2P13) was also constructed in which the expression of tPA was independent of tat by using a plasmid (pL609) in which the tPA gene was expressed from the SV40$_e$ promoter. Methods were developed for using these cell lines in a high volume screen to test possible inhibitors of tat-dependent *trans*-activation. Specific inhibitors of tat would decrease the production of tPA in LT35-tat12 and 1B2L12 but not in 1B2P13.

TABLE 1. Plasmid Titration of Cellular tat[a]

Cell line	pSV2-tat (μg)	LTR-(TAR)CAT (μg)	Acetylation (percent)
IB2L12	—	2	26
	0.1	2	60
	—	5	29
	0.1	5	72
LT35-tat12	—	2	53
	0.1	2	70
	—	5	67
	0.1	5	87

[a] Cells (1×10^6) were transfected with the indicated amounts of tat (pL546) and CAT (pL608) plasmids (not shown) and assayed 48 hours later for CAT activity. Total DNA input (8.0 μg) was equalized with pL545 (a pUC9 derivative). Percent acetylation reflects data from three separate experiments. The titration was also tested at 1 and 10 μg of cat plasmid (data not shown).

REFERENCES

1. FISHER, A. G. *et al.* 1986. Nature **320:** 367-371.
2. DAYTON, A. I., J. G. SODROSKI, C. A. ROSEN, W. D. GOH & W. A. HASELTINE. 1986. Cell **44:** 941-947.
3. SCHUMACHER, G. F. B. & W-B. SCHILL. 1972. Anal. Biochem. **8:** 9-26.
4. VERHEIJEN, J. H., E. MULLAART, G. T. G. CHANG, C. KLUFT & G. WIJNGAARDS. 1982. Thromb. Haemostasis **48:** 266-269.
5. ROSEN, C. A., J. G. SODROSKI & W. A. HASELTINE. 1985. Cell **41:** 813-823.
6. GRINNELL, B. W., D. T. BERG & J. D. WALLS. 1986. Mol. Cell. Biol. **6:** 3596-3605.
7. GRINNELL, B. W., D. T. BERG & J. D. WALLS. 1988. Mol. Cell. Biol. **8:** 3448-3457.

A Rapid Fluorogenic Assay of HIV Protease Inhibitors

EDMUND MATAYOSHI, GARY WANG,
GRANT KRAFFT, DALE KEMPF, LYNN CODACOVI,
AND JOHN ERICKSON

Abbott Laboratories
Abbott Park, Illinois 60064-3500

The 11 kDa protease (PR) encoded by the human immunodeficiency virus 1 (HIV) is required for the processing of viral polyproteins and the maturation of infectious virus, and is therefore a target for the design of selective AIDS therapeutics. To date large scale screening for inhibitors of HIV PR, as well as detailed studies on the enzymology and inhibition of this enzyme, have been difficult due to the lack of a simple, continuous assay for measuring its activity. For this reason, we have developed an assay based on intramolecular fluorescence resonance energy transfer (RET).[1,2] In this assay, continuous data acquisition of substrate hydrolysis is achieved through the use of the quenched fluorogenic substrate DABCYL-Ser-Gln-Asn-Tyr-Pro-Ile-Val-Gln-EDANS (S1). This substrate consists of an octapeptide with a C-terminal fluorophore, EDANS (5-((2-aminoethyl)amino)naphthalene-1-sulfonic acid), and an N-terminal quenching group, DABCYL (4-(4-dimethylaminophenyl)azobenzoic acid). The octapeptide sequence corresponds to the naturally occurring Pr55[gag]p17/p24 cleavage site for HIV PR. The fluorescence of EDANS in S1 is markedly quenched because of intramolecular RET to the DABCYL group; following cleavage of the peptide and concomitant liberation of the DABCYL-linked peptide fragment, the intrinsic fluorescence quantum yield of EDANS is restored. Hence, the kinetics of proteolysis can be obtained by simply recording the increase in fluorescence intensity with time. Incubation of recombinant HIV PR with S1 results in specific cleavage at the Tyr-Pro bond and a 40.0-fold enhancement in fluorescence per mole of substrate cleaved (FIG. 1). The high sensitivity of the assay permits initial rates to be estimated from the hydrolysis of less than 1% total substrate (FIG. 1, inset); and measurements for the evaluation of inhibitors can be performed routinely with 2-5 μM S1, 1 nM HIV PR. Under the high ionic strength assay conditions at 30°C, the hydrolysis of S1 by HIV PR follows Michaelis-Menten kinetics, with $K_m = 103 \pm 8$ μM; assuming the catalytic unit to be a dimer, $k_{cat} = 4.9$ sec^{-1} is calculated.

The continuous nature of the fluorogenic RET assay makes the analysis of protease inhibitors relatively straightforward. The ability of HIV PR to cleave at the amino side of proline residues prompted us to design inhibitors based on the structure of the Phe-Pro dipeptide. In TABLE 1 are listed the inhibitory potencies of a series of compounds in which the C_1 to C_4 dihedral angle is restricted in a manner similar to the tetrahedral intermediate for cleavage of Phe-Pro. The small nonpeptide inhibitor **1** shows significant, albeit weak, activity (IC$_{50}$ = 0.12 mM). Addition of residues at the P2 and P3 subsites to give **3** provides a moderate enhancement in potency (15 μM). Interestingly, the attachment of residues in the P' region (compounds **4** and **5**) has a

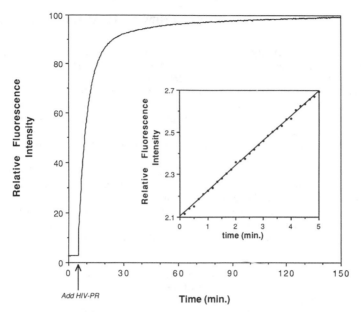

FIGURE 1. Hydrolysis of fluorogenic substrate S1 by HIV PR at 37°C as monitored by steady state fluorescence. The reaction was carried out with 10.7 μM S1 at pH 4.7 in a buffer containing 0.1 M NaOAc, 1 M NaCl, 1 mM EDTA, 1 mM dithiothreitol, 10% dimethylsulfoxide, and 1 mg/mL bovine serum albumin. The arrow denotes the addition of recombinant HIV PR to a final concentration of 35 nM. The final products were subjected to HPLC, amino acid, and fluorescence lifetime analyses. **Inset:** Initial phase of the hydrolysis used for rate determinations. The reaction shown was carried out at 30°C with 20 μM S1, 1.1 nM HIV PR in the buffer described above. The digitized points represent signal-averaging, over 10 s intervals, and the least squares linear fit to the data is indicated by the solid line.

TABLE 1. Inhibitors of HIV-1 Protease

No.	A	B	IC$_{50}$ (μM)
1	H	NH-isopentyl	124[a]
2	AcNH	NH-isopentyl	50
3	Cbz-Leu-Asn-NH	NH-isopentyl	15
4	H	Ile-Ser-Pro-Ile-OMe	> 200[a]
5	H	Val-Val-NH$_2$	> 200[a]
6	Cbz-Leu-Asn-NH	Ile-Ser-Pro-Ile-OMe	1
7	Ac-Val-Val-NH	Val-Val-NH$_2$	0.03
8	Cbz-Leu-Asn-NH	NH-isopentyl	50

[a] C$_4$ configuration is *RS*.

detrimental effect on activity; however, the inclusion of residues at both P and P' ends of **1** to give the modified pol cleavage sequence **6** results in inhibitory activity (IC_{50} = 1 μM), which is superior to "reduced amide" inhibitors of similar size.[3,4] The use of a furan ring rather than cis olefin to more closely resemble the size of a Pro residue results in a loss of potency (compare **8** with **3**). The most significant boost in activity is observed when the P2/P3 residues of pepstatin, a known potent inhibitor of HIV PR, are incorporated at both P2/P3 and P2'/P3' positions (compound **7**). An analysis of the inhibition of HIV PR by **7** indicates that inhibition is competitive, with K_i = 30 nM.

The simplicity, rapidity, sensitivity, and precision of the RET method facilitates its adaption to a variety of uses and formats. In addition to the enzymological and inhibitor studies described above, we have found that the assay can be easily adapted for large-scale screening with an automated 96-well fluorescence plate reader. The RET method may also be used for studying substrate specificity requirements, because the same fluorophore/quencher pair can be employed with virtually any peptide sequence.[5]

REFERENCES

1. LATT, S. A. *et al.* 1972. Anal. Biochem. **50:** 56.
2. CARMEL, A., *et al.* 1973. FEBS Lett. **30:** 11.
3. BILLICH, S. *et al.* 1988. J. Biol. Chem. **263:** 17905.
4. MOORE, M. L., *et al.* 1989. Biochem. Biophys. Res. Commun. **159:** 420.
5. WANG, G. T., E. MATAYOSHI, J. W. ERICKSON & G. A. KRAFFT. 1990. Ann. N.Y. Acad. Sci. This volume.

Sodium Thiophosphonoformate, A Selective HIV RT Inhibitor

Facile Synthesis and Effects in HIV-Infected Cell Culture[a]

C. E. McKENNA,[b] T.-G. YE,[b] J. N. LEVY,[b] T. WEN,[b]
J.-P. BONGARTZ,[b] Y.-C. CHENG,[c,d] M. C. STARNES,[c]
A. BODNER,[e] AND R. KILKUSKIE[e]

[b]Department of Chemistry
University of Southern California
Los Angeles, California 90089-0744

[c]Department of Pharmacology
University of North Carolina at Chapel Hill
Chapel Hill, North Carolina 27541

[d]Department of Pharmacology
Yale University
New Haven, Connecticut 06510

[e]Biotech Research Laboratories
Rockville, Maryland 20850

Sodium thiophosphonoformate (TPFA, 1), a novel sulfur analogue of phosphonoformate (PFA, 2), inhibits the reverse transcriptase (RT) of human immunodeficiency virus (HIV-1), with $IC_{50} = 1$ μM.[1] The inhibition is selective compared to both human DNA polymerase α ($IC_{50} > 100$ μM) and several herpesvirus DNA polymerases ($IC_{50} = 12\text{-}70$ μM for HSV-1, HSV-2, EBV, and HV-6 DNA polymerases). PFA inhibits HIV RT with similar potency ($IC_{50} = 0.7$ μM), but is less selective for pol α ($IC_{50} = 31$ μM) and nonselective for the same herpesvirus DNA polymerases ($IC_{50} = 0.7\text{-}1$ μM). No significant change in 1 (2 mM) was observed by ^{31}P-NMR under the assay conditions.

TPFA is readily obtained by way of[1] conversion of trimethyl PFA 3 to trimethyl TPFA 4 using 2,4-bis(p-methoxyphenyl)-1,3-dithiaphosphetane-2,4-disulfide 5. Direct hydrolysis of 4 to 1 (characterized by ^{1}H-, ^{31}P-, ^{13}C-NMR; IR; UV; C, H, S, Na elemental analyses) is effected by brief exposure to 10 M NaOH. The regioselectivity of 5 in P=O $\rightarrow$ P=S vs. C=O $\rightarrow$ C=S thiation of 3 is usefully manifested in thiation of other phosphonocarboxylate esters.[2] TPFA is stable in solid form for months when stored in a sealed container at 4 °C. In anaerobic aqueous solution, pH 7-8 at 20 °C, it very slowly changes into PFA (^{31}P-NMR) decomposing about 10% after 10 weeks. The transformation proceeds somewhat more rapidly under aerobic conditions (about 40% after 10 weeks).

[a]This research was supported by NIH Grant AI-25697.

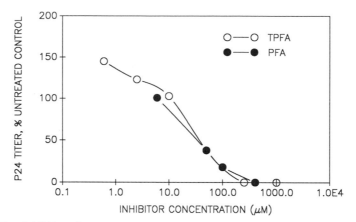

FIGURE 1. Inhibition of p24 expression in HIV-infected H9 cells by added TPFA vs. PFA. H9 lymphocytes (3.5×10^6 cells/mL) were incubated $\pm$ HIV-1 for 1 h at 37 °C. Cells were washed and suspended at 4×10^5 cells/mL in culture medium (RPMI 1640 + 10% fetal calf serum). Aliquots (1 mL) were mixed with 1 mL PFA or TPFA in culture medium and incubated for 3 days at 37 °C. A p24 antigen capture assay (BioTech Research) was used to determine levels of HIV infection.

TPFA and PFA were tested over a range of concentrations as inhibitors of HIV replication in H9 cell culture using a p24 antigen capture assay. TPFA and PFA show similar apparent inhibition-dose dependencies under the assay conditions used (FIG. 1). Both compounds were noncytotoxic ($\geq$ 92% cell survival, uninfected cells) at concentrations giving 0% of control p24.

The chemical fate of 1 in the HIV inhibition experiments was investigated by ^{31}P-NMR. Preliminary data are presented in FIGURE 2. TPFA (2 mM) was completely

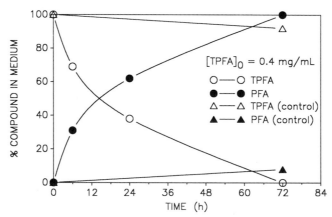

FIGURE 2. Conversion of TPFA to PFA in cell medium. TPFA (400 μg/mL; ca. 2 mM) was incubated in the complete assay mixture, minus HIV, at 37 °C. After 6, 24, and 72 h, aliquots were withdrawn, immediately frozen (dry ice-ethanol bath) and stored at -20 °C. ^{31}P-NMR analysis was carried out on a Bruker WP270-SY NMR spectrometer using multiple FT scans over 14 h at ca. 20 °C. Data are uncorrected for further reaction in the spectrometer.

transformed into 2 after 72 h in the cell culture assay mixture (and also in the medium alone, data not shown) at 37 °C. A control containing only the bicarbonate buffer component of the medium showed < 10% conversion of 1 into 2 after 72 hours. Our HIV RT inhibition studies clearly demonstrate that 1 can function as a direct inhibitor of HIV replication in *in vitro* cell culture. The results in FIGURE 2 raise the interesting possibility that in the latter part of these experiments, TPFA may function as a PFA prodrug.

REFERENCES

1. McKENNA, C. E., T.-G. YE, J. N. LEVY, P.-T. PHAM, T. WEN, J.-P. BONGARTZ, M. C. STARNES & Y.-C. CHENG. 1990. Phosphorus Sulfur Silicon. **49/50:** 183-186.
2. McKENNA, C. E. & P. T. PHAM. In preparation.

Complement-Mediated Enhancement of HIV-1 Infection Reverses the Anti-HIV-1 Activity of Castanospermine

DAVID C. MONTEFIORI,[a]
W. EDWARD ROBINSON, JR.,
ANN MODLISZEWSKI, AND
WILLIAM M. MITCHELL

Department of Pathology
Vanderbilt University Medical School
Nashville, Tennessee 37232

Fresh human serum is required as a source of complement for antibody-dependent enhancement of human immunodeficiency virus type 1 (HIV-1) infection of CD4+ cells expressing complement-receptor type 2 (CR2).[1,2] Further, particulate glycoprotein lacking sialic acid is known to activate complement independent of antibody.[3] Because one of the effects of castanospermine (CS) is to prevent sialylation of glycoprotein carbohydrates,[4] we investigated the effect of fresh human serum on the infectivity of HIV-1 synthesized in the presence and absence of CS using MT-2 cells as targets. When preincubated with 30% heat-inactivated human serum (a process that destroys complement) prior to challenge of MT-2 cells, the number of infectious CS-treated virions per reverse transcriptase (RT) unit was reduced 27-fold (TABLE 1), a result consistent with previously demonstrated anti-HIV-1 activity of CS.[5] When preincubated with 30% fresh human serum, however, infectious virions per RT unit increased 42-fold (TABLE 1). Thus, fresh human serum abolished the anti-HIV-1 activity of CS and actually increased the infectivity of CS-treated virus for MT-2 cells. An increase in viral infectivity was also observed for untreated virions preincubated in 30% fresh human serum (TABLE 1). The effect of fresh human serum on CS-treated virions was not observed in CD4+ cells lacking CR2 (*i.e.*, H9 and CEM cells). Loss of castanospermine's antiviral activity was attributed to the classical complement pathway because drug-treated virions remained attenuated if preincubated in C1q-deficient serum but not if preincubated in factor B-deficient serum (TABLE 2). Reversal of viral attenuation required the OKT4a epitope on CD4 but did not require the complement receptors, CR1 and CR3, or the OKB7 epitope of CR2 (data not shown). These results suggest that some cells may escape the potential therapeutic utility of *N*-glycosylation inhibitors in treatment of acquired immune deficiency syndrome (AIDS).

[a] Address correspondence to David C. Montefiori, Department of Pathology, Room C-3321 MCN, Vanderbilt University, Nashville, TN 37232.

TABLE 1. Effect of Thirty Percent Human Serum on Infectivity of HIV-1 Synthesized in the Presence and Absence of Castanospermine[a]

	Relative increase in infectious virions/RT	
Drug treatment	Heat-inactivated serum[b]	Fresh serum
None	1	27
CS[c] (0.5 mM)	−27	15

[a] Virus was obtained from H9 cells chronically infected with HTLV-III$_B$ and cultured in the presence and absence of CS. Conditioned culture fluids were made cell-free by low-speed centrifugation and filtration (0.45 μm pore size). A portion of the virus-containing fluids was precipitated with polyethylene glycol and assayed for reverse transcriptase (RT) activity as described.[6] Another portion of the virus-containing fluids was mixed with fresh human serum or heat-inactivated (56°C, 1 h) human serum, such that the final serum concentration was 30%. After a 1 h incubation at 37°C the viral preparations were diluted serially into growth medium (RPMI-1640 containing 12% heat-inactivated fetal bovine serum and 50 μg gentamicin/mL) in 96-well microdilution plates. MT-2 cells (40,000 cells in 100 μL of growth medium) were added to each well and the plates incubated at 37°C in a 5% CO_2/95% air environment for 10 days. Twice during this period the cells in each well were reduced by 75% and the medium replaced. Plates were examined by light microscopy after 10 days for syncytium formation in each well. The reciprocal dilution where syncytia were present in less than 50% of wells on day 10 was used as a measure of infectious virions/mL. Normal human serum was shown to be HIV-1 negative by immunofluorescence assay (IFA) as described.[7] Values are given relative to untreated virus preincubated with heat-inactivated serum. Total yields were approximately equivalent (RT activity = 180,000-210,000 cpm/mL) for untreated and CS-treated viral cultures.

[b] Human serum was obtained as a lyophylized powder from Sigma.

[c] Castanospermine (CS) was purchased from Boehringer Mannheim.

TABLE 2. Effect of Fresh Human Serum and Complement Component-Deficient Sera on Castanospermine-Treated HIV-1 Infection[a]

Human serum[b]	Percent IFA positive[c]	Percent CPE	RT activity (cpm × 10^{-4}/mL)
None	5	28 ± 5	24
Fresh, 30%	100	92 ± 4	200
C1q-deficient, 30%	15	47 ± 11	40
Factor B-deficient, 30%	100	95 ± 2	244

[a] HTLV-III$_B$ was prepared and preincubated with various sera as described in TABLE 1. Each serum-treated virus preparation was diluted 5-fold with growth medium and 50 μL added to each of 24 wells of a 96-well microdilution plate containing 100 μL of growth medium/well. MT-2 cells were added and incubated as described above. After 5 days incubation, cytopathic effect (CPE) was measured by vital dye (neutral red) uptake in a portion of remaining viable cells in each well as described.[8] Another portion of remaining cells for each sample was pooled, collected by centrifugation, and used for IFA. In addition, pooled culture supernatants were used for measurement of RT activity.

[b] Human sera were obtained as lyophilized powders from Sigma.

[c] Serum for IFA was from an individual who was positive by Western immunoblot (DuPont) for all major HIV-1 antigens.

REFERENCES

1. ROBINSON, W. E., JR., D. C. MONTEFIORI & W. M. MITCHELL. 1988. Lancet i: 790-794.
2. ROBINSON, W. E., JR., D. C. MONTEFIORI & W. M. MITCHELL. 1989. J. AIDS 2: 33-42.
3. MCSHARRY, J. J., R. J. PICKERING & L. A. CALIGUIRI. 1981. Virology 114: 507-515.
4. ELBEIN, A. D. 1987. Annu. Rev. Biochem. 56: 497-534.
5. MONTEFIORI, D. C., W. E. ROBINSON, JR. & W. M. MITCHELL. 1988. Proc. Natl. Acad. Sci. USA 85: 9248-9252.
6. POIESZ, B. J., F. W. RUSCETTI, A. F. GAZDAR, P. A. BUNN, J. D. MINNA & R. C. GALLO. 1980. Proc. Natl. Acad. Sci. USA 77: 7415-7419.
7. MONTEFIORI, D. C. & W. M. MITCHELL. 1986. Virology 155: 726-731.
8. MONTEFIORI, D. C., W. E. ROBINSON, JR., S. S. SCHUFFMAN & W. M. MITCHELL. 1988. J. Clin. Microbiol. 26: 231-235.

Effect of Imexon on Friend Virus Complex Infection in Rfv-3$^{r/s}$ Genotype-Containing Mice as a Model for AIDS[a]

JOHN D. MORREY, REED P. WARREN,
KEVIN M. OKLEBERRY, ROGER A. BURGER,
ROBERT W. SIDWELL,[c] AND
MICHAEL A. CHIRIGOS[b]

AIDS Research Program
Utah State University
Logan, Utah 84322-5600
[b]*United States Army Medical Research Institute*
for Infectious Diseases
Fort Detrick, Maryland

Acquired immune deficiency syndrome (AIDS) is a difficult disease to treat because of the complex pathogenesis of the disease. Biological response modifiers (BRM), specifically immunomodulators, have been the subject of considerable research effort as an approach for enhancing current antiviral therapies.

Prophylactic treatment, using the BRM imexon (4-imino-1,3-diazobicyclo-(3.1.0)-hexan-2-one), has been shown in a very limited study to be effective in reducing Friend virus complex (FV)-induced splenomegaly in mice.[1] In this report, we have used a murine model recently described[2] for evaluating BRMs for the treatment of retroviral infection. A mouse strain, (B10.A × A/WySn)F$_1$, was used that is capable of eliciting a specific retroviral immune response analogous to that seen in AIDS, that is, viral-specific antibodies are produced soon after viral challenge despite the occurrence of immunosuppression. The production and persistence of the antibodies are correlated with a reduction of infected cells and viremia. Regardless of the virus-specific immune response, the disease is fatal.

Intraperitoneal (ip) imexon treatment initiated on days +1 or +3 after FV inoculation (schedule 1 and 2, respectively) at 110 and 55 mg/kg/day markedly reduced the weight of spleens (p < 0.01) from FV-infected mice compared to placebo-treated mice (TABLE 1). Treatment initiated on day +7 (schedule 3) was less effective in reducing splenomegaly.

In mice treated with the highest dosage (110 mg/kg/day), using schedule 1, the cell-free virus from spleen homogenates and FV-specific RNA/splenocytes were significantly reduced when assayed on day 15 (TABLE 1). Plasma virus titers and viral

[a]This work was supported by NIH contract #NO1-A1-72662.
[c]To whom correspondence should be addressed.

TABLE 1. Effect of Intraperitoneal Imexon Treatment on Disease Parameters in FV-Infected (B10.A × A/WySn)F$_1$ Mice[a]

Treatment	Schedule	No. mice	Dose mg/kg/day	Toxicity controls Mean wt. change (g)	FV Infected				
					Mean spleen wt. (mg ± 2 SE)	Mean splenic IC(log$_{10}$/10^6 splenocytes ± 2 SE)	Mean plasma FV(log$_{10}$FFU /mL ± 2 SE)	Mean cell-free virus(log$_{10}$FFU[d] /mL ± 2 SE)	Mean FV RNA ng(10^{-4})/ splenocyte (± 2 SE)
Imexon	1	10	110	−0.6	86 ± 15[b]	2.28 ± 0.63	1.79 ± 0.34	0.76 ± 12[b]	13.7 ± 0[b]
		10	55	−0.6	277 ± 91[b]	3.11 ± 0.27	1.97 ± 0.56	1.51 ± 0.82[b]	49.5 ± 32
	2	10	110	−1.1	123 ± 29[b]	2.90 ± 0.71	2.28 ± 0.53	2.18 ± 0.89	24.7 ± 16
		10	55	−0.4	285 ± 86[b]	3.54 ± 0.26	2.09 ± 0.38	1.98 ± 0.77	49.5 ± 11.0
	3	10	110	−0.6	232 ± 121[c]	3.44 ± 0.28	2.95 ± 0.88	1.84 ± 0.66[c]	55.0 ± 0
		10	55	−0.2	556 ± 311	3.33 ± 0.85	3.83 ± 1.67	—	66.0 ± 36.0
Saline	1	20	0	—	510 ± 167	3.68 ± 0.36	2.67 ± 0.81	2.74 ± 0.38	60.9 ± 28.0
Normal	—	20	—	+1.0	—	—	—	—	—

[a] Female (B10.A × A/WySn)F$_1$ female mice were injected ip, 3.8 × 10^4 50% infectious dosages (ID$_{50}$), with Lilly Steeves strain B-tropic FV complex.[2] The three treatment schedules used were schedule 1: qd × 13 initiated 1 day; schedule 2: qd × 11 initiated 3 days; and schedule 3: qd × 7 initiated 7 days after FV inoculation. Necropsy for each treatment schedule was terminated at the same time after FV inoculation (day +15) to compare the effect of each treatment schedule. Viral parameters are described in detail elsewhere.[2]
[b] p < 0.01, compared to placebo-treated controls.
[c] p < 0.05, compared to placebo-treated controls.
[d] Fluorescence focal-forming units.

infectious centers (IC)/10^6 splenocytes appeared to be reduced using schedule #1 of imexon treatment, but the differences in the means of imexon- and placebo-treated mice were not statistically significant. Delayed treatments using schedules 2 and 3 were less efficacious in inhibiting these viral parameters. Some sublethal toxicity was apparent in uninfected control mice treated with all schedules and dosages of imexon as evidenced by a mean loss of weight compared to untreated mice that gained weight (TABLE 1).

TABLE 2. Effect of Intraperitoneal Imexon Treatment on Immune Parameters in FV-Infected (B10.A $\times$ A/WySn)F$_1$ Mice[a]

| | | Mean $\pm$ 2 SE | | | |
| | | Imexon Dosage (mg/kg/day) | | | |
Group	Parameters	110	55	Saline	Normal
Toxicity controls	PHA-induced blastogenesis (mean ^{3}H incorporation)	8178 $\pm$ 740[b]	5987 $\pm$ 964	—	7022 $\pm$ 746
	Splenic percentage of total T cell	57 $\pm$ 7[c]	38 $\pm$ 4	—	35 $\pm$ 3
	Splenic percentage of T-helper cell	30 $\pm$ 3[c]	22 $\pm$ 2	—	21 $\pm$ 2
	Splenic percentage of T-suppressor cell	25 $\pm$ 3[c]	18 $\pm$ 2	—	16 $\pm$ 1
	Splenic percentage of B cell	26 $\pm$ 4[c]	39 $\pm$ 3	—	42 $\pm$ 2
FV infected	PHA-induced blastogenesis (mean ^{3}H incorporation)	8033 $\pm$ 604[c]	6347 $\pm$ 791	5084 $\pm$ 700	—
	Splenic percentage of total T cell	62 $\pm$ 11[c]	45 $\pm$ 3	43 $\pm$ 4	—
	Splenic percentage of T-helper cell	30 $\pm$ 4[c]	23 $\pm$ 2	20 $\pm$ 2	—
	Splenic percentage of T-suppressor cell	31 $\pm$ 5[c]	22 $\pm$ 2	21 $\pm$ 2	—
	Splenic percentage of B cell	26 $\pm$ 7[c]	37 $\pm$ 3	38 $\pm$ 2	—

[a] qd $\times$ 13 beginning on day +1. Refer to TABLE 1 for design of experiments. Immune parameters are described by Morrey *et al.*[2] PHA-induced blastogenesis was performed on splenic cells. Subpopulations of splenic cells were enumerated with a fluorescence-activated cell sorter by using the following panel of fluorescein isothiocyanate-labeled antibodies: anti-Thy 1.2 (total T cells), anti-L3T4 (helper-T cells), anti-Lyt 2 (suppressor/cytotoxic T cells), and anti-mouse IgG (total B cells).
[b] p < 0.05, compared to placebo-treated or normal controls.
[c] p < 0.01, compared to placebo-treated or normal controls.

Phytohemagglutinin (PHA)-induced blastogenesis was depressed in placebo-treated, infected mice compared to the response of uninfected mice (TABLE 2). This viral-induced depression was prevented using imexon treatment at both dosages when treatment was initiated at either day +1 (TABLE 2), +3, or +7 (data not shown). In the uninfected mice treated with 110 mg/kg/day using schedule 1, PHA-induced blastogenesis was elevated to above-normal values.

In uninfected toxicity control mice and FV-infected mice, imexon treatment using schedule 1 significantly increased the percentage of total T, T-helper, and T-suppressor/ cytotoxic cells and decreased the percentage of B cells (TABLE 2). Natural killer cell activity was not significantly affected (data not shown).

In conclusion, imexon treatment, if started 1 or 3 days after FV inoculation, significantly reduced spleen weights and viral parameters. T-cell subsets and function, as determined by PHA-induced blastogenesis, appeared to be enhanced with imexon treatment. These results indicate that imexon should be studied further as a possible drug for the treatment of HIV infection.

REFERENCES

1. BICKER, U. 1978. *In* Immune Modulation and Control of Neoplasia by Adjuvant Therapy. M. A. Chirigos, Ed. Raven Press. New York.
2. MORREY, J. D., R. P. WARREN, K. M. OKLEBERRY, R. A. BURGER, M. A. JOHNSTON & R. W. SIDWELL. 1990. J. AIDS **3:** 500-510.

Structure-Activity Correlations of Pyrimidine and Purine Dideoxynucleosides as Potential Anti-HIV Drugs

MOHAMED NASR, CHARLES LITTERST, AND
JOHN McGOWAN

Division of AIDS
National Institute of Allergy and Infectious Diseases
National Institutes of Health
Rockville, Maryland 20892

The Developmental Therapeutics Branch, Division of AIDS, National Institute of Allergy and Infectious Diseases (NIAID), has established a computerized database with the capacity to analyze the structure-activity relationships for active and inactive anti-HIV compounds. The following are the results of analysis of data accumulated so far on *in vitro* anti-HIV testing of more than 350 dideoxynucleosides (ddN) and analogues.

Compounds that have shown promising activity against HIV are 2',3'-dideoxypyrimidine and purine nucleosides[1] (TABLES 1-3) and to a lesser extent acyclonucleoside analogues[2] (FIGURES 1 and 2). Only 3'- or 2'- azido (TABLE 4) or -fluoro (TABLE 5) substitution has shown anti-HIV activity. 3'-Azido or 3'-fluoro enhanced the activity of the dideoxypyrimidine nucleosides[3] but not dideoxypurine nucleosides. Unsubstituted sugar is optimal for activity of purine ddNs.

3'-Substitution with amino, alkyl, cyano, alkoxy, thioalkyl, thiocyanato (SCN), isothiocyanato (NCS), and 3'-halo other than fluorine gave inactive compounds. 3'-Acetylenic groups or pseudohalogens have not been reported in the literature.

Introduction of a 2'-ara-fluoro substituent retained the activity of the purine ddN and to a lesser extent the pyrimidine ddN, whereas 2'-erythro fluoro inactivated both purine and pyrimidine ddN. Threo 3'-fluoro gave inactive compounds, whereas erythro 3'-fluoro gave active compounds, particularly with pyrimidine ddN.

Introduction of a 2'-OH in 3'-azidopyrimidine ddN abolished activity.

A 2',3' double-bond inactivated purine, but not pyrimidine, ddN (TABLE 6). No ddN with 3',4', or 1',2'-3',4' double bonds have been reported.

5-Halogen-substituted pyrimidine ddN are active[4] (TABLE 7). This was attributed to the larger size of Cl, Br, and I but not F, which may approach the size of a methyl group, so increasing the affinity of these compounds to thymidine kinase.

Only one isocytidine ddN has been reported and has anti-HIV activity.

Monomethylation of the 6-amino group in ddA or the 4-amino group in ddC may have enhanced the activity of these compounds, whereas introduction of ethyl, two methyl groups, or benzyl abolished the activity.

Carbocyclic purine ddN but not pyrimidine analogues have anti-HIV activity.

TABLE 1. 2′,3′-Unsubstituted Dideoxypyrimidine Nucleosides[a]

Compound	R	R1	in vitro Activity
5-F-ddC	F	NH$_2$	+
ddC	H	NH$_2$	+
ddT	Me	OH	+
5-Me-ddC	Me	NH$_2$	+ −
5-Et-ddU	Et	OH	−
5-Et-ddC	Et	NH$_2$	−
ddU	H	OH	−
5-Br-ddU	Br	OH	−
5-I-ddU	I	OH	−
5-Br-CH=CH-ddU	CH=CHBr	OH	−
5-Br-ddC	Br	NH$_2$	−

[a] 2′,3′-Dideoxycytidine (ddC) is the most potent. Introduction of a methyl group at the 5 position of dideoxyuridine (ddU) enhanced the antiviral activity. Similarly, introduction of a methyl group at the 5 position of ddC retained antiviral activity, whereas a 5-ethyl substitution reduced activity. Introduction of bromine and iodine at the 5 position in ddU had no effect on activity.

TABLE 2. 2′,3′-Unsubstituted Dideoxypurine Nucleosides[a]

Compound	R	R1	*in vitro* Activity
ddA	NH$_2$	H	+
ddDAPR[b]	NH$_2$	NH$_2$	+
ddG	OH	NH$_2$	+
ddI	OH	H	+
Me-ddA	NHMe	H	+
2-Br-ddA	NH$_2$	Br	+ −
2-F-ddA	NH$_2$	F	+ −
2-Cl-ddA	NH$_2$	Cl	+ −
ddClP	Cl	H	+ −
ddBnA	NHBn	H	+ −
ddEtA	NHEt	H	−
ddMe$_2$A	NMe$_2$	H	−
ddP	H	H	−

[a] 2′,3′-Dideoxy-*N*6-methyladenosine (ddMeA) had greater antiviral activity than ddA. This enhanced activity could be related to its resistance to deamination. The 2-halo derivatives of ddA demonstrate reduced anti-HIV activity, but greater toxicity than ddA.
[b] DAPR = diaminopurine.

TABLE 3. Sugar-Substituted Dideoxypurine Nucleosides[a]

Compound	R	R1	in vitro Activity
3'-N$_3$ddDAPR	NH$_2$	NH$_2$	+
3'-N$_3$ddG	OH	NH$_2$	+
3'-FddDAPR	NH$_2$	NH$_2$	+
3'-FddG	OH	NH$_2$	+
2'-FddAraA	NH$_2$	H	+
3'-FddA	NH$_2$	H	+
2'-N$_3$ddAraA	NH$_2$	H	+
3'-N$_3$ddA	NH$_2$	H	+ −
3'-N$_3$ddA(threo)	NH$_2$	H	−
2'-N$_3$ddA	NH$_2$	H	−
3'-FddA(threo)	NH$_2$	H	−
3'-OH-2'-dG(threo)	OH	NH$_2$	−
2'-FddA	NH$_2$	H	−

[a] The active compounds in this class are mainly 3'-azido, 3'-fluoro (3'-F), and ara-substituted 2'-F and 2'-azido derivatives. The replacement of 2'-ara-F with 2'-Cl or 2'-Br gave inactive compounds. The configuration of the 2'-F in the ara position is essential for the activity of these compounds.

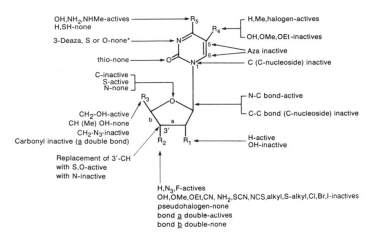

FIGURE 1. Structure-activity relationship of pyrimidine analogues. *Not reported in the literature.

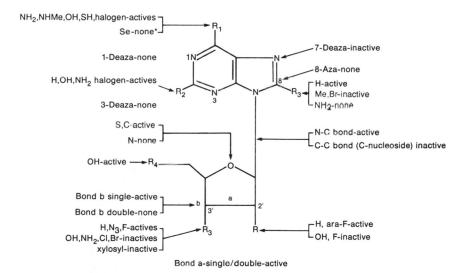

FIGURE 2. Structure-activity relationship of purine analogues. *Not reported in the literature.

TABLE 4. 3'-Azido-2',3'-Dideoxypyrimidine Nucleosides[a]

Compound	R	R1	in vitro Activity
AzddClU	Cl	OH	+
AzddMeC, N4-OH	Me	NHOH	+
AzddMeC-N4Me	Me	NHMe	+
AZT-P-AZT	Me	OH	+
AZT-P-CyE-ddA	Me	OH	+
AZT-P-ddA	Me	OH	+
AZT-P-ddI	Me	OH	+
AZT	Me	OH	+
AzddEtU (CS-85)	Et	OH	+
AzddMeC	Me	NH₂	+
AzddU (CS-87)	H	NH₂	+
AzddC (CS-91)	H	NH₂	+
AzddFC	F	NH₂	+
AzddBrU	Br	OH	+
AzddIU	I	OH	+
AzddFU	F	OH	−
AzddSCNU	SCN	OH	−
AzddNH₂U	NH₂	OH	−
AzddOHU	OH	OH	−

[a] AZT is the most potent analogue. The nature of substitution on the 5 position of dideoxyuridine affects the anti-HIV activity in the following order: methyl, hydrogen, chloro, bromo, fluoro. The replacement of (5-Me) in AZT by CF₃ or propyl abolishes activity. A group of anti-HIV active nucleotide homo- and heterodimers (e.g., AZT-P-ddA, AZT-P-CyE-ddA) represent compounds in which the active nucleoside monomers are connected at the 5' position by a phosphate (P) or cyanoethylphosphate (PCyE) bridge. The anti-HIV activity of these nucleotide dimers is greater than or equal to the combination of the monomers, with AZT and ddA dimers having the most activity. The presence of 2'-OH in AZT, azidoU (AzdU), or AzdC abolishes the anti-HIV activity of these compounds.

TABLE 5. 3′-Halopyrimidine Dideoxynucleosides[a]

Compound	R	R1	*in vitro* Activity
3′-FddClU	Cl	OH	+
3′-FddU	H	OH	+
3′-FddT	Me	OH	+
3′-FddBrU	Br	OH	+
3′-FddEtU	Et	OH	−
3′,3′-diFddT	Me	OH	−
3′-I-ddEtU	Et	OH	−
3′-Cl-ddT	Me	OH	−
3′-Br-ddT	Me	OH	−
3′-I-ddC	H	NH$_2$	−
3′-I-ddU	H	OH	−
3′-I-ddT	Me	OH	−

[a] 3′-Fluorodideoxythymidine (3′-FddT) is the most potent antiviral analogue, but it also has high toxicity. The replacement of the 5-Me group in 3′-FddT by an ethyl group abolishes antiviral activity. The introduction of a second fluorine at the 3′-lyxo position in 3′-FddT abolishes all antiviral activity. The replacement of the 3′-fluoro in ddU and ddT by Cl, Br, and I abolishes antiviral activity.

TABLE 6. 2',3'-Didehydro-2',3'-Dideoxynucleosides[a]

Compound	B	in vitro Activity
D4T	Thymine	+ +
D4C	Cytosine	+ + +
D4MeC	5-Me-cytosine	+ +
D4A	Adenine	−
MeD4A	N-Me-adenine	−
D4G	Guanine	−
D4U	Uracil	−
ddeDAPR	2,6-Diaminopurine	+ +
D4EtU	5-Ethyluracil	−
2-ClD4A	2-Cl-adenine	+ −

[a] This class of compounds is less active than the parent dideoxynucleosides (ddN). Pyrimidine analogues are the most active, whereas the purine analogues are the least active. Replacement of the methyl group in D4T by ethyl (as in D4EtU) or by H (as in D4U) abolishes the activity of both compounds. Replacement of H at the 5 position in D4C by Me (as in D4MeC) retains activity.

Of the acyclonucleosides studied so far the purines but not the pyrimidines have shown activity. Active acyclic purine nucleosides have a 9-phosphonylmethoxyethyl or a 9-(4'-hydroxy-1',2'-butadienyl) side chain.

Replacement of 3'-CH of the sugar with S or O, but not N, gave active ddN. Anti-HIV activity has been reported for ddN with four-membered sugar rings and its carbocyclic analogues, whereas ddN with six-membered sugar rings (*e.g.*, 2',3'-dideoxy or dideoxydidehydrohexopyranosyl analogues) have not been investigated.

Dideoxynucleosides in which the ring size of the purine or pyrimidine bases was modified or the nitrogens replaced by S or O have not been reported.

TABLE 7. Compounds Selected from Data Base Sorted in Order of MuLV ED_{50} *in Vitro*

Compound	MuLV ED_{50}^a	PBM ED_{50}	MT-4 ED_{50}	MT-4 SI^b	ATH8 ED_{50}	ATH8 TI^c
AZT	0.02	0.002	0.006	666	2.4	19
3'-N₃-5-Br-ddU	1.5	1.04				
D₄T	2.5	0.009	0.01	120	4.1	27
3'-N₃-5-I-ddU	3.0	1.14				
D₄C	3.7	0.005	0.13	61	0.3	100
ddC	4.0	0.011	0.046	128	0.2	175
3'-N₃ddU (CS-87)	52.0	0.2	0.36	677		
3'-N₃ddC	58.0	0.66	3.1	11		
3'-N₃-5-Me-ddC	100.0	0.08	1.8	555		
ddT	100.0	0.17	0.20	625	100.0	20

[a] 50% effective dose or dose required to protect 50% of the HIV-infected cells.
[b] Ratio of CD_{50} (50% cytotoxic dose, not shown in Table) to ED_{50}.
[c] Therapeutic index.

The aza and deaza purine and pyrimidine ddN analogues have not been fully investigated.

REFERENCES

1. MITUSYA, H. & S. BRODER. 1986. Proc. Natl. Acad. Sci. USA **83**: 1911-1915.
2. PAUWELS, R. & J. BALZARINI. 1988. Antimicrob. Agents Chemother. **32**: 1025.
3. CHU, C. K., R. F. SCHINAZI *et al.* 1989. J. Med. Chem. **32**: 612.
4. DE CLERCQ, E. 1989. Antiviral Res. **12**:1.

Differential Effect of Cyclic Nucleotide Modulators on HIV Replication

MOSTAFA NOKTA AND RICHARD POLLARD

Department of Internal Medicine
Division of Infectious Diseases
The University of Texas Medical Branch
Galveston, Texas 77550

It has been previously reported that viruses such as measles virus and cytomegalovirus were sensitive to certain agents that alter either intracellular cAMP or cGMP alone or both.[1-3] Intracellular levels of cyclic nucleotides (CN) can be manipulated by using specific pharmacological agents that are known to exert their effect directly by activating the enzymes adenylate cyclase or guanylate cyclase to synthesize cAMP and cGMP, respectively. An example of the former is forskolin (FK) and of the latter sodium nitroprusside (NaNP). Intracellular levels of cAMP and cGMP can also be increased by phosphodiesterase inhibitors (PDI), such as papaverine (PAP) and isobutylmethylxanthine (IBMX). Such agents indirectly increase the intracellular levels of CN by inhibiting the respective phosphodiesterases responsible for their metabolism.[4] The present study was conducted to determine the effect of CN modulators on the *in vitro* propagation of HIV.

As shown in TABLE 1, FK enhanced the RT activity and P_{24} antigen levels of HIV in culture supernatants in a dose-dependent fashion. FK, at the doses used to enhance HIV replication, also increased cAMP in MT-4 cells. These data suggest that high levels of cAMP favor HIV replication. NaNP had a variable effect that was less prominent, despite its effect on increasing intracellular cGMP levels (data not shown). This suggests that HIV replication may be relatively independent of cGMP levels in contrast to cAMP. Next, agents that have been reported to increase cAMP by other mechanisms were investigated for their effect on HIV replication. As shown in FIGURE 1, PAP inhibited HIV replication. The inhibition appeared dose-dependent and by day 4 postinfection, doses of 10 μM and 30 μM inhibited RT enzyme activity by 67 and 94% and P_{24} Ag by 78 and 99%, respectively.

To determine if the inhibition of HIV replication was a feature characteristic to PDI or was unique to PAP, the sensitivity of HIV replication to other PDI was examined. In contrast to PAP, IBMX, at doses of 30 μM and 100 μM, enhanced HIV replication by 4- and 7-fold, respectively. Thus the mechanism of PAP-induced inhibition of HIV replication appeared independent from its functional ability to increase intracellular CNs. From the results reported above it would seem that agents that enhance intracellular cAMP also enhanced HIV replication except for PAP. Because PAP has been shown to diminish intracellular calcium concentrations ($[Ca^{2+}]_i$) in other cells, it would seem possible that HIV replication could be a Ca^{2+}-dependent event. To test this hypothesis, the effect of TMB-8 on HIV replication was examined.

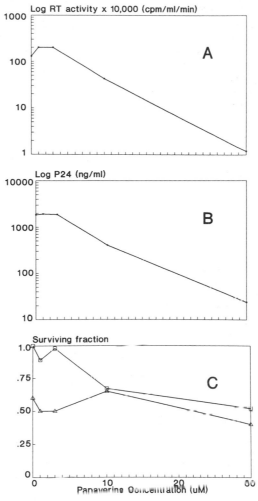

FIGURE 1. Effect of PAP on HIV replication in MT-4 cells. Infection and culture conditions are the same as described in the footnote for TABLE 1. **A:** Reverse transcriptase activity of PEG precipitated culture supernatants. **B:** HIV-P_{24} Ag of inactivated culture supernatants determined by antigen capture assay using Coulter Kits. **C:** Ratio of cell survival in the presence and absence of PAP in uninfected (□) and infected (△) MT-4 cells. PAP at the above doses increased intracellular levels of cAMP 2-2.8-fold above the control level.

TMB-8 is an agent that has been shown to inhibit the mobilization of Ca^{2+} from endoplasmic reticulum to the cytoplasm. The TMB-8 enhanced HIV replication in a dose-dependent manner. At doses of 10 μM, RT activity was enhanced 12-fold. These data suggest that HIV replication may require a low Ca^{2+} environment. Thus PAP would appear to inhibit HIV replication by a mechanism that is unrelated to its currently reported pharmacological mechanism of action.

In conclusion, these data suggest that CN modulators have a differential effect on HIV replication, and that HIV replication appears to require an intracellular physiologic environment that has a relatively high level of cAMP and a low level of $[Ca^{2+}]_i$.

TABLE 1. Effect of Forskolin on HIV Replication in MT-4 cells

HIV	Forskolin[a] (μM)	RT activity[b] (cpm/mL/min)	Fold increase	P_{24} Ag[b] ng	Fold increase
+	—	2×10^3	—	15	—
+	0.1	1.6×10^2	0.08	7	0.5
+	0.3	1.6×10^3	0.8	13	0.9
+	1	6.8×10^3	3.4	29	2
+	10	1.4×10^4	7	31	2
+	100	1.5×10^5	75	153	10

[a] A pharmological agent that specifically activates adenylate cyclase. The doses indicated increased intracellular levels of cAMP by 2.2-3.4-fold above the control, as determined by radioimmunoassay RIA using Amersham Kits.

[b] MT-4 cells were infected with HIV strain HTLV III_B with 0.002-0.005 $TCID_{50}$ per cell for one hour and then incubated in the presence or absence of the indicated dose of FK. HIV replication was determined at day 4 postinfection by measuring RT activity of culture supernatants and by HIV P_{24} Ag by antigen capture assay using Coulter Kits.

REFERENCES

1. NOKTA, M., C. LEE, O. STEINSLAND & T. ALBRECHT. 1984. *In* Herpesvirus. F. Rapp, Ed.: 465-475. Alan R. Liss, Inc. New York.
2. ALBRECHT, T., C. H. LEE, D. J. SPEELMAN & O. S. STEINSLAND. 1987. Proc. Soc. Exp. Biol. Med. **186:** 41-46.
3. YOSHIKAWA, Y. & K. YAMANOUCHI. 1984. J. Virol. **50:** 489-496.
4. BEAVO, J. A. 1988. *In* Advances in Second Messenger and Phosphoprotein Research. P. Greengard & G. A. Robison, Ed. **22:** 1-38. Raven Press. New York.

Interaction of 3'-Deoxythymidin-2'-ene Triphosphate (d4TTP) with Reverse Transcriptase from Human Immunodeficiency Virus[a]

U. PATEL-THOMBRE AND W. H. PRUSOFF[b]

Department of Pharmacology
Yale University School of Medicine
New Haven, Connecticut 06510

3'-Deoxythymidin-2'-ene (d4T),[1-4] 3'-deoxycytidin-2'-ene (d4C),[5,6] and 3'-azido-3'-deoxythymidine (AZT)[7] are potent and selective inhibitors of human immunodeficiency virus (HIV-1) replication, and are phosphorylated to their mono-, di-, and triphosphates by cellular enzymes.[8-11] Once converted to the 5'-triphosphate, they prevent the replication of the virus[1,3-5] by at least two different mechanisms. First, the 5'-triphosphates compete with the appropriate normal nucleoside 5'-triphosphate for incorporation by the reverse transcriptase into the growing DNA chain.[8,12-15] Second, once incorporated, they act as chain terminators because no 3'-OH group is available for further elongation of the chain.[12]

To further understand the mechanism by which these analogues inhibit HIV-1 replication, we have studied the interaction of d4TTP and d4CTP with HIV-1 reverse transcriptase (HIV-1 RT). H9 DNA polymerase α was observed to be several orders of magnitude less sensitive than the viral reverse transcriptase to inhibition by d4TTP, d4CTP, and AZTTP, and these nucleoside triphosphate analogues are therefore selective inhibitors of HIV-1 replication. Initial velocity studies with d4CTP and AZTTP showed competitive inhibition kinetics, whereas d4TTP consistently and unexpectedly demonstrated a noncompetitive profile. A further examination of the interaction of d4TTP with HIV-1 RT showed that D4TTP inhibited the enzyme in a reversible manner in the absence of primer-template poly $r(A)$ oligo $d(T)_{12-18}$. d4TTP also showed concentration-dependent inhibition of HIV-1 RT similar to AZTTP.[12] This decrease in the rate of [³H]dTMP incorporation was partially prevented by the presence of excess primer-template.

[a] This research was supported by Training Grant CA-09085, NCI Grants CA-05262 and CA-45410, AIAID Grant AI-26055, and an unrestricted Grant from the Bristol-Myers Squibb Company.
[b] To whom correspondence should be addressed.

591

REFERENCES

1. LIN, T. S., R. F. SCHINAZI & W. H. PRUSOFF. 1987. Biochem. Pharmacol. **36:** 2713-2718.
2. BALZARINI, J., G. J. KANG, M. DALAL, P. HERDEWIGN, E. DECLERQ, S. BRODER & D. G. JOHNS. 1987. Mol. Pharmacol. **32:** 162-167.
3. BABA, M., R. PAUWELS, P. HERDEWIJN, E. DECLERCQ, J. DESMYTER & M. VANDEPUTTE. 1987. Biochem. Biophys. Res. Commun. **142:** 128-134.
4. HAMAMOTO, Y., H. NAKASHIMA, T. MATSUI, A. MATSUDA, T. UEDA & N. YAMAMOTO. 1987. Antimicrob. Agents Chemother. **31:** 907-910.
5. LIN, T. S., R. F. SCHINAZI, M. S. CHEN, E. KINNEY-THOMAS & W. H. PRUSOFF. 1987. Biochem. Pharmacol. **36:** 311-316.
6. BALZARINI, J., R. PAUWELS, P. HERDEWIJN, E. DECLERCQ, D. A. COONEY, G. J. KANG, M. DALAL, D. G. JOHNS & S. BRODER. 1986. Biochem. Biophys. Res. Commun. **140:** 735-742.
7. MITSUYA, H., K. J. WEINHOLD, P. A. FURMAN, M. H. ST. CLAIR, S. N. LEHRMAN, R. C. GALLO, D. BOLOGNESI, D. W. BARRY & S. BRODER. 1985. Proc. Natl. Acad. Sci. USA **82:** 7096-7100.
8. FURMAN, P. A., J. A. FYFE, M. H. ST. CLAIR, K. WEINHOLD, J. L. RIDEOUT, G. A. FREEMAN, S. N. LEHRMAN, D. P. BOLOGNESI, S. BRODER, H. MITSUYA & D. W. BARRY. 1986. Proc. Natl. Acad. Sci. USA **83:** 8333-8337.
9. AUGUST, E. M., M. E. MARONGIU, T. S. LIN & W. H. PRUSOFF. 1988. Biochem. Pharmacol. **37:** 4419-4422.
10. HO, H. T. & M. J. M. HITCHCOCK. 1989. Antimicrob. Agents Chemother. **33:** 844-849.
11. BALZARINI, J., P. HERDEWIJN & E. DECLERCQ. 1989. J. Biol. Chem. **264:** 6127-6133.
12. ST. CLAIR, M. H., C. A. RICHARDS, T. SPECTOR, K. J. WEINHOLD, W. H. MILLER, A. J. LANGLOIS & P. A. FURMAN. 1987. Antimicrob. Agents Chemother. **31:** 1972-1977.
13. MATTHES, E., CH. LEHMANN, D. SCHOLZ, M. VON JANTA-LIPINSKI, K. GAERTNER, H. A. ROSENTHAL & P. LANGEN. 1987. Biochem. Biophys. Res. Commun. **148:** 78-85.
14. VRANG, L., H. BAZIN, G. REMAUD, J. CHATTOPADHYAYA & B. OBERG. 1987. Antiviral Res. **7:** 139-149.
15. MITSUYA, H. & S. BRODER. 1987. Nature **325:** 773-778.

Synthesis and Liposome Encapsulation of Antisense Oligonucleotide-Intercalator Conjugates

C. PIDGEON, H. L. WEITH, D. DARBISHIRE-WEITH,
M. CUSHMAN, S. R. BYRN, J.-K. CHEN,
J. G. STOWELL, K. RAY, AND D. CARLSON

*Departments of Biochemistry, Medicinal Chemistry and
Pharmacognosy,
and Industrial and Physical Pharmacy
Purdue University
West Lafayette, Indiana 47907*

Antisense oligonucleotides offer the opportunity to deliver biomolecules to specific sequences on HIV RNA, thereby inhibiting template transcription and also leading to digestion of the viral RNA by RNase H. The affinity of the antisense oligonucleotide for viral RNA, as well as binding site selectivity and metabolic stability, may be enhanced by the covalent attachment of intercalating agents through linker chains.

The synthesis of antisense oligonucleotide-benzophenanthridine alkaloid intercalator conjugates is shown in FIGURE 1. Alkylation of the phenolic hydroxyl group to add a linker chain onto fagaronine chloride (1) was desired. The combination of potassium *tert*-butoxide-dimethyl sulfoxide[1] was found to be the most effective medium to achieve this alkylation. Accordingly, fagaronine chloride was alkylated using the 5-ethoxycarbonylpentyl-*p*-toluenesulfonate to give compound 2. Both the ester and the iminium functionalities were reduced with lithium aluminum hydride to provide the dihydrofagaronine alcohol 3.

In contrast to its quaternary ammonium salt, this dihydrofagaronine alcohol 3 can easily be dissolved in most common inert organic solvents. Therefore, compound 3 was reacted with *N,N*-diisopropylaminocyanoethoxychlorophosphine[2,3] in THF in the presence of *N,N*-diisopropylethyl amine to give the corresponding phosphoramidite 4[4]. The final product 5 was assembled with the standard solid-phase phosphoramidite procedure using a Milligen 7500 DNA synthesizer. The dihydrofagaronine was then converted to the iodide salt upon treatment with I_2 in THF/H_2O/pyridine in the oxidation step. Finally, concentrated NH_4OH treatment provided the desired oligonucleotide-fagaronine iodide conjugate 5.

Purification of compound 5 was accomplished by ion exchange HPLC using a Supelcosil LC-Si column (150 mm × 4.6 mm ID, silica coated with polyethyleneimine, cross-linked) in a gradient mode. The oligonucleotide-fagaronine iodide conjugate 5 could be monitored by the absorbance at 390 nm, which is a characteristic absorbance of fagaronine chloride.

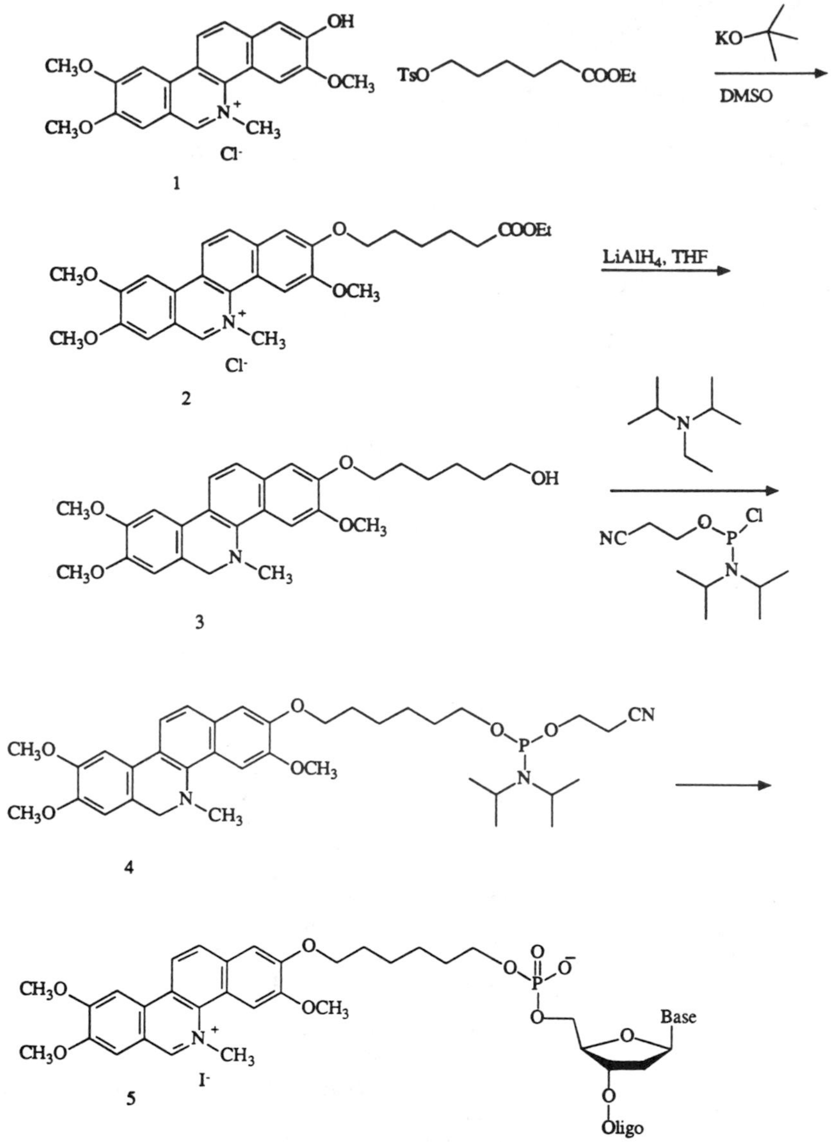

FIGURE 1. Attachment of fagaronine (**1**) to antisense oligonucleotides.

High entrapment in liposomes is critical to efficiently test liposomes as a drug delivery system for oligonucleotide drug conjugates. High drug entrapment usually requires sonication of organic aqueous mixtures to form an emulsion.[5–7] Initial experiments showed that oligonucleotides degraded during sonication even under anaerobic and ice bath conditions. Consequently, we immediately abandoned traditional methods[5–7] to obtain high drug entrapment in liposomes.

Our strategy for optimizing oligonucleotide entrapment in liposomes involves three steps (FIG. 2). Step 1 involves forming planar membranes under mobile phase conditions that favor binding to phosphatidylcholine. Step 2 involves adding excess mobile phase to form closed liposome membranes with most of the nucleotide entrapped. Step 3 involves equilibrating the liposome suspension to the appropriate pH; oligonucleotides adsorbed to the outside surface of the liposome surface will dissociate and not be liposome-associated. This experimental strategy to optimize oligonucleotide entrapment, however, requires sheets of lipid to survive the process of liposome formation. If individual lipid molecules are dispersed, or if the membrane falls apart during step 2, then the oligonucleotide will not have high entrapment in the final liposome population.

We have found that annealing dilaurylphosphatidylcholine (DLPC) lipid films, prior to adding the dispersion buffer (which usually contains the drug), causes the lipids to crystallize into a metastable state. Lipid structural changes occur in the

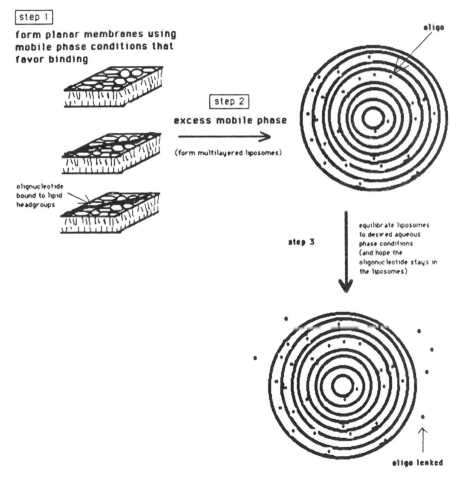

FIGURE 2. Experimental strategy to optimize oligonucleotide entrapment in liposomes.

headgroup phosphate and alkyl chains. These metastable lipid structural changes exist several hours at room temperature in the fully hydrated DLPC liposome suspension. For lipid structural changes generated at low temperature in a lipid film to persist in fully hydrated liposomes, sheets of lipids must survive liposome formation. Thus, incubation of DLPC at low temperature causes sheets of lipid to survive liposome formation. Consequently, this lipid mixture was used for the preliminary studies to entrap oligonucleotides, and entrapment ratios approaching 75% were attained using this procedure. Methods using different lipid mixtures are presently being evaluated.

REFERENCES

1. FIESER, M. & L. FIESER. 1967. Reagents for Organic Synthesis. 1: 914. John Wiley and Sons, Inc. New York.
2. SINHA, N. D., J. BIERNAT, J. MCMANUS & H. KOSTER. 1984. Nucleic Acid Res. 12: 4539.
3. WESTERDUIN, P., G. H. VEENEMAN, J. E. MARUGG, G. A. VAN DER MARAL & J. H. VAN BOOM. 1986. Tetrahedron Lett. 27: 1211.
4. CONNOLLY, B. A. 1987. Nucleic Acid Res. 15: 3131.
5. PIDGEON, C. et al. 1987. Biochemistry. 26: 17.
6. PIDGEON, C. et al. 1986. Pharm. Res. 3: 23-34.
7. SZUKA, F. & D. PAPAHADYAPOULOS. 1978. Proc. Natl. Acad. Sci. USA 75: 4194.

Development of an *in Vitro* Human Monocyte-Derived Macrophage-Based System for Drug Screening against HIV-1

BRUCE POLSKY, PENNY A. BARON,
HOWARD E. GENDELMAN,[a]
JONATHAN W. M. GOLD, T-C CHOU, AND
DONALD ARMSTRONG

Memorial Sloan-Kettering Cancer Center
New York, New York 10021

[a]*The Henry M. Jackson Foundation*
Bethesda, Maryland

The monocyte-macrophage has been recognized as an important reservoir for HIV-1 and may serve a role in the development of latent HIV-1 infection. For these reasons, it may be important to determine whether agents under development for clinical use are active against HIV-1 infection in these cells. We have developed an *in vitro* system based on human monocyte-derived macrophages (MDM) for drug screening against HIV-1. This system is an adaptation of the method previously described by one of us[1] for the isolation of monocytotropic strains of HIV-1 from patients with AIDS and ARC.

MATERIAL AND METHODS

Monocyte-derived macrophage-enriched populations of peripheral blood leukocytes from HIV-seronegative donors were prepared by elutriation and seeded in 96-well plates, preincubated for one hour in the presence of 10-fold dilutions of experimental drugs, infected with a monocytotropic HIV-1 isolate (HIV_{Ada}), and carried in the presence or absence of recombinant human macrophage colony-stimulating factor-1 (rMCSF-1). Culture supernatants were serially assessed for p24 antigen by ELISA-capture.

RESULTS

Zidovudine (AZT), phosphonoformate (PFA), 3'-deoxy-3'-fluorothymidine (FLT), and recombinant interferon alpha$_{2a}$ (α-IFN) strongly inhibited HIV-1 infection in MDM (TABLE 1). No cytotoxicity attributable to the drugs was observed.

CONCLUSIONS

In vitro anti-HIV-1 activity of experimental drugs may be rapidly assessed in this human MDM-based system. HIV-1 infection of MDM is inhibited by concentrations

TABLE 1.

Compound	ED$_{50}$	
	+rMCSF-1	−rMCSF-1
AZT	0.044 μM	0.015 μM
PFA	8.757 μM	5.270 μM
FLT	0.036 μM	0.088 μM
α-IFN	11.772 U/mL	27.758 U/mL

of these drugs similar to those reported in lymphocyte-based systems and is not significantly influenced by the presence of rMCSF-1.

REFERENCE

1. GENDELMAN, H. E., J. M. ORENSTEIN, M. A. MARTIN, ET AL. 1988. Efficient isolation and propagation of human immunodeficiency virus on recombinant colony-stimulating factor 1-treated monocytes. J. Exp. Med. **167:** 1428-1441.

In Vitro Testing of Therapeutics against SIV and HIV

A Comparison[a]

P. R. SAGER,[b] J. C. CRADOCK,[b] C. L. LITTERST,[b]
L. N. MARTIN,[c] K. F. SOIKE,[c] M. MURPHEY-CORB,[c]
P. A. MARX,[d] C.-C. TSAI,[e] A. FRIDLAND,[f]
A. BODNER,[g] L. RESNICK,[h] AND R. F. SCHINAZI[i]

[b]*Developmental Therapeutics Branch*
Division of AIDS
National Institute of Allergy and Infectious Diseases
National Institutes of Health
Bethesda, Maryland 20892

[c]*Delta Regional Primate Research Center*
Tulane University
Covington, Louisiana 70433

[d]*California Primate Research Center*
University of California
Davis, California 95616

[e]*Regional Primate Research Center*
University of Washington
Medical Lake, Washington 99022

[f]*St. Jude Children's Research Hospital*
Memphis, Tennessee 38101

[g]*Biotech Research Laboratory, Inc.*
Rockville, Maryland 20850

[h]*Mount Sinai Medical Center of Greater Miami*
Miami Beach, Florida 33110

[i]*VA Medical Center*
Emory University School of Medicine
Atlanta, Georgia 30032

[a]The work described here was supported in part by Grants UO1-AI25696, UO1-AI25697, and UO1-AI26055, and contracts NO1-AI62526, NO1-AI62559, and NO1-AI62560 from the Division of AIDS, NIAID, NIH.

INTRODUCTION

Simian immunodeficiency virus (SIV), a lentivirus similar to HIV, causes a disease in macaques that is similar to AIDS.[1] Recently, testing of antiretroviral therapies has begun using this model.[2] It will be several years, however, before correlations of efficacy in the SIV-macaque model and humans with AIDS can be made for more than a very few therapies.

SIV also infects a number of human cells and cell lines. This has been used as the basis for *in vitro* systems to measure the efficacy of antiretroviral drugs. In developing these cell-based assays, a number of drugs with known activity against HIV have been tested. These drugs include primarily nucleosides that have been shown to be active against HIV *in vitro*.[3,4] In addition, active and inactive drugs were tested against both SIV and HIV in blinded studies.

As with HIV, the effective concentrations of drugs vary with the specific conditions of the assay, such as cell type and SIV strain. The purpose of this paper is to compare the efficacy of a limited number of drugs against SIV and HIV *in vitro*. Because different cell types and end points have been used, direct quantitative comparisons are not possible. Qualitative and relative comparisons can be made, however.

METHODS

SIV Assay Systems

H9 and HuT78 Cells

Cells were infected with SIV_{MAC251} in culture medium containing the test drug. After 7 days, cultures were assessed for cell growth. Viral expression was assessed by an immunofluorescence assay (IF) using polyclonal antibodies against several viral antigens.

CEM × 174 Cells

The MTT (methylthiozol tetrazolium bromide) assay measures protection, by an antiviral agent, against SIV-induced cell death. CEM × 174 cells (B-cell/T-cell somatic hybrid) were treated with diluted drug just prior to virus inoculation using 100 $TCID_{50}$ of SIV_{MAC251}. After 5 to 7 days, MTT substrate solution was added for 3 to 4 hours. Colored product was quantitated using an ELISA reader (570 nm).

Human PBLs

Human peripheral blood lymphocytes (PBL) were incubated with $SIV_{Delta\ B670}$ for one hour, washed and resuspended in medium containing diluted test compound. Cell viability was assessed at days 3 and 7. Viral replication was measured on day 7 using a p24 antigen capture assay.

HIV Assay Systems

H9 Cells

H9 lymphocytes were incubated with HIV-1 (HTLV-IIIB) at 0.01-0.1 $TCID_{50}$/cell for one hour, and washed and resuspended in culture medium containing test compound. A p24 antigen capture assay was used to determine the level of HIV infection on day 3.[5]

MT-2 Cells

MT-2 cells were infected with HIV (isolate TM) for one hour and resuspended in medium; test compounds were added. Syncytia were counted at day 4.[6]

Human PBMCs

PHA-stimulated peripheral blood mononuclear cells (PBMC) were infected with HIV-1 (LAV-1) and then placed in culture medium containing test compound. After 6 days, RT activity was determined in the culture supernatant.[7]

Data Evaluation

EC_{50}s (50% effective concentrations) were calculated from inhibition data for each drug. Where multiple sets of data were available, the values were averaged.

TABLE 1. EC$_{50}$ μM SIV versus HIV

Drug	SIV				HIV		
	H9 IF	HuT78 IF	CEM ×174 MTT	PBL p24	H9 p24	MT-2 syncytia	PBMC RT
AZT	<0.05	<0.05	<<0.4	0.022	0.02	0.07	0.004
ddA	6	13	4	NT[a]	NT	0.5	0.9
ddC	<0.1	<0.1	2	0.06	0.03	1	0.01
ddI	0.3	12	4.5	4.4	<1	NT	1-4
d4T	0.5	11	2.2	NT	NT	NT	0.009
Foscarnet	<0.1	43	29	1.1-3.3	20	0.33-22	22
Castanospermine	0.1	>100	>100	NT	11	0.5-5.2	>100
IdUR	Uniformly Cytotoxic				Uniformly Cytotoxic		
Mannitol	Uniformly Inactive				Uniformly Inactive		

[a] NT = Not tested.

TABLE 2A. Comparison of Cells or Cell Line

	PBL		H9 Cells	
	SIV	HIV	SIV	HIV
AZT				
EC_{50}	0.022	0.004	$\ll 0.05$	0.02
EC_{90}	<0.12	0.06	<0.05	0.75
ddI				
EC_{50}	4.4	1-4	0.3	<0.1
EC_{90}	10	8-10	≤ 10	10

RESULTS AND DISCUSSION

The efficacy of several drugs against SIV and HIV was determined using *in vitro* assays. The data (EC_{50}s) are summarized in TABLE 1. Most of the drugs tested, AZT (zidovudine), ddA (dideoxyadenosine), ddC (dideoxycytidine), ddI (dideoxyinosine), and d4T (dideoxydidehydrothymidine), are nucleosides. These drugs, along with foscarnet, act by way of inhibition of reverse transcriptase.[8–10] Castanospermine is thought to block viral glycoprotein processing.[11–13]

Because the efficacy of drugs can vary with cell types, perhaps due to differences in intracellular drug metabolism, activity against SIV and HIV was compared in similar cell types (TABLE 2A). For AZT, SIV appeared to be less sensitive than HIV in PBL. In H9 cells, however, SIV appeared to be at least as sensitive to AZT as HIV. The activity of ddI against SIV and HIV appeared to be about equivalent in both PBL and H9 cells. Despite differences in the values for EC_{50}s in different cell types and using different end points, the relative efficacy of drugs, as shown in TABLE 2B, remained fairly constant. There are qualitative similarities in results from *in vitro* testing of SIV and HIV. AZT was the most active drug against SIV and HIV, as measured in several different cell types and with several end points. Other dideoxy nucleosides are generally less active than AZT but showed activity within one or two logs of the effective concentration of AZT. Although d4T was not tested in all systems, its activity varied

TABLE 2B. Relative Efficacy: EC_{50}s[a]

SIV						
H9	AZT	< ddC, Fos, Cas, ddI, d4T	< ddA			
Hu1/8	AZT	< ddC		< d4T, ddI, ddA, Fos	< Cas	
CEM × 174	AZT	< ddC, d4T, ddA, ddI		< Fos		< Cas
PBL	AZT	< ddC		< Fos, ddI		

HIV					
H9	AZT, ddC	< ddI		< Cas, Fos	
MT-2	AZT	< ddA, ddC, Cas, Fos			
PBMC	AZT	< d4T, ddC, ddA, ddI		< Fos	< Cas

[a]IdUR was uniformly cytotoxic; mannitol was uniformly inactive. Fos, foscarnet; Cas, castanospermine.

with cell type, as did the efficacy of foscarnet. Non-nucleosides (castanospermine and foscarnet) varied greatly in their activity against both SIV and HIV. Inactive and cytotoxic control compounds were uniformly inactive against both SIV and HIV. Except for the known cytotoxic drug, idoxuridine (IdUR), the $EC_{50}s$ for all compounds were at least one log less than the concentration that produced toxicity in uninfected cells (data not shown).

Quantitative comparisons of activity against SIV versus HIV are difficult. Confounding factors include cell type used in the assay, relative timing of virus infection and drug addition, and end point measuring viral replication or expression. In addition, it should be noted that most drugs tested were nucleosides; it is not clear that drugs acting by other mechanisms would be equally effective against both HIV and SIV. Despite these limitations, it appears that *in vitro* systems using SIV yield results similar to systems using HIV, and, because few drugs have been used extensively in the clinic, the clinical predictive value of these *in vitro* systems cannot be determined.

REFERENCES

1. BASKIN, G. B., M. MURPHEY-CORB, E. A. WATSON & L. N. MARTIN. 1988. Necropsy findings in rhesus monkeys experimentally infected with cultured simian immunodeficiency virus (SIV)/Delta. Vet. Pathol. **25:** 456-467.
2. WATANABE, M., K. A. REIMANN, P. Q. DeLONG, T. LIU, R. A. FISHER & N. L. LETVIN. 1989. Effect of recombinant soluble CD4 in rhesus monkeys infected with simian immunodeficiency virus of macaques. Nature **337:** 267-270.
3. MITSUYA, H., K. J. WEINHOLD, P. A. FURMAN, M. H. ST. CLAIR, S. NUSINOFF, R. GALLO, D. BOLOGNESI, D. W. BARRY & S. BRODER. 1985. 3'-Azido-3'-deoxythymidine (BWA509U): an antiviral agent that inhibits the infectivity and cytopathic effect of human T-lymphotropic virus type III/lymphadenophathy-associated virus *in vitro.* Proc. Natl. Acad. Sci. USA **82:** 7096-7100.
4. MITSUYA, H. & S. BRODER. 1986. Inhibition of the *in vitro* infectivity and cytopathic effect of human T-lymphotropic virus type III/lymphadenophathy-associated virus (HTLV-III/LAV) by 2',3'-dideoxynucleosides. Proc. Natl. Acad. Sci. USA **83:** 1911-1915.
5. NISHIZAWA, M., T. YAMAGISHI, G. E. DEUTSCHMAN, W. B. PARKER, A. J. BODNER, R. E. KILKUSKIE, Y-C CHEUNG & K-H LEE. 1989. Anti-AIDS Agents. 1. Isolation and characterization of four new tetragalloylquinic acids as a new class of HIV reverse transcriptase inhibitors from tannic acid. J. Nat. Prod. **52:** 762-768.
6. BUSSO, M., A. M. MIAN, E. F. HAHN & L. RESNICK. 1988. Nucleotide dimers suppress HIV expression *in vitro.* AIDS Res. Hum. Retroviruses **6:** 449-455.
7. SCHINAZI, R. F., D. L. CANNON, B. H. ARNOLD & D. MARTINO-SALTZMAN. 1988. Combinations of isoprinosine and 3'-azido-3'-deoxythymidine in human immunodeficiency virus type 1 infected lymphocytes. Antimicrob. Agents Chemother. **32:** 1784-1787.
8. FURMAN, P. A., J. A. GYFE, M. H. ST. CLAIR, K. WEINHOLD, J. L. RIDEOUT, G. A. FREEMAN, S. NUSINOFF LEHRMAN, D. P. BOLOGNESI, S. BRODER, H. HITSUYA & D. W. BARRY. 1986. Phosphorylation of 3'-azido-3'-deoxythymidine and selective interaction of the 5'-triphosphate with human immunodeficiency virus reverse transcriptase. Proc. Natl. Acad. Sci. USA **83:** 8333-8337.
9. MITSUYA, H., R. F. JARRETT, M. MATSUKURA, F. D. VERONESE, A. L. DeVICO, M. G. SARNGADHARAN, D. G. JOHNS, M. REITZ & S. BRODER. 1987. Long term inhibition of human T-lymphotrophic virus type III/lymphadenopathy associated virus (human immunodeficiency virus) DNA synthesis and RNA expression in T cells protected by 2'3'-dideoxynucleosides *in vitro.* Proc. Natl. Acad. Sci. USA **84:** 2033-2037.
10. SANDSTROM, E. G., R. E. BYINGTON, J. C. KAPLAN & M. S. HIRSCH. 1985. Inhibition of human T-cell lymphotropic virus type III *in vitro* by phosphonoformate. Lancet. **i:** 1480-1482.

11. GRUTERS, R. A., J. J. NEEFJES, M. TERSMETTE, R. E. Y. DE GOEDE, A. TULP, H. G. HUISMAN, F. MIEDEMAD & H. L. PLOEGH. 1987. Interference with HIV-linked syncytium formation and viral infectivity by inhibitors of trimming glucosidase. Nature **330:** 74-77.
12. TYMS, A. S., E. M. BERRIE, T. A. RYDER, R. J. NASH, M. P. HEGARTHY, D. L. TAYLOR, M. A. MOBBERLEY, J. M. DAVIS, E. A. BELL, D. J. JEFFRIES, D. TAYLOR-ROBINSON & L. E. FELLOWS. 1987. Castanospermine and other plant alkaloid inhibitors of glucosidase activity block the growth of HIV. Lancet ii: 1025-1026.
13. WALKER, B. D., M. KOWALSKI, W. C. GOH, K. KOZANSKY, M. KRIEGER, C. ROSEN, L. ROHRSCHNEIDER, W. A. HASELTINE & J. SODROSKI. 1987. Inhibition of human immunodeficiency virus syncytium formation and virus replication by castanospermine. Proc. Natl. Acad. Sci. USA **84:** 8120-8124.

Self-Cleaving RNAs (Ribozymes) as New Modalities for Anti-HIV Therapy

NAVA SARVER,[a] ARNOLD HAMPEL,[b]
EDOUARD M. CANTIN,[c] JOHN A. ZAIA,[c]
PAIROJ S. CHANG,[c] MARGARET I. JOHNSTON,[a]
JOHN McGOWAN,[a] AND JOHN J. ROSSI[c]

[a]Division of AIDS
National Institute of Allergy and Infectious Diseases
National Institutes of Health
Bethesda, Maryland 20892

[b]Plant Molecular Biology Center
Northern Illinois University
DeKalb, Illinois 60115

[c]City of Hope
Duarte, California 91010

Studies reported here demonstrate the ability of two distinct ribozymes (catalytic RNAs), "hammerhead"[1] and "hairpin",[2] to precisely cleave human immunodeficiency virus (HIV) RNA sequences. Accurate RNA cleavage occurs in a simple cell-free system and in a complex cellular environment (ref. 3 and Rossi et al., this volume). These results suggest that ribozymes can potentially be used therapeutically to reduce the level of deleterious RNA, be it viral or cellular, involved in human diseases.

The experimental rationale for the present study is based on previous observations that ribozyme-mediated cleavage can occur in *trans* using separate substrate and catalytic RNAs[4] and that RNA sequences containing the cleavage domain can serve as compatible substrates.[5] The ability of hammerhead catalytic RNA to precisely cleave HIV sequences is demonstrated in the following experiment that approximates conditions of HIV infection. CD4$^+$ HeLa cells were transformed with a mammalian expression vector coding for anti-*gag* catalytic RNA. Stable transformants expressing the catalytic RNA were isolated and challenged with HIV-1. Polymerase chain-reaction analysis was performed on total RNA to identify intact and cleaved *gag* sequences as outlined in FIGURE 1. In the absence of cleavage the expected amplified product is a 480 nucleotide (nt) fragment extending from LTR1 to GAG1, encompassing the cleavage site (arrow). A cleavage at that site is expected to reduce the yield of the intact fragment relative to a smaller (200 *nt*) fragment located downstream of the cleavage site. The cleavage fragments representing the region upstream of the cleavage of the substrate site are not detected under these conditions. As shown in FIGURE 1, untransformed cells (A) contain similar levels of the intact substrate and the smaller, 200 nt fragment. By contrast, RNA samples from cells expressing anti-*gag* catalytic RNA contain significantly less of intact *gag* substrate relative to the smaller fragment, indicating that cleavage of the substrate has occurred. This conclusion is supported by the observation that catalyst-positive cells containing predominantly the smaller *gag* sequence secrete 40-fold less p24 (GAG) antigen than HIV-infected, catalyst-negative cells (not shown). In toto, these results demonstrate that catalytic RNAs are expressed and are sufficiently stable in a complex intracellular environment to effect significant cleavage of target RNA sequences. Further, the presence of catalytic RNAs within the cell is not detrimental to cell viability, indicating, albeit indirectly, that cleavage is specific.

Hairpin catalytic RNA is a newly identified ribozyme that differs from hammerhead catalytic RNA in having distinct primary sequence and structural motifs.[2] Although

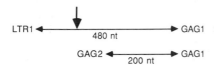

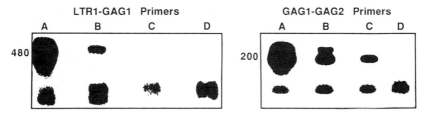

FIGURE 1. Hammerhead catalytic RNA cleaves HIV RNA in mammalian cells. Cleavage site is indicated by the vertical arrow. Three different primers were used in the polymerase chain reaction (PCR) analysis: LTR1 and GAG2 are of the same polarity as HIV-1 RNA; GAG1 is of the opposite polarity. This analysis would yield different ratios of the 200 and 480 nt fragments depending whether the original *gag* RNA substrate was cleaved or uncleaved. Following PCR amplification the products were treated as described[3] and hybridized with a ^{32}P-labeled oligonucleotide probe complementary to sequences between GAG2 and GAG1. Each lane contained DNA amplified from 0.5 μg of total RNA from HIV-infected cells: lane A, untransformed CD4$^+$ HeLa (parental) cells; lane B, cloned cell line expressing the catalytic RNA; lane C, pooled clones expressing the catalytic RNA; lane D, PCR contamination control.

the protective effect of hairpin catalytic RNA has not yet been tested against a challenge virus, it shares many of the features ascribed to hammerhead ribozymes, specifically the ability to cleave substrate RNA in *trans* in a catalytic fashion (FIG. 2). During the course of the reaction there is a reduction in the amount of substrate RNA (S17) concomitant with the emergence of new cleavage products (5'P and 3'P). The level of input catalyst remains constant throughout the reaction. The fact that the catalyst performs multiple cleavage events even in the presence of great excess of substrate indicates that the reaction is indeed catalytic. Native and heterologous RNA sequences, including synthetic HIV-*gag* and HIV-*tat* RNAs, are cleaved by specifically designed hairpin catalysts (not shown).

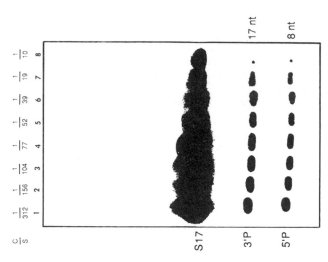

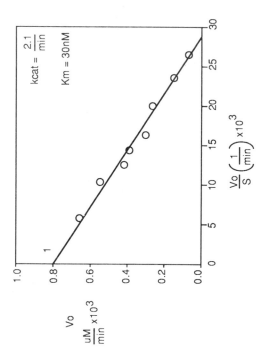

FIGURE 2. Catalytic cleavage by hairpin ribozyme. Catalytic and substrate RNAs were transcribed using T7 RNA polymerase in the presence of alpha [32P]CTP and purified on acrylamide-urea gels as described.[2] Cleavage rates were determined by isolating the gel bands, counting the radioactivity, plotting the data using the Michaelis-Menton method, and calculating the K_m and k_{cat} (number of cleavages per minute). The respective catalyst to substrate ratios (C:S) are shown. The catalytic RNA concentration was constant at 0.3 nM. Reactions were at 37°C for 60 minutes in 12 mM MgCl$_2$, 2 mM spermidine, 40 mM Tris, pH 7.5. S, substrate; 3'P, 3' cleavage product; 5'P, 5' cleavage product. V_0, velocity. The 55 nt catalyst is not detected under these conditions.

In conclusion, hammerhead and hairpin catalytic RNAs can be designed and used to effect cleavage of target RNA sequences. As such, they may constitute a new class of anti-HIV therapeutic agents.

REFERENCES

1. KEESE, P. & R. H. SYMONS. 1987. *In* Viroids and viroid-like pathogens. J. R. Semancik, Ed. CRC Press. Boca Raton, Florida.
2. TRITZ, R. & A. HAMPEL. 1989. Biochemistry **28:** 4929.
3. CHANG, P. S. *et al.* Clin. Biotechnol. **2:** 23.
4. UHLENBECK, O. C. 1987. Nature **328:** 596.
5. HASELOFF, J. & W. L. GERLACH. 1988. Nature **334:** 585.

NIH/NIAID-WHO AIDS Research and Reference Reagent Program

S. STERN,[a] L. MUUL, AND G. MILMAN

Pathogenesis Branch
AIDS Program
NIAID, NIH
Rockville, Maryland 20850

Research on HIV and its interactions with target cells often requires difficult-to-obtain experimental materials. To encourage research on AIDS-related problems, the National Institute of Allergy and Infectious Diseases established the NIH AIDS Research and Reference Reagent Program Repository in January 1988. The United States repository in Rockville is one of three World Health Organization Collaborating Centers in the Global Program on AIDS. Approximately 1400 AIDS researchers worldwide were surveyed to determine which reagents are most critically needed in a repository. Results of the survey guided repository acquisitions.

There is provision in the contract for purchase of reagents, but most have been donated to the program so far. Material has been contributed by scientists at NIH and various companies, but more than 60% of reagents have come from scientists at universities and research institutes. There is a list in the front of the repository catalogue of the sixty-one contributors and a message of gratitude for their participation in the program.

The reagents are available to qualified investigators worldwide—both established and newly recruited—whose research relates to AIDS. Currently available materials include clones of HIV-1, HIV-2 (the AIDS virus found primarily in West Africa), the closely related simian immunodeficiency virus (SIV), other related retroviruses, uninfected cell lines that support the growth of these viruses, cells chronically infected with retroviruses, and plasmids that express viral proteins. The repository also contains standardized reference antisera and monoclonal antibodies to specific viral antigens. Biological response modifiers such as lymphokines, cytokines, and monokines (cellular hormones that influence cell function), and chemicals or drugs used to modulate the immune system will be standardized and distributed to the scientific community.

The repository will distribute standardized protocols for viral isolation, as well as titration and neutralization assays. Standardized biochemical assays for evaluating compounds with antiviral potential will be available.

To foster the free exchange of reagents, materials from the repository are provided for research purposes only. Before obtaining a reagent, the recipient must agree that he or she will not transfer the material to a third party. Donors of a reagent routinely obtain information about each request for the reagent, and acknowledgement as the source of the reagent in published work associated with its use. Reagents are not available for therapeutic use or for commercial purposes. For further information contact Dr. Susan Stern by telephone at (301) 340-0245 or FAX (301) 340-9245.

[a] Address for correspondence: Pathogenesis Branch, AIDS Program, NIAID, NIH, 649A Lofstrand Lane, Rockville, MD 20850.

Computerized Probe Analysis of the Energetically Favored Binding Sites of an Aspartyl Protease

KENT D. STEWART AND PATRICK K. MARTIN

Division of Organic Chemistry
Burroughs Wellcome Company
Research Triangle Park, North Carolina 27709

Medicinal interest in aspartyl proteases has increased in recent years due to the identification of renin and HIV protease (enzymes involved in blood pressure regulation and AIDS virus replication, respectively) as members of this class of hydrolytic enzyme. The aspartyl protease rhizopuspepsin is an enzyme for which detailed structural information is available for the active site both with and without an inhibitor present.[1,2] We have analyzed the active site of this enzyme with the computer program GRID, a computer program that analyzes enzyme active sites for favored positions of binding of small molecules.[3,4] GRID evaluates the energy of binding of the "probe" group, such as methyl, water, or ammonium ion, in the active site as a sum of pairwise interactions between the probe and each atom of the protein taking into account van der Waals, hydrogen bond, and electrostatic interactions.

AMMONIUM PROBE RESULTS

A favorable binding position for the ammonium probe was observed to occur above the central aspartates of the active site. The ammonium probe responded to changes in electrostatic field of the active-site center, and the corresponding energy contours were shifted to lower levels in the bis-ionized state: that is, the ammonium ion is more favored to bind to the bis-ionized enzyme than the mono-ionized enzyme.

WATER PROBE RESULTS

GRID predicted several well-defined positions for bound water molecules to be energetically favorable. GRID located 11 of 22 water molecules, crystallographically found within the first solvation shell of the active site, within the -7 kcal/mol energy contour and 19 of 22 waters within the -4 kcal/mol energy contour.

METHYL PROBE RESULTS

The crystal structure of the peptide inhibitor, D-HisProPheHisPhe[CH$_2$-NH]Phe ValTyr bound in the active site of rhizopuspepsin, shows that the amine group of the reduced peptide bond is located above the aspartates (similar position as that described above for the ammonium probe). The phenyl side chains on either side of the reduced linkage are located in regions that are energetically favored for methyl probe binding, that is, the phenyls bind in what GRID predicts to be hydrophobic binding sites. The valine side chain of the inhibitor is also found in a hydrophobic pocket, although the pocket is much smaller than that predicted for the phenyl side chains.

In conclusion, crystallographically determined water and hydrophobic pocket positions compare favorably with the results of the GRID calculations. The consistency of the experimental and theoretical results lends credibility to this method of analyzing the active sites of enzymes.

REFERENCES

1. SUGUNA, K., E. A. PADLAN, C. W. SMITH, W. D. CARLSON & D. R. DAVIES. 1987. Proc. Natl. Acad. Sci. USA **84:** 7009-7013.
2. SUGUNA, K., R. R. BOTT, E. A. PADLAN, E. SUBRAMANIAN, S. SHERIFF, G. H. COHEN & D. R. DAVIES. 1987. J. Mol. Biol. **196:** 877-900.
3. BOOBBYER, D. N. A., P. J. GOODFORD, P. M. MCWHINNIE & R. C. WADE. 1989. J. Med. Chem. **32:** 1083-1094.
4. GOODFORD, P. J. 1985. J. Med. Chem. **28:** 849-857.

Dipyridamole Potentiates the Activity of Zidovudine and Other Dideoxynucleosides against HIV-1 in Cultured Cells[a]

JANOS SZEBENI,[b] SHARON M. WAHL,[c]
RAYMOND F. SCHINAZI,[d] MIKULAS POPOVIC,[e]
SUZANNE GARTNER,[e] LARRY M. WAHL,[c]
OWEN S. WEISLOW,[f] GURUPADAPPA BETAGERI,[b]
ROBERT L. FINE,[g] JOHN E. DAHLBERG,[h]
EDWARD HUNTER,[h] AND JOHN N. WEINSTEIN[b]

[b]Laboratory of Mathematical Biology
[e]Laboratory of Tumor Cell Biology
[g]Medicine Branch
National Cancer Institute

[c]Laboratory of Microbiology and Immunology
National Institute of Dental Research
National Institutes of Health
Bethesda, Maryland 20892

[f]National Cancer Institute-Frederick Cancer Research Facility
Frederick, Maryland 21701

[d]VA Medical Center
Emory University School of Medicine
Decatur/Atlanta, Georgia 30033

[h]Pan-Data Systems, Inc.
Rockville, Maryland 20850

Dipyridamole (DPM, Persantine), a potent inhibitor of nucleoside transport, is commonly used as a coronary vasodilator and inhibitor of platelet aggregation in the treatment of cardiovascular diseases. For the past few years, there has also been increasing interest in its use in cancer chemotherapy, as a potentiator of the cytotoxic effects of antitumor agents. We have found that DPM also potentiates the antiviral effects of 3'-azido-3'-deoxythymidine (AZT) against HIV-1 in primary cultures of human monocyte/macrophages, in phytohemagglutinin (PHA)-stimulated human T lymphocytes, and in human T-lymphoblastoid (CEM-SS) cells. In the CEM-SS cells, furthermore, DPM decreases the cytotoxicity of AZT.[1]

[a]This work was supported in part by the NIH Intramural AIDS Targeted Antiviral program.

Monocyte-derived macrophages were prepared by purification from mononuclear cells either by adherence or by counterflow centrifugal elutriation. They were infected with HIV-1/NIH/USA/1985/HTLV-III$_{Ba-L}$ and cultivated in the presence of various levels of AZT $\pm$ DPM.[1] At intervals, supernatant samples were analyzed for HIV-1 p24 antigen. Stimulated human T-lymphocytes were obtained by growing mononuclear cells in the presence of PHA (5 μg/mL) for 2 days, followed by exposure to IL-2. After 3 days, the cells were infected with various titers of HIV-1$_{(IIIB)}$ and were treated with the drugs. Ten days later, p24 was measured. CEM-SS cells were infected either with free HIV-1$_{(IIIB)}$ or with HIV-1$_{(RF)}$-infected H9 cells. After 7 days, the tetrazolium salt "XTT" (1 mg/mL) and phenazine methosulfate (0.01-0.02 mM) were added. Photometric measurement of the formazan formed provided an index of cell health.[2]

TABLE 1 shows the effect of AZT-DPM combinations on p24 levels in adherence-purified M/M and in PHA-stimulated T lymphocytes. In the case of M/M (panel A), DPM had little effect by itself, but it significantly enhanced the antiviral efficacy of 0.5 and 2.5 μM AZT. The estimated ID$_{50}$ levels of AZT were decreased by more than 5-fold in the presence of 2 and 10 μM DPM.[1] In M/M purified by centrifugal elutriation, DPM by itself appeared to be inhibitory: p24 expression on day 14 was decreased 30-50% by 0.4-10 μM[1] DPM. Combination of DPM with AZT almost completely suppressed p24 expression at AZT levels $\geq$ 1.6 nM. Such inhibition could be achieved only at 1 μM AZT when it was applied alone.[1] In M/M, DPM also potentiated the antiviral effect of 2',3'-dideoxycytidine and 2',3'-dideoxycytidine-triphosphate.[1] In PHA-stimulated T lymphocytes, DPM by itself inhibited p24 production and potentiated the inhibitory activity of AZT (panel B of TABLE 1). The antiviral effects of these two agents appeared to be strongly synergistic, so that HIV-1 replication was close to baseline levels following combination treatment.

In CEM-SS cells, DPM had no intrinsic effect, but it potentiated the antiviral effect of AZT and, simultaneously, antagonized the cell toxicity of AZT. Thus, the *in vitro* therapeutic index was greatly increased. For example, formazan production, expressed as a percent of uninfected control, increased from $\sim$30% in cells treated only with 10 nM AZT to $\sim$60% in cells treated with 10 nM AZT and 2.5 μM DPM. At the same time, formazan levels remained unchanged in cells treated with 0.1-1 mM AZT together with > 2.5 μM DPM, whereas they significantly decreased (by a factor of > 2) in the absence of DPM.

Concerning the toxicity of DPM-AZT combinations, spontaneous and phorbol-ester-stimulated superoxide production by uninfected M/M, taken as indices of cell function, showed no discernible toxicity for DPM $\pm$ AZT at the concentrations applied in the viral studies.[1] Nor could we detect significant changes in cell counts and viability following combination treatment. The granulocyte-monocyte colony-forming unit (CFU$_{GM}$) assay, performed to test the bone marrow toxicity of AZT-DPM combinations, showed the 50% inhibitory level of AZT on colony formation to be 0.6 $\pm$ 1 μM, and that of DPM to be 10.0 $\pm$ 4.5 μM. The toxic effects of AZT and DPM, however, did not synergize.[1]

To assist in extrapolating from tissue culture DPM levels to studies *in vivo* (DPM strongly binds to plasma proteins), we determined the levels of free DPM in human plasma and in standard tissue culture media.[3] At therapeutically relevant concentrations of DPM (2-10 μM), its free fraction in human plasma was $\sim$2-4%, whereas in culture media containing 10% fetal calf serum the free fraction was 75-100%. These results suggest a factor in the range of 24-55 for the interconversion of *in vitro* and *in vivo* DPM concentrations that provide equivalent levels of free drug. Hence, mean steady state plasma levels of DPM obtained with currently applied oral dosing schedules (3-5 μM), and the maximum tolerated plasma level obtained with iv infusion ($\sim$12 μM), correspond to tissue culture DPM levels of 0.05-0.15 μM and 0.5 μM, respectively. These ranges, particularly the latter one, overlap with the concentration range of DPM that we find effective against HIV-1 in M/M and T-lymphocyte cultures.

As to mechanism of action, it is known that DPM inhibits carrier-mediated transport of physiological deoxynucleosides, including thymidine (dThd), across cell membranes. AZT, on the other hand, enters cells by passive diffusion.[4] Because dThd counteracts the antiviral activity of AZT in numerous cell types, it has been suggested that DPM, by inhibiting dThd uptake in cells, could suppress an antagonistic influence on AZT's antiviral action. To test this hypothesis, we have studied the cellular uptake of [³H]dThd and [³H]AZT in M/M cells and their incorporation into the nucleotide

TABLE 1. Potentiation by Dipyridamole of the Antiviral Effect of AZT in Monocyte-Derived Macrophages (A)[1] and T Lymphocytes (B)[a]

(A) M/M

DPM (μM)	AZT (μM)			
	0	0.1	0.5	2.5
0.0	50.3 ± 1.1[b]	45.2 ± 0.8	33.3 ± 2.8	5.8 ± 1.0
0.08	55.0 ± 0.3	40.7 ± 6.0	16.9 ± 2.9	2.4 ± 0.5
0.4	51.8 ± 0.7	39.2 ± 1.3	22.0 ± 6.7	0.1 ± 0.1
2.0	51.3 ± 1.5	42.3 ± 2.1	4.1 ± 0.7	0.1 ± 0.4
10.0	46.9 ± 2.0	36.1 ± 1.8	3.2 ± 1.3	0 ± 0

(B) T lymphocyte

DPM (μM)	AZT (μM)				
	0	0.16	0.63	2.5	10.0
0.0	635[c]	470	147	19	[d]
0.07	1423	24	6	1	[d]
0.22	1251	9	5	4	[d]
0.67	597	5	2	6	[d]
2.0	255	5	2	5	[d]
6.0	172	1	3	6	[d]

[a] Entries are p24 antigen levels expressed as ng/mL (A) or pmole/well (B).
[b] Means ± SEM of quadruplicate wells.
[c] Means of duplicate wells.
[d] Cell toxicity.

pools. DPM (2 μM) significantly inhibited both the uptake and the phosphorylation of [³H]dThd, whereas it did not influence the uptake and phosphorylation of [³H]AZT.[5] Thus, a differential effect on dThd metabolism may underlie, at least in part, the potentiating effect of DPM on the anti-HIV activity of AZT. DPM has several other cellular actions,[1] however, that could also contribute to the phenomena described here.

In conclusion, because cells of M/M and T-lymphocyte lineage are the main targets for HIV-1 infection *in vivo*, our findings suggest the possibility of using DPM or its analogues in combination chemotherapy of HIV infections. The efficacy and safety of this approach, however, can be determined only in clinical studies.

REFERENCES

1. SZEBENI, J., S. M. WAHL, M. POPOVIC, L. M. WAHL, S. GARTNER, R. L. FINE, U. SKALERIC, R. M. FRIEDMAN & J. N. WEINSTEIN. 1989. Dipyridamole potentiates the inhibition by 3'-azido-3'-deoxythymidine and other dideoxynucleosides of human immunodeficiency virus replication in monocyte-macrophages. Proc. Natl. Acad. Sci. USA **86:** 3842-3846.
2. WEISLOW, O. S., R. KISER, D. L. FINE, J. BADER, R. H. SHOEMAKER & M. R. BOYD. 1989. New soluble-formazan assay for HIV-1 cytopathic effects: application to high-flux screening of synthetic and natural products for AIDS-antiviral activity. J. Natl. Cancer Inst. **81:** 577-586.
3. SZEBENI, J. & J. N. WEINSTEIN. 1989. Dipyridamole binding to proteins in human plasma and in tissue culture media. Submitted for publication.
4. ZIMMERMAN, T. P., W. B. MAHONY & K. L. PRUS. 1987. 3'-Azido-3'-deoxythymidine. J. Biol. Chem. **262:** 5748-5754.
5. BETAGERI, G., J. SZEBENI, K. HUNG, S. S. PATEL, L. M. WAHL, M. CORCORAN & J. N. WEINSTEIN. 1990. Effect of dipyridamole on transport and phosphorylation of thymidine and 3'-azido-3'-deoxythymidine in human monocyte/macrophages. Biochem. Pharmacol. **40:** 867-870.

Fluorogenic Determination of Structural Requirements for HIV Protease Substrates

GARY T. WANG, EDMUND MATAYOSHI,
JOHN W. ERICKSON, AND GRANT A. KRAFFT[a]

Abbott Laboratories
Abbott Park, Illinois 60064-3500

The HIV protease enzyme (HIV-PR) is an 11 kDa protein encoded by HIV. Functioning as a dimer, this aspartic protease processes immature viral polyproteins by catalyzing hydrolysis reactions at a variety of sequences along the polypeptide backbone.[1,2] These hydrolytic cleavages result in the formation of mature structural proteins (p17 and p24) and viral enzymes (reverse transcriptase, and the protease itself). Because HIV protease activity is pivotal in the formation of mature infectious virus, it represents an important target for therapeutic intervention in AIDS. In order to study this enzyme effectively, we have developed novel fluorogenic substrates to measure enzyme kinetic parameters and inhibitor efficacy. In this paper, we describe our efforts to assess the specific structural requirements for efficient substrate activity, and to develop optimized fluorogenic probe molecules for HIV-PR based upon this structural information.

The fluorogenic substrate S1 (FIG. 1), on which our current HIV protease screening assay is based,[3] permitted us to survey the competitive ability of a variety of unfunctionalized peptide sequences that corresponded to known HIV protease cleavage sites, or hybrid sequences of interest. The results of these experiments are shown in TABLE 1. The peptides were evaluated initially with respect to HIV-PR hydrolysis inhibition of S1, and those sequences that exhibited significant inhibitory activity were evaluated with respect to inhibition of S2 hydrolysis. Three sequences, SQNYPIVQ, TATIMMQ-RGE, and RVSFNFPQITR, showed significant inhibitory activity. The latter two peptides were quite effective, consistent with HPLC hydrolysis data for similar sequences.[4-6] A surprising result was the fact that equimolar quantities of the unmodified peptides suppressed only ca. 13-15% of the hydrolysis of the analogous fluorogenic substrates, rather than ca. 50%, which would have been expected for substrates having comparable binding interactions. This significant enhancement of substrate activity by the quenching DABCYL chromophore and EDANS fluorophore might be attributed to altered physical properties (*e.g.*, solubility), enhanced solution conformations of the peptides, or to optimized binding interactions with the protease at the periphery of the active site.

Two sequences that are substrates for the avian myeblastosis virus protease (AMV-PR) showed little or no competitive inhibition of fluorogenic substrate hydrolysis by HIV-PR and served as additional negative control experiments in our studies. The SVVYPVVQ peptide is a hybrid sequence with valines replacing Asn, Gln, and Ile at

[a] Address correspondence to Grant A. Krafft, Abbott Laboratories, Exploratory Molecular Probe Design, Department 9-MN, Bldg. AP9A, Abbott Park, Illinois 60064-3500.

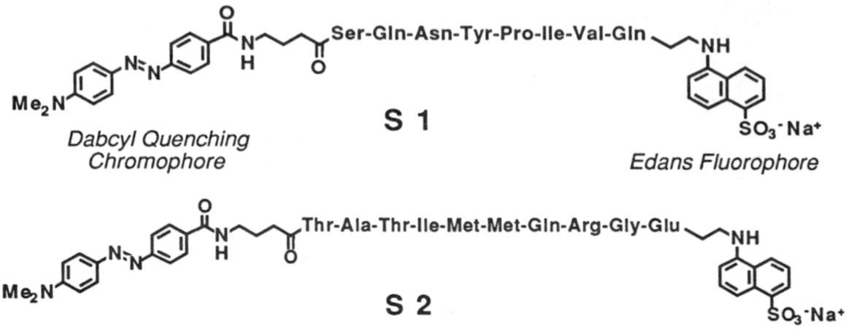

FIGURE 1. Fluorogenic substrates S1 and S2.

P2, P3, and P2′, respectively, of the native SQNYPIVQ, yet these relatively minor changes drastically reduced the substrate capability.

TABLE 2 presents enzyme kinetic data for several HIV-PR and AMV-PR substrates. The fluorogenic substrate S2 with the sequence TATIMMQRGE has the lowest K_m of the HIV substrates, but is only slightly more effective as a substrate than S1, indicating that its k_{cat} is likely to be lower than for S1. A similar situation exists for the AMV-PR substrates that we evaluated. The SVVYPVVQ fluorogenic substrate has a very low K_m, but has a V_{max} 7-fold lower than the TFQAYPLRGA substrate, derived from a native AMV sequence.[7,8] It is clear for both retroviral proteases that hydrophobic residues near the cleavage site afford good binding as evidenced by the low K_m values for the TATIMMQRGE and SVVYPVVQ substrates, but this good binding does not necessarily orient the substrate optimally in the active site to undergo efficient hydrolysis.

TABLE 1. Competitive Inhibition of HIV Protease Cleavage of Fluorogenic Substrates by HIV Peptides[a]

Peptide	Cleavage Site	Inhibition of S1	Inhibition of S2
SQNYPIVQ	p17/p24	15.0%	8.7%
TATIMMQRGE	p24/p15	24.6%	12.7%
RVSFNFPQITR	p12 NT	29.6%	22.6%
ATLNFPISQE	p66/p51	4.8%	—
IRQANFLRGA	hybrid	8.0%	—
TFQAYPLRGA	AMV	1.3%	0%
SVVYPVVQ	hybrid	1.3%	—

[a] Assay protocol: Equal volumes (5.0 μL) of fluorogenic substrate solution (1.0 mM in DMSO) and peptide solution (10 mM in DMSO) were mixed in 100 μL of 0.1 M NaOAc buffer (pH 4.7) containing 1.0 M NaCl, 4 mM EDTA, and 1.0 mg/mL of BSA, incubated at 37°C, and monitored to obtain a baseline fluorescence intensity. Final peptide and/or fluorogenic substrate concentration was 46 μM. Addition of 5.0 μL HIV-1 protease solution (recombinant) initiated hydrolysis of the fluorogenic substrate. The resulting increase of fluorescence intensity was monitored, and initial velocities were determined. Control reactions were run without peptide (5.0 μL DMSO) to give baseline reaction rates for the protease and fluorogenic substrate. All data shown represent at least three separate determinations. Variability among identical reactions was <5%.

TABLE 2. Kinetic Parameters for Fluorogenic Substrates of HIV and AMV Proteases[a]

Substrate	Enzyme	K_m (μM)	V_{max} (nM/min)	(k_{cat}/K_m) relative[b]	(k_{cat}/K_m) relative[c]
Dab-Gab-SQNYPIVQ-Ed	HIV-PR	103	164	1.0	<0.01
Dab-Gab-SQNYPIVQ-LY[d]	HIV-PR	—	390	—	—
Dab-Gab-TATIMMQRGE-Ed	HIV-PR	5.9	180	1.02	<0.01
Dab-Gab-TFQAYPLRQA-Ed	AMV-PR	46	548	<0.01	1.00
Dab-Gab-SVVYPVVQ-Ed	AMV-PR	2.2	80	<0.02	0.43

[a] Initial rates were determined as described in TABLE 1. At least six substrate concentrations were used for K_m and V_{max} determinations, and all hydrolysis reactions were run in triplicate. All substrates manifested typical Michealis-Menten kinetics.

[b] These ratios refer to HIV-PR activity and were estimated from ratios of intial cleavage rates of the fluorogenic substrates at constant enzyme and substrate concentrations. Under these conditions, $V_1 : V_2 = (k_{cat}/K_m)_1 : (k_{cat}/K_m)_2$. These ratios provide a relative scale of substrate efficiency for these molecules. Studies to determine the k_{cat} for each of these substrates are in progress.

[c] Data refer to AMV protease activity and were determined as described in footnote *a*.

[d] LY = Lucifer yellow.

These studies have provided valuable correlates between structure and substrate efficiency, facilitating the design of more effective protease substrates. These studies also illustrate the great utility of these new fluorogenic substrates in fundamental kinetic studies of protease enzymes.

REFERENCES

1. KRAUSSLICH, H.-G. & E. WIMMER. 1988. Annu. Rev. Biochem. **57:** 701 754.
2. LEIS, J. *et al.* 1988. J. Virol. **62:** 1808-1809.
3. MATAYOSHI, E. *et al.* 1990. Ann. N.Y. Acad. Sci. This volume.
4. KRAUSSLICH, H.-G. *et al.* 1989. Proc. Natl. Acad. Sci. USA **86:** 807-811.
5. DARKE, P. L. *et al.* 1988. Biochem. Biophys. Res. Commun. **156:** 297-303.
6. BILLICH, S. *et al.* 1988. J. Biol. Chem. **263:** 17905-17908.
7. KOTLER, M. *et al.* 1989. J. Biol. Chem. **264:** 3428-3435.
8. SKALKA, A. 1989. Cell **50:** 911-913.

The Cellular Metabolism of AzdU

Correlation with *in Vitro* Anti-HIV and Cytotoxic Activities

G. J. WILLIAMS,[a] C. B. COLBY,[a] R. F. SCHINAZI,[b]
J-P. SOMMADOSSI,[c] C. K. CHU,[d] D. G. JOHNS,[e] AND
H. MITSUYA[e]

[a]*Triton Biosciences Inc.*
Alameda, California 94501

[b]*Veterans Administration Medical Center and*
Emory University School of Medicine
Atlanta, Georgia

[c]*University of Alabama*
Birmingham, Alabama

[d]*University of Georgia*
Athens, Georgia

[e]*National Cancer Institute*
National Institutes of Health
Bethesda, Maryland

INTRODUCTION

Both 3'azido-2',3'-dideoxyuridine (AzdU) and 3'-azido-3'-deoxythymidine (AZT) have been shown to inhibit HIV replication *in vitro*. The anti-HIV effects, however, of AzdU in PHA-stimulated human peripheral blood mononuclear (PBM) cells and in CEM and ATH8 human cell lines vary depending on the cell type used. When the cytotoxicity of AzdU was compared to that of AZT in human bone marrow cell cultures, AzdU was found to be at least 20-fold less toxic than AZT. To explain these disparities, experiments were conducted to examine the inhibitory effects of AzdU-triphosphate (AzdUTP) and AZT-triphosphate (AZTTP) on HIV reverse transcriptase (HIV RT) and cellular DNA polymerases α, β, and γ, as well as examine the accumulation of AzdUTP and/or AZTTP in these cell types. Results of these experiments suggest that the *in vitro* anti-HIV activity of AzdU is dependent on how AzdU is metabolized by various cell types. By contrast, differences in the cytotoxicity of AzdU and AZT in bone marrow cell cultures appears to be dependent on the differences of inhibitory effects of AzdUTP and AZTTP on cellular DNA polymerases as well as the amount of these triphosphates formed in bone marrow-derived cells.

TABLE 1. Anti-HIV Activity of AzdU and AZT in Various Cell Types

	EC$_{50}$ (μM)	
	AzdU	AZT
CEM	0.013	0.002
PBM	0.180	0.002
ATH8	> 100	0.320

RESULTS

The effects of AzdU and AZT on HIV replication have been compared in a variety of human cells. Regardless of cell type, AzdU was consistently less potent than AZT (TABLE 1 and data not shown). Because the activity of AzdU varies from cell type to cell type, however, the difference in anti-HIV potency between AzdU and AZT ranged from as much as 300-fold to as little as 6-fold. When the amount of AzdUTP formed in three different cell types was compared, it was found that CEM cells accumulated two times more AzdUTP than human PBM cells and at least 30 times more than ATH8 cells (FIG. 1). The differences in AzdUTP formation in these cell types correlated well with the *in vitro* anti-HIV activity observed for these cells (see TABLE 1).

Because the anti-HIV and cytotoxic effects of many nucleoside analogues are attributable to their triphosphates, the effects of AzdUTP and AZTTP on HIV RT and cellular DNA polymerase α, β, and γ were compared. The HIV RT inhibitory activity

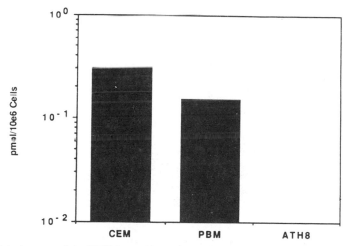

FIGURE 1. Amount of AzdUTP formed in various cell types. Cell lysates were prepared from cultures treated with 0.5 μM [^{3}H]AzdU or [^{3}H]AZT for 24 hours and analyzed by HPLC.

TABLE 2. Inhibition of HIV Reverse Transcriptase and Cellular DNA Polymerase by AzdU- and AZT-5'-Triphosphate

Polymerase	AzdUTP K_i (μM)	AZTTP K_i (μM)
HIV RT	0.27	0.073
DNA polymerase α	250	46
DNA polymerase β	75	6.8
DNA polymerase γ	9	2.4

of AzdUTP was found to be 3- to 4-fold less than that of AZT (TABLE 2, data supplied by Yung-Chi Chang, Yale University), suggesting that most of the observed differences in anti-HIV activity between AzdU and AZT *in vitro* are not due to differences in the ability of the triphosphates of AzdU and AZT to inhibit HIV replication, but in fact are due to a lesser amount of AzdUTP formed in certain cell types (FIG. 1). In addition, AzdUTP was found to be 4- to 11-fold less inhibitory to cellular DNA polymerases than AZTTP, suggesting that AzdU would be less cytotoxic than AZT (TABLE 2).

To test this hypothesis, *in vitro* cytotoxicity assays were performed using human bone marrow-derived cells. Results showed that AzdU was 20-fold less toxic to progenitor bone marrow cells than AZT. When the cellular metabolism of these agents was examined in bone marrow cell cultures, it was found that although comparable levels of unchanged, mono- and diphosphate AzdU and AZT were formed, at least 8-fold more AZTTP than AzdUTP accumulated in these cells (FIG. 2). These results,

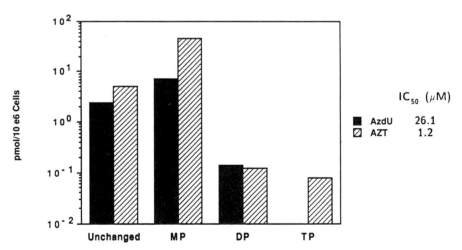

FIGURE 2. Metabolites of AzdU and AZT formed in human bone marrow cell cultures. Cell lysates were prepared from cultures treated with 10 μM [^{3}H]AzdU or [^{3}H]AZT for 24 hours and analyzed by HPLC.

in combination with the cellular enzyme studies suggest that the differences in cellular cytotoxicity of AzdU and AZT in bone marrow-derived cell cultures are due to the greater inhibitory effects of AZTTP on cellular DNA polymerases as well as the formation of higher intracellular levels of AZTTP than AzdUTP in bone marrow-derived cells. In addition, the results suggest that AzdU will be less myelosuppressive than AZT *in vivo.* Two phase 1 AzdU clinical trials, one at the University of California at Los Angeles and another at the NIH, have been initiated.

Computer-Assisted Design of Antiviral Agents Directed against Human Immunodeficiency Virus Reverse Transcriptase as Their Target[a]

JANARDAN YADAV,[b] PREM NARAYAN YADAV,[c]
SWAMY LAXMINARAYAN,[b] LESLIE MICHELSON,[b]
EDWARD ARNOLD,[d] AND MUKUND J. MODAK[c]

[b]Division of Academic Computing Services
Department of Information Services and Technology

[c]Department of Biochemistry
New Jersey Medical School
University of Medicine and Dentistry of New Jersey
Newark, New Jersey 07103

[d]Center for Advanced Biotechnology and Medicine
and Department of Chemistry
Rutgers University
Piscataway, New Jersey 08854-5638

INTRODUCTION

Reverse transcriptase (RT) is an integral part of many oncogenic viruses, including those from human leukemia and human AIDS viruses.[1] It is absolutely essential for viral replication. Thus, one of the most promising strategies for the treatment of retroviral diseases is to inhibit the process of reverse transcription. Obviously, this enzyme has been one of the most desired targets for antiviral agents.[2-7] Nucleoside analogues that lack the 3'-hydroxyl group have been extensively considered as potential therapeutics against human immunodeficiency virus type 1 (HIV-1), the causative agent of acquired immunodeficiency syndrome (AIDS) and AIDS-related complex (ARC). Some well-recognized anti-AIDS agents, namely, 3'-azido-3'-deoxythymidine (N_3ddT), also known as azidothymidine (AZT); dideoxycytidine (ddC), and dideoxyinosine (ddI); and other analogues are inhibitors of HIV RT. Nucleoside 5'-triphosphates are the active substrates of RT. N_3ddT (AZT) is converted to N_3ddTTP by

[a]Parts of this research work were supported by Grants from the National Institutes of Health (AI-27690 to E. Arnold and AI-26652 to M. Modak), the New Jersey Commission on Science and Technology, and the Center for Biotechnology and Medicine.

thymidine kinase and thymidylate kinases of the host cells.[8] N_3ddTTP competes with the natural substrate, thymidine 5'-triphosphate (dTTP), for binding to RT. The uptake of the N_3ddTTP in the DNA chain that is being synthesized results in chain termination because of the inability to form the 3',5'-phosphodiester link to the next nucleotide.

Furthermore, the different analogues differ greatly in anti-HIV activity levels. The differences in the antiviral activity may be caused by differences in the binding to RT or by different rates of phosphorylation. As of today, no definite answer has been found to whether chain termination is required or whether the reversible competitive binding of the nucleotide analogue to RT would be sufficient for activity. Nonetheless, correlation of activity with structural information and intermolecular interactions are important factors for determining the molecular basis of the activity of these compounds.

These agents, however, have significant problems, and thus more work is needed to develop optimal therapeutics against AIDS. Furthermore, development of virus mutants that exhibit resistance to these agents as well as host cell toxicity considerations require that better inhibitors for this enzyme be constructed. An important consideration in the construction of newer agents will require clarification of the structural and electrostatic interactions between the antiviral agent and its binding site(s) or target (receptor). The ability to predict these interactions leads to the possibility of designing new inhibitors that could prove useful as research tools for building novel drugs. Three-dimensional molecular modeling studies, which include conformational analyses, electrostatic potential calculations, interactive graphics, and receptor mapping techniques, can help to elucidate the structural and electrostatic requirements for predicting the possible inhibitors and provide a rational approach for design of new inhibitors. The three-dimensional atomic level model of human immunodeficiency virus (HIV) reverse transcriptase will act as a springboard for development of effective intervention strategies against HIV infection and disease. There will be great potential for rational design of specific antiviral agents directed against AIDS once the structure and activity of the enzyme is known and better understood. The structure determination of HIV RT by X-ray diffraction is being worked on in the laboratory of one of the authors (E. Arnold). We have undertaken the computer-assisted three-dimensional studies of known potent anti-HIV RT agents to (1) explore the conformational, steric, and electrostatic properties of agents that inhibit RT, (2) map the RT polymerization active site based on complementarity with inhibitors, and (3) use the receptor model to guide the design of new inhibitors. A large number of experimental structure determinations of RT inhibitors have already been reported, and these results have been used by Van Roey *et al.*[6,7] and others[8,9] in an attempt to correlate conformational preferences with inhibitory activity. As a first step towards this goal, we have begun to compare structures and structure-related properties of known RT inhibitors, using SYBYL molecular modeling software,[10] to develop an interaction model for the design of new inhibitors for RT. This communication describes our current results on 3'-azido-3'-deoxythymidine (AZT), 3'-azido-2',3'-dideoxy-5-ethyluridine (CS85), 3'-azido-2',3'-dideoxyuridine (CS87), dideoxycytidine (ddC), and dideoxythymidine (ddT).

MOLECULAR MODELING AND COMPUTATIONAL DETAILS

The Cartesian coordinates for nucleosides were taken for B-DNA from Dr. R. Srinivasan of the Chemistry Department of Rutgers University. The AZT, CS85, and CS87 coordinates were taken from crystal structure work of Van Roey *et al.*[6] These coordinates were read into SYBYL[10] molecular modeling software, and the rest of the hydrogens were generated, as the coordinates of all hydrogen atoms were not reported in the crystal structure studies.[6] The new molecules so generated were subjected to MM2 minimization[9] to produce the realistic hydrogen locations and to provide uniform treatment of all molecules going into the structural comparisons. It is important to note that the nonhydrogen framework of the MM2-minimized structures did not change significantly from the input crystal structures.[6] The minimized coordinates were again read into SYBYL to perform superposition studies and volume calculations. The MM2 minimization was carried out on a Hewlett/Packard HP9000 series 840 technical computer. The molecular modeling with the SYBYL program was carried out using IRIS workstation.

STRATEGIES OF SELECTING ATOM PAIRS FOR SUPERPOSITIONS

AZT is at this time the most commonly used drug for the treatment of AIDS patients. Therefore, we selected it as the reference molecule for superposition. The geometry of the glycosyl link, the rotation about the exocyclic C4'-C5' bond, and the puckering of the sugar ring are three important considerations in the conformational flexibilities of nucleosides and their analogues. Thus, the superposition studies were carried out for four sets in the pairs of atoms. The first pair of atoms includes C2, N3, and C4. The second set of atoms consists of C1', N1, and C2. The third and fourth pair of atoms are O4', C1', N1 and C3', C4', and C5', respectively. These sets were considered to assess the fittings of atoms of both the bases and the sugar rings. The numbering scheme is shown in FIGURE 1. The fitted structures along with their intersection volumes are depicted in FIGURE 2.

RESULTS AND DISCUSSION

From an examination of the superpositions depicted in FIGURE 2, it is clear that the selection of different reference atoms for the superposition leads to different results. None of the choices is adequate for considering changes at all substituent positions. Different classes of substituent modifications, however, can be sensibly examined by using different reference atoms for the superpositions. For example, the set that uses the pyrimidine atoms C2, N3, and C4 (FIG. 2a) for superposition shows a sterically allowable map for the substituents on the pyrimidine ring based on the molecules included in these studies. Inclusion of more representative pyrimidine nucleoside inhibitors of RT will allow a more generalized mapping of the steric, electronic, and chemical requirements for the substitution on the ring.

Likewise, examination of the superpositions that use the sugar atoms as reference (FIGURES 2c and 2d) gives some insight into variations in the sugar ring conformations in the current set of RT inhibitors. As also pointed out by Van Roey *et al.*,[6,7] the majority of the sugar ring conformations are of the C2'-endo/C3'-exo class. More study is required to determine what mode(s) of superposition will most meaningfully guide design efforts. In terms of a global superposition for the current set of inhibitors studied, perhaps the reference set C1',N1,C2 (FIG. 2b) provides the best overall matching. Another possibility that we are pursuing is to enforce similarities at the major internal torsion angles in the sugar ring and the glycosyl linkage to provide more similar conformations for comparisons. In view of the latter strategy, it is conceivable that the RT active site enforces conformational similarity upon the triphosphate forms of these inhibitors during the polymerization process.

Also illustrated in FIGURE 2 is the volume of intersection of the inhibitors considered in this study resulting from each of the four superpositions. The intersection volume highlights the spatial similarities of regions of the inhibitor molecules and presumably indicates spatial requirements for the enzyme active site. As more inhibitors become included in this study, this approach should yield a "receptor map" (Yadav *et*

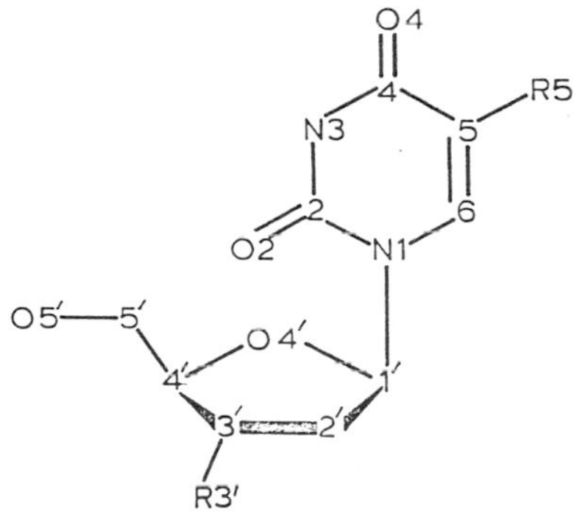

FIGURE 1. Schematic diagram and numbering scheme used for thymidine analogues.

al.[11]) that is complementary to the RT polymerization active site. The utility of such a receptor map might be to eliminate candidate inhibitors for chemical synthesis that do not conform to the RT enzyme's requirements. On the other hand, candidates that fit within the receptor map would be deemed very favorable candidates for synthesis.

CONCLUDING REMARKS

A three-dimensional atomic model of RT will greatly enhance the rational design of improved RT inhibitors. In the meantime, we are applying the receptor mapping technique to identify the common features of available effective inhibitors. Extension of the current results will provide receptor maps for RT inhibitors that will include more of the relevant features (*e.g.,* triphosphate conformations and modifications;

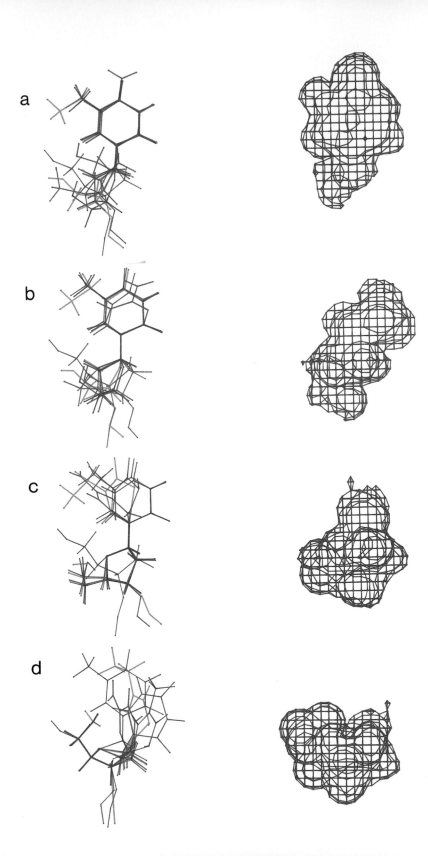

purine versus pyrimidine nucleoside analogues; and sugar modifications, including acyclic derivatives). Because experimental structural studies of RT inhibitors are being frequently reported, this will permit the construction of more accurate receptor maps based on a larger set of structures. Critical examination of the receptor maps may facilitate the synthetic design of more potent and more selective inhibitors of HIV RT.

Computer-assisted three-dimensional molecular modeling, and in particular the technique of receptor mapping, has been applied to help predict which steric and electronic features of a selected set of human immunodeficiency virus reverse transcriptase inhibitors best correlate with activity. Structural superpositions about the glycosyl bond and the exocyclic bond were carried out to ascertain the structural similarities and the differences among the molecules. The fitted structures were then used to obtain their intersection volumes in an effort to help define the acceptable range of inhibitor substituents at the C3' and C5 positions. The results may have potential use in guiding the design of new inhibitors for human immunodeficiency virus reverse transcriptase enzyme.

ACKNOWLEDGMENTS

We thank Dr. R. Srinivasan of the Chemistry Department of Rutgers University for providing us the Cartesian coordinates of B-DNA nucleosides. E. Arnold wishes to thank Dr. Manfred Weigele at Hoffmann-La Roche, for support of this work. J. Yadav is personally grateful to Professor Tamara Gund for allowing him to use her molecular modeling facilities to complete a part of this work and to Dr. P. Van Roey for helpful discussions and for providing results in advance of publication.

REFERENCES

1. GALLO, R. C. & F. WONG-STAAL. 1989. Retrovirus Biology and Human Disease. Marcel Dekker, Inc. New York and Basel.
2. CHANDRA, P., A. VOGEL & T. GERBER. 1985. Cancer Res. (Suppl.) **45:** 4677s-4684s.
3. MITSUYA H. & S. BRODER. 1986. Proc. Natl. Acad. Sci. USA **83:** 1911-1915
4. MITSUYA, H. & S. BRODER. 1987. Nature **325:** 773-778.
5. LIN, T. S., J. Y. GUO, R. F. SCHINAZI, C. K. CHU, J. N. XIANG & W. H. PRUSOFF. 1988. J. Med. Chem. **31:** 336-340.

FIGURE 2 a. Structural superposition and the corresponding intersection volume of nucleoside analogues around C2-N3-C4. **b.** Structural superposition and corresponding intersection volumes of nucleoside analogues around C1'-N1-C2. **c.** Structural superposition and corresponding intersection volume of nucleoside analogues around 04'-C1'-N1. **d.** Structural superposition and corresponding intersection volume of nucleoside analogues around C3'-C4'-C5'.

6. VAN ROEY, P., J. M. SALERNO, W. L. DUAX, C. K. CHU, M. K. AHN & R. F. SCHINAZI. 1988. J. Am. Chem Soc. **110:** 2277-2282.
7. VAN ROEY, P., M. SALERNO, C. K CHU & R. F. SCHINAZI. 1989. Proc. Natl. Acad. Sci. USA **86:** 3929-3933.
8. WAQAR, M. A., M. J. EVANS, K. F. MAULY, R. G. HUGHES & J. A. HUBERMAN. 1984. J. Cell Physiol. **121:** 402-408.
9. BURKERT, U. & N. L. ALLINGER. 1982. Molecular Mechanics. ACS Monograph 177. American Chemical Society. Washington DC.
10. SYBYL Molecular Modeling Software. Tripos Associates. St. Louis, MO 63117.
11. YADAV, J. S., M. HERMSMEIER & T. GUND. 1989. Int. J. Quant. Cnem. Quant. Biol. **16:** 101-117.

Index of Contributors